GLENCOE

Medical Laboratory Procedures

Physician's Office Laboratory · POL

Tom Palko
M.Ed., M.C.S., MT(ASCP)
Director, Medical Assistant and Medical
Technology Programs
Professor of Allied Health Sciences
Arkansas Tech University

Hilda Palko
B.S., MT(ASCP), CMA

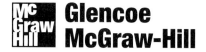

Glencoe McGraw-Hill

New York, New York   Columbus, Ohio   Woodland Hills, California   Peoria, Illinois

Dedicated to the memory of Oran and Lovie West and George and Grace Palko, our parents and the grandparents of James, Carl, and Mark

Contributor
Mark Palko, M.S.
Assistant Director, Math Resources and Tutoring Center
University of Arkansas, Fayetteville

Library of Congress Cataloging-in-Publication Data
Palko, Tom.
    Glencoe medical laboratory procedures / Tom Palko, Hilda Palko.
        p.   cm. — (Glencoe allied health series)
    Rev. ed. of: Laboratory procedures for the medical office/Tom
Palko, Hilda Palko. ©1996.
    Includes bibliographical references and index.
    ISBN 0-02-80214-6 (student text). — ISBN 0-02-802015-4
(instructor's guide)
    1. Diagnosis, Laboratory—Handbooks, manuals, etc. 2. Medical
assistants—Handbooks, manuals, etc.   I. Palko, Hilda.   II. Palko,
Tom.   Laboratory procedures for the medical office.   III. Title. IV. Series.
    [DNLM: 1. Diagnosis, Laboratory—methods.   QY 25 P163g 1999]
RB38.2.P35   1999
616.07'56—dc21
DNLM/DLC
for Library of Congress   97-46117
                                                                CIP

Glencoe/McGraw-Hill

A Division of The **McGraw·Hill** *Companies*

Send all inquiries to:
Glencoe/McGraw-Hill
8787 Orion Place
Columbus, Ohio 43240-4027

ISBN   0-02-802014-6 (Student Text)
ISBN   0-02-802015-4 (Instructor's Manual)

        4 5 6 7 8 9   024   04 03 02

WARNING NOTICE: The clinical procedures, medicines, dosages, and other matters described in this publication are based upon research of current literature, consultation with knowledgeable persons in the field, and the authors' experience. To the best of the authors' knowledge, the procedures and matters described in this text reflect currently accepted clinical practice. However, this information and the authors' recommendations cannot and should not be relied upon as necessarily applicable to a given individual's case. Accordingly, each person must be separately diagnosed to discern the patient's unique circumstances. Likewise, the manufacturer's package insert for current drug product information should be consulted before administering any drug. Authors and publisher disclaim all liability for any inaccuracies, omissions, misuse, or misunderstanding of the information contained in this publication. Authors and publisher caution that this publication is not intended as a substitute for the professional judgment of trained medical personnel.

Preface

There has never been a more challenging time than the present to enter the clinical laboratory profession. The enactments of the Clinical Laboratory Improvement Amendment (CLIA 1988) and the Occupational Safety and Health Administration (OSHA) regulations, which now cover clinical laboratory personnel, have brought changes and new demands to the profession. The effects of CLIA 1988 and OSHA are already felt in the physician's office laboratory. The CLIA regulations are concerned with quality control of POL testing, including proficiency testing. OSHA regulations are concerned with POL safety of both laboratory workers and physicians' patients. OSHA's guidelines for Universal Precautions address the spread of the hepatitis B virus (HBV) and the virus that causes AIDS (HIV). These guidelines are given in Appendix A. We address both CLIA 1988 and OSHA regulations throughout this book. Compliance on the part of the medical laboratory worker will result in a more effective, more accurate, and safer laboratory. We hope this book will help you meet the challenges brought about by these recent measures.

This book can serve you in the following ways:

- as a textbook in the clinical laboratory portion of the curriculum for students of allied health, especially those in medical assisting programs.

- as a reference source for the medical assistant who is employed in the clinical laboratory of a medical office (physician's office laboratory).

- as a learning resource and reference for persons who will be trained as on-the-job workers to perform laboratory procedures in the physician's office laboratory (POL).

To be an effective laboratory worker, you must understand the theory behind each test you perform. We have, whenever possible, incorporated the laboratory procedure with the theory and pathology of each test. When you know about the conditions and diseases that alter test results, you will find your job more meaningful and also more enjoyable.

Medical laboratory instrumentation has been developed to a more simplified technology, making it practical to run many laboratory tests in the POL. The technology has advanced to the point where subtle changes in amounts of various substances in the body can be tested with a high degree of accuracy. Both basic, manual laboratory procedures and automated methods are explained in the book. The manual procedures usually give a better understanding of the principle or theory of the tests than do the automated methods. All automated (or instrumental) methods are adaptations of manual methods.

Because of the volume of tests performed in a hospital laboratory setting, it is necessary to departmentalize the laboratory. As a result, a laboratory worker who works in a hospital's hematology department would generally not be called upon to perform procedures in blood chemistry. In the POL, however, a lab worker will be required to function as a generalist. Most POLs have only from one to three workers, who must therefore be proficient in all areas of testing in their laboratory.

It is the physician's responsibility to utilize laboratory test results for both diagnosis and treatment of the patient. It is the responsibility of the POL worker, however, to be certain that all test results are accurate as reported. The more knowledge the POL worker has about the clinical laboratory, the greater the chance that his or her performance will be accurate. A POL worker who does not understand the theory of a laboratory procedure cannot function as effectively as one who understands, especially in the area of quality-control management. Good quality-control management is mandated under the CLIA regulations. Quality control is emphasized throughout the text.

As a professional laboratory worker in the POL, you will be responsible for the accuracy of results. If you understand the theory or principle of the test and if you have good technique and follow good quality-control procedures, your work will be accurate and reproducible.

———————————————————— ♦ ♦

ORGANIZATION OF THE BOOK

Medical Laboratory Procedures is a competency-based textbook and reference that functions also as a workbook and laboratory manual. The chapters in the book are grouped into five units.

Unit I, Introduction to the Physician's Office Laboratory, includes an informative chapter on laboratory safety. The quality assurance and quality-control chapter in this unit provides a good foundation for the POL worker.

Unit II, Urinalysis, first gives students an understanding of the anatomy and physiology of the urinary system, then takes them through all parts of a urinalysis. The student is also introduced to automated urine chemistry, a topic not covered in other medical assisting laboratory texts.

Unit III, Hematology, begins by teaching the student about blood-collection methods and goes on to cover all aspects of a complete blood count. The unit includes advanced hematology procedures with the pathology that alters results. Presented in this book, and not available in other medical assisting texts, is a complete explanation of the three types of automated hematology instruments presently used in the POL.

Unit IV, Blood Chemistry, gives students an understanding of how blood chemistry analyzers work using the principles of photometry. There is a complete discussion of the three most common blood chemistry analyzers currently used in the POL. Chapter 24's topic, blood chemistry, is not found in other medical assisting texts. It provides the reader with an understanding of the physiology of blood chemistry and its relationship to pathology.

Unit V, Immunology and Microbiology, includes a chapter on immunology tests, discussing the body's immune system and the tests relating to antigen/antibody reactions. The microbiology chapter gives students the basic theory and practical applications needed to function in this area of the POL. The Appendices provide additional helpful information.

Each chapter includes learning objectives, performance objectives, and medical terminology. Chapter content revolves around theory, patient precautions, OSHA requirements, and appropriate quality-control measures. You will also find in each chapter relevant procedures, and an outcome assessment in the form of a chapter review section. The chapter reviews each offer more than 30 questions. (Answers are at the end of the book.) Types of assessment questions include Using Terminology, Acquiring Knowledge, and Applying Knowledge—On the Job, which give students the opportunity to learn from mini case studies.

The accompanying Instructor's Manual includes teaching strategies and resources, along with transparency masters. The test for each chapter is based on the extensive chapter review questions in the text. An answer key for all questions is included.

The laboratory procedures discussed in the text will give students a good background in the area of laboratory testing for the certification examination. Both the Certified Medical Assistant (CMA) examination, administered by the American Association of Medical Assistants (AAMA), and the Registered Medical Assistant (RMA) examination, administered by the American Medical Technologists (AMT), include an area on medical laboratory testing. Mastery of each procedure in this text will give students entry-level competency for that task or skill.

Following are some of the job-entry level skills for which this textbook prepares students:

- Complying with safety requirements of OSHA and Universal Precautions.

- Keeping legal records mandated by CLIA 1988 for quality control.

- Performing complete urinalysis and other urine tests using proper collection techniques.

- Performing blood collections (both capillary and venipuncture).

- Performing hematology tests, including CBC, erythrocyte sedimentation rate, bleeding time, and prothrombin time.

- Understanding the theory of instrumentation, including automated hematology cell counters and blood chemistry analyzers.

- Performing the latest immunology tests of antibody-antigen reactions, including pregnancy, strep screening, mononucleosis, and others.

- Performing microbiology procedures recommended for the POL, including maintaining aseptic technique and collecting and processing specimens.

ACKNOWLEDGMENTS

We wish to express our deepest appreciation to the individuals and companies that contributed materials and information used in the development of this book. We thank you for your time, expertise, and ideas. They are:

- Abbott Laboratories, Diagnostics Division, Abbott Park, IL
- Becton Dickinson and Company, Rutherford, NJ
- Boehringer Mannheim Corporation, Indianapolis, IN
- Stanley C. Bradley, M.D.—Millard-Henry Clinic, P.A., Russellville, AR
- Eastman Kodak Company, Rochester, NY
- Fisher Scientific Company, Pittsburgh, PA
- Helen M. Free, M.A., Miles Inc., Diagnostics Division, Elkhart, IN
- Lucia Johnson, M.A., MT(ASCP), SBB, Director, Medical Technology Program, Research Medical Center, Kansas City, MO
- Douglas Martin, RMT, ISCLT, Laboratory Manager, Millard-Henry Clinic P.A., Russellville, AR

- POLYMEDCO, Inc., Cortland Manor, NY
- Melanie Posey, B.S., MT(ASCP), Ashcraft-Monfee Medical Clinic, P.A., Russellville, AR
- Barbara Watson, Medical Assistant, Clarksville Medical Group, Clarksville, AR
- Jerry West, President, DANAM Electronics, Inc., Dallas, TX

We also thank Tommy L. Mumert, M.A., Director of News Bureau, Arkansas Tech University, and Mark Palko, M.S., Assistant Director of Math Resource and Tutoring Center, University of Arkansas, Fayetteville, for their many photographs used throughout the book. Additional thanks to Mark Palko for his contribution of Chapter 4, Math in the POL, and Chapter 5, Statistics in the POL.

We thank the reviewers for their professional assistance. Their critiques, comments, suggestions, and ideas were helpful in molding this book. We appreciate their time and involvement: Jeanette Girkin, Ed.D., CMA, Tulsa Junior College; Sharon Paff, RMA (AMT), Platt College; Janet Sesser, RMA (AMT), CMA, Bryman School; Pat V. Thompson, M.A., HT (ASCP), CMA, Wingate College; Pamela Huber, MT (ASCP), Erie Community College; and Geraldine Todaro, B.S., CMA, Clplb, Stark Technical College.

Needless to say, this project would not have been possible without guidance, support, encouragement, and an occasional gentle nudge from the various professional staff at Glencoe/McGraw-Hill. We especially want to thank Teri Zak, Editorial Director; Ed Parker, Executive Editor; Molly Kyle, Editor; and Sue Diehm, Production Editor, for their involvement with the project.

Contents

UNIT II   URINALYSIS   131

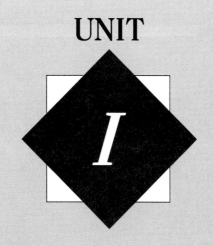

UNIT

I

Introduction to the Physician's Office Laboratory

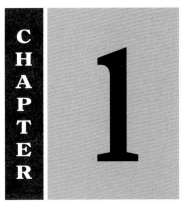

CHAPTER 1

Safety in the Laboratory

COGNITIVE OBJECTIVES

After studying this chapter, you should be able to
- use each of the vocabulary terms appropriately.
- identify the agencies primarily responsible for regulating lab safety.
- list three major types of laboratory hazards and give examples of each.
- identify four types of control methods used to promote lab worker safety and describe one example of each.
- discuss the role of HBV vaccination in promoting lab worker safety.
- describe how lab workers are evaluated and the follow-up after exposure to a biohazard in the lab.
- Explain how biohazardous materials can be safely disposed of in laboratories.
- discuss the role of good housekeeping practices in maintaining a safe work environment in the lab.
- describe the areas in which lab workers should be educated in order to be safe on the job.
- identify four safety tips for using lab chemicals.
- describe how reagents should be labeled and stored.
- explain why acids and bases pose special risks for lab workers.
- describe how to prevent injury from electrical, fire, weather, and personal hazards.
- explain why a professional attitude is important for safety in the lab.
- list seven reasons for lab accidents that are related to worker characteristics.
- discuss steps that can be taken to alleviate stress on the job.

PERFORMANCE OBJECTIVES

After studying this chapter, you should be able to
- plan a lab safety orientation program for new employees.
- devise a waste-disposal plan for a physician's office laboratory.
- develop an accident-proofing program for the lab.
- plan fire and severe weather drills for lab workers.
- design posters that remind lab workers to follow important safety guidelines and procedures.
- evaluate a lab on campus for safety and prepare a report listing ways in which safety can be enhanced.

TERMINOLOGY

acid: a chemical that donates hydrogen ions (H^+), lowers the pH of solutions, and reacts with bases to form water and chemical salts.

aerosolization: the conversion of a liquid, such as blood or blood products, or a solid, such as a powdered chemical, into a fine mist that travels through the air.

autoclave: a device utilizing steam under pressure to sterilize medical instruments and laboratory specimens.

base: a chemical that yields hydroxide ions (OH^-) when dissolved in water (e.g., sodium hydroxide). Bases raise the pH of a solution and react with acids to form chemical salts and water.

biohazard: a biological specimen containing blood or other body fluid that has the potential for transmitting disease.

biological specimen: a specimen that originates from a living organism. Examples are blood, blood products, other body fluids such as cerebrospinal fluid or urine, biopsy samples, bacterial smears, and bacterial cultures.

CDC: Centers for Disease Control and Prevention.

caustic: burning or corrosive; usually destructive to living tissue.

chain of transmission: the unbroken line of transmission of a disease from one host with the disease to a new host.

chemical hazard: a source of danger from exposure to chemicals.

contamination: the pollution of an area or substance with unwanted extraneous material such as pathogens or hazardous chemicals.

disinfection: any practical procedure for reducing the pathogen contamination in the inanimate environment, as in the air, on work counters, or on equipment.

engineering control: a device that keeps biohazards away from laboratory workers.

exposure incident: a situation in which a laboratory worker is exposed to a potentially hazardous substance, such as blood or a toxic chemical.

hazardous chemical list: a list maintained by OSHA that identifies toxic chemicals used in laboratories. It may be consulted to determine the toxicity of a chemical.

HBV (hepatitis B virus): the virus that causes hepatitis B, a type of severe hepatitis transmitted by sexual contact, by needle sharing, or through contaminated blood, blood products, or other body fluids.

HIV (human immunodeficiency virus): the virus that causes AIDS (acquired immunodeficiency syndrome).

ICP (infection-control program): a program that provides the maximum protection for health care workers against occupational sources of disease.

OSHA (Occupational Safety and Health Administration): a federal agency within the U.S. Department of Labor. OSHA works to assure the safety and health of workers.

pathogen: disease-causing microorganism.

physical hazard: a source of danger in the environment, such as shock, housekeeping accidents, and falls.

POL: physician's office laboratory.

post-exposure evaluation: a set of procedures required by OSHA as a follow-up to exposure incidents in the lab.

PPE (personal protective equipment): clothing and other equipment that shield workers from outside contaminants. PPE includes gloves, uniforms, fluid-proof aprons, masks, and eye-shields.

specimen: a small amount of body tissue (e.g., urine, blood, or tumor biopsy) taken for purposes of examination. The sample is assumed to represent the whole and to provide meaningful results for the total individual.

STD: sexually transmitted disease.

toxic: poisonous.

Universal Precautions: a set of recommendations formulated by the CDC to protect workers against HIV and other pathogens. The precautions impose isolation of all specimens of blood, blood products, and other body fluids capable of transmitting pathogens.

vector: an animal, such as an insect, that carries a pathogen.

work-practice control: a method that incorporates safety into laboratory procedures.

● ● ● ● ● ● ● ● ● ● ● ● ● ● ● ●

Safety in the **POL**, physician's office laboratory, is an essential part of all laboratory work. No laboratory procedure is complete unless it includes controls against infection, chemical toxicity, and physical hazards.

WORKING TOWARD A SAFE LABORATORY

Laboratory safety requires knowledge of laboratory procedures, equipment, and reagents, as well as constant watchfulness for danger. One careless worker can undo all the safety practices followed by coworkers in the lab.

♦♦ *Regulating Lab Safety*

Today, there is more concern than ever before about the safety of medical laboratory workers. This concern stems largely from the recent epidemic of AIDS, a fatal blood-borne disease that poses a risk to lab workers. New legislation to enforce laboratory standards of safety has been passed. As a result, clinical laboratories are probably safer now than they were in the past, when disease prevention received less emphasis. In fact, the chances of lab workers being exposed to danger today are probably greater on the commute to work than in the lab, as long as good safety practices are followed.

Two government agencies have had primary responsibility in monitoring medical lab safety—CDC, **Center for Disease Control and Prevention,** and **OSHA,** the **Occupational Safety and Health Administration,** within the U.S. Department of Labor. These two agencies have researched and formulated detailed guidelines for laboratory safety. OSHA has established procedures for avoiding biological and chemical hazards. The CDC has developed a set of principles called **Universal Precautions,** which heighten awareness of the potential risk that medical laboratory **specimens** pose to the workers who handle them.

♦♦ *Hazards*

Potential hazards in POLs fall into three categories:

- **Biohazards** are sources of danger from living ("bio") specimens, including blood and other body fluids, microbiology specimens, and cultures.
- **Chemical hazards** are sources of danger from exposure to laboratory chemicals, including immediate and long-term effects on the health of workers.
- **Physical hazards** are sources of danger in the environment, including electrical shock, housekeeping accidents, and falls.

The federal government mandates addressing all three types of potential hazards in the procedure manuals of POLs. You should familiarize yourself with the procedure manual in any lab where you work. The rest of this chapter describes potential dangers and how to deal with them for each of these three types of hazards.

BIOHAZARDS

Lab specimens sometimes contain disease-causing microorganisms, called **pathogens.** Exposure of lab workers to pathogens is likely to vary from one medical practice to another. A small rural family practice will have a much different patient population with different health problems than will a specialty practice in a large metropolitan area. Nonetheless, general principles of hygiene and safety should be followed in all POLs to decrease the risk of disease transmission.

♦♦♦ Safety and ♦♦♦ Procedure Manuals

Specific safety procedures addressed in POL procedure manuals includes the following:

- safe workplace practices
- disinfection
- hepatitis vaccine
- avoiding and reporting needle stick injuries
- spills and cleanups
- labeling of hazardous materials
- waste disposal
- hygienic practices
- OSHA accident log (for reporting accidents)
- safety education
- storage, inventory, and handling of chemicals
- first aid
- fire presention and use of fire blankets

♦♦♦ Biohazards ♦♦♦

Potentially infective biospecimens encountered in clinical laboratories include the following:

- blood
- body tissue biopsies
- urine
- exudates (pus, mucus, sputum)
- bacterial smears
- bacterial cultures

❖❖ How Diseases Are Transmitted

To know how to avoid disease transmission in the lab, you first must understand how diseases are transmitted. Most infectious disease pathogens gain entry to the body through one of the body's systems, most commonly the skin, respiratory system, or gastrointestinal tract (see Table 1.1). In order to cause disease in a susceptible person, the pathogen must leave the first host and enter an uninfected individual in an unbroken **chain of transmission**. Pathogens in test specimens and on contaminated equipment may infect laboratory workers who handle them. To prevent infection in the lab, barriers must be maintained between workers and biohazardous material, thereby breaking the chain of transmission.

❖❖ Disease Risks in the Lab

Because blood is so frequently encountered, blood-borne diseases are a special risk for lab workers, but almost any type of infection can pose a risk for those who work in a medical lab (see Figure 1.1).

Blood-Borne Infections. Even though they usually cannot survive for long outside body fluids or tissues, blood-borne pathogens pose the greatest potential risk to lab workers. Most important of these are **HIV, human immunodeficiency virus,** which causes AIDS, and **HBV, hepatitis B virus.** They are usually transmitted by the direct contact of body fluids, such as blood or semen, from one person to another in some manner, most often through sexual activity or use of

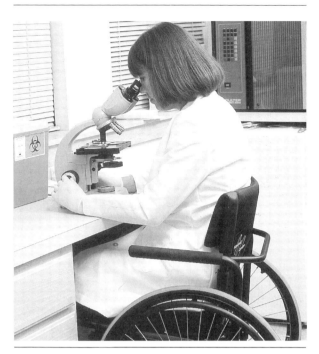

Figure 1.1. To reduce the risk of infection in the POL, keep it clean and orderly at all times. Photo by Matt Meadows.

contaminated needles. Both viruses may cause infections in which the virus is present in body tissues and fluids even though the patient has no symptoms of disease. Because clues may not be apparent from patients or specimens to warn the laboratory workers of infection, all **biological specimens** should be considered potentially infectious and handled as such. Nee-

---

TABLE 1.1 Major Routes of Disease Transmission

Type of Contact*	Infections
Direct skin contact	Staph, strep, measles, colds, influenza, tuberculosis
Mucus-to-mucus contact	Strep, syphilis, gonorrhea, herpes, HIV, other **STDs**
Aerosols and dust	Colds, influenza, measles, tuberculosis, chicken pox
Food and water	Food poisoning, typhoid, hepatitis A, cholera, intestinal parasites
Blood and other body fluids	HIV, HBV
Animal **vectors**	Tularemia, malaria, Rocky Mountain spotted fever, Lyme disease

*This list is not inclusive. For example, rabies can be transferred by a rabid animal's bite or by infected tissue in surgical transplants.

dle sticks are the leading cause of blood-borne infections of lab workers. Improper handling of sharps, such as broken glass tubes, slides, or lancets, may result in cuts to lab workers.

The actual number of people contracting HIV through work in clinical laboratories is thought to be very small. There are only a few documented cases of HIV being transmitted through occupational exposure of health workers.

The number of people infected with HIV remains high, so exposure of health workers is still a concern. In 1996, the U.S. Public Health Services reported that 286,459 persons in the United States were living with HIV infection and with AIDS. AIDS, the disease caused by HIV, results when the virus damages the immune system, allowing other diseases to ravage the body. At this time, there is no cure for AIDS, so preventive measures must be 100 percent effective to ensure the safety of lab workers.

There is a much higher rate of infection of health workers with HBV. According to a CDC survey, between 8,000 and 12,000 health care workers contracted HBV in 1988 alone. Fortunately, there is now a vaccine available to prevent HBV infection.

Other Disease Risks. Diseases that are not blood-borne can also be transmitted in laboratories, especially where cultures are grown and analyzed. They include influenza, tuberculosis, typhoid, strep, and staph. Many pathogens, such as flu virus, travel from host to host on droplets in the air expelled during coughing, sneezing, and talking. In labs, spattering and misting of infectious material can result in infection of workers. Some pathogens, such as tuberculosis and staph, travel on contaminated objects like tissues, clothes, hair, jewelry, and pencils. Practices like putting objects or fingers in the mouth may introduce such agents into the gastrointestinal and respiratory systems.

♦ ♦

WORKING SAFELY WITH BIOHAZARDS

Although hazards such as disease-contaminated biospecimens must always be part of laboratory work, they need not pose a serious threat to the safety of lab workers. Personal protective equipment, if properly worn, is an important safeguard. In addition, automation has greatly reduced the need to handle contaminated specimens and toxic chemicals. Prefabricated tests using very small amounts of specimens and chemicals also make clinical laboratories safer.

OSHA has established medical laboratory guidelines and procedures to reduce the risk of infection from biohazards. OSHA's Infection Control Program details procedures to be used in the following areas, each of which is addressed in the remainder of this section:

- control methods
- HBV vaccination
- post-exposure evaluation and follow-up
- disposal of infectious waste and biohazardous material
- housekeeping practices
- worker education

♦♦ *Control Methods*

Control methods refer to procedures and devices meant to eliminate or prevent **exposure incidents** in POLs. They include Universal Precautions, engineering controls, work-practice controls, and personal protective equipment.

Universal Precautions. The CDC's Universal Precautions are based on the premise that all body fluids and tissues are potentially infected with HIV, HBV, or other pathogens and that lab workers are safe only when they are completely isolated from direct contact with biological specimens. The precautions help ensure that all human blood and other potentially infectious materials are adequately isolated to protect workers from infection.

The Universal Precautions are a departure from past practices. Traditionally, only specimens from patients with diagnosed diseases were isolated. In this era of AIDS, it is realized that only when all biological specimens are treated as contaminated and potentially infectious can there be total protection of lab workers from exposure to biohazards.

Engineering Controls. Devices that provide a safer laboratory environment are called **engineering controls**. They are meant to eliminate or minimize worker exposure to biohazards. They may enclose the biohazard completely, shield the biohazard from aerosolization and spattering, clean and disinfect contaminated equipment, or identify and enclose hazardous waste. It is imperative for worker safety that all engineering-control devices be inspected on a regularly scheduled basis and repaired or replaced as needed.

◆ ◆ ◆ Body Fluids and Disease ◆ ◆ ◆

Body fluids capable of transmitting HIV and HBV include the following:

- blood and blood products
- semen
- vaginal secretions
- spinal fluid
- synovial fluid
- peritoneal fluid
- pericardial fluid
- amniotic fluid

Some body secretions, such as urine, saliva, sputum, and tears may be capable of transmitting HIV if they contain blood. It is important to remember that minute amounts of blood in body fluids may not be obvious or easily detected. These body fluids may carry other pathogens as well. The fact that the body fluid is being tested in a clinical laboratory suggests that it is likely to have a higher than average probability of disease.

Following are descriptions of some engineering controls that you should employ to ensure safety in the medical lab:

- *Specimen containment.* Confine and transfer body fluids within closed containers whenever possible. Place specimens in well-constructed containers with secure lids to prevent leakage during mailing or transport. Do not contaminate either the laboratory request form or the outside of the container during collection.

- *Prevention of aerosolization.* When minute amounts of body fluids or bacterial cultures are sprayed or swept into the air by spillage, laboratory procedures, or wind currents within the room, aerosols are formed. Aerosol droplets cannot be seen by the naked eye, but they can carry disease and penetrate to the depths of the respiratory tract, causing infection of lab workers. Avoid aerosolization of biohazards by covering all specimens. Cap or cover urine containers and tubes of blood when they are not undergoing actual testing.

- *Vented hoods or biohazard cabinets with filters.* Use this equipment when working with bacteria or hazardous material that may generate aerosols. Always inoculate microbiological specimens onto culture media and streak and isolate cultures inside a hood or biohazard cabinet because minute amounts of microscopic organisms may be infectious.

- *Safe use of centrifuges.* Stopper or cap specimens and centrifuge them with the lid closed. An open lid is unsafe because of occasional accidental breakage. Flying glass fragments and spattering or aerosolization of biological specimens can result in both cuts and contamination at once. Never stop centrifuges by hand or open them before spinning down because these actions encourage spattering and aerosolization of contents.

- *Barriers between body fluids and laboratory technicians.* In addition to the engineering control devices that completely enclose blood and other biological materials, other devices serve as shields between laboratory workers and the biohazard. Devices that remove test tube stoppers prevent aerosols from escaping and eliminate direct handling of contaminated stoppers (Figure 1.8). Needle shields provide distance from sharp needles and permit lab workers to remove contaminated needles for disposal without touching the needles or risking needle-stick injury. Plexiglass shields also can be placed as needed between the specimens and technicians. Figures 1.2 and 1.8 show examples of barrier devices.

- *Safe pipetting.* Pipetting by mouth is unsafe because of the danger of aspirating contaminated body fluids and hazardous chemicals. Instead, use mechanical suction devices to uptake and release fluids from pipettes.

- *Disposable equipment.* The less often contaminated equipment is handled, the less likely there is exposure to disease organisms. Disposable equipment, which does not have to be washed and disinfected for reuse, provides a safer laboratory environment. Using disposables is also usually cheaper than cleaning and sterilizing used equipment. A wide variety of disposable products is available, including glassware, needles, lancets, and transfer pipettes.

Work-Practice Controls. Any technique or procedure that makes lab work safer falls into this category. Most **work-practice controls** are simple but proven methods of protecting oneself from disease. All require self-discipline if they are to be effective. To keep yourself as safe as possible in the lab, you should follow these important rules:

- *Wash your hands frequently with a disinfectant soap.* This is especially important when working with biohazardous material. If your skin comes into direct contact with blood or other body fluid, wash the area immediately and thoroughly (see Figure 1.3). **Apply lotion after drying your hands.**

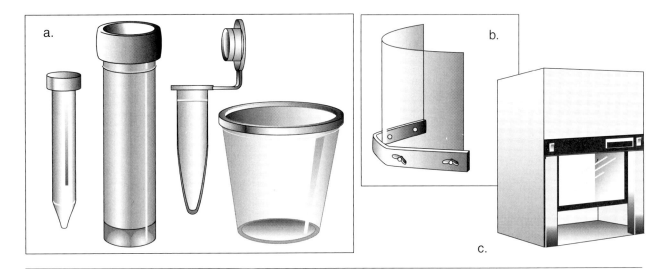

Figure 1.2. Enclose laboratory test fluids in covered containers and place them behind barriers whenever possible for tests. This will result in a safer laboratory. a. Containers should have covers to contain biohazards and prevent spills. b. Shields provide protection from spattering. c. A hood will contain toxic fumes and aerosols.

- *Keep objects away from your face.* The mouth is the entrance to the body's digestive and respiratory systems. The mucous membranes of the nose and eyes also are pathways for infection. Absentmindedly chewing on pencils or fingernails, rubbing your face, or putting on makeup in the lab

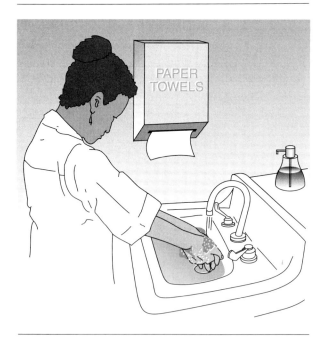

Figure 1.3. Wash your hands thoroughly between patients, after handling hazardous chemicals, between laboratory and nonlaboratory activities, and before and after using the restroom.

can breach the barrier between pathogen and worker. In order to avoid possible contamination with biospecimens and chemicals, do not store or consume food and drink in the laboratory. Take coffee breaks and meals outside the laboratory after washing your hands.

- *Keep personal items in storage.* A closet or locker near the laboratory should house personal effects, such as jewelry and purses or extra clothing worn to and from work. Carrying such personal items into and out of the lab increases the risk of spreading pathogens and other hazards outside the lab environment.

- *Clean up spills immediately.* In the case of potentially infectious spills, pour a 1:10 bleach solution liberally, cover the spill with paper towels to prevent spreading, and allow the spill to soak for 5 minutes before wiping it up. If glass is broken, never pick up the pieces by hand because of the danger of cuts. Instead, scoop broken glass into a dustpan or box and dispose of it in a puncture-proof container (see Figure 1.4). Dispose of items used in the wipe-up, including gloves, aprons, and other barrier items, in another plastic bag. Label these bags with a biohazard indicator. Always wash your hands after cleaning up a spill.

- *Decontaminate equipment.* Decontaminate equipment such as centrifuges that come into contact with blood or other body fluids on a daily basis with disinfectant, such as a 1:100 bleach solution. Equipment that may corrode from daily wiping with a bleach solution may be wiped with alcohol.

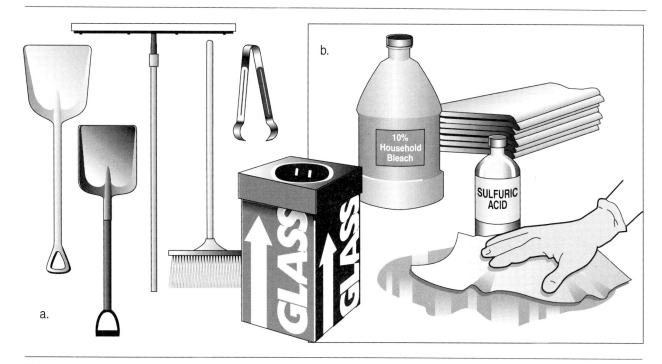

Figure 1.4. a. Clean up broken glass with tools—never with your hands. Place the glass in a stiff cardboard container that will not permit the glass to penetrate. b. Remove spills immediately with absorbent towels or pads. A freshly made solution of 10% household bleach may be used to sanitize the area.

- *Prevent splashing or spraying of materials.* Analyze all procedures for better ways to control mishaps that may contaminate equipment or the lab environment.

Personal Protective Equipment (PPE). PPE (personal protective equipment) refers to specialized clothing and other gear that help shield laboratory workers from contaminants. Examples include fluid repellant, high-collar laboratory jackets and coats, vinyl or latex disposable gloves (see Figure 1.5), fluid-proof aprons, enclosed shoes, face shields, masks, and goggles. PPE should be exchanged for street clothing before lab workers leave the medical office and placed in a designated area for storage, laundry, decontamination, or disposal. OSHA stipulates that medical labs must provide these items and that the equipment must be replaced or repaired when necessary to maintain its effectiveness.

Always wearing disposable, protective gloves is especially important when working with biohazardous material. Wearing gloves helps prevent the entrance of pathogens into abrasions, which may not be obvious if they are very small. Gloves used in venipuncture and laboratory procedures should be discarded after specimen processing. Gloves also should

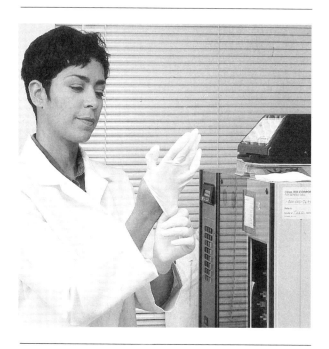

Figure 1.5. Wear clean, disposable protective gloves to reduce the risk of infection. Photo by Matt Meadows.

be changed after each patient contact, and hands should be washed thoroughly between each glove change. Gloves should not be disinfected and reused because disinfected gloves may disintegrate and allow fluid to pass through undetected holes. At the end of the day, gloves should be discarded and hands washed again before lab workers leave the office.

❖❖ HBV Vaccination

Although there is no proven vaccine to prevent HIV infection, a safe and effective vaccine is available for the prevention of HBV infection. This vaccine is recommended for laboratory personnel who are at risk of HBV infection. It is offered free of charge on a voluntary basis by all employers.

❖❖ Post-Exposure Evaluation and Follow-Up

Even when control measures are followed, exposure accidents sometimes occur. If you receive a needle stick or other exposure to potentially hazardous biomaterial, you should submit a written report of the incident to your employer. As a **post-exposure evaluation** and follow-up, your employer must then do the following:

- Track the exposure incident to blood or other potentially infectious material.
- Report the injury on the OSHA 200 Occupational Injury and Illness Log if medical treatment, such as gamma globulin, hepatitis B immune globulin, or hepatitis B vaccine, is prescribed and administered by licensed medical personnel.
- Record HBV or HIV exposure if the infection can be traced to an injury or other biohazard exposure incident.

- Make available to the exposed worker a confidential medical evaluation and follow-up.
- Document the route of exposure, the HBV and HIV status of the source patient, if known, and the circumstances of the exposure.
- Notify the source patient of the incident and ask for consent to collect and test his or her blood for the presence of HIV and HBV.
- Collect blood samples from the worker as soon as possible after exposure for HIV and HBV testing.
- Repeat HIV testing for the exposed worker at 6 weeks, 12 weeks, and 6 months after the exposure.
- Provide counseling to the exposed worker and medical evaluation of any acute febrile illness occurring within 12 weeks after exposure.

This system of record keeping and data collection ensures that exposed workers receive the best possible treatment for potential health problems relating to the accident. It is required by OSHA to increase our knowledge of the dangers of laboratory procedures relating to such diseases as HIV and HBV. OSHA compiles similar information on the incidence of chemical exposures and other laboratory accidents.

❖❖ Disposal of Biohazardous Material

One of the most important aspects of safe handling of biohazardous material is appropriate decontamination and/or disposal of contaminated equipment, especially sharp instruments, and of used biospecimens and other contaminated waste. The laboratory waste-disposal system should provide safe, quick disposal of all items used in collecting and testing body specimens, following federal, state, and local regulations. The aim is to prevent contamination of the lab environment and possible infection of lab workers.

Bagging, Tagging, and Labeling Biohazardous Materials. To protect themselves from possible infection, all lab workers must be aware of the location of biohazardous materials—whether they are blood samples, dirty glassware, or used needles. To this end, it is crucial that biohazards be marked with the word *biohazard*, the red or orange biohazard symbol (see Figure 1.6), or simply color coded red or orange. The identifying mark must be recognizable from a distance of 5 feet. If you use identifying tags or labels, fasten them as closely as possible to the hazard with

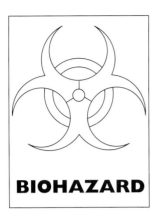

BIOHAZARD

Figure 1.6. This symbol in orange or red permits quick identification of biohazardous material.

string, wire, or adhesive to prevent their loss or unintentional removal. Before you work in any lab, it is important to familiarize yourself with the location of all biohazardous materials. You must be constantly aware of biohazards as you work. In addition, maintenance crews and other nonmedical personnel should be instructed on proper safety and handling of lab wastes.

Cleaning or Disposal of Contaminated Equipment. Reusable pieces of equipment such as hema-

cytometers and pipettes should be placed immediately after use in a suitable disinfectant, such as household bleach. This reduces risk of further **contamination** and makes the equipment easier to clean. Larger pieces of equipment should be washed by hand or in an automatic washer and then disinfected with bleach or sterilized in a drying oven. Contaminated disposable supplies like plastic tubing should be disinfected with germicide or bleach prior to disposal.

Disposal of Sharp Instruments. All disposable sharp instruments, including needles, lancets, and syringes, should be placed in a sharps container immediately after use. The sharps container should be located where these items are most often used. The container should be disposed of when the fill line has been reached. If a sharps container is not available, a substitute container may be used. It should be puncture proof, opaque, **autoclavable,** and tamper proof.

You should be especially careful when discarding contaminated needles. A significant number of infections of lab workers have been documented from needle sticks received while discarding needles. If it is necessary to remove used needles, use a needle remover, a pair of forceps, or clamps—never fingers (see Figure 1.7).

Disposal of Biohazardous Waste. Discarded lab specimens, blood, and other contaminated waste

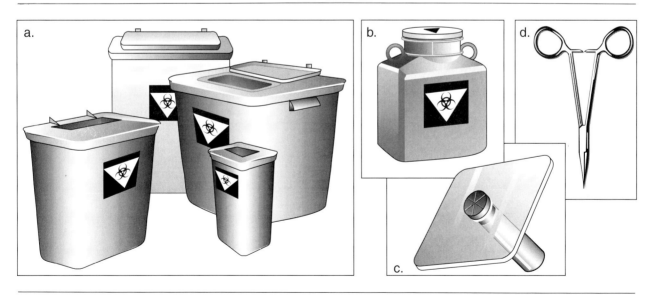

Figure 1.7. These laboratory safety devices are designed to help laboratory workers avoid skin puncture from contaminated needles, lancets, and other sharp objects. a. Sharps containers accommodate different needs in the laboratory. b. This sharps container has a lid designed to remove needles from syringes. c. A needle sheath holder allows removal of special needles that are not disposable. d. In the absence of other devices, use forceps to manipulate sharps and hold them away from the hands.

must be placed in containers or bags that are sturdy and leak proof. They also must be labeled, tagged, or color coded so that the danger of their contents is apparent to anyone who may handle them. If the outside of the bag is contaminated with blood or other potentially infectious material, the waste must be double bagged—one bag inside another. Contaminated waste that will be placed in a landfill must be autoclaved or incinerated first.

♦♦ *Housekeeping Practices*

Safe medical laboratories have smooth, seamless surfaces on floors and countertops so that they are easily washed and disinfected. Floors should be covered with vinyl, not carpeting, to facilitate thorough cleaning and disinfection. The entire laboratory should be well lighted and well ventilated, with plenty of room for work areas and storage of supplies and equipment. Cleaning should be scheduled as often as necessary to maintain a sanitary workplace. When cleaning, workers should use appropriate PPE, including gloves.

Disinfection. For general cleanup, an approved hospital disinfectant, a chemical germicide that is tuberculocidal, or a fresh bleach solution should be used each day on counters, work surfaces, and accessible machine parts that are subject to contamination. Because bleach solutions lose their potency over time, they should be made up daily. A 1:100 dilution of household bleach, such as 5 percent sodium hypochlorite in water, is effective against HIV and other pathogens. A 1:10 dilution should be used for porous surfaces that cannot be physically cleaned before **disinfection.**

Laundry. Laundry that is contaminated with blood or other potentially infectious material should be treated as if it were HBV or HIV infectious and handled as little as possible, with a minimum of agitation. It should be bagged at the location where it is used and transported in biohazard-identified bags. A solution of 1:10 to 1:100 bleach can be used to disinfect the garments before laundering. Many laboratories use disposable lab coats, but these are expensive.

♦♦ *Worker Education*

Training and education of employees are required by law for everyone whose work exposes them to blood or other potentially infectious materials. An education program should include maintenance crews who do general after-hours cleaning and/or repairs. The program must explain the following:

- epidemiology, transmission, and symptoms of HBV and HIV
- effectiveness, safety, and benefits of HBV vaccination
- employer's **ICP, infection-control program,** including procedures to follow if an exposure incident occurs and labeling of biohazards
- methods of control that may prevent or reduce exposure to biohazards, including Universal Precautions, engineering controls, work-practice controls, and personal protective equipment

---
♦♦

WORKING SAFELY WITH CHEMICAL HAZARDS

Safety in POLs requires knowledge of and respect for chemicals. The current trend is using very small amounts of premixed chemicals embedded in plastic or dissolved in some other medium in order to eliminate most mixing and handling of reagents. Test kits with these small amounts of chemicals are not hazardous if used correctly.

Unfortunately, hazardous chemicals cannot be eliminated entirely from medical labs. Chemicals such as methyl alcohol and acetone are required as preservatives, stains, drying agents, and cleaners. These and other lab chemicals may be flammable, caustic, carcinogenic, or **toxic** in other ways. This is true of their fumes as well as their liquid or solid forms. Therefore, it is important to be familiar with the rules of safety concerning lab chemicals.

♦♦ *Safety Tips for Using Lab Chemicals*

Lab workers should assume that all chemicals are harmful until they learn otherwise and should never taste or sniff an unknown chemical in order to identify it. OSHA maintains a list of toxic chemicals used in medical labs that may be checked if there is any question about toxicity. OSHA also requires chemical manufacturers and distributors to furnish a Material Safety Data Sheet (MSDS) with all shipments of hazardous chemicals. The MSDS provides usage precautions, among other information. For safety's sake, familiarize yourself with all precautions for chemicals that you use in the lab.

When using hazardous chemicals, it is especially important to keep your work station free of excess reagents and equipment. This will help prevent spills and mistakes. Manipulate chemicals that generate fumes or a cloud of powder under a vented hood. Avoid direct contact of lab chemicals with skin or clothes, and wash your hands after each use.

Always lay covers from reagent containers top down on a clean counter to prevent contaminating both the counter and reagent container cover. Replace the cover and return the reagent to its storage place as soon as possible.

When heating chemicals in a test tube, be sure to turn the test tube so that the opening is pointed away from you and coworkers. Heat the test tube gently in the flame, starting at the top of the liquid and moving toward the bottom. If heated from the bottom up, the fluid may expand quickly and rise to the top, forcing hot liquid and steam out of the tube.

Reagents may be safely flushed down the laboratory sink unless otherwise specified. Place these directly into the drain to prevent spattering and flush with plenty of water.

•• Labeling and Storing Reagents

OSHA requires that all reagent containers be clearly and prominently labeled with the chemical's name and pertinent information about hazards, such as toxicity and flammability. The date of receipt or

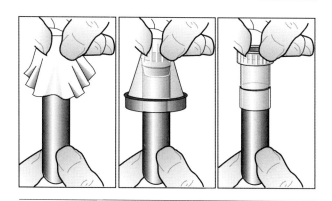

Figure 1.8. When removing stoppers from test tubes, use a disposable cover, either improvised or purchased, to prevent spattering and aerosol contamination in the laboratory.

preparation of chemicals, their expiration date, and any special storage requirements also should be noted. Discard reagents with missing or unreadable labels to prevent potential misuse. As an extra safety measure, it is a good idea to label all caustic reagents with a brightly colored sticker or easily recognized symbol.

All reagents should be stored away from heat and sunlight in a dry location because heat, light, and moisture often cause chemicals to react. Reagents may be stored at room temperature unless storage directions indicate the need for refrigeration. Reagents that react together should be stored in isolation from one another, and flammable reagents should be stored in a fireproof metal cabinet. The smallest amount of all necessary chemicals should be kept in stock to keep the potential for contamination and injury at a minimum.

•• Acids and Bases—Special Concerns

Two groups of chemicals requiring special caution are **acids** and **bases**. Both are **caustic**, generate heat when they come into contact with water, and react quickly with other chemicals and each other. Even the fumes of acids and bases react together. Acids and bases are prone to spattering and can cause serious burns to the eyes and skin. Protective eye wear is recommended when working with acids, bases, and other chemicals that may spatter.

Acids always should be added to water—not water to acids—because there is less chance of spattering and burns. When water is added to acid, it remains on top because it is less dense. There, it reacts and generates heat, potentially spattering the work station and lab workers.

Acids and bases neutralize each other; therefore, a base is used to neutralize acid spills and an acid to neutralize base spills. A large amount of weak base will neutralize a strong acid as effectively as a smaller amount of stronger base but in a safer manner. Similarly, a large amount of weak acid is safer to neutralize a strong base than is a stronger acid.

•• First Aid for Chemical Spills

No matter how careful laboratory workers are, the possibility of an accident with hazardous chemicals still exists. Therefore, every laboratory should have a designated sink where chemical spills can be washed off quickly. An eyewash station should be installed at

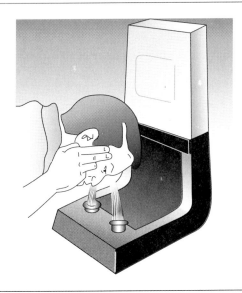

Figure 1.9. An eyewash station is an instant source of water for a quick rinse when an accident occurs. A quick response can be crucial.

a sink that is quickly accessible (see Figure 1.9). Check your lab's manual for more explicit procedures to follow when chemical spills occur.

SAFETY FROM PHYSICAL HAZARDS

Physical hazards such as slippery floors and falling objects may present risks to workers in most workplaces, but are especially dangerous in laboratories where biohazardous materials are at hand. Good housekeeping and time management are important to help prevent accidents of this nature. The best way for lab workers to avoid injury from physical hazards is to follow basic rules for physical safety. These are described next for electrical, fire, weather, and personal hazards.

✦✦ *Electrical Hazards*

Always use common sense when using electricity. For example, always unplug electrical appliances before changing bulbs or servicing. Be careful to keep water and chemicals away from outlets and electrical equipment to avoid dangerous shorts that can start fires and cause electrocution.

The electrical wiring system of the laboratory should be adequate for the amount of electricity used—extension cords and multiple tap plugs are not safe and usually indicate an inadequate electrical wiring system. There should be safety devices such as grounded plugs, current breakers or fuses, and a master switch that is accessible in case of emergency.

Any malfunctioning electrical equipment should be checked by a professional. If the malfunction is major, unplug the machine until it can be repaired or replaced. Often, suppliers loan out another machine in the interim. Check cords periodically for breaks and frays.

✦✦ *Fire Hazards*

Any situation that is a potential fire hazard should be remedied before an accident occurs. For example, long hair or loose clothing presents a fire hazard around open flames such as Bunsen burners. Situations like this are easily avoided.

Even when precautions are taken to prevent fires, fires may still occur. Every lab worker should know how to report a fire. Each lab should have a small, multiple-use fire extinguisher mounted on a wall ready for use. Know how to use it. The fire extinguisher should be in good condition and checked periodically. A fire blanket at a convenient location is essential to smother flames.

The POL manual should include a fire escape plan. Dual exits should be included in the plan in case one exit is blocked by fire. Exits to be used as fire escapes should be clearly marked and accessible at all times during work hours.

✦✦ *Weather Hazards*

In some parts of the country, weather emergencies are relatively common. For example, hurricanes are a potential risk in the Southeast and tornadoes in the Midwest. The places to take cover in case of severe weather in your area should be described in the POL manual. Learn where they are.

✦✦ *Personal Hazards*

Wherever you work, you should analyze your work environment for personal safety hazards such as theft and assault. To maximize your personal safety in the lab, in the parking lot, and on route to and from work, follow these safety tips recommended by police:

- When you arrive at work, park in a well-lighted area and lock your car.

- At work, keep your purse or other valuables out of sight, preferably in a locked place, such as a desk or filing cabinet.
- Avoid working alone, especially at night.
- When you leave work, particularly after dark, stay alert, leave the building with coworkers, have your keys handy, and drive on well-lighted streets.

WORKER CHARACTERISTICS AFFECTING LAB SAFETY

Safety rules and regulations and specialized equipment and gear cannot ensure lab safety unless workers use care and common sense on the job everyday.

Worker Attitudes

In POLs, as elsewhere, worker attitudes can contribute to an unsafe work environment. Workers who take shortcuts and are inconsiderate of others may undermine everyone's safety. Attitudes that may contribute to a safer laboratory, on the other hand, include awareness of potential danger, willingness to learn and use safe methods, and concern for the welfare of coworkers. Professionalism in medical laboratories is a combination of positive attitudes that puts a high priority on worker safety.

Risk Taking

To ensure safety on the job, lab workers should avoid taking unnecessary risks. Sometimes, even experienced workers take risks that can cause lab accidents. Indeed, experienced workers sometimes take unnecessary risks because they have performed risky tasks without incident so many times in the past. Other common reasons for lab accidents include:

- hurrying to meet deadlines or goals
- carelessness and fatigue
- preoccupation with nonwork matters
- excessive stress

Keep in mind that working under these conditions may lead to accidents.

Chronic Injury to Muscles and Bones

Muscles and bones, if overused over a period of time, can develop chronic injuries classified as occupational diseases. Two examples are carpal tunnel syndrome of the wrist, which affects keyboard operators, and neck torsion disorder, which may occur from long periods of microscope use.

The following suggestions can help you prevent these injuries. Examine your work activities, furniture, and lighting for stressful elements. Use good posture, comfortable chairs, good lighting, large, padded grip and handle surfaces, and cushioned hand/wrist rests. Alternate between high- and low-risk activities and take brief breaks to stretch muscles during tedious tasks. Try to eliminate awkward or stressful motions, such as reaching beyond your usual reach. Use minimal, not excessive, force to operate keyboards and instruments. If the microscope is not at a comfortable height, try placing books under it to raise it to a level that does not require you to bend your neck tightly.

More About Stress

While some stress may be helpful in maintaining alertness, too much stress may cause work quality to deteriorate and lead to accidents on the job. Stress may originate off the job—a too busy life-style, for example—or work conditions may be the cause. It is not uncommon for lab workers to feel pressure to work faster. Whatever the cause, excessive stress should be brought under control before injury or ill health results. Following are some ways to help control job-related stress:

- Prioritize your job tasks each day and schedule your work assignments by the day, week, and month. Work piling up on your desk may create job stress. If you develop a plan to deal with all of the work, you will feel less stressed.
- Try to resolve job-related stress by first discussing problems with your supervisor. For example, be realistic with your time. Tell your supervisor if you have more work than you can handle.
- Develop a personal wellness program—eat a well-balanced diet, get plenty of rest, and exercise regularly.

PROCEDURE

Hand Washing

- Wash your hands before gloving and working with hazardous laboratory procedures and also after such procedures.

Goal

- After successfully completing this procedure, you will be able to wash your hands with soap and running water to sanitize your skin prior to gloving before hazardous laboratory procedures and also after completing such procedures.

Completion Time

- 2 minutes

Equipment and Supplies

- a sink with running water
- liquid soap in a dispenser (preferably an antiseptic soap)
- paper towels in a dispenser
- hand lotion

Instructions

Read through the list of equipment and supplies you will need and the steps of the procedure. Be sure you understand each step correctly and in the proper order.

S = Satisfactory U = Unsatisfactory	S	U
1. Remove all jewelry such as rings (except for a plain gold band), bracelets, and your wristwatch because these may harbor microorganisms in the crevices. Wristwatches worn at work in the POL should be sanitized separately.		
2. Turn on the faucet and regulate the water temperature to a desired warm temperature. Soap will suds better in warm water.		
3. Wet your hands with water. Hold your hands lower than your elbows to prevent water running past your elbows. Microorganisms and debris will be washed away into the sink instead of traveling up your arms.		

4. Apply approximately one teaspoon of liquid soap to your hands and arms up to your mid forearm. Suds the soap with about ten circular motions of your hands.

5. Use friction along with the circular motions to suds your palms, the backs of your hands, and your forearms.

6. Wash your fingers with ten circular motions, interfacing your fingers and rubbing them back and forth with friction and circular motions.

7. Rinse your hands well, making sure to hold your hands lower than your elbows. Then rinse your wrists and forearms until no soap remains.

8. Repeat the soaping and rinse process to be sure that your hands are clean.

9. Dry your hands gently and thoroughly with paper towels. Drying your hands well will help prevent chapping, which causes crevices and breaks in skin.

10. Turn off the water using a paper towel. The faucet handles are considered contaminated.

11. Inspect your hands for cuts and abrasions. Cover any hangnails or open wounds with bandages.

12. Put lotion on your hands.

13. If this is your last hand wash of the day before leaving work, clean your nails thoroughly with an orange stick. Nails harbor microorganisms in the debris lodged underneath them.

14. If work is to continue with hazardous material, put on nonsterile latex gloves.

15. Wipe the sink area with a paper towel to remove water and debris. Keep the paper towel between your hands and the sink. The sink is considered contaminated.

OVERALL PROCEDURAL EVALUATION

Student's Name _____

Signature of Instructor _____ **Date** _____

Comments

> ## Note
>
> Frequent hand washing dries and cracks the skin. Always use hand lotion after washing your hands, to help maintain skin integrity.

PROCEDURE

1.2 Practicing Lab Safety

Goal

- After successfully completing this procedure, you will be able to handle and use biohazardous materials safely in the lab.

Completion time

- 45 minutes

Equipment and Supplies

- disposable latex gloves
- hand disinfectant
- surface disinfectant
- paper towels
- biohazard container
- sharps container
- pipette and suction device
- personal protective gear
- bags and tags for biohazardous waste
- needle and needle remover or forceps
- tap water

Instructions

Read through the list of equipment and supplies you will need and the steps of the procedure. Be sure you understand each step before you begin. Then complete each step correctly and in the proper order. If your completion time is too long, repeat the procedure until you increase your speed.

S = Satisfactory U = Unsatisfactory	S	U
1. Collect or locate the appropriate equipment.		
2. Wash your hands thoroughly with hand disinfectant.		
3. Dry your hands completely.		

4. Put on disposable latex gloves.

5. Assemble and put on correctly a complete outfit of personal protective gear.

6. Remove all gear, except the latex gloves, and return it to storage.

7. Use the pipette suction device to pipette a small amount of tap water into a disposable pipette.

8. Empty the pipette and repeat step 7.

9. Pour a small amount of tap water on the floor to simulate a biohazardous spill.

10. Pour surface disinfectant liberally on the spill. Cover the spill with paper towels to prevent spreading, and let the spill soak for 5 minutes.

11. Wipe up the spill thoroughly with paper towels.

12. Dispose of the paper towels in a plastic bag. Label the bag with a biohazard indicator.

13. Remove your gloves, wash your hands with disinfectant, dry your hands, and put on clean gloves.

14. Thoroughly wipe a piece of equipment such as a centrifuge with disinfectant or alcohol and paper towels.

15. Dispose of the paper towels in a plastic bag and label the bag with a biohazard indicator.

16. Remove your gloves, wash your hands with disinfectant, dry your hands, and put on clean gloves.

17. Using a needle remover or forceps, carefully remove a needle from a syringe.

S = Satisfactory	U = Unsatisfactory	S	U
18. Dispose of the needle in the sharps container.			
19. Discard disposable equipment.			
20. Disinfect other equipment and return it to storage.			
21. Clean the work area following the Universal Precautions.			
22. Remove your gloves, wash your hands with disinfectant, and dry them.			

OVERALL PROCEDURAL EVALUATION

Student's Name _____

Signature of Instructor _____ Date _____

Comments

CHAPTER 1 REVIEW

Using Terminology

Define the following terms as they apply to laboratory safety.

1. Aerosolization: _____

_____

2. Biohazard: _____

_____

3. Biological specimen: _____

_____

4. Chain of transmission: _____

_____

5. Engineering control: _____

_____

6. Exposure incident: _____

_____

7. Material Safety Data Sheet: _____

_____

8. HBV (hepatitis B virus): _____

_____

9. HIV (human immunodeficiency virus): _____

_____

10. ICP (infection-control program): _____

_____

11. OSHA (Occupational Safety and Health Administration): _____

_____

12. PPE (personal protective equipment): _____

_____

13. Universal Precautions: _____

_____

14. Work-practice control: _____

_____

Acquiring Knowledge

Answer the following questions in the spaces provided.

15. How do the Universal Precautions protect laboratory workers against infection?

_____

_____

16. List five medical problems or diseases that may be encountered in a laboratory.

_____

_____

_____

17. Discuss appropriate ways to manage a high level of stress at work.

_____

_____

_____

_____

_____

18. How should you apply the rule of placing a barrier between you and the possible source of contamination or disease in the laboratory? Give examples for:

Pipetting _____

_____

_____

Disposing of used needles and lancets _____

_____

_____

Working with biohazards that may splatter _____

_____

_____

19. Why are biohazards labeled with an easily read label, whether they are test specimens or waste material?

_____

_____

20. Why do the Universal Precautions dictate that all biospecimens be regarded as hazardous?

_____

_____

21. Which of the following may transmit HIV?

_____ a. blood

_____ b. amniotic fluid

_____ c. semen

_____ d. synovial fluid

22. What protection against HBV is available to laboratory workers?

_____

_____

23. What records are kept of reported laboratory accidents involving biohazards and toxic chemicals?

_____

_____

24. List seven ways to prevent exposure to toxic chemicals in the laboratory.

_____

_____

_____

_____

_____

_____

_____

25. In a safety education program provided by the employer, what information should be provided to new lab workers?

_____

_____

_____

_____

26. What are some physical hazards in the laboratory and how are they best controlled?

_____

_____

_____

_____

_____

27. What is an acceptable dilution of household bleach prepared daily for the purpose of decontaminating counters, equipment, and floors?

_____

28. What part does attitude play in laboratory safety?

_____

_____

_____

29. When should laboratory workers wash their hands?

_____

30. What rule should laboratory workers follow regarding facial contamination?

_____

31. How should laboratory workers dispose of waste contaminated with biohazards or chemicals?

_____

_____

_____

32. Why should fire escape routes be posted and exits not blocked with supplies or furniture?

_____

_____

33. How can lab workers avoid being exposed to needle sticks from contaminated needles?

_____

34. When should lab workers wear gloves in the laboratory?

_____

Applying Knowledge—On the Job

Answer the following questions in the spaces provided.

35. Mary and Jane were working as a team in the POL. The schedule for that day was very busy. Mary had just drawn blood. As she attempted to dispose of the contaminated needle into the sharps container, Jane reached for a reagent and was accidentally stuck. Write the report that Jane must submit to her employer and list the post-exposure procedure steps that her employer must follow.

_____

_____

_____

_____

_____

36. A patient infected with HIV is having a blood test in the POL. What precautions should you take when you draw his blood? When you perform the blood test?

_____

_____

_____

_____

_____

37. Joseph, a student, is instructed to visit a lab to see how safety rules are being observed. Make a list of at least eight safety rules that Joseph could easily observe being followed or disobeyed when he visits the lab.

_____

_____

_____

_____

_____

_____

_____

_____

38. Susan, a lab worker, performs the following tasks in the following order. After which tasks should she wash her hands?

_____ a. entering the lab for her work shift

_____ b. putting on disposable gloves

_____ c. performing a test using a test tube of blood

_____ d. removing gloves

_____ e. taking the lab report to the receptionist

_____ f. putting on gloves

_____ g. drawing blood from a patient for a blood test

_____ h. performing the blood test

_____ i. removing the gloves

_____ j. putting the cover on the microscope

_____ k. making a phone call

_____ l. going to the waiting room to call a patient to come to the lab for a timed blood test

_____ m. verifying that the test request is for the right patient

39. A laboratory fails a fire safety inspection only because an exit in the lab is partially blocked. List three other safety requirements that it must have met.

_____

_____

_____

2 *The Microscope*

COGNITIVE OBJECTIVES

After studying this chapter, you should be able to

- use each of the vocabulary terms appropriately.
- describe the parts of the compound microscope.
- explain how the lens system of the microscope works.
- explain the difference between low-power and high-power objectives.
- explain the difference between magnification and resolution.
- illustrate how specimens are illuminated for visibility under the microscope.
- list the steps in focusing a specimen under various objectives.
- identify safety precautions to protect the microscope from damage.
- list the attributes of a good microscope for the medical lab.
- identify the causes and remedies of common microscope problems.

PERFORMANCE OBJECTIVES

After studying this chapter, you should be able to

- focus a slide under the 10X, 45X, and 100X objectives.
- demonstrate how to clean the microscope.
- design a poster for use in a medical lab to show how to protect a microscope from damage.

TERMINOLOGY

adjustable ocular: usually, the eyepiece on the left. It can be adjusted to correct the focus for the individual's visual acuity.

aperture: in a microscope, the opening through which the light passes such as in the stage or iris diaphragm.

artifact: an extraneous, nontissue feature that contaminates specimen slides.

binocular: literally, pertaining to two eyes; a microscope with two eyepieces, one for each eye.

coarse adjustment: the first step in focusing, in which the distance between the specimen and the lens (working distance) is covered very quickly, either by lowering the objective or raising the stage.

condenser: also called the substage. Located just below the opening in the mechanical stage and above the light source, the condenser controls the amount of light.

eyepiece: *see* ocular.

fine adjustment: the step in focusing in which only small changes are made in the working distance between the lens and the specimen.

iris diaphragm: located in the condenser, the iris diaphragm is the aperture that controls the amount of light entering through the opening in the stage by contracting or enlarging like the iris of the eye.

mechanical stage: a platform that holds the slide. The mechanical stage can be moved in four directions, so that any part of the slide may be viewed.

microscope: an instrument that uses a lens or combination of lenses to enlarge very small objects for viewing.

microscopy: the use of a microscope.

monocular: literally, pertaining to one eye; a microscope in which there is only one eyepiece.

nosepiece: a rotating, circular apparatus on the microscope, which holds the objectives and moves them into position as needed.

objective: the lens of the microscope that collects the image from the slide, magnifies it, and transmits it to the eyepiece lens, or ocular.

ocular: also called eyepiece. The ocular lens collects the image from the objective lens and magnifies it 10X in most oculars.

oil-immersion objective: the lens with the highest power of magnification (about 100X). The oil-immersion objective clarifies the image by using a layer of oil between the specimen and the objective to refract the light into the lens.

reagent: a substance used to produce a chemical reaction.

resolution: the ability of a set of lenses to distinguish fine detail; the most important gauge of a microscope's quality.

rheostat: a device that controls the amount of current entering an electrical circuit. A rheostat controls the light on a microscope.

stage: the platform on a microscope that supports the glass slide and specimen for viewing. The stage may move up and down for focusing.

stationary ocular: usually, the eyepiece for the right eye. It is adjusted for focus first using the coarse and fine adjustment knobs.

visual acuity: clarity of vision.

working distance: the distance between the specimen and the objective. It is important to check this distance frequently to avoid bringing the lens into contact with the slide.

● ● ● ● ● ● ● ● ● ● ● ● ● ● ●

This chapter describes why the **microscope** is an important tool in medical laboratories and how the microscope works. It also explains how to use, care for, and select a microscope.

MICROSCOPY

Microscopes are used in all POLs to obtain valuable information about patients by viewing structures invisible to the naked eye. Many abnormalities in blood and other body tissues and many types of disease-causing microorganisms can be identified when they are viewed under the magnification of a microscope.

◆◆ *The Role of the Microscope*

Lab workers use the microscope (see Figure 2.1) often for a diversity of tasks. They may test blood for anemia or leukemia, which requires them to magnify a blood specimen so that they can recognize blood-cell maturation stages. To identify a particular type of microorganism, such as bacteria, lab workers must magnify specimens to see their shape, size, and stain and growth characteristics.

◆◆ *Quality Control*

As valuable as it is, **microscopy** is the most variable aspect of laboratory testing because of problems with quality control. For example, slide specimens require special preparation, which may produce variable results unless timing and quality of **reagents** are monitored closely. Slides may be contaminated with **artifacts** that mimic biological structures. Interpreting slides may be difficult, requiring lab workers to recognize complicated patterns of blood-cell structure, urine-sediment composition, and microorganisms. These and other factors may introduce error in test results.

◆◆ *Mastering the Microscope*

Mastering the essentials of microscope use takes practice. It is not as easy as it looks. The microscope requires extended training to utilize its different functions. In addition, identifying differences among microorganisms and cell structures takes much study and practice viewing them under magnification.

HOW THE MICROSCOPE WORKS

Before learning how to use the microscope, it is important to understand how the microscope works.

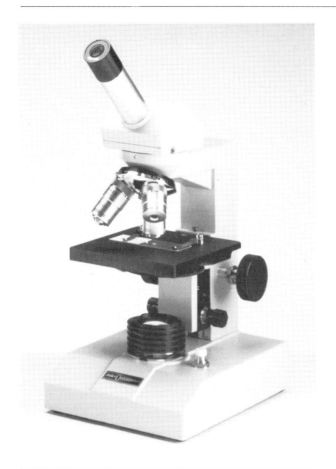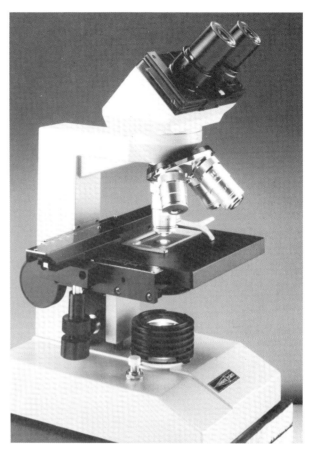

Figure 2.1. Two styles of microscope. a. Micromaster Monocular Microscope. Note that this does not have a mechanical stage. It has stage clamps to hold the slide in place. b. Micromaster Binocular Microscope with a built-in graduated mechanical stage and four objectives—4X, 10X, 40X, and 100X. Courtesy of Fisher Scientific.

This section describes the different features of the microscope and the role that they play in magnifying specimens. While reading this section, refer to Figure 2.2, which shows the microscope and its parts.

All of the following parts of the microscope are mounted in a stand, which consists of an arm and a base. The stand must be sturdy enough to resist vibrations and jars. It supports the lens system, the accessories needed to operate it, and the **stage** upon which the specimen is mounted on its slide. The base usually contains the light source necessary to operate the microscope.

◆◆ *The Lens System*

The compound microscope, which is the type most commonly used in POLs, has two lenses mounted on opposite ends of a closed tube, called the barrel.

These two lenses, the **ocular** and the **objective,** work together to magnify the specimen.

Ocular. The lens nearest the eye is called the ocular, or eyepiece. **Monocular** microscopes have one eyepiece, **binocular** microscopes have two. Most oculars magnify the specimen by a power of ten (10X), meaning that the ocular increases the diameter of the specimen to ten times its actual size.

Objectives. The lens farthest from the eye and closest to the specimen is called the objective. A microscope may have three or four objectives offering different powers of magnification (usually 4X, 10X, 45X, and 100X). Only one objective is used at a time. The objectives are screwed into a circular **nosepiece,** which is revolved by hand until the objective with the desired magnification is reached and clicked into place. Each objective is stamped with its power of magnification. It also has a different-colored band around it for quick identification.

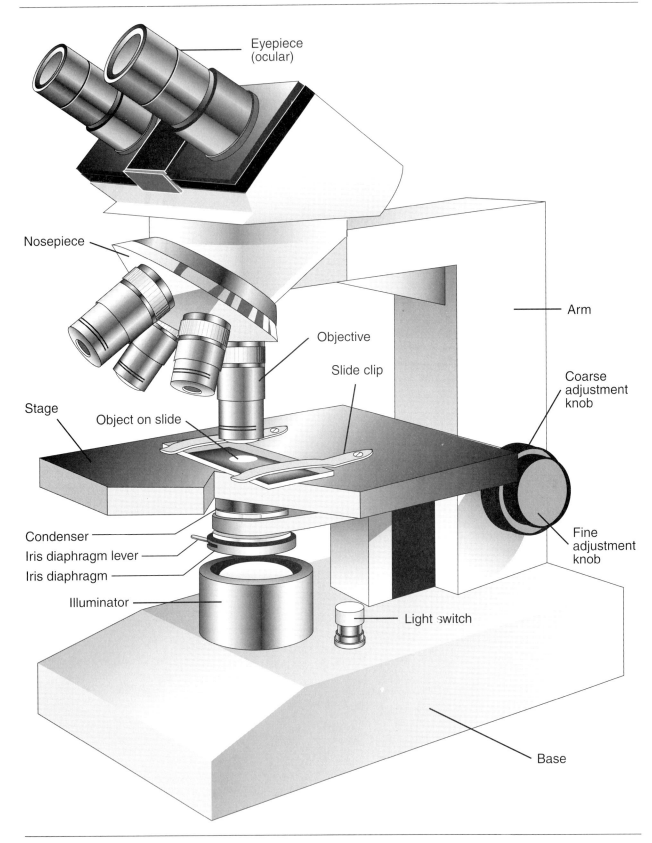

Figure 2.2. The parts of a microscope.

The 4X objective is used for scanning a slide for areas to examine under higher magnification. The 10X objective is referred to as low power, and it is used extensively in the initial steps of focusing, to count cells, and to scan urine sediment. The 45X (40X or 43X on some microscopes) objective is referred to as high power. It is used extensively for red and white blood-cell counts, scanning differential smears, and viewing urine sediment. The 4X, 10X, and 45X objectives are called dry lenses because they do not require oil to assist in magnification. In fact, if oil touches these objectives, it should be removed immediately because it softens the cement that holds the lenses in place.

The 100X (95X or 97X on some microscopes) is an **oil-immersion objective,** which uses a layer of oil between the specimen and the objective to refract light into the lens. Because this oil is a relatively dense medium, with about the same refractive index as glass, the light rays do not diffuse through it as they do through air, which is less dense. The 100X oil-immersion objective has the greatest power of magnification. Only under this objective are the identifying characteristics of the different types of bacteria and white blood cells revealed. Blood-differential smears are routinely counted under the oil-immersion objective. The oil should be wiped from the 100X objective after each slide is viewed to prevent the oil from damaging the cement around the lens.

Magnification and Resolution. Total magnification of a microscope is the product of the magnification of the ocular and the magnification of the objective. If the ocular magnifies 10X and the objective 10X, for example, the total magnification is 100 times actual size (10X × 10X = 100X). A 10X ocular with a 43X objective would give a total magnification of 430 times actual size (10X × 43X). With the 100X objective, the magnification would be 1000 times actual size (10X × 100X).

The **resolution** of the microscope is its ability to distinguish fine details. This ability depends on not only the power of magnification but also the quality of the microscope. For the same level of magnification, a better quality of microscope will have higher resolution. Resolution can best be assessed by viewing a familiar slide and noting the details discernable with different microscopes.

✦✦ *The Stage*

The stage is the platform that holds the slide to be viewed. The stage provides a secure grip on the slide, which is placed over a circular or oval hole in its center. The hole allows light to enter from below, passing through the specimen to the lens system. On some microscopes, the platform stage may be raised or lowered to focus the specimen with the objective. On other models, the stage is stationary, and the objective moves up and down instead.

Fastened onto the platform stage, a smaller optional stage allows movement of the slide in four directions along the x and y axes. This smaller stage is usually referred to as the **mechanical stage.** Etched markings on a scale on the mechanical stage denote the position of a field on the slide.

✦✦ *Light*

In order for the microscope to work, light must pass upward through the material being viewed and into the objective lens. Then, the light must travel to the ocular lens and to the eyes of the lab worker viewing the specimen. The light is changed by the lens of the microscope so that the rays reaching the eyes show a magnified image of the specimen.

The light source usually is located in the base of the microscope stand. It has a filter to change wavelengths. Generally, blue daylight is used because it provides the most comfortable viewing, but other filters may be used for special purposes. Light intensity may be controlled with a **rheostat.** The **condenser,** also called the substage, is located just below the opening in the mechanical stage and above the light source. It controls the stream of light. The condenser may be lowered or raised and its aperture narrowed or widened to control the amount of light passing through to the specimen on the slide. The **aperture** in the condenser is called the **iris diaphragm** because it resembles the iris of the eye.

Because the light shines up through the specimen to the viewer (see Figure 2.3), the specimen must be transparent, that is, thin enough to allow light to pass through it without being diffused. This also is why specimens are always viewed on glass slides. In addition, there must be enough contrast in light and dark shades and different colors among structures for the structures to be visible. Most specimens do not have the natural level of contrast or color needed for effective viewing; therefore, stains and dyes are used to prepare specimens. Also, the specimen must be only one cell-layer thick in order to show cellular structures clearly.

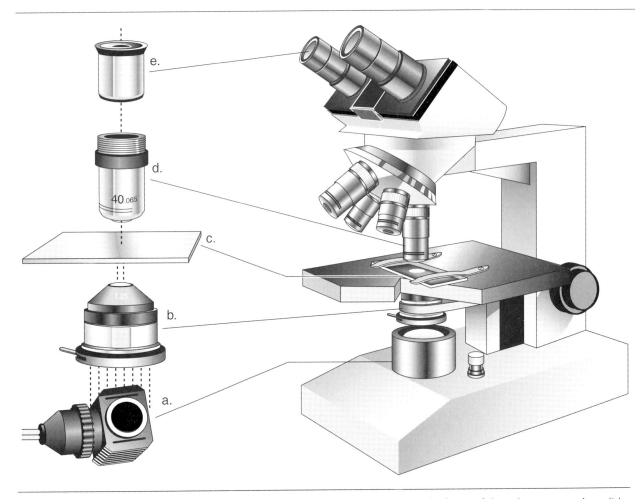

Figure 2.3. The path of light through the microscope. a. The light originates at the base of the microscope, where it is adjusted with a rheostat. A lens directs it upward to the condenser. b. The condenser concentrates the light into an intense cone of light. It may be raised or lowered. The iris diaphragm, part of the condenser, will open and close to control the light. c. The light passes through the glass slide and specimen and into the objective. d. The objective magnifies the image on the glass slide and passes the image into the eyepiece. e. The eyepiece again magnifies the image, which enters the user's eye.

HOW TO USE A MICROSCOPE

Using a microscope primarily involves focusing the image by moving the objective closer to the specimen (or the specimen closer to the objective) and attaining the correct level of illumination from the light source. Although this chapter describes focusing and adjusting the light source, they actually are done together as part of the same process.

❖❖ *Focusing*

Focusing the microscope is done by moving the objective up or down relative to the stage (or the

stage relative to the objective). Movement of the objective (or stage) is controlled by round knobs, usually located on both sides of the microscope and near enough to the base of the microscope to permit resting your arms on the table while focusing.

Working Distance. The distance between the specimen on the stage and the objective lens is referred to as the **working distance.** The working distance is longest at lower magnification (4X and 10X) and gets shorter as the magnification increases. With the 100X objective, the working distance is very small, about the same thickness as a piece of heavy paper. At this distance, the oil on the oil-immersion lens touches both the glass slide and the objective. Because the objective is so close to the slide under high-power magnification, you should check the working distance by looking at the microscope from the side when changing from 45X to 100X. If you move the objective too close to the stage, you can grind it into the slide and ruin the lens.

Coarse and Fine Adjustments. The **coarse adjustment** focus knob moves the objective quickly; that is, it moves the objective a great distance with one revolution. This knob is used first to bring the specimen into approximate focus. The **fine adjustment** focus knob then brings the specimen into sharper focus. It moves the objective much more slowly because the knob moves the objective only a short distance with one revolution.

In order to prevent damage to the lens, it is especially important to use the fine adjustment knob at high power when the objective is close to the slide. For the same reason, the specimen should be focused first under the 4X or 10X objective, because on most microscopes, these low-power objectives usually cannot touch the slide even when they are moved as close as possible to the stage. Only then should the objective be changed to 45X or 100X, when further focusing should require only a partial turn of the fine adjustment focus knob.

❖❖ Eyepiece Adjustment

When using a binocular microscope, it is necessary to adjust the eyepieces to your own eye span and **visual acuity.** A gentle push inward or pull outward will adjust the distance between the eyepieces to accommodate your eye span.

To adjust the eyepieces to the visual acuity of each of your eyes, first bring the specimen into focus with the **stationary ocular.** The stationary ocular is usually on the right, and you should look through it with your right eye, your left eye closed. Use the coarse and fine adjustment knobs on low power to obtain a clear image with the right eye. Then, close your right eye and use your left eye on the **adjustable ocular.** The latter will have a collar of ridges or beads around it. Adjust this eyepiece to correct the focus for the visual acuity of your left eye. Then, check the focus using both eyes. Repeat these steps if necessary until you obtain a clear focus when viewing the specimen through both oculars simultaneously.

❖❖ Light Adjustment

The right level of light is essential for a clear image. Too little light will obscure details in darkness, while too much light will produce a blinding glare

without the contrast necessary to distinguish features. As a general rule, less light is required at lower levels of magnification. As higher power objectives are used, the light must be increased accordingly. Some specimens also require more light than others. A darkly stained slide requires more light than does an unstained one.

The level of light is adjusted by raising or lowering the condenser, narrowing or widening the iris diaphragm, or adjusting the rheostat. The higher the condenser and the wider the iris, the greater the level of light.

♦ ♦ ♦ Note ♦ ♦ ♦

Never force the leaves of the diaphragm.

❖❖ Putting It All Together

To focus the microscope for lab work using the 10X objective:

- With the maximum distance between the stage and objective, clamp the slide on the stage, specimen side up, to prevent it from moving.
- Turn on the light (or, with a student microscope, adjust the mirror to reflect light from an outside source up through the condenser).
- Raise the condenser to its highest position with the control knob and open the iris diaphragm to its maximum extent.
- Looking at the microscope from the side, not through the oculars, rotate the lowest power (10X) objective into viewing position in the center of the stage.
- Still looking at the microscope from the side and using the coarse adjustment knob, lower the objective until it nears the stage or stops.

♦ ♦ ♦ Note ♦ ♦ ♦

When handling slides of biospecimens, such as blood smears, remember to follow the Universal Precautions and other biohazard safety procedures to prevent possible contamination. Remember to coverslip liquid specimens of urine to prevent damage to the objectives and biohazardous contamination of the POL.

- Look through the eyepiece and reverse the direction of the coarse focus adjustment knob until the slide comes into focus.
- Still looking through the eyepiece, turn the fine focus adjustment knob back and forth until you attain the clearest possible image.
- Adjust the condenser and light source until the image is clear and the light level is comfortable.
- Adjust the oculars for your eye span and visual acuity.
- Scan the slide to observe the entire specimen, using the knobs on the mechanical stage to move the slide in four directions (on a student microscope, you may have to do this manually).

To focus the microscope for lab work using the 45X objective:

- Again viewing the microscope from the side, rotate the 45X objective into place.
- Looking through the eyepiece, turn the fine adjustment focus knob to focus clearly.
- Adjust the condenser and light source until the image is clear and the light level is comfortable.
- Scan the slide to observe the entire specimen, using the mechanical stage to move the slide.

To focus the microscope for lab work, using the 100X objective:

- Return to the side view and rotate the 100X power objective into position.
- Look through the ocular and turn the fine focus adjustment knob to focus clearly.
- Adjust the condenser and light source until the image is clear and the light level is comfortable.
- Rotate the oil-immersion objective slightly out of the way. Taking care that the 45X objective does not touch the oil, add one drop of oil to the center of the slide over the condenser.
- Carefully rotate the 100X lens back into place over the slide.
- Turn the fine focus adjustment knob back and forth a fraction of a turn, until the image is clear. If you lose the focus, you must return to the 10X objective and start focusing all over again.
- Scan the slide to observe the entire specimen, using the mechanical stage to move the slide.

MICROSCOPE CARE

The microscope is a delicate, expensive instrument that is easily damaged by dust, excess oil and light, vibrations, and falls. It must be located in a safe place, cleaned carefully after each use, and otherwise treated as the sensitive device it is. If properly cared for, most microscopes require very little service and work well for years.

♦♦ *Service and Parts*

As with any other piece of expensive equipment, records should be kept of routine maintenance and other service procedures performed on the microscope. The microscope should be cleaned and serviced annually by a professional microscope service company. Likewise, only a professional should disassemble the microscope or try to clean the back of the objectives or adjust any interior part of the microscope.

Because parts may differ from one manufacturer to another, they should be purchased from the original manufacturer whenever possible. For example, only the bulb and illuminator recommended by the microscope's manufacturer should be used—others may produce too much heat. Use only recommended brands of immersion oil, never cedar wood oil.

♦♦ *Location and Storage*

The microscope should be assigned a permanent space on a counter where it is not likely to vibrate or be knocked off. It should be kept away from extremes of heat and cold and sudden temperature changes because these may injure the lens cement and damage the alignment of the lens system. The microscope should not get wet or sit in liquid on the counter—electric shock could result.

When not in use, the microscope should be kept in a cabinet or under a plastic cover. This will help protect it from dust and excess light, both of which may damage the lenses. This also will lessen the likelihood of its being struck by other objects or knocked over. Security precautions should be taken to prevent theft of the microscope, such as keeping the cabinet or room where it is housed locked when not in use.

♦♦ *Cleaning*

Use a magnifying glass if necessary to examine the lenses when cleaning them. Blow dust from the glass surfaces with an infant's ear syringe or a similar device that does not touch the lens.

Clean only the outside surfaces of the lenses, using a circular motion from the center outward. Use a piece of lens paper slightly moistened with 70 percent isopropyl alcohol or lens cleaning solution. Never substitute Kimwipes or other tissues to clean the lenses—they may leave behind a residue or scratch the lenses. Many microscope warranties may be voided by the manufacturer if lens paper is not used. Do not use Xylene to clean the lenses because it is toxic and may loosen the lens cement. If you used the 100X objective, take special care to clean the oil from the objective and all other parts of the microscope immediately after use.

❖❖ *After Using the Microscope*

After using the microscope, you should follow these steps in cleaning and storing it:

- Looking at the microscope from the side, rotate the 10X power objective back into place in the center. Take care that the 45X objective does not touch the oil if the 100X objective was used.

- Remove the slide from the microscope. If it is to be saved, wipe it with a piece of lens paper to remove the oil.

- Clean the outside of all the lenses with lens paper, taking particular care to remove all traces of oil from the 100X lens.

- Clean the stage, condenser, and other accessible parts of the microscope.

- Using the coarse adjustment focus knob, move the 10X objective to the lowest position in preparation for the next use of the microscope.

- Cover the microscope with a plastic cover or return it to its storage cabinet. See Figure 2.4 for instructions for carrying a microscope.

- Follow the procedures outlined in Chapter 1 to clean and disinfect the work area, other equipment that was used, and your hands.

SELECTING A MICROSCOPE

There are several important considerations in selecting a microscope for the POL. A demonstration

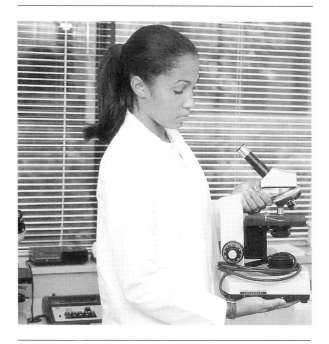

Figure 2.4. When carrying a microscope, always support it underneath with one hand and grasp the arm fully with the other hand. Photo by Matt Meadows.

before purchase is essential. A familiar slide should be used to test the quality of the microscope by focusing and viewing its features. Differentiation of detail, that is, the microscope's resolution, is the most important criterion for microscopic work in medical labs.

While monocular microscopes are sometimes used in schools because they cost less, binocular microscopes are preferred in labs because viewing a magnified specimen with both eyes (through two eyepieces) is less stressful. This is an important consideration in POLs, where much time is spent studying specimens through a microscope. For the same reason, eyepieces should be in a comfortable position and focusing adjustments should allow the arms to rest comfortably on the table.

Other criteria to consider when selecting a microscope for the POL include:

- objectives in the powers of 10X, 45X, and 100X.

- parfocal objectives for easy focusing.

- a mechanical stage (on the platform stage) that moves easily and enables methodical, efficient viewing of specimens.

- a built-in light source.

♦ ♦ ♦ Troubleshooting ♦ ♦ ♦

Following are nine common microscope problems. For each problem, the probable cause or causes and remedies are given.

- *Problem:* the light will not come on. *Probable cause:* the light bulb may be burned out or the light may not be plugged in. *Remedy:* check the light bulb and plug.

- *Problem:* the bulb burns out often. *Probable cause:* the bulb may not be a standard bulb or the voltage switch of the light does not match the local mainline voltage. *Remedy:* use a bulb recommended by the manufacturer or replace the voltage switch.

- *Problem:* the lamp flickers or goes off and on. *Probable cause:* the lamp may be about to burn out or there may be a loose electrical connection. *Remedy:* change the light bulb or check the electrical connections.

- *Problem:* the light is too bright or too dark and cannot be adjusted. *Probable cause:* the line voltage switch may not be suitable for the local mainline voltage. *Remedy:* change the selector switch.

- *Problem:* the field of vision remains too dark after increasing the voltage. *Probable cause:* the condenser may not be high enough or it may not be positioned correctly. *Remedy:* raise or reposition the condenser.

- *Problem:* the field of vision is dark even with the light switched on. *Probable cause:* the iris diaphragm may be closed. *Remedy:* open the diaphragm.

- *Problem:* too much contrast of the image. *Probable cause:* the condenser may be too low. *Remedy:* raise the condenser.

- *Problem:* the image cannot be focused without blurs. *Probable cause:* the lenses may not be clean. *Remedy:* clean the lenses with lens paper and alcohol.

- *Problem:* dust is visible on the lens. *Probable cause:* the lenses may not be clean. *Remedy:* blow dust away with an infant ear syringe. If dust specks remain, wipe the lens with lens paper dampened in lens cleaner.

PROCEDURE

2.1

Focusing the Microscope

Goal

- After successfully completing this procedure, you will be able to focus the microscope at 10X, 45X, and 100X magnification.

Completion Time

- 10 minutes

Equipment and Supplies

- disposable latex gloves, impermeable apron, lab jacket, or gown
- hand disinfectant
- surface disinfectant
- paper towels and tissues
- biohazard container
- microscope, accessories, and immersion oil
- blood differential smear
- lens paper
- 70% isopropyl alcohol or lens cleaner

Instructions

Read through the list of equipment and supplies that you will need and the steps of the procedure. Be sure that you understand each step before you begin. Then complete each step correctly and in the proper order. If your completion time is too long, repeat the procedure until you improve your speed.

S = Satisfactory	U = Unsatisfactory	S	U
1. Wash your hands with disinfectant, dry them, and put on gloves, apron, jacket, or gown.			
2. Follow the Universal Precautions.			
3. Collect and prepare the appropriate equipment.			

4. Clean the ocular and objective lenses with lens paper slightly moistened with 70% isopropyl alcohol or lens cleaner.

5. Observing the microscope from the side:

   a. Raise the condenser to its highest position by turning its control knob.

   b. Open the diaphragm to the maximum extent and turn on the light.

   c. Increase the distance between the stage and objective.

   d. Secure the slide on the stage with the specimen side up and fasten it with clips to prevent movement.

   e. Rotate the lowest power objective into viewing position in the center of the stage.

   f. Turn the coarse adjustment focus knob to decrease the distance of the slide to the objective until it stops or is just above the slide.

6. Looking through the eyepiece:

   a. Reverse the direction of the coarse adjustment focus knob, increasing the distance between the objective and the stage until the slide comes into focus.

   b. Use the fine adjustment focus knob by turning it back and forth for short distances until you obtain the best image.

   c. Adjust the condenser and light controls until the image is clear and the level of illumination is comfortable for viewing.

   d. Adjust the ocular lenses to each eye.

   e. Scan the slide using the stage controls to move it in four directions.

	S	U

7. Observe the microscope from the side and rotate the 45X objective into place.

8. Look through the eyepiece and repeat steps 6b, 6c, and 6e.

9. Observe the microscope from the side and rotate the 100X objective into place.

10. Look through the ocular lenses, and repeat steps 6b, 6c, and 6e.

11. Observe the microscope from the side, and rotate the 100X objective slightly out of the way. Add one drop of oil to the center of the slide over the condenser, and then carefully rotate the 100X lens back into place over the slide.

12. Look through the ocular lenses, and repeat steps 6b, 6c, and 6e.

13. Rotate the 10X objective back into place in the center, taking care that the 45X lens does not touch the immersion oil.

14. Remove the slide from the microscope, wiping it with a piece of lens paper to remove the oil if the slide is to be saved.

15. Clean the lenses with lens paper, including the oculars and all objectives, going from lowest to highest power.

16. Clean the 100X oil-immersion lens with lens paper to remove all traces of oil.

17. Clean the stage, condenser, and other parts of the microscope.

18. Move the 10X objective to the lowest position in preparation for the next use of the microscope.

19. Cover the microscope with a plastic cover or place it in its cabinet and return it to storage.

20. Discard disposable supplies.

21. **Disinfect and return other equipment to storage.**

22. **Clean your work area following the Universal Precautions.**

23. **Remove your gloves and apron, jacket, or gown; wash your hands with disinfectant, and dry them.**

OVERALL PROCEDURAL EVALUATION

Student's Name _____

Signature of Instructor _____ **Date** _____

Comments

CHAPTER 2 REVIEW

Using Terminology

Match the terms in the right column with the appropriate definition in the left column.

_____ 1. eyepiece of microscope

_____ 2. rotates the objectives

_____ 3. controls the amount of light

_____ 4. moves a shorter distance

_____ 5. microscope with two eyepieces

_____ 6. determines the quality of a microscope

_____ 7. has the highest magnification

a. binocular
b. condenser
c. fine adjustment focus knob
d. nosepiece
e. ocular
f. oil-immersion lens
g. resolution

Acquiring Knowledge

Answer the following questions in the spaces provided.

8. Label the parts of the microscope in Figure 2.5 as indicated.

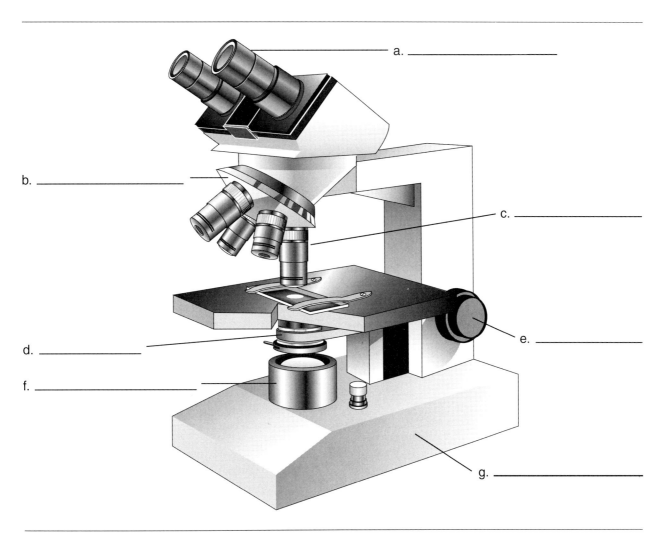

a. _____

b. _____

c. _____

d. _____

e. _____

f. _____

g. _____

Figure 2.5. A microscope.

9. Explain why you must be careful when focusing the oil-immersion objective.

_____

_____

10. What pretreatment of specimens makes the features of microscopic structures more visible?

_____

_____

11. How many lens in the compound microscope act together as one to make a clear image of a magnified specimen?

_____

12. What easy formula gives the total magnification of a specimen?

_____

13. Name the type of compound microscope that has two oculars (eyepieces) and is therefore less tiring and preferred for lengthy viewing of specimens.

_____

14. Where is the lens magnification system of the compound microscope mounted?

_____

15. What result is obtained when the power of the objective you are using is multiplied by the power of the eyepiece of the microscope?

_____

16. In order to receive the best quality and best fitting replacements, what specification should you include when ordering light bulbs and other replacements for the microscope?

_____

17. What is the total magnification of a red cell in a urine specimen viewed under a 10X ocular and a 45X high dry objective?

_____

18. In order for you to view a microscopic specimen clearly, what quality must the specimen have in regard to the passage of light?

_____

19. Staining a specimen allows you to distinguish the details more clearly. Name the two qualities that staining enhances.

_____

_____

20. When you view a prepared slide under the microscope, how many layers can you see clearly with distinct details?

_____

21. When you focus a slide under the microscope, why should you alternate between looking through the oculars and looking at the objectives from the side of the microscope?

_____

22. What is the technical term for the hole in the microscope stage that permits light to pass from the condenser to the objective?

_____

23. When using the microscope, you must always be aware of the space between the objective and specimen in order to prevent damage to the objective. What term describes this space?

_____

24. Which focus adjustment knob should you use to begin the focusing process?

_____

25. Which focus adjustment knob should you always use finally to adjust the details of a fuzzy focus?

_____

26. Which focus adjustment knob should you always use to focus the oil-immersion lens?

_____

27. In which direction, up or down, must the stained side of a glass slide face on the microscope stage in order to bring the specimen into focus?

_____

28. What objective has a very short working distance and therefore requires the fine focus adjustment knob for focusing?

_____

29. Why must you always use special lens paper for cleaning the microscope lenses instead of ordinary facial tissue?

_____

30. How and when do you clean a microscope lens in order to keep the microscope in good order?

_____

_____

_____

_____

31. How and where should you store a microscope when it is not in use?

_____

_____

_____

Directions: Place a + in the space at the left of each true statement. Place a 0 at the left of each false statement. Rewrite each false statement so that it is true.

_____ 32. A rheostat is a device that controls the size of the magnification of an objective.

_____

_____

_____ 33. A microscope specimen consists of a part or product of the human body or a microbe. A specimen is examined microscopically in order to learn about the health of the whole body.

_____

_____

_____ 34. The oil-immersion objective has a very high power of magnification and therefore requires oil to produce a clear image of the specimen.

_____

_____

_____ 35. The working distance is the distance between the oculars and the specimen.

_____

_____

_____ 36. Lab workers using the microscope must learn to recognize complicated patterns of blood-cell structures, urine-sediment composition, and microorganisms.

_____

_____

_____ 37. Most microscopes require very little maintenance except for routine care and a yearly inspection by a professional microscope technician.

_____

_____

_____ 38. In the term 45X, the X means times or magnification.

_____

_____

_____ 39. A mechanical stage is attached to the platform stage.

_____

_____

_____ 40. Resolution refers to the fact that when objectives are changed, the object in the center of the magnified field should remain centered in the field of view.

_____

_____

_____ 41. A darkly stained slide requires more light than does a lightly stained or unstained slide.

_____

_____

_____ 42. Located in the condenser, the rheostat controls the amount of light entering through the aperture in the stage.

_____

_____

_____ 43. The higher the magnification, the more light is required for viewing a specimen.

_____

_____

_____ 44. The higher the magnification, the longer the working distance.

_____

_____

_____ 45. The fine focus adjustment knob causes the objective to move farther for each complete turn of the knob.

_____

_____

_____ 46. With a mechanical stage, you can control much more easily the direction of the slide movement.

_____

_____

_____ 47. When moving from the 45X objective to the oil-immersion objective, you should remove your eyes from the oculars and look from the side at the microscope objectives.

_____

_____

_____ 48. There is no need to keep service records on the microscope.

_____

_____

_____ 49. On a mechanical stage, the range of motion between the x axis and the y axis permits movement in four directions.

_____

_____

_____ 50. If you lose your focus on a higher powered objective, you must return to the 10X objective and start the focusing process from the beginning.

_____

_____

_____ 51. Immersion oil is used with the 100X objective because this oil has about the same refractive index as glass and therefore prevents light rays from diffusing.

_____

_____

Applying Knowledge—On the Job

Answer the following questions in the spaces provided.

52. Melissa performs some blood-cell differential counts under the oil-immersion objective of the laboratory's binocular microscope. She has to leave the microscope, and while she is gone, Susan (a coworker) views urines under the 10X and 45X objectives. When Melissa tries to resume her blood-cell

differential work, she finds that she cannot bring one of the oculars into focus. What is the problem? How can it be solved?

_____

_____

53. Joyce looks over the service records of the microscope at the laboratory where she has begun work. The microscope does not focus well and she finds that a professional has not inspected it for several years. What should she do?

_____

54. Brenda observes that her coworker does not coverslip the urine-sediment specimen when she views it under the microscope. Is this practice acceptable? If not, what should Brenda do about it?

_____

55. One of your coworkers has placed the POL's microscope next to the centrifuge and near the laboratory entrance for convenience. There is a sturdy table that would accommodate the microscope in the back of the laboratory. Should you mention this to your supervisor? Why or why not?

_____

56. Your coworker, Jamie, is trying to focus the microscope onto a urine-sediment specimen, but all that she can see is a black hole down the oculars. What advice would you give Jamie?

_____

_____

57. In the laboratory where you work, a blood smear is focused under the oil-immersion lens by a coworker. She asks you why the slide is dark with indistinct cells. What do you tell her?

_____

_____

58. Tim is counting and identifying the white blood cells on a stained blood smear under a microscope with a mechanical stage. Several of the white cells are abnormal, so he lays the slide aside until later, when the doctor will be in and can view them. When he reinserts the slide, he has to search for ten minutes to find the blood cells that he had viewed before. How could Tim have found the cells quickly on the second viewing?

_____

_____

59. Patricia, a worker in the laboratory, wipes the oculars of the microscope with her laboratory coat sleeve to clean them. She does not bother to clean the objectives between uses. What long-term effects will this type of care have on the microscope?

_____

_____

3 Other Laboratory Equipment and Supplies

COGNITIVE OBJECTIVES

After studying this chapter, you should be able to

- use each of the vocabulary terms appropriately.
- identify the kinds of equipment used in POLs.
- explain the use and care of different kinds of glass and plastic ware, including slides, test tubes, and pipettes.
- describe the use and care of equipment for temperature maintenance.
- list the different types of centrifuges and describe their functions.
- specify how to maintain a supply inventory.
- describe techniques to ease the transition to a new workplace or new technology.

PERFORMANCE OBJECTIVES

After studying this chapter, you should be able to

- clean and store glassware without breakage.
- demonstrate how to read the meniscus in volumetric flasks, pipettes, and graduated cylinders.
- measure and dispense liquids from pipettes and other glassware.
- maintain temperature regulation equipment.
- light a Bunsen burner and adjust the flame.
- heat fix smears on glass slides using a Bunsen burner.
- centrifuge samples in test tubes and microhematocrit tubes.
- maintain inventory-control records.
- devise a plan to learn how to use a new piece of equipment.

TERMINOLOGY

agar: an extract of red algae used as a culture medium; not digested by most bacteria.

autoclave: a pressurized steam cabinet used to sterilize reusable supplies.

beaker: a deep glass container with a wide mouth, often with a lip for pouring.

Bunsen burner: a small gas burner with an open flame that is used to heat fix slides.

centrifuge: a machine that uses centrifugal force to separate materials into different layers according to weight.

colorimetric: analysis based on comparing the color of a liquid with a standard color.

coverslip: a small square of glass used to cover liquid specimens on slides to protect the microscope and stabilize the specimen. A special coverslip is manufactured for use on the hemacytometer.

cuvette: a clear glass container, manufactured to exact optical standards, used to hold fluids for photometric and colorimetric analysis.

cylinder: a tall, round container with a broad base to provide stability; commonly graduated for measuring liquids.

flask: a container with a broad base and a narrow neck for holding liquids or mixing reagents.

heat fixing: quickly passing the bottom of a slide over the tip of a Bunsen burner flame to coagulate a smear and seal it on the slide so that the smear will not wash off during staining.

hemacytometer: a "blood-cell meter" or counting chamber; a glass slide used to count cells, such as red or white blood cells.

hematocrit: the volume of red blood cells packed by centrifugation in a given volume of blood; expressed as a percentage of total blood volume.

incubator (bacterial): a cabinet that provides the right temperature and humidity for bacteria to thrive.

meniscus: the downward curve formed at the surface of a liquid in a container, due to the attraction of molecules of liquid to the side of the container. The bottom of the curve always is used for reading the amount of liquid in the container.

petri dish: a flat, round, clear glass or plastic dish with a fitted cover, which contains a semisolid medium on which bacteria are implanted for growth and observation.

phlebotomy: blood drawing.

photometric: analysis based on measuring the intensity of light.

pipette: an instrument that is used for measuring small, accurate quantities of laboratory samples or reagents.

supernatant: the liquid portion of a fluid that has been centrifuged. The solid heavier matter separates into a bottom layer.

TC: to contain; a designation printed on a pipette, indicating that the pipette delivers the volume indicated when blown out or rinsed.

TD: to deliver; a designation printed on a pipette, indicating that the pipette delivers the volume indicated when allowed to drain.

volumetric flask: a flask with a fill line etched on the neck, manufactured to contain a very exact quantity.

wire loop: a slender rod about 8 inches long with a small loop on one end used to transfer bacterial growths from one area to another.

• •

Medical labs of the nineties are increasingly automated and technically sophisticated, relying on costly, specialized equipment and supplies. The equipment in today's labs generally uses smaller samples and requires less handling of the samples. For example, in the past, test tubes of blood used to be separated into cells and serum and then tested in multistage procedures involving measuring, weighing, and mixing reagents. Today, a single drop of blood can be added to a test strip and read by machine. Although lab workers have to keep up with the new technology, their jobs are safer and easier because of it.

──────────────────────────────── ♦ ♦

TYPES OF EQUIPMENT AND SUPPLIES

As the size and test profiles of POLs differ, so do the instruments with which they are equipped and the supplies that they must keep in inventory. Nonetheless, certain basic supplies and pieces of equipment are found in virtually all POLs. Many of these items are described in this chapter. Others are described in later chapters where they are more relevant.

In addition to the microscope, which was the subject of Chapter 2, virtually all POLs have an assortment of glass and plastic ware (such as slides, test tubes, and pipettes), supplies for blood collection (including vacutainer tubes, blood-collection tubes, and tourniquets), urinalysis supplies and equipment (such as disposable specimen cups and urinometers), refrigerators and freezers, thermometers, centrifuges, cleaning equipment, and drying and sterilizing ovens. Many POLs also have bacterial incubators, automated cell counters, automatic test-strip analyzers, glucometers, and photometers. Some of this equipment is shown in Figure 3.1.

Figure 3.1. The equipment found in POLs varies with the size of the clinic, the specialties of the practices, and the availability of nearby reference laboratories. a. Ready-prepared packets of sterile swabs and media are convenient for collecting throat cultures and other cultures. They may be forwarded to a reference laboratory or processed in the POL. b. Loops, either plastic disposable ones or resterilized wire ones, are used to isolate and inoculate bacterial specimens. c. Glass slides are used for a variety of microscopic studies, including blood smears, urine sediment, and stained bacterial smears. d. A hood prevents infectious aerosols from contaminating the laboratory. e. Petri dishes are used for bacterial cultures. f. An incubator is maintained at body temperature (37 degrees C) for optimal growth of bacteria. g. A thermometer is used to check the temperature of the incubator, refrigerator, and room daily. h. A colorimeter of some type is usually found in POLs. Colorimeters vary from the hand-held glucometer that measures blood glucose to automated multitest machines that test whole blood and print out test results. i. Fibrometer systems perform coagulation tests such as prothrombin time on plasma. j. Laboratory refrigerators and freezers, along with a thermometer for daily temperature checks, are required for preservation of specimens and reagents. k. Laboratory ovens dry and sterilize glassware.

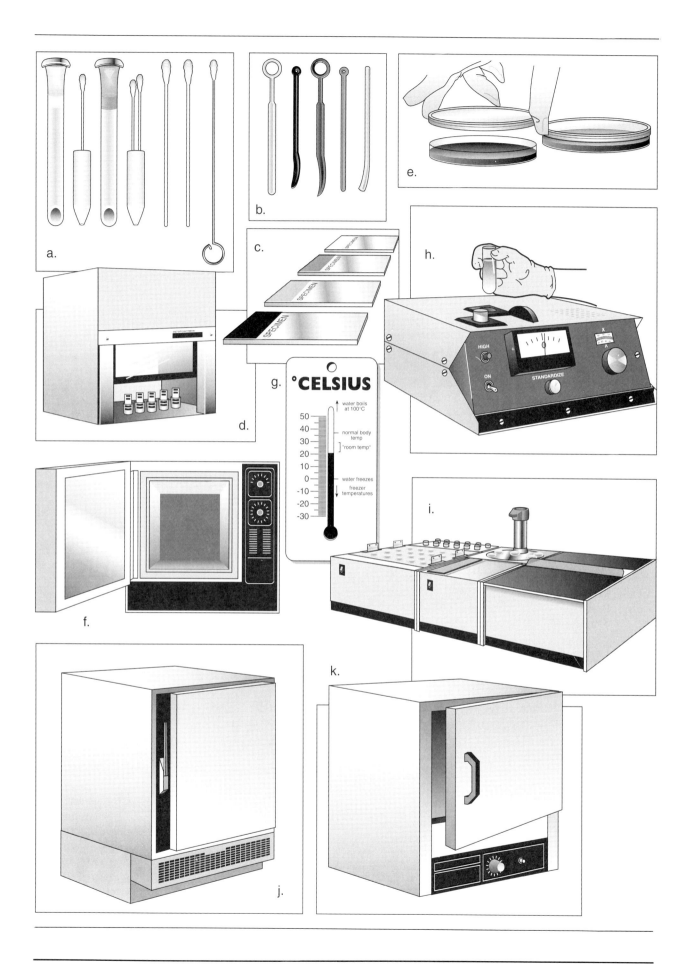

GLASS AND PLASTIC WARE

Most of the glass and plastic ware in POLs is used to measure, mix, store, or hold specimens and reagents. Specific items include glass slides, blood-collection tubes, pipettes, beakers, and flasks. Glass is much more expensive than is plastic and requires extra equipment and labor to keep it clean. It also requires special care to prevent scratches and breakage. For these reasons, disposable plastic ware should be used whenever possible.

Glass Slides

Plain glass slides are used for viewing bacteria, blood, and parasites under the microscope. Specialized glass slides are used for viewing urine sediment and other liquids. There are slides with multiple concave depressions to hold urine specimens, for example, and others with circles of plastic to hold liquids for serological tests where the liquid is scrutinized for precipitation. Plain glass slides are usually disposable and bought in bulk. Specialized slides generally require cleaning and reuse due to their high cost.

Coverslips are small, disposable squares of glass placed over liquid specimens on slides to prevent the microscope objective from coming into contact with the specimen and to keep the specimen from moving on the slide. Coverslips are used in microscopic examinations of urine sediment and fresh microbiology specimens.

Test Tubes

Test tubes are usually disposable, eliminating the labor of cleaning and the risk of exposure to hazardous materials. The general-purpose test tube has a rounded bottom and comes in different sizes. It serves most purposes in POLs. Several types of specialized test tubes are suited for particular purposes. For example, centrifuge tubes have conical ends that permit better concentration of sediment. Stoppered sterile tubes with swabs are used to collect smears from the throat and other body areas. Screw-capped bottles, with the same general contour as test tubes, are used to grow bacteria in liquid cultures.

Cuvettes

Cuvettes are small, optically ground glass containers, rectangular or round in shape, which are used to hold test fluids for **photometric** or **colorimetric** analysis. They are precisely ground to transmit the maximum amount of light. Great care should be taken to protect cuvettes from scratches, because scratches may cause biased readings of test fluids. Cuvettes should not be laid down or mixed with other glassware, for example, and they should be wiped only with a soft cloth or tissue.

Petri Dishes

Petri dishes are flat, round, clear covered dishes of glass or disposable plastic used for bacterial cultures. They may be purchased already prepared with a sterile **agar** culture medium, which must be kept refrigerated until the agar is inoculated with patient smears. The flat, round shape of these dishes allows the bacteria to spread over a thin, semisolid surface where they can be examined easily. Because petri dishes are used for bacterial growth, soiled ones are biohazardous. They must be handled with care and disposed of as biohazardous waste.

Beakers, Flasks, and Cylinders

Many different types of glass and plastic containers are used for mixing and measuring liquids in POLs, including beakers, flasks, and cylinders (see Figure 3.2). **Beakers** are deep glass containers with

---

✦✦✦ The Metric System ✦✦✦

All glass and plastic ware used for measuring in POLs are labelled in metric units. In fact, POLs rely exclusively on the metric system because metric units are more appropriate for the very small quantities usually measured. Weight usually is measured in grams, length in millimeters, and fluid volume in milliliters.

- 1 gram = 0.03527 avoirdupois ounces
- 1 millimeter = 0.03937 inches
- 1 milliliter = 0.0338 fluid ounces

✦✦✦ How to Use a ✦✦✦ Volumetric Flask

Mix the solute with a small amount of solvent in the flask. Then add the rest of the solvent until it reaches the fill line on the neck of the flask. Read the final measurement at eye level with the bottom of the meniscus directly on the fill line.

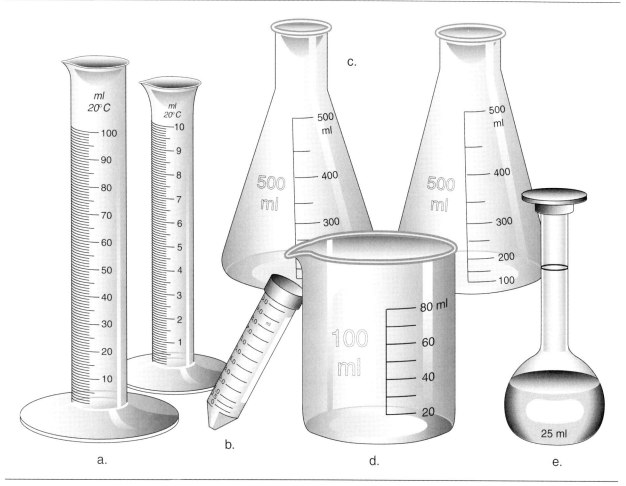

Figure 3.2. Laboratory containers for mixing and measuring fluids. a. Graduated cylinders can measure various quantities of fluid within their capacity. b. Covered centrifuge tubes with graduated measurements are often useful. c. Erlenmeyer flasks have a large base and are therefore very stable. d. Beakers come in various sizes and are all-purpose containers. e. Volumetric flasks are manufactured for the purpose of measuring total volume very accurately.

◆ ◆ ◆ Meniscus ◆ ◆ ◆

The word **meniscus** comes from the Greek word meaning crescent. It refers to the downward curve formed at the surface of liquids in containers like flasks and pipettes. The downward curve is due to the attraction between the molecules of liquid and the container wall. Precise measurements of liquids in the laboratory, with few exceptions, are taken at the bottom of the meniscus (see Figure 3.3). This measurement ensures consistency among workers and labs.

wide mouths, often with a lip for pouring. They are used when measuring is not necessary. **Flasks** are containers with broad bases and narrowed necks for holding liquids and mixing reagents. **Volumetric flasks** have fill lines etched on the neck. Each is manufactured to hold a very exact quantity, so they are used when precise measurements are needed. Volumetric flasks marked with a large *A* are the most accurate and are used for preparing standards and controls. **Cylinders** are tall, round containers with a broad base for greater stability. They are usually graduated for measuring liquids that do not require great accuracy. For example, 24-hour urine samples are generally measured in a large graduated cylinder.

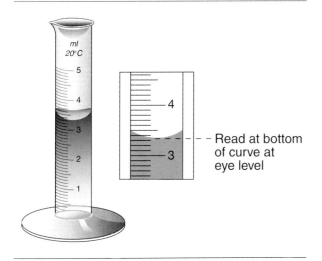

Figure 3.3. Always read a meniscus at eye level at the bottom of the curve. An erroneous reading will result from any other angle or part of the curve.

A smaller cylinder without graduations is used to float a specific gravity meter in urine.

✦✦ *Pipettes*

While flasks and cylinders usually are used to measure large amounts, **pipettes** are used for measuring small quantities. The word *pipette* comes from the French word for "little pipe," a good description of the traditional pipette.

✦ ✦ ✦ Note ✦ ✦ ✦

Never pipette by mouth! Always use a suction device or mechanical pipette to prevent accidental ingestion of biohazardous material or toxic reagents.

Both plastic and glass pipettes are available. Pipettes are differentiated by their markings and shapes. Graduated pipettes have markings similar to those on a metric ruler, but these pipettes are not accurate enough to measure standards or serum. Vol-

---

✦ ✦ ✦ TD or TC? ✦ ✦ ✦

Always note if the pipette that you are using is marked **TD** or **TC**. These markings designate two distinct types of pipettes which must be used quite differently.

- *TD.* This pipette is designed "to deliver" varying amounts of fluid. It should be held vertically against the inside of the container while draining. Never blow out the remaining fluid that clings to the inside of a pipette marked TD.

- *TC.* This pipette is designed "to contain" a specified amount of fluid. The liquid in pipettes marked TC always should be blown out. In the case of very small TC pipettes, the remaining fluid should be rinsed out.

- Some pipettes are marked with opaque rings. Two rings mean that the pipette is both TD and TC—it has two fill marks. One ring means that the pipette is TC.

---

umetric pipettes measure only one predetermined amount. They are more accurate and used to measure serum. Volumetric pipettes marked with a large *A* have been manufactured to the highest standards of accuracy. They are used to prepare controls and standards. The recommended type of pipette for a particular procedure always should be used, following manufacturer's instructions.

Pipette Safety. The epidemic of HIV infection over the past decade has increased awareness of the need for safe pipetting. Pipetting was traditionally done by mouth, and this posed the risk of accidentally ingesting the fluid being pipetted. Mechanical pipettes have replaced many of the traditional pipettes in today's POLs (see Figure 3.4). Although the initial cost is greater, mechanical pipettes offer the advantages of speed and accuracy in addition to safety.

A large variety of pipetting devices, like rubber bulbs that fit over glass pipettes to ensure safety, also are available. Mechanical pipettes with disposable plastic tips measure very small amounts, and pumps dispense premeasured amounts of reagent without contaminating the reagent bottle. These devices make

---

Figure 3.4. Pipettes. a. The traditional glass/plastic pipettes are always pipetted with a suction device to avoid exposure to pathogens and toxic chemicals. b. Graduated pipettes, available in different sizes, can measure varying amounts of liquid. c. Volumetric pipettes, available in different sizes, measure only total amount, but very accurately. One is shown attached to a pump. d. Disposable Pasteur pipettes and other droppers deliver semiquantitative amounts by controlling the size and number of drops.

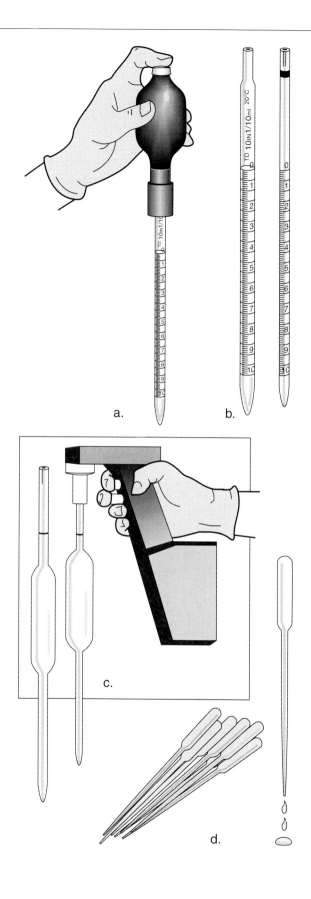

a.

b.

c.

d.

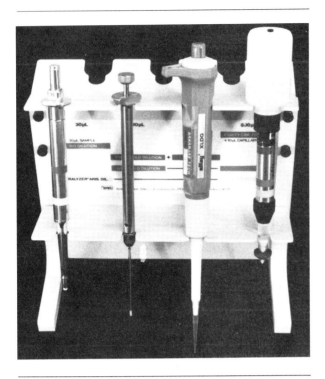

Figure 3.5. Automatic pipettes dispense fluids accurately, safely, and conveniently. Photo by Mark Palko.

pipetting quicker, more accurate, and safer than it was in the past (see Figure 3.5).

Pipettes should always be stored where they are safe from dust and damage. Glass pipettes are extremely fragile, especially their tips, so handle them with great care. Discard pipettes with chipped tips, because they are inaccurate and dangerous to handle.

◆◆ *Cleaning Glass and Plastic Ware*

Most glassware and some plastic ware are expensive, so they are used repeatedly and cleaned after each use. Follow these guidelines for cleaning:

- As soon as possible after use, soak glass or plastic ware in a disinfectant solution, such as dilute bleach. This will make it much easier to clean.
- Wash small pipettes in an automatic pipette washer and very large pipettes in a cylinder washer. Always follow the manufacturer's instructions for loading and using automatic washers.
- For hand washing, use a commercial laboratory detergent, rinse the pipettes thoroughly in tap water to remove all the detergent, and then rinse them in distilled water to remove any chlorine or other chemicals in the tap water (traces of detergents or

chemicals can produce inaccurate test results by interfering with chemical reactions).

- After washing and rinsing, dry the pipettes thoroughly, one or two hours in a dry heat oven or, for delicate pieces, in an autoclave. This renders the equipment sterile.

◆◆

TEMPERATURE MAINTENANCE

Temperature plays an important role in medical testing—low temperatures preserve specimens and reagents for future testing; body temperature (37 degrees Celsius) is required to grow bacterial cultures and for tests like enzyme levels and prothrombin times. High temperatures sterilize and dry equipment. It is not surprising, then, that POLs contain several pieces of equipment for monitoring and regulating temperature.

◆◆ *Thermometers*

Many pieces of equipment in POLs, ranging from refrigerators to incubators, have thermometers, which are always in Celsius. The Celsius scale also is called Centigrade, referring to the 100 divisions, or degrees, between the freezing and boiling points of water on this scale. In Celsius, the freezing point of water is 0 degrees (32 degrees Fahrenheit), and the boiling point is 100 degrees (212 degrees Fahrenheit). Normal body temperature of 98.6 degrees Fahrenheit is 37 degrees Celsius, which is the required temperature for many lab tests and chemical reactions.

◆◆ *Refrigerators and Freezers*

Refrigerators and freezers to preserve and store specimens and reagents are essential in every POL. The refrigerator should have a constant temperature of 4 degrees Celsius, which can be monitored with a thermometer in a sealed bottle of water kept on an upper shelf. The temperature should be recorded daily. The refrigerator, especially its handle, should be disinfected routinely, as it comes into contact with biohazardous materials. All containers in the refrigerator should have their contents labeled clearly. Food and drink never should be kept in the lab refrigerator because of potential contamination with specimens and reagents.

The freezer temperature should be maintained at −20 degrees Celsius. The freezer thermometer should be checked and the temperature recorded daily. All containers used in the freezer should be plastic because glass contracts and may break when it freezes. All stored frozen reagents and specimens should be labeled clearly.

❖❖ Microbiology Incubators

Incubators are cabinets used to keep bacterial cultures warm (usually at body temperature, 37 degrees Celsius). The incubator thermometer should be kept in a sealed container of water, and the temperature should be monitored and recorded daily. Another container of water in the incubator, this one without a cover, helps keep the cultures from drying out by maintaining humidity in the range of 40 to 80 percent. Incubators and other equipment surfaces should be disinfected according to the safety guidelines explained in Chapter 1.

❖❖ Autoclaves and Drying Ovens

All POLs have **autoclaves** to decontaminate biohazardous material. The autoclave also may be used by the clinical staff. Autoclaves use steam under pressure to sterilize. To avoid burns from steam and hot instruments, always let the autoclave cool before opening.

POLS also have dry heat ovens with very high temperatures to dry and sterilize nondisposable pipettes and other glassware. To prevent burns, let the contents of the oven cool before handling them. A schedule that allows overnight cooling is best.

❖❖ Water Baths and Heat Blocks

Some tests require that specimens and reagents be kept at a constant temperature. Water baths keep containers of reagents and specimens bathed in warm water. A disinfectant is added to the water if biohazardous products are being heated. Heat blocks serve the same purpose as water baths but do not contain water. Always check the temperature of water baths and heat blocks before use.

❖❖ Electric Incinerators

An electric incinerator is used to sterilize equipment used in bacterial testing, including the necks of culture bottles and the **wire loops** used to transfer bacteria from patient specimens to culture media.

❖❖ Bunsen Burners

Open flames from **Bunsen burners** are used in POLs to heat fix smears for microscopic examinations.

Bunsen burners burn natural gas. If the ratio of air to gas is correct, the flame will be blue and will burn quietly without sputtering. The ratio can be adjusted by letting more or less air into the gas stream at the base of the burner. In some labs, natural gas is un-

---

❖❖❖ Heat Fixing ❖❖❖
Microbiology Smears

Before a microbiology slide is stained for viewing under the microscope, it may require **heat fixing**, passing the bottom of the slide quickly over the tip of a Bunsen burner flame, coagulating the specimen, and sealing it on the slide. Heat fixing prevents the smear from washing off during staining.

---

available and alcohol lamps may be used instead of Bunsen burners.

Bunsen Burner Safety. Knowing how to use Bunsen burners safely is mandatory for all workers in POLs. The heat of a Bunsen burner flame is intense, and the burner should be used with the same care as is used with any other open flame. Long hair and loose clothing, for example, may be hazardous when working around the open flame of a Bunsen burner. Bunsen burners also should not be used around flammable reagents like acetone or ether. Any glassware heated over a Bunsen burner must be heat-resistant or it may shatter.

OTHER BASIC EQUIPMENT AND SUPPLIES

Numerous instruments and other types of supplies are used routinely in POLs—ranging from hemacytometers, which count cells, to patient test kits that detect strep infections among other conditions.

❖❖ Hemacytometers

The **hemacytometer**, also called a counting chamber, is a very precise glass slide for the microscope, made of heavy glass and manufactured according to

National Bureau of Standards specifications. The word *hemacytometer* literally means "blood-cell meter." It is used to count cells in blood, including red blood cells, white blood cells, platelets (thrombocytes), and eosinophils (granular leukocytes). Cells in urine, spinal fluid, synovial fluid, and semen are also counted on the hemacytometer.

The working surface of the hemacytometer has depressions, called moats, in the form of the letter *H*. Two ruled counting areas are located on either side of the horizontal bar of the *H*, and each is divided into nine equal squares of 1 square millimeter each.

The working surface of the hemacytometer is covered with a glass plate called the coverslip. Two raised areas on either side of the *H* hold the coverslip in place, exactly 0.1 mm above the ruled counting areas. This ensures that when the counting chambers are filled and the coverslip is in place, the sample examined will be a uniform 0.1 mm deep.

Filling and Using the Hemacytometer. Fill the hemacytometer with fluid to be analyzed by touching the tip of a pipette to the edge of the coverslip. This is called charging the hemacytometer. The fluid flows under the coverslip by capillary action. It should flow smoothly with a constant stream. Be careful not to overfill the chamber or to allow fluid to flow into the moats—otherwise, an incorrect count will result.

After the chamber is filled, count the cells. This part of the procedure is described in a later chapter. Then, clean and dry the chamber and coverslip.

Cleaning the Hemacytometer. To fill a hemacytometer and to count cells properly, be sure that the hemacytometer is completely free of dirt and oil. Wash both the hemacytometer and coverslip with soap and warm water or clean them with 70 percent alcohol. Disinfect them for both bacteria and viruses with a 1:10 dilution of household bleach, followed by clear water rinses. Use soft tissue or lens paper to dry both the hemacytometer and coverslip to avoid scratching the surfaces. After drying, position the coverslip so that it covers both ruled areas of the counting chamber.

Storing the Hemacytometer. The hemacytometer is an expensive piece of laboratory equipment that you should handle carefully. Hold it only by the sides or bottom to avoid getting fingerprints on the ruled counting area. Hold the coverslip by the edges for the same reason. Store both hemacytometer and coverslip in a container or area that is free of dirt and dust. A petri dish cover may be placed over the hemacytometer to help keep it clean.

⁂ Centrifuges

Centrifuges separate materials into different layers according to weight by spinning them at high speed (see Figure 3.6). Dissolved or suspended solid materials are usually heavier and settle to the bottom, while the liquid portion, called the **supernatant,** rises to the top. When blood is centrifuged, for example, it separates into layers of red cells, white cells, and platelets, above which is either plasma or serum as the supernatant fluid. When urine is centrifuged, cells, crystals, casts, and debris concentrate into the sediment on the bottom of the tube. The supernatant fluid is poured off and the sediment is examined under the microscope. Because centrifuges are used with biological specimens like blood and urine, they should be disinfected daily.

Centrifuges work because of centrifugal force—the outward force created by the fast spinning action.

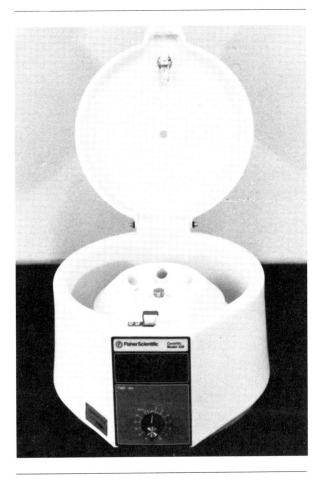

Figure 3.6. A centrifuge spins tubes of fluid to separate the components. It is used to obtain urinary sediments and blood serum and plasma. Photo by Mark Palko.

The greater the speed (the more revolutions per minute) and the larger the diameter of the centrifuge, the greater the centrifugal force. The size and speed of the centrifuge and the length of time required for centrifuging are specified for each test. This helps standardize test results.

Two types of centrifuges are usually found in POLs—the tube centrifuge and the microhematocrit centrifuge. The tube centrifuge spins test tubes of larger specimens, while the microhematocrit centrifuge spins microhematocrit capillary tubes. Some electronic test instruments also have built-in centrifuges.

Microhematocrit Centrifuge. This centrifuge is used to spin capillary tubes to separate out cells from plasma. The tubes are open at both ends for blood collection. For centrifuging, the outer end is sealed with clay or a plastic cap to prevent leakage. The sealed tubes are then placed in the centrifuge against a rubber gasket that cushions them as they spin. An inner metal cover screws tightly over them to prevent movement.

Each microhematocrit tube is placed in a numbered slot with a matched specimen from the same patient placed opposite it in the centrifuge. The tubes are arranged from the center outward, like the spokes of a wheel. The test result is the **hematocrit,** or the percent of packed red cells to total blood volume.

Centrifuge Safety. For safety's sake, the centrifuge always must be closed when in operation. An outer microhematocrit centrifuge lid with a secure lock folds over the metal tube cover for extra protection. Be aware that the centrifugal force may shatter weak tubes or tubes not placed on the rubber gasket. Remember to use stoppered or covered tubes for any biohazardous or toxic material. Always balance the test tubes in a centrifuge by placing tubes of similar weight opposite each other. If equally weighted containers of test material are not available, you can use tubes of water for balance. (See Chapter 1 for additional centrifuge safety tips.)

♦♦ *Mixers*

For certain tests and reagents, thorough mixing of solutions to a uniform consistency is crucial. Most POLs have a variety of mixers, vibrators, and shakers to rapidly and conveniently mix solutions. No mixers require special care—just routine cleaning.

One type of mixer consists of a rotating electromagnetic field inside a base. A small stirring magnet is placed in the container of liquid to be mixed, and the container is placed on the base of the mixer. The electromagnetic field causes the stirrer to move rapidly through the container, thoroughly mixing the liquid. Another type of mixer is a rapid vibrator block. When a test tube is touched to the block, the contents are mixed instantly. A third type of mixer shakes the contents of red and white blood-cell pipettes before counts are made.

♦♦ *Electronic Test Instruments*

POLs rely increasingly on specialized, high technology instruments, many of which are described in later chapters where they are most relevant. Common sense rules for operating electronic instruments apply to these machines—keep them away from vibrations, jars, strong electrical fields, spilled liquids, and extremes of heat and cold. Although most electronic instruments require little maintenance, they must be serviced at the factory or by a factory representative. If servicing takes several days or weeks, the medical supply company usually provides a replacement instrument.

♦♦ *Test Kits*

Most POLs perform several medical tests using prepackaged kits, each containing all the instructions, supplies, and controls needed for one patient test. Pregnancy, strep infections, and rheumatoid arthritis are among the many conditions that now can be diagnosed using test kits. The kits are generally convenient, easy to use, and accurate. Many require refrigeration. Check the manufacturer's instructions for storage and always check the expiration date.

♦♦ *Specimen-Collection Station and Supplies*

A specimen-collection station is an essential part of every POL. Because it is used primarily for blood drawing (**phlebotomy**), a sturdy seat with an armrest is part of the basic equipment (see Figure 3.7). Special blood-collection chairs are not mandatory, but they are convenient and safer for patients. A specimen-collection chart to guide lab workers should be displayed prominently at the specimen-collection station. It should show both the procedures and the supplies needed for every type of specimen collection routinely done in the POL.

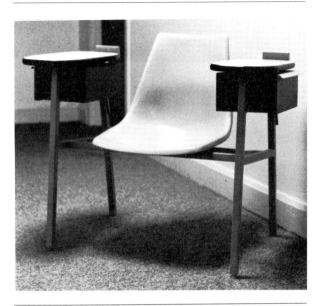

Figure 3.7. Blood-collection chairs are convenient and safe.

Each specimen-collection procedure requires specific supplies. For example, supplies for blood drawing include needles, vacutainer tubes, gauze, alcohol, and tourniquets. For specimens that are forwarded to reference laboratories, special supplies are required, including mailing tubes and boxes, leak-proof specimen containers, and, for microbiology cultures, special culture media.

INVENTORY CONTROL

All POLs have a system of inventory control to ensure that adequate supplies are maintained. The inventory maintained depends on the size of the POL, the storage space available, the type of medical practice, and access to medical suppliers. An isolated, rural, general practice POL, for example, may need to maintain a larger inventory than does a specialty practice POL in an urban area near medical suppliers.

✦✦ *Inventory Files*

Although everyone who uses supplies in POLs should note when particular items are getting low, it is most efficient if one lab employee is responsible for keeping track of inventory and ordering supplies. That individual should maintain two files:

- A file of ordering instructions, costs, and manufacturers' addresses for all supplies used.

- A schedule or calendar showing when to reorder or check inventory for all supplies usually kept in stock.

A calendar and a list of suppliers also may be kept near the phone for convenience in placing routine orders.

To compile an ordering schedule or calendar, the person doing the ordering must have an estimate of how quickly each item usually is depleted. Having either too few or too many of a particular item in inventory can create problems. Lack of a critical supply can seriously hamper the operation of the entire POL, so it is important to keep on hand supplies adequate for the lab's day-to-day operation. On the other hand, space is generally limited and some supplies have expiration dates or may become obsolete, so it is also important to avoid overstocking. These two constraints place limits on how much of a particular item should be ordered or kept in stock.

✦✦ *After an Order Arrives*

Whenever an order arrives, check it for discrepancies against the purchase order and invoice. If there is a discrepancy or any other problem with the order, call the supplier, making sure all necessary information is close at hand before you place the call. You should have handy the invoice number, the date of the purchase order, the name of person who placed the order, and the nature of the problem. If you used a catalog to place the order, have it opened to the page where the problem item is located.

Only when you are satisfied that the order received is correct should you add the new items to the inventory list and shelve them. Store most supplies close to where they are needed but away from risk of contamination or damage. Many supplies must be protected from light, heat, moisture, and air. Always follow the manufacturer's guidelines.

ADAPTING TO A NEW LAB OR NEW EQUIPMENT

New equipment and procedures can be frustrating, whether the lab worker is a new employee learning the POL routine from scratch or an experienced lab worker adapting to a new instrument or test procedure. Lab manuals provide detailed information about procedures and equipment and are useful sources when questions arise, but practical demonstrations and hands-on experience are crucial to

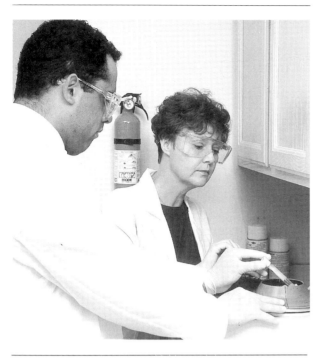

Figure 3.8. The best way to become proficient with a piece of equipment is to ask questions. Photo by Matt Meadows.

make the procedures familiar and the equipment comfortable and easy to use (see Figure 3.8). Follow-

ing are some other ways to help make the transition to a new work place or new technology easier:

- *Study and practice.* Study the instructions, reading and rereading them until they are clear. Spend time working through the procedures and getting acquainted with the equipment.

- *Ask and learn.* Compile a list of any questions that you have as you work through the procedures; ask questions when demonstrations are given; attend training sessions and workshops; study manuals; call hot lines; and use any other means available to increase your knowledge and understanding of the new technology or procedure. Keep a collection of familiar textbooks handy as your own personal reference library.

- *Tickle your memory.* Keep a notebook for "tickler files," items to jog your memory for details about the new procedures and equipment. Use your notebook to personalize the procedures and instructions so that they are more comprehensible and meaningful to you.

- *Anticipate change.* Most workers today will change jobs several times during their work lives, necessitating adjustment to new procedures and equipment. Be aware of the need to be flexible and do not expect your training and education to be over once you receive your degree and land your first job.

PROCEDURE

3.1

Using Glassware, the Centrifuge, and the Bunsen Burner

Goal

- After successfully completing this procedure, you will be able to measure fluids in a variety of glassware safely and accurately, use a centrifuge to spin down urine specimens, and use a Bunsen burner to heat fix microbiology smears.

Completion Time

- 45 minutes

Equipment and Supplies

- disposable latex gloves, impermeable apron, lab jacket or lab coat
- hand disinfectant
- surface disinfectant
- paper towels and tissues
- biohazard container
- beaker and several different flasks, cylinders, and pipettes
- tap water
- paper and pen
- microbiology smear on a glass slide (obtained from swabbing students' mouths or throats)
- Bunsen burner
- fresh urine specimen
- centrifuge
- disposable centrifuge tubes

Instructions

Read through the list of equipment and supplies that you will need and the steps of the procedure. Be sure that you understand each step before you begin. Then complete each step correctly and in the proper order. If your completion time is too long, repeat the procedure until you increase your speed.

1. Wash your hands with disinfectant, dry them, and put on gloves. Don your personal protective equipment such as an apron or lab jacket.

2. Follow the Universal Precautions.

3. Collect and prepare appropriate equipment.

4. Fill different sized flasks and graduated cylinders with tap water.

5. Place the glassware on a level surface and read the meniscus at the lowest point for each container.

6. Record the measurements on a sheet of paper and save the samples of tap water until your instructor can check your work.

7. Following your instructor's example, use a pipette suction device to pipette several different amounts of tap water from a beaker.

8. Read the levels in the pipettes and record the measurements. Save the samples until your instructor can check your work.

9. Verify identification of the urine specimen and label the container.

10. Use a glass rod to thoroughly mix the specimen.

11. Pour about 10 to 15 milliliters of urine into a disposable centrifuge tube.

12. Label and stopper the tube, and place it in the centrifuge tube holder.

13. Balance the test tubes in the centrifuge by placing tubes of similar weight opposite each other. If equally weighted tubes of urine are not available, use tubes of water for balance.

14. Close the centrifuge and lock the lid.

15. Following the manufacturer's instructions, centrifuge the specimen for five minutes at 1,500 to 2,000 rpm.

16. After centrifuging, dispose of the urine specimen appropriately as a biohazard.

17. Verify the identification of the smear on the glass slide.

18. Following the tips for Bunsen burner safety given in the text, light the Bunsen burner.

19. Correct the ratio of air to gas in the Bunsen burner by letting more or less air into the gas stream at the base of the burner, following your instructor's example. The flame should be blue and should burn without sputtering.

20. Quickly pass the bottom of the slide over the tip of the Bunsen burner flame to coagulate the smear and to seal it on the slide.

21. After heat fixing the smear, dispose of the slide appropriately as a biohazard.

22. Discard disposable equipment.

23. Disinfect other equipment and return it to storage.

24. Clean the work area following the Universal Precautions.

25. Remove your gloves and other personal protective equipment; wash your hands with disinfectant, and dry them.

OVERALL PROCEDURAL EVALUATION

Student's Name _____

Signature of Instructor _____ **Date** _____

Comments

CHAPTER 3 REVIEW

Using Terminology

Match the terms in the right column with the appropriate definition in the left column.

_____ 1. allow to drain

_____ 2. rises to the top

_____ 3. downward curve

_____ 4. bacteria container

_____ 5. used for exact measurement

_____ 6. used for heat fixing smears

_____ 7. blow or rinse out

_____ 8. transfers bacteria

_____ 9. used in photometry

_____ 10. sterilizes supplies by steam

_____ 11. source of dry heat

a. petri dish
b. volumetric flask
c. meniscus
d. TD
e. TC
f. cuvettes
g. autoclave
h. oven
i. Bunsen burner
j. wire loop
k. supernatant

Define the following terms.

12. Beaker: _____

_____

13. Flask: _____

_____

14. Meniscus: _____

_____

15. Pipette: _____

_____

Acquiring Knowledge

Answer the following questions in the spaces provided.

16. How does an autoclave sterilize instruments?

_____

17. What is used to dry glassware in POLs?

_____

18. Describe how to heat fix a bacterial smear.

_____

_____

19. Explain how a wire loop is used in POLs.

_____

_____

20. Why is the Celsius temperature scale also called Centigrade?

_____

21. What temperature should the thermometer read in the POL refrigerator?
                                            freezer?
_____

22. What temperature is maintained in a bacterial incubator? Why?

_____

23. What is the difference between graduated and volumetric containers?

_____

24. What type of containers should be used for measuring in tests of controls and standards? Why?

_____

_____

25. Why should you never pipette by mouth?

_____

26. What type of test tube is used for separating out sediment from urine?

_____

27. What type of container is used to culture bacteria?

_____

28. When is a cylinder used in POLs?

_____

29. Describe how glassware should be cleaned in POLs.

_____

_____

_____

30. Identify the roles that temperature plays in POLs.

_____

_____

_____

31. What optically precise container used for photometric test reading must be kept scratchfree?

_____

32. How is the hemacytometer filled?

_____

_____

_____

Applying Knowledge—On the Job

Answer the following questions in the spaces provided.

33. Martha works in a POL that she feels is badly managed. Lab workers sometimes must stay late to wash glassware that has been allowed to dry dirty, reagents often must be discarded because they are out of date, and disinfecting the lab has fallen behind schedule. The physician who owns the practice has asked for suggestions to make the POL more efficient. What should Martha tell the doctor?

_____

_____

_____

_____

_____

34. Dr. DesMarais has an isolated practice in a small town 100 miles from the nearest medical laboratory or source of medical supplies. Recently, the doctor's lab was unable to perform some routine tests because needed supplies had run out unexpectedly. How can this situation be prevented in the future?

_____

_____

_____

_____

35. Victoria's supervisor observed her using a kind of pipette not listed in the directions for the procedure she was doing. After the supervisor pointed out the discrepancy to her, Victoria retorted that it did not matter what pipette she used as long as she measured out the quantity called for. The supervisor replied that Victoria never should change test procedures in any way, no matter how insignificant the change might seem. The supervisor added that if Victoria had suggestions for improving the lab's protocol, she should take them up with her supervisor, not implement them on her own. How should this situation have been handled?

_____

_____

_____

_____

36. Jan has been hired on a trial basis in a POL. She really needs the job and wants to make a success of it. The details seem overwhelming—so many procedures and pieces of equipment that she is not familiar with! Her coworkers seem to think that giving her directions once is enough. What advice would you give Jan?

_____

_____

_____

_____

37. Rob has been reprimanded by his supervisor for several things that Rob feels are trivial—letting the hemacytometer dry before cleaning it, placing unbalanced tubes in the centrifuge, and tossing pipettes into the soaking cylinder. Is the supervisor correct to criticize Rob for these actions, or is she being unduly harsh with him?

_____

_____

_____

4 *Math in the POL*

COGNITIVE OBJECTIVES

After studying this chapter, you should be able to

- use each of the vocabulary terms appropriately.
- distinguish among numbers expressed as fractions, decimals, and percents, and list ways in which each type of number is used in the POL.
- give examples of equivalent fractions and explain why they are equal.
- explain how and why scientific notation is used.
- identify the differences between the English and metric systems of measurement and explain why the metric system is preferred for use in the POL.
- give examples of metric units used in the POL.
- list the steps that lab workers should take if they are having problems with math in the POL.

PERFORMANCE OBJECTIVES

After studying this chapter, you should be able to

- multiply, divide, add, and subtract fractions.
- find common denominators and simplify fractions.
- convert fractions to decimals, round correctly, and calculate with decimals.
- measure length, mass, and volume in metric units.
- solve simple POL formulas.
- prepare solutions and dilutions as described in procedures and manufacturer's instructions.

TERMINOLOGY

colorimeter: an instrument for measuring intensity of color. It identifies the wavelengths of colored light in nanometers.

common denominator: a common multiple of the denominators of two or more fractions.

concentrate: a substance, either liquid or solid, that is strong because it has had fluid removed from it.

concentration: the strength of a chemical in a solution.

decimal: any number expressed in base 10, or a fraction in which the denominator is a power of 10.

denominator: the part of a fraction that is at the bottom of a fraction. It functions as a divisor.

diluent: an agent that reduces the strength of a substance to which it is added.

dilution: a solution that has been weakened by addition of a diluent.

dividend: a number to be divided.

divisor: the number by which a dividend is divided.

English system: the foot–pound–ounce system of units of measurement that most of us use every day.

equation: a mathematical statement that expresses equality between two expressions on either side of an equals sign.

equivalent fractions: fractions that look different but have the same quantity.

exponent: a symbol written above and to the right of a number. An exponent indicates how many times the number is multiplied by itself.

formula: a rule written in mathematical symbols and numbers. A formula expresses the relationship between two or more quantities.

fraction: a numerical representation of the quotient of two numbers.

gram (g): the basic metric unit for weight or mass. A gram equals 0.03527 ounces in the English system.

inverse: opposite or reverse. The inverse of a fraction is created by turning it upside down.

kilogram (kg): the metric unit of weight or mass that is equal to 1,000 grams and to 2.2 pounds in the English system.

kilometer (km): the metric unit of length that equals 1,000 meters. A kilometer equals 0.62137 miles in the English system.

liter (L): the basic unit of volume in the metric system. A liter equals 1.0567 quarts in the English system.

meter (m): the basic unit of length in the metric system. A meter equals 1.0936 yards in the English system.

metric system: the system of measurement based on the meter, in which each unit is related to a basic unit of volume, length, or mass by a power of ten.

milligram (mg): the metric unit of weight or mass obtained by dividing the gram by 1,000.

millimeter (mm): the metric unit of length obtained by dividing the meter by 1,000.

numerator: in any fraction or ratio, the number at the top of a fraction.

quotient: the number resulting from the division of one number by another.

percent: "out of a hundred"; a fraction with 100 as the denominator.

ratio: the relationship in size or quantity between two things.

reconstitute: to add liquid to a dried powder to return it to its original liquid form.

scientific notation: a system of writing decimals. In scientific notation, 10 raised to some power is used to specify where the decimal should be placed.

simplify: to express a fraction as a ratio between smaller numbers.

solute: the substance dissolved in a liquid to form a solution.

solution: the liquid containing a dissolved substance or substances.

solvent: the liquid in which substances are dissolved to form a solution.

total volume: the amount of a solution, including both solute and solvent.

● ● ● ● ● ● ● ● ● ● ● ● ● ● ● ● ●

Because of recent advances in medicine and engineering, today's POLs are technological marvels. Fortunately, as POL technology has become more complex, the job of lab technicians generally has become simpler. One area where simplification is a great boon is mathematics. Lab workers no longer need to perform lengthy calculations to obtain test results. By and large, manufacturers of instruments, controls, and reagents have done the math. POL workers need only to use a calculator or computer to evaluate simple formulas.

This chapter reviews basic math, outlines how to use formulas, introduces the metric system, and explains how to calculate solutions and dilutions. You may want to skip the first section if you already feel comfortable using fractions, decimals, and percents. If math is not your strong point, however, read on and take time to work through the examples to make sure that you understand the material.

REVIEW OF BASIC MATH

Fractions, decimals, and **percents** are different ways of expressing the same thing, a proportion or ratio. The same quantity, say half an inch, can be expressed using a fraction ($\frac{1}{2}$ inch), a decimal (0.5 inch), or a percent (50 percent of an inch). Most people have enough familiarity with math to realize that $\frac{1}{2}$, 0.5, and 50 percent are equal, but they may not know how to figure out the decimal and percentage equivalence of fractions such as $\frac{8}{9}$ or $\frac{11}{32}$. The next sections demonstrate how to convert from fractions to decimals and percents and how to use these different quantities.

✦✦ *Fractions*

Many people find fractions difficult. The following discussion should help clarify them for you.

What a Fraction Is. A fraction is a way of expressing the **ratio**, or relationship in size or quantity of two things. The ratio of 3 to 4, for example, is the fraction $\frac{3}{4}$. The bar (/) represents division, so the fraction $\frac{3}{4}$ really means 3 divided by 4. It may also be written as $3 \div 4$, or as 3/4. In any fraction or ratio, the number at the top is called the **numerator** and the number at the bottom is called the **denominator** (see Figure 4.1). In the case of $\frac{3}{4}$ the numerator is 3 and the denominator is 4.

Most people are familiar with fractions as parts of wholes. If a pie is divided into six pieces, for example, the part of the pie represented by three of the pieces is three-sixths, written as the fraction $\frac{3}{6}$, or in words, three out of six. As another example, the ratio of two chapters in a book to the total of 20 chapters would be represented by the fraction $\frac{2}{20}$. In these two examples, the fractions $\frac{3}{6}$ and $\frac{2}{20}$ each represent a part of the total. In other words, each of these fractions is less than one.

Because fractions are ratios between any two numbers, they also can have values greater than one. Whenever the numerator is larger than the denominator, the value of the fraction is greater than one. The larger the numerator relative to the denominator, the greater the value of the fraction. When the numerator and denominator of a fraction are the same, as in $\frac{2}{2}$ or $\frac{3}{3}$, the value of the fraction is one. This is because any number divided by itself equals one. Use your calculator and several different numbers to verify that this is true.

Multiplying and Dividing Fractions. Multiplying and dividing fractions are easier than you might think if you follow a few simple rules. To multiply two fractions, just multiply the two numerators and then the two denominators, as in the following example:

$$\frac{1}{2} \times \frac{3}{4} = \frac{1 \times 3}{2 \times 4} = \frac{3}{8}$$

This rule also applies to multiplication of fractions by whole numbers. For example:

$$\frac{1}{2} \times 20 = \frac{1}{2} \times \frac{20}{1} = \frac{1 \times 20}{2 \times 1} = \frac{20}{2} = 10$$

---

numerator

denominator

Figure 4.1. Parts of a fraction.

Dividing fractions requires an additional step. To divide one fraction by another, you first must change the **divisor** (the denominator, or the one being "divided into" the other) into its **inverse**, or opposite. To change a fraction into its inverse, simply flip-flop the fraction. For example, the inverse of $\frac{3}{4}$ is $\frac{4}{3}$, the inverse of $\frac{4}{5}$ is $\frac{5}{4}$, and the inverse of $\frac{1}{2}$ is $\frac{2}{1}$.

To divide two fractions, multiply the dividend fraction by the inverse of the divisor fraction, as in the following example:

$$\frac{1}{2} \div \frac{3}{4} = \frac{1}{2} \times \frac{4}{3} = \frac{1 \times 4}{2 \times 3} = \frac{4}{6} = \frac{2}{3}$$

Equivalent Fractions and Common Denominators. Because $\frac{3}{3}$ and $\frac{2}{2}$ both equal one, these two fractions are **equivalent fractions;** they are two different ways of writing the same quantity. Common sense tells us that three out of six pieces of pie is half a pie—in other words, $\frac{3}{6}$ equals $\frac{1}{2}$—but it is not so easy to tell if other fractions are equal. For example, is the fraction $\frac{2}{3}$ equal to $\frac{4}{6}$? Is $\frac{3}{4}$ equal to $\frac{9}{12}$? Is $\frac{3}{8}$ equal to $\frac{12}{32}$?

In order to compare any two fractions to determine if they are equivalent, you must rewrite them so that they have the same denominator, called a **common denominator.** A common denominator is also required for adding and subtracting fractions. Take the example of $\frac{2}{3}$ and $\frac{4}{6}$. It is easy to see that if you multiply the denominator of $\frac{2}{3}$ by 2, it will be 6, the same as the denominator of $\frac{4}{6}$. To write $\frac{2}{3}$ as a fraction with denominator of 6, you also must multiply the numerator by 2. This is because the denominator was multiplied by 2, and, to preserve the value of the fraction, both numerator and denominator must be multiplied by the same number. In other words, the fraction $\frac{2}{3}$ must be multiplied by the fraction $\frac{2}{2}$, producing $\frac{4}{6}$.

For more difficult fractions, you can find a common denominator by multiplying the denominator of one fraction by the denominator of the other. Take the fractions $\frac{2}{3}$ and $\frac{4}{6}$ again. Their denominators are 3 and 6, respectively. Multiplying 3×6 yields a common denominator of 18. To write $\frac{2}{3}$ as a fraction with denominator of 18, multiply the numerator by 6 to preserve the value of the fraction:

$$\frac{2}{3} \times \frac{6}{6} = \frac{2 \times 6}{3 \times 6} = \frac{12}{18}$$

To change $\frac{4}{6}$ to a fraction with a denominator of 18, multiply the denominator of 6 by 3. Also multiply the numerator by 3:

$$\frac{4}{6} \times \frac{3}{3} = \frac{4 \times 3}{6 \times 3} = \frac{12}{18}$$

Now that $\frac{2}{3}$ and $\frac{4}{6}$ have the same denominator, 18, you can see that they are equivalent—both equal the same amount, $\frac{12}{18}$.

Adding and Subtracting Fractions. To add and subtract fractions, make sure that they have the same denominator. Once they do, adding and subtracting is simple. To add two or more fractions with the same denominator, just add the numerators, as follows:

$$\frac{3}{4} + \frac{2}{4} = \frac{5}{4}$$

To subtract fractions with the same denominator, just subtract the numerators:

$$\frac{3}{4} - \frac{2}{4} = \frac{1}{4}$$

Simplifying Fractions. You can multiply the numerator and denominator of a fraction by the same number without changing the value of the fraction when you wish to compare fractions or to add or subtract them. Sometimes it is useful to divide the numerator and denominator of a fraction by the same number to **simplify** it (to express a fraction as a ratio between smaller numbers).

Consider the fraction $\frac{10}{20}$. Are there any numbers that will divide the numerator of 10 and the denominator of 20 without producing a remainder? Three numbers, 2, 5, and 10, will:

$$\frac{10 \div 2}{20 \div 2} = \frac{5}{10}$$

$$\frac{10 \div 5}{20 \div 5} = \frac{2}{4}$$

$$\frac{10 \div 10}{20 \div 10} = \frac{1}{2}$$

Because the value of the fraction $\frac{10}{20}$ is unchanged when you divide both its numerator and its denominator by the same number (2, 5, or 10), $\frac{10}{20}$ has the same value as $\frac{5}{10}$, $\frac{2}{4}$, and $\frac{1}{2}$. For most purposes, $\frac{1}{2}$, which is the most simplified form of the fraction $\frac{10}{20}$, is preferred.

◆◆ Decimals

Everyone is familiar with decimals, whether they realize it or not, because our money system works on the decimal principle. *Decimal* means "based on the number 10," that is, divided into units of 10 (or 100 or some other power of 10). A dollar is divided into 100 cents, and dollar amounts are expressed using a decimal point. Half a dollar, for example, is written as $0.50, and one dollar and seventy cents is written as $1.70. From your experience with money, you know that anything to the right of the decimal point is less than one, while anything to the left of the decimal point is one or more.

Studying the fractions and decimal equivalents will help you understand decimal notation. The first position to the right of the decimal place is tenths, the second position hundredths, the third position thousandths, and so on (see Table 4.1). Each time you increase the denominator of a fraction by a power of ten, you add a zero to the right of the decimal point. The more zeros to the right of the decimal point in front of a digit, the smaller the number.

◆◆◆ Note ◆◆◆

To reduce errors in reading and transcribing decimal numbers of less than one, always add a zero to the left of the decimal point. For example, .5 should be written as 0.5 to avoid errors.

Converting Fractions to Decimals. Every fraction can be converted to a decimal. Two obvious examples are $\frac{1}{2} = 0.5$ and $\frac{1}{4} = 0.25$. Some are not so obvious, like $\frac{255}{425}$. Fortunately, converting fractions to decimals is easy with a calculator. Just remember that the bar in the fraction represents division. To convert

TABLE 4.1 Decimal Equivalents

Fraction	Decimal Equivalent
$\frac{1}{10}$	0.1
$\frac{1}{100}$	0.01
$\frac{1}{1,000}$	0.001
$\frac{1}{10,000}$	0.0001
$\frac{1}{100,000}$	0.00001
$\frac{1}{1,000,000}$	0.000001

$\frac{255}{425}$ to a decimal, divide 255 by 425 on your calculator. You should get 0.6 for the answer. Convert the following fractions to decimals using your calculator to be sure that you understand the method:

$$\frac{79}{85} = 0.93$$

$$\frac{22}{345} = 0.06$$

$$\frac{3}{999} = 0.003$$

Rounding. In each of the examples just given, the answer on your calculator actually was a longer number than the answer shown above. For example, when you divided 79 by 85 on your calculator, your answer should have been 0.9294117. Round this off to 0.93, meaning that you express it with fewer digits to the right of the decimal point. Calculators usually carry out division (and most other calculations) to more digits than are needed for the answer, so rounding is a procedure that is done repeatedly in POL work. It is crucial for standardizing results that everyone rounds off the same way. When rounding off numbers, always follow these rules:

- Never express an answer with more digits than the original measurements contain. For example, if you multiply the numbers 0.788 and 2.334, your answer should have three digits to the right of the decimal point (1.839). To include more digits in the answer than in the original measurements suggests a degree of precision that is bogus. The answer cannot be more precise than the numbers entered into the calculation.

- Always round up if the next digit is 5 or greater, and always round down if it is 4 or less. For example, to express 2.82513 with just two digits to the right of the decimal point, look at the third digit to the right of the decimal point (in this case 5) and round up if it is 5 or more (as here) and down if it is 4 or less.

To be sure that you understand how to round off numbers, convert the following fractions to decimals, each with just two digits to the right of the decimal point. You should get the same answers as those given here:

$$\frac{2}{45} = 0.04$$

$$\frac{31}{669} = 0.05$$

$$\frac{75}{59} = 1.27$$

Calculating With Decimals. You should convert difficult fractions to decimals, rounding when necessary, before doing further calculations. This greatly simplifies subsequent work. Follow these guidelines when adding decimals:

- Write the numbers in a column, lining up the decimal points. Put a decimal point on the right of any whole number.
- Add the numbers.
- Bring the decimal point straight down into the answer.

$$\begin{array}{r} 1.3 \\ +0.25 \\ \hline 1.55 \end{array}$$

Follow these guidelines when subtracting decimals:

- Write the numbers in a column, lining up the decimal points. Put the larger number on top.
- If necessary, add zeros as place holders.
- Subtract.
- Bring the decimal point straight down into the answer.

$$\begin{array}{r} 1.3 \\ -0.25 \\ \hline \end{array} = \begin{array}{r} 1.30 \\ -0.25 \\ \hline 1.05 \end{array} = 1.05$$

Follow these guidelines when multiplying decimals:

- Multiply the numbers.
- Count the total number of places to the right of each decimal point. Add them together.
- Count off this total number of decimal places in the answer. Count from right to left.

$$\begin{array}{rl} 1.3 & \text{1 place} \\ \times 0.25 & \text{2 places} \\ \hline 65 & \\ 26 & \\ \hline .325 & \text{3 places} \\ .325 = 0.325 \end{array}$$

Follow these guidelines when dividing decimals:

- Make the divisor a whole number by moving the decimal point to the right of the last digit.
- In the **dividend**, move the decimal point to the right the same number of places.

- Place the decimal point directly above in the **quotient,** or answer.
- Divide.
- Round off if necessary.

$$
\begin{array}{r}
5.2 \\
.25.\overline{)1.30.} \\
1\,25 \\
\hline
50 \\
50 \\
\hline
\end{array}
$$

See Figure 4.2.

◆◆ **Note** ◆◆◆

If the answer is less than 1, add a zero to the left of the decimal point.

Scientific Notation. Expressing very small quantities with decimals can lead to error. Numbers with many zeros after the decimal point, such as 0.000000001, are difficult to read and transcribe. It is easy to misplace decimal points and change values by a power of ten or more. To help reduce errors, a system of writing decimals called **scientific notation** is often used with very small and very large numbers.

Scientific notation uses **exponents,** which are symbols written above and to the right of a number. Exponents tell how many times the number is to be multiplied by itself. For example, the number 10^2 is 10×10, or 100. The number 10^3 is $10 \times 10 \times 10$, or 1,000. The notation 10^{-1} is the inverse of 10^1. It means $1/10^1$, which is 1/10 or 0.1. The number 10^{-2} is the inverse of 10^2, or $1/10^2$, which is 1/100 or 0.01. Using scientific notation, the number 0.1 is expressed as 1×10^{-1}, 0.01 as 1×10^{-2}, and 0.001 as 1×10^{-3}.

Here is an easy way to convert numbers to their equivalents in scientific notation, using as an example the number $0.000001234 = 1.234 \times 10^{-6}$.

- Place the decimal point to the right of the first nonzero digit: 1.234.

---

quotient

divisor $\overline{)}$ dividend

Figure 4.2. Parts of a division problem.

◆◆◆ **More About** ◆◆◆
Exponents

Any number raised to the zero power, that is, with an exponent of zero, equals one. A number raised to the first power, that is, with an exponent of one, equals itself. A fractional exponent takes a root of a number. For example, the exponent $\frac{1}{2}$ takes the square root and the exponent $\frac{1}{3}$ takes the cube root.

To multiply or divide exponents, make sure that they have the same base, such as 5^2, 5^4, or other exponents of the base number 5. To multiply these numbers, simply add the exponents: $5^2 \times 5^4 = 5^6$. To divide them, subtract the exponents: $5^2 - 5^4 = 5^{-2}$. Use your calculator to perform the calculations to verify to yourself that the method produces correct answers.

- Multiply this number by 10: 1.234×10.
- Use as the exponent of 10 the number of places the decimal point was moved in step one: 1.234×10^6.
- The exponent is positive if you moved the decimal point to the left and negative if you moved it to the right: 1.234×10^{-6}.

◆◆ *Percents*

Percent literally means "out of a hundred," so a number expressed as a percent is a fraction with 100 as the denominator. Fifty percent, also written 50%, means 50 out of 100 or $\frac{50}{100}$. Likewise, 10 percent means 10 out of 100, or $\frac{10}{100}$. Because the denominator is always 100, it is easy to convert percents to decimals and decimals to percents even without a calculator. Just remember that any number followed by the word *percent* or the percent sign, %, is divided by 100.

Study the following examples to be sure that you understand the relationship between percents, fractions, and decimals:

- $50\% = \frac{50}{100} = 0.50$
- $6\% = \frac{6}{100} = 0.06$
- $99.5\% = \frac{99.5}{100} = 0.995$
- $0.1\% = \frac{0.1}{100} = 0.001$.

In general, to convert numbers from percents to decimals move the decimal point two places to the left and drop the percent sign. To convert numbers from decimals to percents, move the decimal point two places to the right and add a percent sign.

USING FORMULAS

Formulas are rules that are written in mathematical symbols and numbers. They express the relationship between two or more quantities, such as temperature in Celsius and temperature in Fahrenheit. Most formulas are written in the form of **equations,** which are mathematical statements that express equality between two expressions on either side of an equal sign, such as $C = \frac{5}{9}(F - 32)$, which is the formula for converting temperature in Fahrenheit, represented by the letter F, into temperature in Celsius, represented by the letter C. The left side of an equation (everything to the left of the equal sign, =) is always equal to the right side of the equation (everything to the right of the equal sign).

In addition to temperature conversion, formulas are used in POLs to calculate cell counts, calibrate instruments, and establish quality control limits, among other uses. The best way to learn how to use POL formulas is by working through them. Knowledge of algebra is not necessary if you follow the instructions step by step and remember these three rules about all mathematical equations:

- If part of an equation is enclosed in parentheses, as in the temperature conversion equation above, complete that part before solving the rest of the equation.

- In order to preserve the equality of expressions on both sides of the equal sign, treat both sides of any equation equally. For example, if you multiply the right side of an equation by 2, you also must multiply the left side of the equation by 2 to preserve the equality.

- When you solve equations, always use and carry through with the correct units of measurement (for example, degrees or mm^3). If you do, your answer should be in the correct units; if it is not, then you may have made an error in your calculations.

Work through the following two examples for a better understanding of how to use formulas:

- The formula for converting Fahrenheit to Celsius was given above as:

$$C = \tfrac{5}{9} \times (F - 32°)$$

where:

C = temperature in Celsius
F = temperature in Fahrenheit.

Calculate the temperature in Celsius when it is 72 degrees Fahrenheit. Substitute 72 degrees for F into the formula:

$$C = \frac{5}{9} \times (72° - 32°), \text{ or}$$

$$C = \frac{5}{9} \times 40° = \frac{200°}{9} = 22°$$

- The formula for calculating platelet counts is:

$$\text{Platelet count} = \frac{\text{Avg. no. of platelets} \times \text{Depth factor} \times \text{Dilution factor}}{\text{Area counted}}$$

Assume that the values to be substituted into the formula for the platelet count are:

Avg. no. of platelets = 170
Depth factor = 10
Dilution factor = 100
Area counted = 1 mm^3

Substituting into the formula, you get:

$$\text{Platelet count} = \frac{170 \times 10 \times 100}{1 \text{ mm}^3}$$
$$= 170,000/\text{mm}^3$$

THE METRIC SYSTEM

In your day-to-day life, most of you use the **English system** of measurement. For example, you measure length in inches and feet, weight in ounces and pounds, and volume in cups and quarts. The English system has two major drawbacks for use in POLs. One drawback is that it lacks precise units for measuring very small quantities, which are required for medications, transfusions, and accurate test procedures. The second drawback is that it is very difficult to convert from one unit of measurement to another. For example, there are 12 inches in a foot, 16 ounces in a pound, and 4 cups in a quart. Because the English system evolved over many generations of practical use, it has no systematic basis.

The **metric system** in contrast, is ordered, methodical, and easy to use. It was designed by scientists in the late eighteenth century in Europe to replace the confusing patchwork of measuring systems then in use. The basic original metric units include the **meter** (m) for length, the **gram** (g) for weight, and the **liter** (L) for volume. All other units are obtained by multiplying or dividing these basic units by ten or some power of ten (one hundred, one thousand, one million, and so on). These derived units are distinguished

TABLE 4.2 Prefixes in the Metric System

Power of Ten	Prefix	Abbreviation
1,000,000	mega-	M
1,000	kilo-	k
100	hecto-	h
10	deka-	dk
0.1	deci-	d
0.01	centi-	c
0.001	milli-	m
0.000001	micro-	μ
0.000000001	nano-	n
0.000000000001	pico-	p
0.000000000000001	femto-	f

by prefixes, and each has its own abbreviation (see Table 4.2).

Converting from one unit to another is easy with the metric system, and some units are extremely small, making the metric system particularly useful for POLs.

♦♦♦ Comparison of the ♦♦♦ English and Metric Systems of Measurement

1 centimeter = 0.3937 inches
1 meter = 1.0936 yards
1 kilometer = 0.62137 miles
1 cubic centimeter = 0.061 cubic inch
1 gram = 0.03527 ounces
1 kilogram = 2.2046 pounds
1 liter = 1.0567 quarts

Some examples will help clarify how metric prefixes are used. Multiplying the gram by 1,000 produces a unit called the **kilogram (kg)**. Dividing the gram by 1,000 produces a unit called the **milligram (mg)**. Similarly, multiplying a meter by 1,000 produces the **kilometer (km)**, and dividing a meter by 1,000 produces the **millimeter (mm)**. For very small units, scientific notation usually is used to express the power of ten. For example, the prefix *micro-* can be expressed as 10^{-6}, *nano-* as 10^{-9}, *pico-* as 10^{-12}, and *femto-* as 10^{-15}.

♦♦♦ Examples of POL ♦♦♦ Metric Measurements

- Most cylinders, beakers, flasks, syringes, and test tubes measure fluid in milliliters.
- Large flasks measure fluid in liters.
- Pipettes measure fluids in milliliters or microliters.
- Solid reagents are measured in grams.
- The hemacytometer has a fluid depth of 0.10 millimeter.
- Erythrocyte sedimentation rate tubes are read in millimeters.
- The **colorimeter,** an instrument for measuring intensity of color, identifies the wavelengths of colored light in nanometers (nm).

In 1960, the **International System of Units** (SI) modernized the metric system to include newer scientific measurements, such as the candela, which measures light intensity, and the ampere, which measures electric current. Other changes also were introduced at that time, including substitution of the kilogram for the gram as the basic unit of weight and capitalization of the abbreviation for liter (L). Since medical laboratories have not completed the change-over to SI yet, some tests are reported in both metric and SI units in some textbooks.

Because the metric system is used exclusively in POLs, you will need to convert between English and metric systems only when you move into the clinical setting. You may need to convert a patient's body weight from pounds to kilograms to calculate drug doses, for example, or to convert doses of medications from milliliters to teaspoons. For situations such as these, it is most convenient to use a metric conversion chart, which may be found in a medical dictionary or similar reference. To feel at ease using the metric system, practice measuring with the pipettes, flasks, and cylinders in your student laboratory and use the metric side of your ruler for measuring length.

◆ ◆

SOLUTIONS AND DILUTIONS

Preparing **solutions**, liquids containing dissolved substances, to exact specifications is a task that is done repeatedly in the POL. Most solutions are prepared in one of two ways:

- making a weaker solution from a stronger one, that is, making a **dilution.**

- adding liquid to **reconstitute** a dried powder, that is, to return it to its original liquid form.

Dilution refers to the strength, or **concentration,** of a chemical in a solution, not to the volume of the solution. For example, a very small amount of solution, measured in microliters, and a very large

---

◆ ◆ ◆ Solution and ◆ ◆ ◆ Dilution Terminology

- **Concentrate:** a substance, either liquid or solid, that is strong because it has had the fluid removed from it.

- **Diluent:** an agent that reduces the strength of a substance to which it is added.

- **Dilution:** a solution that has been weakened by addition of a diluent.

- **Solute:** the substance that is dissolved in a liquid to form a solution.

- **Solution:** the liquid containing a dissolved substance.

- **Solvent:** the liquid in which substances are dissolved to form a solution.

- **Total Volume:** the amount of a solution, including both solute and solvent.

---

amount, measured in liters, may have the same concentration of chemicals and therefore the same dilution. The phrase "make a dilution" often is seen in manufacturers' directions, and many dilutions are used in test procedures.

Specimens for manual blood-cell counts require dilution in order to be seen under the microscope. Blood, serum, or plasma are diluted with chemical solutions to produce colored reactions that are measured by a colorimeter.

The concentration of a solution may be specified in one of two equivalent ways—as a ratio or as a percent. Ratios are used for dilutions. For example, a 1 to 10 (or $1:10$ or $\frac{1}{10}$) dilution and a 10 percent solution both describe the same concentration. In either case, the amount of solute is represented by the numerator and the total volume of the solution, not the amount of solvent, by the denominator.

Whenever a dilution is used to specify the concentration of a solution, the numerator is set equal to one. When a percent is used, the denominator is 100 units of volume. The numerator may be measured as weight for solids or volume for liquids in a percent but only as volume in a dilution ratio. Consider these two examples:

- 0.2 L of 100 percent bleach is diluted up to a total volume of 2 L. This is expressed as a $1:10$ solution: $\frac{0.2}{2} = \frac{0.1}{1} = 0.1$.

- 0.20 grams of solute is diluted to a total volume of 2 mL. This is expressed as a 10 percent solution: $\frac{0.2}{2} = \frac{0.1}{1} = 10\%$.

ᐧᐧ *Making Solutions*

To calculate the amount of solute needed for a particular solution, you need to know the concentration and total volume required. Assume you are to prepare a 1:7 dilution with a total volume of 20 mL. Use this formula, in which the amount of solute required is represented by the letter *x*:

$$\frac{x}{20 \text{ mL}} = \frac{1}{7}.$$

◆ ◆ ◆ **Note** ◆ ◆ ◆

When making solutions and dilutions, always follow the manufacturer's instructions on the package insert. Using different methods may produce solutions with different concentrations and introduce error to test results. (See also Figure 4.3.)

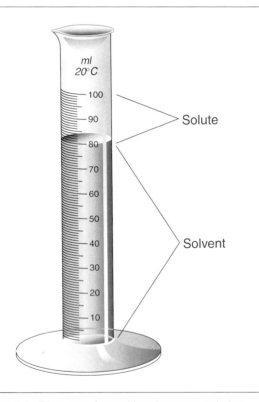

Figure 4.3. Directions for making the same solution may vary from one procedure to another and from one manufacturer to another. Twenty mL of solute added to 80 mL of solvent can be expressed as a dilution of 1:5, a ratio of 1:4, solute to solvent or a 20 percent solution.

This equation means that the solution represented by $\frac{x}{20}$ mL has an unknown amount of solute, a total volume of 20 mL, and a concentration of 1:7.

To solve for *x*, or the amount of solute needed, you must change the equation so that *x* appears by itself on one side of the equal sign. Do this by multiplying both sides of the equation by 20 mL. Recall that to preserve equality you must treat both sides of the equation equally.

$$x = \frac{20 \text{ mL}}{7}$$

Then, rewrite $\frac{20 \text{ mL}}{7}$ as a decimal by dividing 20 by 7:

$$x = 2.9 \text{ mL}$$

In words, 2.9 mL of solute are required to produce a 1:7 solution with a total volume of 20 mL.

◆ ◆ ◆ **Note** ◆ ◆ ◆

When the solute and solvent are both liquids, they must be in the same units of measurement unless otherwise specified.

ᐧᐧ *Making Dilutions*

To dilute a solution from a stronger to a weaker one, use this formula:

$$C_1 \times V_1 = C_2 \times V_2$$

where,

C_1 = concentration of solution 1
V_1 = volume of solution 1
C_2 = concentration of solution 2
V_2 = volume of solution 2

Three out of the four factors in this formula must be known to solve for the fourth. Consider the following examples:

EXAMPLE 1: Determine how much 100 percent bleach is needed to make 500 mL of 10 percent bleach solution.

SOLUTION 1: Substituting in the above formula, you get:

$$100\% \times V_1 = 10\% \times 500 \text{ mL}$$

Solve for V_1 by dividing both sides of the equation by 100%:

$$V_1 = \frac{10\%}{100\%} \times 500 \text{ mL}$$

Simplify the right side of the equation:

$$V_1 = 0.1 \times 500 \text{ mL, or } V_1 = 50 \text{ mL}$$

In words, 50 mL of 100 percent bleach are needed to make a 500 mL solution of 10 percent bleach.

EXAMPLE 2: Determine how much of a 1:10 solution is needed to make a 50 mL solution with a 1:50 concentration.

SOLUTION: For ease in calculation, first convert the ratios to percents:

$1:10 = \frac{1}{10} = 0.10 = 10\%$; $1:50 = \frac{1}{50} = 0.02 = 2\%$

Then substitute into the above formula:

$$10\% \times V_1 = 2\% \times 50 \text{ mL}$$

Solve for V_1:

$$V_1 = \frac{2\%}{10\%} \times 50 \text{ mL}$$

Simplify:

$$V_1 = 0.20 \times 50 \text{ mL, or } V_1 = 10 \text{ mL}$$

WHEN THINGS GO WRONG

Calculations in POLs must be accurate. Life-or-death decisions may depend upon them. You always should ask if the answers you calculate are logical and reasonable. For example, are the figures in the expected units and in the expected range? If not, check and recheck for errors. Misplaced decimal points are common errors that are easy to detect if you use common sense and good judgment.

Never proceed with calculations that you do not understand completely or that are producing illogical results. Use the following steps when you run into problems:

- Reread the instructions, several times if necessary.
- If the method still is unclear, look for an explanation in the appropriate POL manual or reference book or ask a qualified individual for assistance. Use diplomacy and follow the line of authority in your lab. Do not bypass your supervisor by getting information from an outside source.
- To be sure that you thoroughly understand the explanation, write it down, read it back, and see if it makes sense. Then enter the new information in the POL manual or your personal notebook so that you will be prepared the next time you do the procedure or calculation. Be sure to phrase the explanation in clear, understandable terms that you can decipher later.

PROCEDURE

4.1 Measuring and Mixing With Metric

Goal

- After successfully completing this procedure, you will be able to use metric equipment to measure and to calculate and mix solutions.

Completion Time

- 30 minutes

Equipment and Supplies

- metric ruler
- colorimeter
- sedimentation rate tube
- suction device for pipettes
- graduated flasks, cylinders, and pipettes in assorted sizes
- scale
- Celsius thermometer
- Fahrenheit thermometer
- paper clip
- table salt (NaCl)
- tap water (ice water, tepid water, and boiling water)
- calculator
- pen and paper

Instructions

Read through the list of equipment and supplies that you will need and the steps of the procedure. Be sure that you understand each step before you begin. Then complete each step correctly and in the proper order. If your completion time is too long, repeat the procedure until you increase your speed.

		S	U
S = Satisfactory	U = Unsatisfactory		

1. Collect and prepare appropriate equipment.

2. Use the metric ruler to draw straight lines of 6, 10, 15, and 25 millimeters.

3. Reading the sedimentation rate tube from the top down, find these same markings, which are typical readings for erythrocyte sedimentation rates.

4. Inspect the colorimeter to see how wavelengths of light are designated and write the length of the shortest and longest wavelengths listed.

5. Convert the wavelength measurements into meters, using scientific notation. (*Possible answer:* 240 nanometers = 240×10^{-9} meters.)

6. Using tap water and an appropriate flask, cylinder, or pipette, measure each of the following amounts. Always read the measurement at the bottom of the meniscus and use the suction device to pipette.

    a. One liter in a cylinder—this amount of household bleach might be measured to prepare a dilution for general-purpose disinfecting in the lab.

    b. One half liter in a flask—this amount of reagent might be measured to prepare a dilution for patient tests.

    c. One milliliter in a pipette—this amount of blood might be measured for a serological test.

    d. One microliter in a pipette—this amount of blood might be measured for a red blood-cell count.

7. Weigh samples of 1 and 10 grams of table salt.

8. Weigh a paper clip and record your answer in grams: _____.

9. Place both thermometers in ice water and record their temperatures:
C _____; F _____
Caution: Do not put thermometers directly into boiling water from ice water or vice versa—they may shatter.

10. Place both thermometers in tepid water and record their temperatures:

    C _____ ; F _____

11. Place both thermometers in boiling water and record their temperatures:

    C _____ ; F _____

12. Mix a 10 percent solution of table salt and tap water.

13. Mix a 1:10 dilution of table salt and tap water.

14. Discard the disposable equipment.

15. Wash the other equipment and return it to storage.

OVERALL PROCEDURAL EVALUATION

Student's Name _____

Signature of Instructor _____ **Date** _____

Comments

CHAPTER 4 REVIEW

Using Terminology

Match the terms in the right column with the appropriate definition in the left column.

_____ 1. 1×10^{-6}

_____ 2. bottom of fraction

_____ 3. one millionth

_____ 4. one thousandth

_____ 5. per 100

_____ 6. metric unit of length

_____ 7. metric unit of weight

_____ 8. metric unit of volume

_____ 9. weakens solution

_____ 10. strength

a. concentration

b. scientific notation

c. denominator

d. diluent

e. gram

f. liter

g. meter

h. milli-

i. micro-

j. percent

Match the units of measurement in the left column with the correct abbreviation in the right column.

_____ 11. liter

_____ 12. kilogram

_____ 13. gram

_____ 14. microliter

_____ 15. milliliter

_____ 16. femtoliter

_____ 17. meter

_____ 18. millimeter

_____ 19. centimeter

a. cm

b. fL

c. g

d. kg

e. L

f. m

g. mL

h. mm

i. μL

Define the following terms in the spaces provided.

20. Concentrate: _____

_____

_____

21. Diluent: _____

_____

_____

22. Dilution: _____

_____

_____

23. Solute: _____

_____

_____

24. Solvent: _____

_____

_____

25. Total volume: _____

_____

_____

Acquiring Knowledge

Answer the following questions in the spaces provided.

26. What metric unit would you use to measure a person's body weight? The wavelengths of light? The POL disinfectant? A blood specimen?

_____

_____

_____

27. Arrange the following prefixes in order from large to small: deci-, kilo-, micro-, milli-, centi-, femto-. For each prefix, give the multiple or fraction that it represents.

_____

_____

_____

28. Change these dilutions to percent solutions: 1:8, 1:4, and 1:10.

_____

_____

_____

29. Using prefixes, change the following measurements into the simplest, easiest to use units. How is the new unit abbreviated?

0.002 grams _____

0.000015 liter _____

$\frac{15}{1,000}$ liter _____

30. What equation is used to calculate a larger volume of a solution of the same strength? Which variable should be solved for?

_____

_____

_____

31. What equation is used to calculate a dilute solution from a concentrated solution?

_____

_____

_____

32. Why is it important to round off decimal fractions after multiplying or dividing?

_____

_____

_____

33. What conventions should be followed in rounding? Why?

_____

_____

_____

34. What fractions are the same as the following powers of ten: 10^{-2}; 10^{-3}?

_____

35. What is the best way to learn and become comfortable with the metric system?

_____

_____

36. What is the easiest way to add the following fractions: $\frac{1}{2}$, $\frac{1}{4}$, $\frac{1}{10}$, $\frac{1}{20}$, and $\frac{1}{25}$? What is their sum?

_____

_____

_____

37. Which of the systems, English or metric, is the most accurate, especially for small amounts? Why?

_____

_____

_____

38. What are the three original basic units in the metric system? What does each measure? How are prefixes used with them?

_____

_____

_____

_____

39. How can a more dilute solution be made from a concentrated solution?

_____

Applying Knowledge—On the Job

Answer the following questions in the spaces provided.

40. A test often performed in POLs is an erythrocyte sedimentation rate (ESR). It measures the tendency of red cells to settle together at the bottom of a column of blood. While it is not specific for any one disorder, it gives valuable information when combined with a patient's physical symptoms. Patient A had an erythrocyte sedimentation rate (ESR) of 39 mm/hr. Patient B had an ESR of 9 mm/hr. What does the unit "mm" signify? What is each patient's rate in meters? What is the difference in their rates? Use your school library or your own reference books to determine which patient's result is normal and which is abnormal.

    _____

    _____

    _____

41. Mr. Dugal had a reticulocyte count that resulted in 4 reticulocytes for 500 red blood cells (RBC). Using the following formula, calculate the percent of reticulocytes on the stained blood smear:

    $$\text{Percent retic.} = \frac{\text{No. of reticulocytes counted} \times 100}{\text{No. of RBC counted}}$$

    _____

    _____

42. A while ago, your laboratory supervisor assigned you the task of calibrating the spectrophotometer with a new batch of reagents. She went through the procedure with you and you understood it at the time. The old batch of reagents is almost gone, and the supervisor has reminded you that it is time to recalibrate. You feel a little shaky about the task. What should you do?

    _____

    _____

    _____

43. You have calculated a patient's data with a test formula. The answer you get for the patient's test result is abnormal. It is a very busy day. What should you do?

    _____

    _____

    _____

44. In the POL where you work, you have been asked to give a tour to a group of students. You are to explain to them why the POL relies solely on metric measurements. What should you say?

    _____

    _____

    _____

45. You have been instructed to take a blood sample from an infant for a microbilirubin test. The pipette measures a very small amount. You will use a heel stick to obtain the specimen. What metric unit will you use to measure the amount of blood collected?

    _____

5 *Statistics in the POL*

COGNITIVE OBJECTIVES

After studying this chapter, you should be able to

- use each of the vocabulary terms appropriately.
- define *mode, median,* and *range.*
- explain why the mean is the preferred measure of location.
- explain how the standard deviation is used to assess variation within a sample of test results.
- discuss how the coefficient of variation can be used to assess precision and accuracy of procedures and instruments.

PERFORMANCE OBJECTIVES

After studying this chapter, you should be able to

- calculate the mean, standard deviation, and coefficient of variation for a sample of test results.
- assess which of two procedures or instruments is more accurate based on their coefficients of variation.

TERMINOLOGY

coefficient of variation (CV): also called the relative standard deviation; the standard deviation expressed as a percent of the mean.

index: the small *i* under the summation sign. The index indicates the range over which the summation is to be performed.

mean: the arithmetic average of a sample of values.

median: the middle value in an ordered sample of values, with the same number of values below and above it.

mode: the value that occurs most often in a sample.

range: the difference between the largest and smallest values in a sample.

sigma (Σ, σ): the eighteenth letter in the Greek alphabet; used in statistics to represent the standard deviation (lowercase, σ) or summation (uppercase, Σ).

standard deviation (s or σ): a measurement of the variation from the mean in a sample of values.

statistics: the branch of mathematics that deals with the collection, analysis, and interpretation of numerical data.

summation: represented by uppercase sigma, Σ; indicates addition of the numbers or variables that follow.

• • • • • • • • • • • • • • • • • • •

Statistics is one of the newest and fastest growing fields of mathematics and one of the most important tools in science and medicine. It is difficult to read a medical journal or text without encountering statistics. POLs rely heavily on statistics to organize and compare data. Without organized data, POLs could not classify test results and assess the accuracy of test controls and patient tests.

This chapter introduces you to three of the most widely used statistical measures in POLs—the mean, standard deviation, and coefficient of variation. Although you will learn how to calculate these important measures here, when doing statistical calculations in the POL, you should use a calculator or computer so that you will save time and effort and will reduce the chance for errors. Research laboratories and manufacturers often supply POLs with graphs and computer programs for calculating standard deviations and coefficients of variation that are based on their own statistical studies.

THE SUMMATION SIGN, Σ

In order to understand the statistical formulas in this chapter, you need to be familiar with the **summation** sign, Σ, which is the Greek letter **sigma**. The summation sign tells you to add the numbers or variables that follow it. To add the numbers 1 through 4, for example, write:

$$\sum_{i=1}^{4} i = 1 + 2 + 3 + 4 = 10$$

The small i under the summation sign is called the **index.** The small numbers, 1 and 4, indicate the **range** over which summation is to be performed. Most often, the index starts with 0 or 1, but it may start at any number. Consider these additional examples:

$$\sum_{i=2}^{4} (3 + i) = (3 + 2) + (3 + 3) + (3 + 4) = 18$$

$$\sum_{i=0}^{3} 2^i = 2^0 + 2^1 + 2^2 + 2^3 = 15$$

The index often is used to distinguish numbers in a set of numbers, such as in a sample of test results. Then, it is written as a subscript, x_i, read "x sub-i." When $i = 1$, $x_i = x_1$, the first number in the sample. Assume that in a sample of test results, the first test had a result of 23, the second had a result of 14, the third had a result of 5, the fourth had a result of 2, and the fifth had a result of 10. This is written:

$$x = (23, 14, 5, 2, 10)$$

For this sample, x_1 refers to 23, x_2 refers to 14, and so on.

To calculate basic statistical measures like the mean for any sample, such as this one, first add up the test results. Represent addition of the numbers in this sample as:

$$\sum_{i=1}^{5} x_i = 23 + 14 + 5 + 2 + 10 = 54$$

MEASURES OF LOCATION

To interpret any set of test results, first figure a statistic of location or central tendency, which is a single representative value that describes the entire sample. A measure of location gives a general sense of where the results fall. There are three such measures—the mode, the median, and the mean. The **mode** is the test result that occurs most often, such as 5 in the set 3, 4, 5, 5, 6, 7. The **median** is the value that falls in the middle of all of the values obtained, which is again 5 in the set 3, 4, 5, 5, 6, 7. The **mean** is the arithmetic average, calculated by summing all of the individual test results and dividing by the number of tests. The symbol for the mean is $\overline{x}$, read "x bar," and the formula for the mean is:

$$\overline{x} = \frac{\sum_{i=1}^{n} x_i}{n}$$

where,

n = the number of observations in the set

x_i = the individual observations

Returning to the set of values 3, 4, 5, 5, 6, 7, calculate the mean as:

$$\overline{x} = \frac{(3 + 4 + 5 + 5 + 6 + 7)}{6} = \frac{30}{6} = 5$$

In this example, the mode, median, and mean are the same, but this is not always the case. Consider an actual example. In a series of blood-glucose tests, the readings were 60, 90, 90, 91, 92, 93, and 94. The mode is 90, the median is 91, and the mean is 87. Because the mean weights all of the values equally, it is pulled down by the lowest value of 60. The mode and median, on the other hand, are unaffected by the extremely low end value. For this reason, the mean usually is the preferred measure of location for describing test results in POLs.

MEASURES OF DISPERSION

To adequately describe a sample of test results, you need more than just the mean because the mean does not tell much about the distribution of a sample; that is, the mean does not tell how the results are spread around it. Compare the following hypothetical samples of blood-glucose test results:

SAMPLE 1: 87, 88, 89, 90, 90, 91, 92, 93

SAMPLE 2: 80, 80, 81, 85, 95, 99, 100, 100

Both samples have the same mean, 90, but the test values have very different distributions. The values for the first sample are bunched around the mean, while the values for the second sample are much more spread out. A measure of dispersion describes each sample and reflects this difference in distribution. Measures of dispersion are important in POLs for evaluating procedures and instruments. The more variation in test results, the less accurate and less precise the results are likely to be.

◆◆ Range

The simplest measure of the dispersion is the range, the difference between the largest and smallest values in the sample. The problem is that the range depends solely on two observations. An unusually extreme value can greatly influence the results. A better measure of dispersion uses all of the observations and therefore is less sensitive to one or two values. The standard deviation fits the bill.

◆◆ Standard Deviation

The **standard deviation** (s or σ) is the most frequently used statistical measure for describing the dispersion of a sample around its mean.

The standard deviation is calculated as the average difference of each of the observations from the mean value. Generally speaking, the larger the standard deviation, the greater the spread of values around the mean, or the greater the sample's variability. The formula for the standard deviation is:

$$s = \sqrt{\frac{\sum_{i=1}^{n}(x_i - \bar{x})^2}{n - 1}}$$

In other words, the formula for standard deviation tells you first to find the difference between each observation and the mean. Some of the differences will be negative and some will be positive. In fact, the negative and positive differences will cancel each other out. To avoid this, square the differences, because any number squared, even a negative one, is positive. Then add the squared differences and divide by the number of observations minus one to find the average squared difference. Finally, take the square root to return the answer to the original units of measurement. For ease in calculation, the formula for standard deviation is often written as:

$$s = \sqrt{\frac{\sum_{i=1}^{n}x_i^2 - \frac{(\sum_{i=1}^{n}x_i)^2}{n}}{n - 1}}$$

Work through the following example to be sure that you understand how to calculate the standard deviation:

$$x_i = (3, 5, 7, 2)$$

$$\sum_{i=1}^{n}x_i = 3 + 5 + 7 + 2 = 17$$

$$\left(\sum_{i=1}^{n}x_i\right)^2 = (17)^2 = 289$$

$$\sum_{i=1}^{n}x_i^2 = 3^2 + 5^2 + 7^2 + 2^2 =$$
$$9 + 25 + 49 + 4 = 87$$

$$s = \sqrt{\frac{87 - \frac{289}{4}}{3}} = \sqrt{\frac{87 - 72.25}{3}} =$$
$$\sqrt{\frac{14.75}{3}} = \sqrt{4.9167} = 2.2.$$

Many hand calculators include statistical functions such as the mean and standard deviation. If your calculator has these functions, the manual will explain how to use them. The standard deviation also can be estimated from the range if the sample contains between twenty and forty observations, using the formula:

$$s = \frac{range}{4}$$

The standard deviation is used to set limits on the range of values within which test results are considered to be normal. Most often, test results that fall within two standard deviations on either side of the mean ($x \pm 2s$) are considered to be close enough to the mean to be normal. This use of standard deviation is explained more fully in Chapter 6.

❖❖ *Coefficient of Variation*

Both the mean and the standard deviation are measured in centimeters, grams, degrees, or in whatever units are used to measure the original data. For most situations, the original units are the most convenient and meaningful to work with. A problem arises, however, when you wish to compare the amount of variation in two samples that are measured in different units or that have very different means. A 2 mm standard deviation is much more important when the mean is 4 mm, for example, than when the mean is 4 cm. A measure of dispersion must take into account differences in mean values and units of measurement among different samples.

One such measure is the **coefficient of variation** (**CV**), also called the relative standard deviation. The coefficient of variation is the standard deviation relative to the mean for the same sample. It is calculated as follows:

$$CV = \frac{s}{\bar{x}} \times 100$$

The coefficient of variation is expressed as a percent and is unitless. It is just a number. The units in the mean and standard deviation cancel each other out when they are divided. Because the coefficient of variation has been standardized for the mean, any two coefficients of variation can be compared meaningfully, even when they represent samples with very different means.

The coefficient of variation is used commonly in POLs as a measure of precision. It may be used to check the precision of two different methods for the same substances, or it may be used to check the precision of a given procedure using two different instruments. Most manufacturers of lab instruments provide the coefficient of variation of their instruments compared with instruments from other manufacturers. In general, the larger the coefficient, the poorer the precision; the smaller the coefficient, the greater the precision. Consider the following example:

METHOD 1: Mean = 100 mg/dL; s = 2.4 mg/dL

METHOD 2: Mean = 92 mg/dL; s = 2.8 mg/dL

Which method produces results with less variation; that is, which method is more precise? Compare the coefficient of variation for each sample:

METHOD 1: $CV = \dfrac{2.4}{100} \times 100 = 2.4\%$

METHOD 2: $CV = \dfrac{2.8}{92} \times 100 = 3.0\%$

Method 1 has a smaller coefficient of variation. Because it produces less variation, it is more precise.

PROCEDURE

5.1 Computing the Mean, Range, and Standard Deviation With a Calculator

Goal

- After successfully completing this procedure, you will be able to use a calculator to compute the mean, range, and standard deviation for any small sample of test results.

Completion Time

- 30 minutes

Equipment and Supplies

- statistical function calculator
- calculator manual
- pen or pencil

Data

The following results were obtained in repeated tests on a control specimen in the POL:

| 78 | 82 | 89 | 91 | 88 | 89 | 95 | 75 | 88 | 93 |
| 93 | 86 | 78 | 89 | 90 | 91 | 92 | 92 | 94 | 95 |

Instructions

Read through the list of equipment and supplies that you will need and the steps of the procedure. Be sure that you understand each step before you begin. Then complete each step correctly and in the proper order. If your completion time is too long, repeat the procedure until you increase your speed.

Select a partner to work with on this procedure. Each of you should do the calculations independently and then check your answers against each other's. If there are discrepancies, work through the calculations together to find the error. If necessary, ask your instructor for assistance.

S = Satisfactory	U = Unsatisfactory	S	U

1. Familiarize yourself with the mean and standard deviation functions on your calculator. Refer to the manual if necessary.

2. Enter the data on the calculator. Be sure that the calculator is in the statistical mode.

3. Following the steps outlined in the calculator manual, compute the sample mean.

4. Following the steps outlined in the calculator manual, compute the standard deviation.

5. Calculate the range of the sample by subtracting the lowest value from the highest value.

6. Estimate the standard deviation from the range using the formula $s = \dfrac{range}{4}$ (applicable because n is between 20 and 40).

OVERALL PROCEDURAL EVALUATION

Student's Name _____

Signature of Instructor _____ Date _____

Comments

Using Terminology

Define the following terms in the spaces provided.

1. Mode: _____

_____

2. Coefficient of variation *(CV)*: _____

_____

3. Median: _____

_____

4. Index: _____

_____

5. Sigma (Σ, σ): _____

_____

6. Mean: _____

_____

7. Summation: _____

_____

8. Range: _____

_____

9. Standard deviation (s or σ): _____

_____

10. Statistics: _____

_____

Acquiring Knowledge

Answer the following questions in the spaces provided.

11. When a test result falls more than two standard deviations from the mean, how should you interpret it?

_____

_____

_____

12. What term tells you where the middle of a set of samples falls?

_____

13. Calculate the range of the following samples: 88.3, 88.9, 88.9, 88.2, 98.1, 93.3, 98.2.

_____

14. What two values must you calculate in order to set limits for the normal range of test results?

_____

15. Write the inverse of the following exponents and express each inverse as a fraction or whole number: 10^2 and 10^{-3}.

_____

_____

16. Why are exponents used in POLs?

_____

_____

_____

17. What is sigma? What does it mean in statistics?

_____

_____

18. How is the mean represented? How is it calculated? What is the math symbol for the term *mean?*

_____

_____

_____

19. Why is the range not used to measure variation of test results in POLs?

_____

_____

20. What units are used for the mean and standard deviations?

_____

21. What is the formula for the coefficient of variation?

_____

22. What is the purpose of calculating the coefficient of variation?

_____

23. What is another term for the coefficient of variation?

_____

24. In what mathematical measurement is the coefficient of variation reported in the laboratory?

_____

25. What do these symbols mean? Σ; n; $\bar{x}$; $\sqrt{}$

_____

_____

Match the terms in the right column with the appropriate definition in the left column.

_____ 26. x bar ($\bar{x}$)

_____ 27. relative standard deviation

_____ 28. middle value

_____ 29. Greek letter

_____ 30. large variation

_____ 31. data analysis

_____ 32. most frequent

_____ 33. y^3

a. mean

b. mode

c. sigma

d. three standard deviations

e. statistics

f. median

g. CV

h. exponent

Applying Knowledge—On the Job

Answer the following questions in the spaces provided.

34. Your laboratory supervisor has assigned you the task of calculating the mean, standard deviation, and coefficient of variation for a new procedure being considered as a replacement for an older, more complicated procedure. You have not done these calculations in a long time, and you are not sure that you remember how to do them. What should you do?

_____

_____

_____

_____

35. Anne, a coworker in the POL, says that she sees no point in doing the extra work of calculating coefficients of variation. "Why not just compare standard deviations?" she asks. Explain to Anne why comparing coefficients of variation is more valid than is comparing standard deviations.

_____

_____

_____

_____

36. A novice coworker in your POL is having trouble understanding standard deviation. He cannot understand how the working formula for standard deviation can give the same result as the "regular" formula. How would you explain it to him?

_____

_____

_____

_____

37. Your lab supervisor has given you the following two samples of test results and asked you to find the coefficient of variation for each. Without working through the calculations, show how you would set up the problem.

    SAMPLE 1:   98, 99, 88, 85, 93, 96

    SAMPLE 2:   79, 84, 86, 90, 91, 80

_____

_____

_____

_____

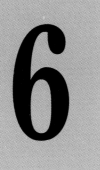

CHAPTER 6

Quality Assurance and Quality Control

COGNITIVE OBJECTIVES

After studying this chapter, you should be able to

- use each of the vocabulary terms appropriately.
- discuss why accurate laboratory test results are necessary for quality patient treatment.
- explain how a daily record of work done in the laboratory contributes to accuracy of test results.
- describe how accuracy in test results is enhanced by continuous comparisons to known standards.
- explain how quality controls may be used to test the work skills of the laboratory staff.

PERFORMANCE OBJECTIVES

After studying this chapter, you should be able to

- show how information is compiled in POLs to satisfy legal requirements.
- calculate the mean, standard deviation, and upper and lower limits of acceptability for quality-control test results.

TERMINOLOGY

accuracy: freedom from error. In POLs, accuracy is assessed by comparing test results of the sample with certified and highly researched standards from research laboratories or by comparing results from the same lab (relative accuracy).

analyte: a substance that is analyzed in a laboratory procedure for its presence or quantity in a patient or quality-control specimen.

assay: a test.

bias: the skewing of test results away from the true value.

calibration: standardization of an instrument as required and recommended by the manufacturer.

calibration standard: a freeze-dried or liquid solution with a very accurate concentration that is used to set an instrument to a certain range of readings.

calibrator: a known solution of an analyte obtained from a medical supply house or professional organization and used as a measuring stick to set instruments to read correctly.

control: a sample used to maintain accuracy and quality in a procedure. Its concentration is known within very accurate limits and its variability is ascertained by the manufacturer.

external control: a check of reagents, test procedures, and/or equipment involving an outside agency to maintain quality control.

in control: a term used to indicate that the quality-control tests that measure the accuracy of a procedure are within acceptable limits.

intralaboratory control: a check of reagents, test procedures, and/or equipment within a POL itself to maintain quality control.

Levey–Jennings chart: a chart on which control values are plotted daily. It is divided into areas of acceptable, low, and high values, enabling lab workers to assess easily the normalcy of test results.

linearity: a measure of an instrument's ability to measure test results in an accurate manner. Test results plotted in a straight line on a graph indicate accuracy.

out of control: the description given to a quality-control procedure when test results are beyond the upper or lower limits of the accepted range or when they are on only one side of the mean, showing a shift or trend pattern.

precision: the closeness of test results from the same sample. Precision must be present in accurate measurements, although precision is possible without accuracy in biased measurements.

primary standard: a quality-control sample that is of the highest possible quality and accuracy.

proficiency testing: a component of quality control that tests the accuracy of laboratory procedures and staff.

quality assurance: a set of policies implemented to give patients the very best medical care possible. Quality assurance covers every aspect of medical care.

quality control (QC): any measure that ensures consistent laboratory procedures and accurate test results.

random error: unpredictable error with no obvious pattern.

reference values: also called normal, or expected, values; the range of values that are expected in a healthy person. About 95 percent of healthy individuals will test in this range.

reliability: the accuracy and precision of a testing procedure or instrument.

reproducibility: the ability to repeat test results.

secondary standard: a quality-control sample that is developed in comparison with a primary standard.

split specimen: a specimen that is divided into two parts and analyzed in two different laboratories as a check on proficiency and accuracy.

standard: a rule by which test results are measured; a quality-control sample manufactured and analyzed to very exact measurements.

standard deviation (s or σ): a measurement of the viariation from the mean in a sample of values.

systematic error: a noticeable pattern of errors.

target value: the value given by the manufacturer of a quality-control sample as the expected quality-control result.

true value: the value for a test result that is based on the results obtained from the best qualified laboratories using the purest reagents, the most refined methods, and the best technology.

variability: the tendency for objects and procedures to change, or deviate, from their original state or from some standard.

• • • • • • • • • • • • • • • • • •

♦ ♦ ♦ Reminder ♦ ♦ ♦

The abbreviation for standard deviation is not standardized. SD, S.D., sd, s, and σ are used as abbreviations for standard deviation.

Quality assurance is the pledge of health professionals to work to achieve the highest degree of excellence in the health care given every patient. It includes all aspects of health care, from the best possible clinical treatment to accurate financial billing. In order to assure quality in health care, there must be well established, widely accepted criteria of quality health care. There also must be a way of assessing how well the care given to a particular individual measures up to the criteria: a way of comparing "what is" to "what should be."

♦ ♦

QUALITY CONTROL

POLs play a vital part in quality assurance because patient treatment is often based on or reinforced by results of laboratory tests. To achieve the **accuracy,** or freedom from error, necessary for quality assurance, a system of monitoring the laboratory, known as **quality control (QC),** has been developed. Quality-control measures ensure consistent laboratory procedures and accurate test results. Quality-control measures also provide laboratory staff with an early warning of developing problems.

Without a quality-control program, laboratory error is difficult to detect unless physicians notice test results inconsistent with patients' history or clinical condition. Undetected lab errors may harm patients by delaying appropriate treatment or leading to inappropriate treatment. The result could be aggravation of the condition, unnecessary time off from work, hospitalization, and a malpractice suit.

General guidelines for maintaining an effective quality-control program include:

- **calibration,** or standardization, of instruments as required and recommended by the manufacturer.
- daily testing of control samples.
- proficiency testing of lab workers.
- accurate record keeping.
- correct patient preparation, such as fasting.
- proper specimen handling, including collection, identification, and preparation, as well as elimination of specimens unsuitable for analysis.

Even with a good quality-control program, errors may still occur. When an error is discovered, it is important to take immediate action by:

- putting a hold on use of the procedure until the cause of the problem has been identified.
- notifying the physician who received the erroneous report.
- investigating what, if any, erroneous results have been reported for other patients and notifying the physician accordingly.

◆◆ *Legal Requirements*

The Clinical Laboratory Improvement Amendment of 1988, CLIA 1988, mandates that all POLs meet acceptable standards of quality. Test results of patients and quality controls must be recorded daily and must be kept on file for inspection. POLs also must enroll in an approved **proficiency-testing** program and receive unknown samples for analysis every three months. These samples are **assayed,** or tested, and the results are sent back to the agency. The test results are then compared to those of other laboratories using the same methodology. To pass proficiency-testing requirements, a laboratory must achieve results that fall within an accepted value range.

The following agencies offer certified proficiency testing:

- American Association of Bio-Analysts
205 West Levee
Brownsville, TX 78520
- American Society of Internal Medicine
1101 Vermont Avenue, NW, Suite 500
Washington, DC 20005
- College of American Pathologists
5202 Old Orchard Road
Skokie, IL 60067

◆◆ *The Role of Lab Workers*

The most important factor affecting quality control in POLs is the laboratory staff. The welfare of patients depends on the care and responsibility of lab workers, who must be dedicated to achieving the highest accuracy in performing lab tests and recording and reporting results. Lab workers also must have the honesty and courage to admit errors when they occur. Lab workers should speak out if test results are questionable. If their work schedule is too fast paced to guarantee care and accuracy, it is up to lab workers to inform their supervisors.

The knowledge and skill of lab workers have a great impact on the accuracy of test results. New workers usually receive initial on-the-job training in all aspects of the lab work in which they will be involved. This is likely to include specimen collection and preparation, laboratory safety, record keeping, equipment operation and care, and test reporting. Competency in these areas may be tested quarterly. New employees should keep a special lab notebook for any questions that they may have about laboratory procedures.

It is a good idea to record more detailed descriptions of procedures than are outlined in lab manuals. Procedures that seem complicated and difficult to you as a new lab worker may seem boringly routine to your lab supervisor or instructor. With practice, they will seem that way to you, too. In the meantime, do not be afraid to ask questions if instructions are not clear.

◆◆

VARIABILITY

Unfortunately, variability is an innate part of laboratory testing as it is of any scientific research. **Variability** is the tendency for objects and procedures to change or deviate from their original state or from some **standard.** Variability in labs refers mainly to variability in test results. The same test done on the same patient on different days, for example, can show variable results. The reasons could range from changes in the state of the patient to differences in the skill of lab workers.

Consider something as simple as taking a blood-pressure reading. Several factors may vary in taking a blood-pressure reading from one time to another, including the sphygmomanometer and its accuracy, the patient's state, and the hearing acuity and training of the individual taking the reading.

Clinical test procedures are affected by many more patient and testing factors. Test results for glucose levels, for example, may vary greatly because of patient diet. A fasting specimen of blood glucose will give a very different reading than a glucose level measured thirty minutes after eating a sugary dessert. The test result also is affected by the manner in which the blood was collected and held prior to testing. A blood-glucose determination on whole blood may be falsely low if collected by capillary tube from a cut that was not bleeding freely. If the glucose determination is on plasma, the plasma must be separated from the red cells soon after collection. Otherwise, red cells that are still alive may deplete the plasma glucose, using it for food. A urine-glucose determination may be falsely low due to outside bacterial contamination occurring at collection or afterward because bacteria digest urine glucose for food.

For many different lab tests, variation in temperature of the testing instruments and the room where the test is performed may affect test results. Worn or failing instrument parts can be a major source of variation in readings. Worker error and contaminated or decomposed reagents and standards also can affect results.

The role of a quality-control program is to monitor such variability in test results, assessing whether the degree of variability is too great to be acceptable. An "acceptable" degree of variation can be attributed to random factors, such as lab worker hearing acuity in the case of blood pressure, that are not clinically significant in producing the results.

To assess the variability of patient test results, you first need to know the **true value** for the control test you are monitoring. The true value is based on the results obtained from the best qualified laboratories using the purest reagents, the most refined methods, and the best technology. An accurate result of a test on a control is one that is in agreement with the true value. The question that you must answer is how much variation away from the true value can be allowed without affecting patient treatment. A variation in a red blood-cell count, for example, of a few cells will not affect patient care. But how much variation will? The permissible variation from the true value must be defined.

◆ ◆

THE STATISTICAL BASIS OF QUALITY CONTROL

The answer lies with statistics. For any given test or procedure, you can use statistics to predict, with a given likelihood, the range of variation within which

most results from multiple analyses of one control test sample will fall. Variability within this range can largely be ignored. Such test results are said to be **in control,** that is, within a range of accuracy that permits physicians to use them in making a proper diagnosis and treatment decision. Test results outside of this range are said to be **out of control.**

As seen in Chapter 5, the standard deviation is a summary measure that describes the extent to which the values are scattered around the mean. If control test results vary only randomly, then they should show a normal distribution. If you plotted the number of times each value resulted when the control test was performed, you would get a bell-shaped curve (see Figure 6.1). This is the ideal, which is only likely in a very large number of repetitions of the test. For a normally distributed sample of test results, one standard deviation on both sides of the mean incorporates about 68 percent of test results. About 95 percent of test results fall within two standard deviations around the mean, and about 99 percent fall within three standard deviations around the mean.

The **standard deviation** can be used to establish an acceptable range of values around the mean. Control

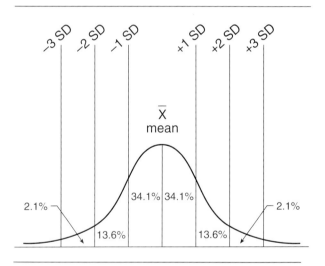

Figure 6.1. Normal distribution. The bell-shaped curve shows the ideal, or expected, distribution of test results from a single lot of control serum. Test results with properly functioning procedure, equipment, and reagents will fall within the acceptable limits of ± 2 standard deviations 95 percent of the time. x̄ = x bar = mean (arithmetic average of test results); SD = standard deviation; −SD = standard deviation less than the mean; +SD = standard deviation greater than mean; ±SD = standard deviation on both sides of mean; ± is read as "plus or minus."

test results falling within this range are considered by the manufacturer or reference laboratory to be near enough to the mean to be useful for clinical purposes. A lab also may compute its own acceptable control test range using the standard deviation formula.

The acceptable range of values is usually considered to be the range between two standard deviations above and two standard deviations below the mean value ($\overline{x} \pm 2$ s). Note that this use of the term *range* is different from its use as the difference between the highest and lowest values in a sample. Values within this range are referred to as **reference values.** Most healthy individuals will have test results within the range of reference values. Keep in mind, however, that age, gender, activity levels, and other factors may have a profound effect on an individual's test result and whether or not it falls within the range of reference values.

◆◆ *Other Statistical Concepts Related to Quality Control*

Precision, bias, reliability, and reproducibility are other important concepts related to quality control. **Precision** is the closeness of test results from multiple analyses of the same sample. While accurate results are always precise, there may be precision without accuracy. This would occur, for example, if faulty equipment or improper technique led to a consistent overestimate or underestimate of the true value of a test. All of the test results would be inaccurate, but they still would be precise if they were close in value. This is an example of **bias,** which is the skewing of test results away from the true value. Bias, a measure of the amount of inaccuracy of a procedure, is apparent when values repeatedly fall on only one side of the mean of the quality-control values. Potential causes of bias include contaminated controls and weak reagents. Figure 6.2 illustrates the concepts of precision and bias. When test results show extreme variability, they are both inaccurate and imprecise.

Reliability is the accuracy and precision of a testing procedure or instrument. It is closely related to **reproducibility,** the ability to repeat test results. Reproducibility is the most important attribute of a clinical procedure. Without reproducibility, the data are useless because they cannot be trusted.

---◆◆

TOOLS AND TECHNIQUES OF QUALITY CONTROL

Maintaining a successful quality-control program requires special tools and techniques. You must become familiar with these before you know how to apply quality-control measures in the lab.

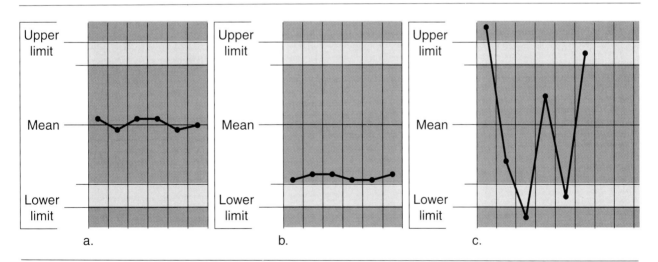

a.   b.   c.

Figure 6.2. The concepts of accuracy, precision, and bias are demonstrated by the first two examples of daily quality-control test-value plottings on Levey–Jennings charts. a. The quality-control daily test results have close proximity to the desired mean value. They show both accuracy and precision. b. The test results are all far below the mean and are therefore inaccurate. However, they are precise, because there is little variation. c. Extreme variability indicates that the test results are both inaccurate and imprecise. The values range out of control from above the upper limit to below the lower limit.

◆◆ Controls, Calibrators, and Standards

Intralaboratory controls are checks of reagents, test procedures, and equipment within a POL itself to maintain quality control. There are also **external controls**, which involve outside laboratories. There are two types of external controls—proficiency-testing programs and split-specimen testing. Many laboratories are enrolled in private proficiency-testing programs, in which unknown specimens are sent to participating labs by professional associations and agencies that sponsor the programs. Each laboratory analyzes the samples and compares its own results to those published by the proficiency-testing program. The testing results also are compared to those of other laboratories participating in the program. In **split-specimen** testing, the POL sends part of a sample to another laboratory, usually a hospital or reference laboratory, for analysis. The remainder of the sample is kept in the POL and analyzed by the usual testing methods. A range of 15 percent variation between the two labs generally is considered acceptable.

Calibrators are known solutions of **analytes**, substances being analyzed, obtained from a medical supply house or professional organization and used as measuring sticks to set instruments to read correctly. The actual amount of the analyte is printed or read directly from many of the newer instruments. In the case of older instruments, a graph is drawn from the readings of known quantities of the analyte. Readings of patient tests tested by the same procedure can be assumed to have the same concentration indicated on the graph. Recalibration of instruments is performed at intervals recommended by the manufacturer and whenever a new lot of reagent is introduced

into the test procedure. The date of calibrations should be entered into the master laboratory log (see Figure 6.3).

Quality-control samples may be purchased from commercial vendors or professional associations. The purest **controls** available are expensive, but they are certified to have a purity in excess of 99 percent. Control samples may come in either of two forms. Lyophilized (freeze-dried) controls are powdered and must be liquified with a carefully measured amount of distilled water. Liquid controls are ready-to-use control materials. Quality-control samples should not be purchased in excessive amounts. Reagents that deteriorate or expire before use are wasteful, expensive, and inefficient to store. On the other hand, purchasing a large supply of the same lot of a QC reagent will prevent time-consuming restandardization due to frequent changing of the QC lot. See Figure 6.4 for a quality-control chart for urinalysis reagent strips.

> ◆◆◆ **Note** ◆◆◆
>
> Quality-control samples should be treated as biological hazards because they may contain human body fluids.

Standards are quality controls for a particular method of analysis. **Primary standards** are of the highest possible quality and accuracy. **Secondary standards** are controls that are developed in comparison with primary standards. **Target values** (see Figure 6.5) are the values given by the manufacturer as the expected control-test result. Actual values attained in POLs will cluster around the target value

MASTER LABORATORY LOG

SPECIMEN IDENTIFICATION RECORD					PROCESSING AND RESULTS RECORD									
Date Rec'd	Date and Time Collected	Patient Name Control Sample	Patient ID	Comments	Test Name	Result	Test Name	Result	Test Name	Result	Date Done	Time	Tech	Comments and Check/Refer Results

Figure 6.3. A master laboratory log has forms for recording the laboratory test information required to satisfy legal regulations. Courtesy of Miles, Inc., Diagnostics Division.

URINALYSIS DAILY QUALITY CONTROL CHART

Reagent Strip Name _____

Control Name _____

Date	Control		Reagent Strip		LEU	Nitrite	pH	Protein	Glucose	Ketone	Urobili.	Bili.	Blood	SG	Tech	Comments
	Lot #	Exp. date	Lot #	Exp. date												

Figure 6.4. A quality-control chart. All quality-control tests must be entered into permanent records. Courtesy of Miles, Inc., Diagnostics Division.

rather than duplicate it exactly. The manufacturer will usually specify the acceptable range of variation for particular test procedures using their quality-control samples. Variability may be expressed as percentages or as standard deviations. This information is usually based on extensive testing of the quality-control product by the manufacturer.

The ability of an instrument or procedure to produce accurate test results can be assessed by measuring the **linearity** of the results. High-value and low-value control samples are tested, and a midpoint sample, made by mixing the high and low value samples half and half, is also tested. Graded specimens with more dilutions may be made. Linearity check

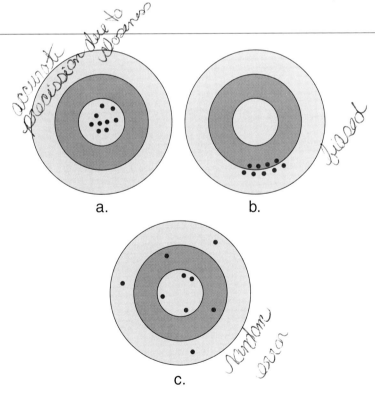

Figure 6.5. Target values. The desired target value is represented by the bull's-eye in the target center. a. The test values show good quality control. b. The test values are biased and inaccurate. They show a consistent pattern of an error that is being repeated. c. The test values show a pattern of random error. The quality is "out of control."

samples also can be purchased from commercial supply houses. The control samples are each tested three times a day for five days, yielding a total of fifteen values for each control sample. These values are plotted on graph paper. A line connecting the pools of high and low values should be straight, and the pool of midpoint values should fall halfway between the high and low values. There is bias in the instrument or procedure if the midpoint is closer to either the high or low value.

Urine and blood specimens with accurate but abnormally low or high test values sometimes are saved or are obtained from larger laboratories and inserted into groups of patient tests being processed. Without the expense of additional standards, their readings provide an additional guarantee that instruments, procedures, and workers are performing correctly.

◆◆ *Instrumentation*

Most lab procedures require some sort of instrument or instruments, so the correct use and upkeep of lab instruments is another important aspect of quality control.

Instrument Maintenance. Well-functioning instruments are essential for accurate laboratory procedures. Instrument maintenance should be the responsibility of one person, preferably the one who is most familiar with the instrument.

The steps suggested by the manufacturer for preventive maintenance should be followed. If the instrument malfunctions, the manufacturer or service company should be called. The person who usually maintains the instrument should make the call. The warranty, model and serial numbers, and maintenance records should be accessible during the phone call. These are most likely listed in the operator's manual for the instrument. Model numbers of replacement parts such as light bulbs also should be recorded there. The call should be made from a phone placed near the instrument, if possible, so that the lab worker can check or manipulate the instrument as needed while talking on the phone. All breakdowns and repairs should be recorded in an instrument-maintenance log. Figure 6.6 is an example of an instrument maintenance record.

Using New Instruments. When a new instrument is purchased, the manufacturer usually provides the assistance of a technical representative who explains the use of the instrument and its capabilities. On-site training, a thorough explanation of the operator's manual, and a day-to-day plan for using the instrument should be provided. The operator's manual should contain detailed descriptions of procedures, including routine maintenance, troubleshooting, and the technical support that is available for problems. The manual also should explain the use of quality control. Software may be available to calculate the

MAINTENANCE, REPAIR, AND PROBLEM RESOLUTION RECORD
Testing System _____ **Page No.** _____

Date	Initials	Test	Description: problem identification and resolution, actions taken, service and repairs done

Figure 6.6. An instrument-maintenance record.

mean, standard deviation, and other quality-control measures, for example, or quality-control analysis may be built into the instrument. While the manufacturer's representative is at the lab, both patient and quality-control samples should be assayed to test the instrument and familiarize the lab workers with the procedures.

Before using the new instrument routinely, another twenty to thirty patient specimens that span the analytical range from low to high should be tested. These may be obtained from a reference lab, if necessary. By the time these specimens are tested, lab workers should feel comfortable with the equipment. During this time, a manufacturer's representative should be available by phone for consultation if any questions or problems arise. If the manufacturer does not provide such assistance free of charge, another manufacturer should be selected. Some manufacturers even provide free proficiency testing on new instruments and reagents. It is also a good idea to check references. Ask for the name of a local POL using the new piece of equipment and call that lab. Arrange for a visit, at their lab's convenience, to see the equipment. Also, get the opinions of the staff who use the equipment.

◆◆ Record Keeping

Accurate record keeping is essential to quality control. A variety of forms, such as the master laboratory log, are used to record lab data. Each procedure performed in the POL requires a separate quality-control record. Every record, for patients and for quality-control results, must be entered into the master laboratory log with dates clearly shown. Every day that patient tests are performed there also must be quality-control tests performed. The results of calibration tests and dates when new control vials are begun must be entered as well. Expiration dates of controls also should be recorded.

Dated quality-control records along with patient reports establish proof that clinical tests are performed in a reliable and valid manner. The records must be retained for a period of years, the exact number specified by state laws and CLIA 1988 mandate. Under no circumstances should out-of-control results be omitted from the records. Other pertinent information that should be included in the records are:

- the date of introduction of new lots of reagents.
- the initials of staff members performing each test.
- the remedies that were instigated for out-of-control results.
- the dates of instrument maintenance.

The results of each quality-control test may be plotted as a daily point on specially printed graph paper called a **Levey–Jennings chart,** on which is printed the mean and the high and low ends of the acceptable range of variation around the mean, usually ± two standard deviations (see Figure 6.7). The graph also may be handdrawn. Usually, two controls a day are tested and recorded for each procedure, one a normal value and the other an abnormal value. Forms for plotting test results for both values on the same page make the procedure more convenient. Use of a Levey–Jennings chart greatly simplifies the record keeping and mathematics of quality control.

◆◆

PUTTING QUALITY CONTROL TO WORK

The purpose of quality-control measures is to detect errors in test results that are significant enough to affect patient care. Any errors must be diagnosed and corrected immediately to prevent reporting of inaccurate patient results.

> ◆◆◆ **Note** ◆◆◆
>
> Whenever quality-control test results are questionable, you should not report patient-test results until the problem is resolved.

◆◆ Errors

Use of a Levey–Jennings chart makes it easy to see when results are out of control. Values for a quality-control test should fall uniformly on both sides of the mean when plotted. The more test results that appear on one side of the mean than the other, the greater the likelihood that the deviation is due to problems of bias, such as defective reagents, defective controls, defective instruments, or errors in staff performance. As explained, quality-control results should fall within ± two standard deviations of the mean 95 percent of the time. The farther away from the mean, the greater the error of that individual test and the more unacceptable the results.

A complete investigation of error is required if any of the following events occur because their individual probabilities are very low in an accurate test series:

- five consecutive test results fall on one side of the mean.

CONTROL VALUE GRAPH

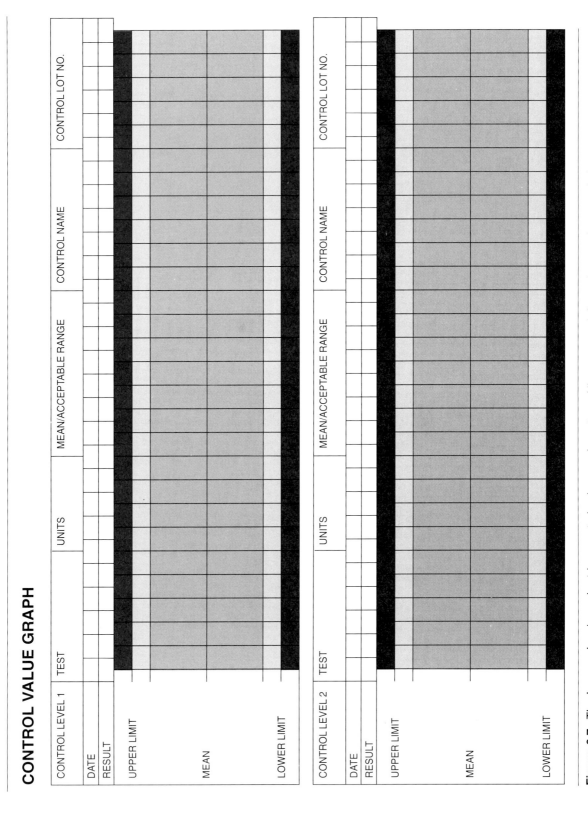

Figure 6.7. The Levey–Jennings chart is a control-value graph system. All necessary information can be recorded conveniently on one page. Daily results of both normal and abnormal quality-control test serums (past and present) are plotted at their appropriate distance from the mean, making it easy to analyze variations from the mean. Courtesy of Miles, Inc., Diagnostics Division.

- two consecutive test results fall outside two standard deviations.
- one test result falls outside three standard deviations.

Three types of error are readily identified using Levey–Jennings charts: random errors, shifts, and trends. Shifts and trends are examples of systematic errors (see Figure 6.8).

Random Errors. Random error is unpredictable error with no obvious pattern. It is characterized by large deviations from the mean. Random errors may have many different causes, including:

- operator inattention due to boredom or fatigue.
- interfering substances in reagents.
- electronic or optical variations in instruments.
- manufacturer's defects in pipettes or other equipment.
- clerical errors, such as misidentification, delays in testing, mislabeling, incorrect transcriptions, and faulty transfers of results. Clerical errors are al-

most entirely preventable if the staff is well trained.

Systematic Errors. Systematic error, a noticeable pattern of error, is evident when test results vary from the mean value in one direction or the other, although the results may not extend past the upper or lower acceptable limits. Systematic error may be caused by differences among staff members in performing a specific function, such as reading the meniscus or rounding off numbers. There are two types of systematic error:

- Shifts show a sudden move away from the mean and then continue in a line parallel to the mean. They may be due to a sudden change in some aspect of the procedure that remains permanent afterward, such as a change in the instrument or reagent.
- Trends show a pattern of moving continuously farther away from the mean in just one direction. Trends often indicate a failing instrument or part or a deteriorating reagent.

❖❖ *Finding the Source of Error*

When quality-control test results are out of control, a systematic method of analyzing the components of quality control is the most efficient approach to finding the source of the error. A checklist such as the following should be used:

STEP 1: Clerical errors.
  a. Was the correct sample tested?
  b. Were letters or numbers omitted or transposed when they were copied into the record?
  c. Were the results entered for the correct test and for the correct control-sample level?

STEP 2: Reagent errors—refer to the package insert and written test procedure.
  a. Were the control samples reconstituted and prepared as directed?
  b. Was the temperature at the recommended level?
  c. Were any reagents, calibrators, or controls past their expiration date?

STEP 3: Procedural errors.
  a. Were written procedures followed exactly?

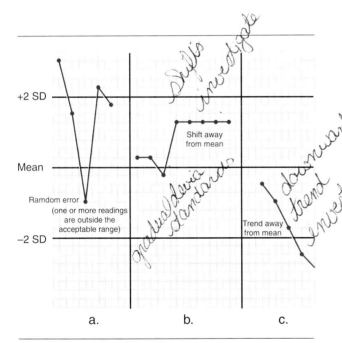

Figure 6.8. Errors that can be identified on Levey–Jennings charts include (a) random errors, where one or more readings are outside the acceptable range specified by the manufacturer or calculated in the POL; (b) a shift, where the values are consistently higher or lower than the mean or target value; and (c) a trend, where the values move farther and farther away from the target value specified by the manufacturer or the mean calculated in the POL.

b. Is the type of error listed in the troubleshooting section of the instrument manual?

If steps 1 to 3 do not identify the problem, then proceed to step 4.

STEP 4: Retest the control sample and record the new result in the master laboratory log and the quality-control journal. If the test result is satisfactory, report the patient-test result and stop here. If the test result is not satisfactory, do not record the test result and go to step 5.

STEP 5: Recalibrate the instrument and test a fresh control sample. Record the new quality-control result if satisfactory, noting that the instrument was recalibrated. Retest the patient specimen and report the result. If the quality-control result is unsatisfactory, however, do not report the patient result and go to step 6.

STEP 6: Test a fresh control sample using fresh reagent. Record the result in the master laboratory log and quality-control journal, noting that fresh reagent was used. If the quality-control test is satisfactory, retest the patient sample and report the result. Otherwise, proceed to step 7.

STEP 7: Contact a source of technical support, such as the lab director or advisor, a reference laboratory, or a hot line of the instrument or reagent manufacturer. Do not report patient test results until the problem is resolved.

—————————————————— ••
CONSTRUCTING A LEVEY–JENNINGS CHART—A WORKED EXAMPLE

This example assumes that two different samples have been tested for glucose concentration. One sample is a normal control and the other is an abnormally high control. Although manufacturers usually provide the mean, standard deviation, and upper and lower limits for their quality-control products, some labs calculate their own values. Calculating values will help you better understand the statistical basis of quality control. For each control sample, you will calculate the mean, standard deviation, and upper and lower limits, constructing a Levey–Jennings quality-control chart for use in testing patient samples.

•• *Samples and Test Results*

The normal control was Lot # 02091, with expiration date April 1995. The mean value supplied by the manufacturer was 91 mg/dL, with a standard deviation of 7, an upper limit of 105 ($\bar{x} + 2$ s), and a lower limit of 77 ($\bar{x} - 2$ s). The following test results were obtained in the POL for the normal control: 91, 91, 93, 88, 88, 106, 84, 85, 80, 92, 91, 96, 91, 92, 95.

The abnormal control was Lot # 020951, with expiration date April 1995. The mean value supplied by the manufacturer was 302 mg/dL, with a standard deviation of 15, an upper limit of 332 ($\bar{x} + 2$ s), and lower limit of 272 ($\bar{x} - 2$ s). For the abnormal control, the test results obtained in the POL were: 334, 249, 303, 322, 300, 297, 305, 315, 307, 282, 287, 303, 311, 292, 325.

•• *Inspecting and Recording the Data*

First, scan the test results to see if they appear reasonable. A value of 5 for the normal control and of 500 for the abnormal control, for example, would be unreasonable. Also, check the calculated values to see if they are logical. The mean cannot be greater or less than all of the test values. A check for logical values is the best protection against clerical errors in calculations.

A visual inspection of the test results shows that all of the normal control tests are within the expected range except one (106), which deviates by only 1 mg/dL. For the abnormal control, on the other hand, the first two test results (334 and 249) are outside the acceptable range. The second test result is very far from the recommended range and assumed to be subject to random error. As a consequence, you will discard that result when calculating the mean and standard deviation. Note that in an already established quality-control procedure, this marked deviation would require a complete investigation using the preceding checklist. However, discarding very deviant control-test results creates a tighter control for future tests because it leads to a smaller standard deviation and narrower limits of acceptability. On the other hand, using such a deviant value to calculate the mean and standard deviation leads to a larger standard deviation and wider limits of acceptability, producing greater tolerance of imprecision and inaccuracy. When the test results in a POL have much more variation than the manufacturer's recommended guidelines, the POL must "tighten up" the precision or use a different and more precise test.

•• Calculating the Mean and Standard Deviation

The mean and standard deviation can be calculated by hand, as here, or with a calculator or computer. The mean, $\bar{x}$, is the sum of the test results for each sample, divided by the number of tests. For the normal control, the sum of test results is 1,363. The number of tests is 15. The mean is therefore $\frac{1,363}{15} = 91$ mg/dL. The mean for the abnormal control, calculated in the same way, is 306. Perform these calculations yourself to verify that you understand the

method if you are unsure. Do not forget to discard the second test result for the abnormal sample.

To calculate the standard deviation, use the following formula, which was introduced in Chapter 5:

$$s = \sqrt{\frac{\sum_{i=1}^{n} (x_i - \bar{x})^2}{n - 1}}$$

where,

$\bar{x}$ = the mean

x_i = each of the individual test results

n = the number of test results

In words, subtract each individual test result from the mean for that sample and square the result. Then add the differences and divide the sum by the number of tests less one ($n - 1$).

For the normal sample, the sum of squared differences is 496 and $n - 1 = 14$. The standard deviation for this sample is 5.9. For the abnormal sample, the sum of squared differences is 2,777 and $n - 1 = 13$. The standard deviation is 14.6. Using Figures 6.9 and

Control Level _____   Test _____   Lot # _____   Units _____

Manufacturer's
Mean/Acceptable Range _____   Expiration Date _____

Test Results	Deviation	Deviation squared
1. _____	_____	_____
2. _____	_____	_____
3. _____	_____	_____
4. _____	_____	_____
5. _____	_____	_____
6. _____	_____	_____
7. _____	_____	_____
8. _____	_____	_____
Totals _____	_____	_____

Figure 6.9. A chart for recording data.

$\bar{x}$ (mean) = summation of test results ÷ number of tests

$$\bar{x} = \underline{\hspace{2cm}}$$

$$SD = \sqrt{\frac{\Sigma(x_i - \bar{x})^2}{n-1}} \qquad\qquad SD = \sqrt{\underline{\hspace{2cm}}}$$

$$SD = \underline{\hspace{2cm}} \qquad\qquad SD \times 2 = \underline{\hspace{2cm}} = \pm\, 2\,SD$$

Figure 6.10. A chart for calculating the standard deviation.

6.10 as worksheets, perform these calculations to be sure that you understand the method. Then plot the mean and standard deviation for each sample on the Levey–Jennings chart in Figure 6.11.

❖❖ *Setting Upper and Lower Limits*

Next set upper and lower limits of acceptability on the range of test values for each sample by calculating $\bar{x} \pm 2$ s. For the normal sample, the calculation is $91 \pm 2(5.9)$, or 79.2 mg/dL for the lower limit and 102.8 mg/dL for the upper limit. For the abnormal sample, the calculation is $306 \pm 2(14.6)$, or 276.8 mg/dL for the lower limit and 335.2 mg/dL for the upper limit. Plot the upper and lower limits for both

samples on the Levey–Jennings chart in Figure 6.11.

Compare the results of your calculations with the manufacturer's recommended guidelines. The POL's range of acceptable values for the normal control is tighter than the manufacturer's. The POL's range of acceptable values for the abnormal control is about 4 mg/dL wider than the recommended values.

> ❖ ❖ ❖ **Note** ❖ ❖ ❖
>
> The answers in these standard deviation problems may vary slightly due to rounding of the figures during calculation.

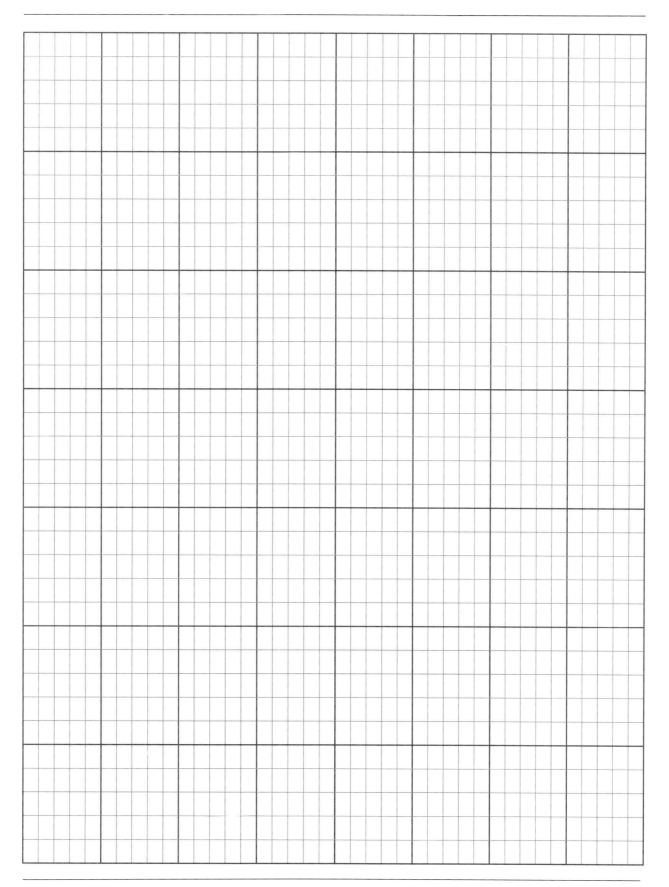

Figure 6.11. A graph for constructing a Levey–Jennings chart.

6.1 Control-Sample Statistics

Goal

- After successfully completing this procedure, you will be able to calculate control-sample statistics and construct a Levey–Jennings quality-control chart for use in testing patient samples.

Completion Time

- 30 minutes

Equipment and Supplies

- calculator
- pen and paper
- graph paper (optional)

Data

Normal Control

- Lot number: 12245
- Expiration date: January 1995
- POL test results: 90, 95, 89, 88, 106, 85, 86, 81, 92, 91

Abnormal Control

- Lot number: 12583
- Expiration date: February 1995
- POL test results: 340, 288, 303, 324, 301, 317, 306, 315, 308, 285

Instructions

Read through the list of equipment and supplies that you will need and the steps of the procedure. Be sure that you understand each step before you begin. Then complete each step correctly and in the proper order. If your completion time is too long, repeat the procedure until you increase your speed.

1. Collect the needed equipment and supplies.

2. Scan the test results to see if they appear reasonable. Omit any that are far out of range.

3. Make a recording chart and a Levey–Jennings chart.

4. Copy the lot numbers and expiration dates onto the charts, which should show both the normal and abnormal control results on the same page for easy comparison.

5. Calculate the mean.

6. Calculate the standard deviation using the following formula:

$$s = \sqrt{\frac{\sum_{i=1}^{n} (x_i - \bar{x})^2}{n - 1}}$$

7. Record the mean and standard deviation for both samples on the charts.

8. Set upper and lower limits of acceptability on the range of test values for each sample by calculating $x \pm 2\ s$.

9. Plot the upper and lower limits for both samples on the Levey–Jennings chart.

OVERALL PROCEDURAL EVALUATION

Student's Name _____

Signature of Instructor _____ **Date** _____

Comments

CHAPTER 6 REVIEW

Using Terminology

Match the terms in the right column with the appropriate definition in the left column.

_____ 1. amount of variance

_____ 2. normal values

_____ 3. calibration

_____ 4. departure from accuracy

_____ 5. extremely accurate

_____ 6. federal law

_____ 7. known concentration

_____ 8. monitoring of quality control

_____ 9. records and manuals

a. reference values
b. CLIA 1988
c. laboratory documentation
d. instrument standardization
e. proficiency testing
f. primary standard
g. standard deviation
h. bias
i. quality-control standard

Define the following terms in the spaces provided.

10. Accuracy: _____

_____

11. Calibration: _____

_____

12. Primary standard: _____

_____

13. Secondary standard: _____

_____

14. Precision: _____

_____

15. Out of control: _____

_____

Acquiring Knowledge

Answer the following questions in the spaces provided.

16. Under CLIA regulations, how often is proficiency testing required in POLs? What does it entail?

_____

_____

_____

17. What percent of test results fall into the following ranges:
$\bar{x} \pm 1\ SD$? _____ $\bar{x} \pm 2\ SD$? _____ $\bar{x} \pm 3\ SD$? _____

18. Arrange the following terms into pairs that are opposite in meaning: *precision, deviation, variability, bias, accuracy, mean.*

_____

_____

_____

19. Give the formula calculating the standard deviation of a sample of test results.

_____

_____

20. Describe the Levey–Jennings charts used to record quality-control results. Why are they so useful?

_____

_____

_____

21. Identify the types of errors that are quickly noted on a Levey–Jennings chart.

_____

_____

_____

22. Discuss legal regulation of quality control in POLs.

_____

_____

_____

Applying Knowledge—On the Job

Answer the following questions in the spaces provided.

23. Your laboratory supervisor informs you that there is too much bias in your quality-control test results although your precision is excellent. What does she mean?

24. Your coworker wants to post the quality-control test results weekly instead of daily in order to save time. Why is this not a good idea?

25. Quality-control results for a POL test that you perform regularly have always indicated accurate test results. One day, you get a control result that is more than three standard deviations from the mean. What might cause this reading and what should you do?

26. Mrs. Smith, a patient who is prone to worry, questions the accuracy of lab tests performed "just in the doctor's office" instead of in a "big, fancy lab." What do you say?

27. On various days, three different workers in your POL perform the same quality-control test and record the results. Worker A is consistently nearest the mean, Worker B is consistently a little above the mean, and Worker C has results that vary widely both above and below the mean. How would you explain these results?

28. A senior coworker has a heavy work load at the clinic as well as heavy home responsibilities. She suggests that both of you take shortcuts and fabricate an occasional quality-control result. What is your response?

29. Dr. Tataglia, your employer, informs you that she will monitor the quality control of the POL chemistry tests by inserting occasional split-sample tests into the work load. What does she mean by this statement?

30. You have been working in a small POL for just a few months. Suddenly, you find yourself responsible for the entire POL due to your supervisor's serious illness. The colorimeter is not functioning properly. What should you do?

_____

_____

_____

_____

31. Dr. Arewa, your employer, has decided to purchase another machine to perform blood chemistries. He is considering two options: (a) an inexpensive, off-brand, used machine without a guarantee, and (b) a new, more expensive machine with extended quality control and service support from the manufacturer. Which machine do you believe is the better buy? Why?

_____

_____

_____

32. A coworker in the POL is in the process of reconstituting a dehydrated control with distilled water. She accidentally adds an extra drop or two of water from the volumetric pipette into the bottle of control. What should she do?

_____

_____

_____

_____

Record Keeping in the POL

COGNITIVE OBJECTIVES

After studying this chapter, you should be able to

- use each of the vocabulary terms appropriately.
- list several reasons why written records are necessary in POLs.
- explain how written records meet the legal requirements of accuracy, safety, and confidentiality.
- discuss how the use of quality-control records safeguards the accuracy of laboratory-test results.
- describe the role of written instructions in assuring accurate and reliable test results.
- explain how the master laboratory log is used as a backup record of all laboratory functions.
- list the contents of a typical requisition form and explain how requisitions are used.
- identify several manuals used in the POL and describe the information and records contained in each.

PERFORMANCE OBJECTIVES

After studying this chapter, you should be able to

- design a plan to orient new lab employees to the record-keeping system of a POL.
- trace the path of a patient's test requisition through the laboratory to the posting of the result in the patient's chart.

TERMINOLOGY

action value: also called panic value; a patient-test result requiring immediate medical attention.

Action values fall outside the normal test-value range, although not all abnormal values require immediate action.

general-policy manual: a laboratory manual that contains the overall policies for every aspect of laboratory operation, particularly as they relate to employees, their qualifications, job duties, and job benefits.

instrument-calibration and -maintenance manual: a laboratory manual that contains instructions and dated records of laboratory instrument calibration and maintenance.

inventory-control manual: a laboratory manual that contains a file of supply house addresses and orders and a calendar for keeping a daily tally of supplies on hand.

manual: a laboratory handbook that contains instructions and recording forms for a particular aspect of laboratory work. Examples include safety and quality control.

master laboratory log: a daily, chronological journal of all work done in a lab, into which patient-test results, quality-control test results, and calibrations are entered. It serves as a backup file for information recorded elsewhere.

policy: a management plan based on the goals of the lab or of particular aspects of lab work. Policies guide decision-making and plans of action.

procedure: test instructions; a detailed written description of a testing process, meant to standardize the manner in which a test is performed so that the same outcome is assured regardless of who does the test and where and when the test is done.

proficiency-testing manual: a permanent record of proficiency-test results that augment the quality-control record.

quality-control manual: a laboratory manual that contains written descriptions of quality-control procedures and records of quality-control test results, the latter usually recorded on Levey–Jennings charts.

records: a written account of a procedure or past event.

requisition: a printed form used by a physician to request a laboratory test for a patient.

safety manual: a laboratory manual containing safety regulations, safety procedures, and policies, particularly as they relate to biological and chemical hazards, exposure incidents, and waste disposal.

specimen-collection manual: a laboratory manual containing all of the information needed to collect specimens for the various tests performed in the POL or its referral laboratory, including the types of collection apparatus required for each test and special handling requirements for specimens. The same information is often found in a chart posted near the specimen-collection site.

standard operating procedure (SOP) manual: a lab manual containing instructions for each procedure performed in the POL.

● ● ● ● ● ● ● ● ● ● ● ● ● ● ● ● ● ●

All POLs must maintain written **policies** (management plans), **procedures** (test instructions), and **records** (written accounts) of patient-test results, quality-control measures, and other aspects of laboratory work. The use of written policies and instructions is necessary to ensure that testing complies exactly with the correct protocol and to ensure safety and accuracy. Written records of patient- and quality-control test results provide legal documentation that they were performed correctly.

───────────────────────── ◆ ◆

LEGAL AND ETHICAL CONSIDERATIONS

Laboratory-test records of patients are subject to the same laws of confidentiality that apply to other medical records. Only the patient's physician has the right to receive and interpret the results of lab tests. The results can be released to other authorized persons with the written permission of the patient, but a patient should not be given the test results directly. If patients ask about the meaning of their laboratory-test results, they should be referred to the physician. Discussing test results with patients risks potential accusations of illegally practicing medicine. Nor should similar cases be discussed with patients. This may infringe on other patients' privacy or be misinterpreted. For the same reasons, laboratory records, especially those that identify individual patients, never should be left in public areas, where they may be read by unauthorized persons.

The federal government requires that POLs maintain and make available upon request their records of quality control, proficiency testing, occupational safety, and Medicare and Medicaid reports and charges. Because federal regulations in this area are subject to change, professional medical organizations sponsor workshops, and government agencies publish documents to keep lab workers abreast of current requirements.

In the event of a malpractice suit, lab records can be used to establish that proper procedures were used for collecting and testing specimens, reporting the results, and assuring accuracy through quality-control measures. If such records do not exist, there is no way to prove that the laboratory was not negligent. State-level statute-of-limitation laws define the length of time that a physician is liable to malpractice suits after treating patients. All laboratory records should be kept for at least that long.

In sum, the records kept in POLs are valuable legal documents that must be protected from fire, theft, and other potential means of destruction or loss. For this reason, it is important to store backup copies of lab records in an area different from the area where the day-to-day records are used.

───────────────────────── ◆ ◆

HOW RECORDS ARE KEPT

While most laboratory records still are written by hand, computers are becoming more important in POLs because of the ease, speed, and convenience they bring to record keeping. Oral transmission of information should be avoided whenever possible.

◆◆ *Computerized Records*

Some POLs use microcomputers to store and print out patient-test results and identify data as well as quality-control results and calibration records. These are easy to retrieve when stored in the computer. **Manuals** are much easier to revise if their contents are saved on computer files. Just how computers are utilized varies from one lab to another, so their specific functions must be learned on the job. Students should strive for computer literacy and be familiar with word-processing and data-base programs because their future employment is likely to require these skills.

❖❖ *Oral Records*

Although it is commonplace to receive oral requests from physicians, any form of written report is preferable to an oral report. Whenever oral messages are received, they should be written down immediately to verify the verbal message. A notepad and pen always should be kept by the phone for this purpose. The confidentiality of patients may be compromised if a verbal message is overheard. Without a backup written record, the accuracy of oral reports may be compromised because of misunderstandings or memory lapses. A test result that is reported verbally and not recorded may be forgotten and never available for future reference.

TYPES OF RECORDS

Records and other written documents in POLs can be divided into three types, each of which is described below: master laboratory log, patient requisitions, and laboratory manuals.

❖❖❖ Types of Records ❖❖❖ in POLs

The following types of records are found in POLs:

- master laboratory log
- patient requisitions
- laboratory manuals
    general-policy manual
    standard operating procedure manual
    safety manual
    specimen-collection manual
    quality-control manual
    proficiency-testing manual
    instrument-calibration and -maintenance
        manual
    inventory-control manual

❖❖ *Master Laboratory Log*

The **master laboratory log** is a daily, chronological journal of all work done in a lab. Into this log are entered all patient-test and quality-control test results, calibrations, and proficiency-sample test results. It shows the day-to-day flow of lab operations and serves as a backup file for information recorded elsewhere—such as in patient charts or lab manuals.

Consider patient testing as an example. The data recorded in the log include the patient's name and chart number, the time at which the specimen to be tested was collected, the type of sample, the type of collection procedure and tube, the test results, and any unusual findings. Also noted for each patient as necessary are repeat tests and referrals of specimens to other laboratories.

❖❖ *Patient Requisitions*

Requisitions are preprinted forms used by physicians to request laboratory tests for patients. Only the patient's physician has the right to requisition lab tests for the patient. A patient cannot order his or her own tests. This is regulated by state laws.

Depending on the size and specific operating procedures of the POL, there may be just one requisition form, which lists all of the tests performed in the POL, or several different forms, each for a different category of tests. After the requested test is completed, the requisition form is posted in the patient's chart. Other copies of the form may be filed elsewhere for backup or financial records.

The requisition form should be filled out accurately, completely, and legibly. It should contain two types of information—(1) information about the patient and specimen and (2) information about the test and its result. The requisition should record the patient's name, chart number or other identifying number such as Social Security number, type of test requested, date and time the test was ordered, and physician giving the order. Also noted should be the date and time the specimen was collected, the name of the individual who collected the specimen, and the date and time the test was completed. The timing of specimen collection and testing is especially important in some tests, such as blood-glucose and fasting blood chemistries. Unusual observations about the patient or test specimen also should be entered onto the requisition form. For example, if blood appears jaundiced, this should be noted. The form should show normal values for the test and have a space for the individual patient's test result.

◆◆ *Laboratory Manuals*

There are several different laboratory manuals that each contain the information, detailed instructions, and records necessary for the day-to-day operation of a particular aspect of laboratory work. There are manuals on safety, specimen collection, quality control, and proficiency testing, among others. The contents of the manuals for a POL are the responsibility of the physician(s) or lab director, who should review them periodically, usually every six months, to confirm that they accurately reflect current policies and procedures. Lab consultants and supply companies may offer workshops and instructions for mastering lab manuals.

Lab manuals are excellent means of educating new employees, but even experienced workers should refer to them to ensure that they are following exactly all laboratory procedures. Some manuals also contain troubleshooting sections that help locate equipment malfunctions and clerical and procedural errors.

Manuals help POLs meet government regulations by providing up-to-date sources of lab policies and procedures and a record of test results and other relevant data. For example, by federal mandate, daily quality-control records must be kept for three years. This information as well as descriptions of quality-control procedures, is recorded in the lab's **quality-control manual.** Part of a government inspection of the lab may include a review of the standard operating procedure manual. OSHA requires that safety regulations, procedures, and policies be accessible to all lab personnel. These can be found in the lab's **safety manual.**

Laboratory manuals usually are kept in three-ring notebooks with removable, laminated pages that are waterproof to protect them from spills and washing. Several manuals may be placed together in one large notebook or each may be maintained separately for convenience. The contents should be typewritten for legibility. An index is a necessity to make retrieval of information easier. Each new subject or procedure should begin on a new page, which should be tabbed for ease in locating it. Manual contents must be dated as to when data were entered and procedures revised.

General-Policy Manual. This manual states the overall policies, or management plans, for every aspect of laboratory operation, particularly as they relate to employees, their qualifications and expectations, job duties, and job benefits. The **general-policy manual** should contain a listing of the technical expertise and personal characteristics expected of em-

ployees. Dress code and professional behavior in the office may be included. The employer's policies with regard to salary reviews, paid holidays and vacation, sick leave, insurance and medical benefits, and hiring and firing procedures also should be explained.

The general-policy manual provides the background necessary to understand the job, particularly as it relates to work in the lab. Some policy manuals are broader in scope, familiarizing the employee with the overall operation of the office or clinic. The contents of the manual and the records and written instructions that the employee is responsible for vary with the size and complexity of the physician's office. The clinical assistant in a small, one-physician office, for example, may be responsible for all the clinical records and laboratory records entered into the patients' charts. The laboratory assistant in a large practice with several physicians, on the other hand, may have only a few types of specialized laboratory-test records and quality-control entries to coordinate with other records.

Standard Operating Procedure (SOP) Manual. The **standard operating procedure (SOP) manual** provides written instructions for each laboratory procedure performed in the POL. The SOP manual incorporates several other records, including quality control, safety, proficiency testing, and instrument maintenance. For example, quality-control and calibration procedures are either described in the SOP or referenced to their location in other manuals. Wherever calculations are necessary, formulas and explanations are included. Manufacturers' instructions may be substituted for typewritten instructions where applicable, as long as any irrelevant text is deleted. Each procedure should begin on a new page and be dated with its most recent revision or review.

> ### ◆ ◆ ◆ Note ◆ ◆ ◆
> No lab worker, no matter how experienced, should rely on memory for the wide variety of laboratory procedures used in POLs. Always refer to the SOP.

SOP manuals include:

- the name of each procedure
- necessary patient preparation
- the requirements of specimen collection and handling

- the size of specimen needed
- a brief description of the method
- reagents required to complete the procedure
- a step-by-step sequence of the procedure
- the normal range of values
- **action values** (abnormal patient-test results requiring immediate medical attention)
- the criteria for ruling a specimen unsuitable for testing (such as a nonfasting blood specimen for a fasting blood-glucose test)
- refrigeration requirements
- centrifugation guidelines
- time limitations
- special precautions

Safety Manual. New employees are required by law to be oriented to safety concerns in the lab. The safety manual provides this orientation. It contains a description of biological and chemical hazards, infection-control methods, and procedures for reporting exposure incidents. Safety tips and legal waste-disposal requirements also are outlined, as are emergency procedures, such as those for fire and severe weather.

The employer is required to keep several employee records relating to safety and occupational exposure to hazards. These include records of employee training sessions in HIV and HBV control and employee HBV vaccination status, with dates of HBV vaccinations.

Specimen-Collection Manual. The **specimen-collection manual** provides the information needed to collect specimens for the various tests performed in the POL or its referral laboratory. It includes a list of names of the tests and their synonyms, types of collection apparatus required for each test, and a description of any special collection techniques. Also included are special handling requirements and transportation and storage needs for each type of specimen. Often, this information is presented in a large, easily read chart, which is posted above the specimen-collection site. The information given in the chart should be complete enough to enable lab workers to collect any specimen shown using the appropriate technique.

Quality-Control Manual. This manual contains written descriptions of quality-control procedures and records of quality-control test results. The accuracy of test results is monitored daily by analyzing artificial specimens with known values of the tested substance. Usually, two control samples are ana-

lyzed, one in the normal range and the other with an abnormally high or low value. If the test results fall within an acceptable range, as provided by the manufacturer in the package insert, then the system of instruments and reagents used in the test procedure are presumed to function properly. If the control sample falls outside the accepted range, on the other hand, then the cause must be determined.

Test values of control samples are recorded on graphs in the quality-control manual. They also are recorded in the master laboratory log. The graphs provide a quick and easy way of observing quality-control results over time and spotting any values that fall outside the acceptable range. Federal law requires that these graphs be kept for three years. They also must be produced at on-site inspections if requested. Daily temperature controls of the freezer, refrigerator, and bacteria incubator are also maintained. The records support the assertion in case of inspection or lawsuits that specimens received proper storage.

Proficiency-Testing Manual. The **proficiency-testing manual** is a permanent record of proficiency-test results that augment the quality-control record. Unlike quality-control procedures that test known controls, proficiency testing uses unknown samples. Proficiency testing may involve an agency-run proficiency-testing program or split-specimen testing. Both types of testing provide a check of the quality of testing procedures, reagents, and lab workers' skills. Proficiency-test results and split-specimen test results are plotted on graphs with colored zones that indicate acceptable and unacceptable ranges of results.

Instrument-Calibration and -Maintenance Manual. The **instrument-calibration and -maintenance manual** contains instructions and dated records of laboratory-instrument calibration and maintenance. Although most lab instruments are easy to use, many are complex systems that must receive regular maintenance to prevent wear and reduce instrument failure. Manufacturers provide written guidelines for periodic maintenance of their instruments. The guidelines help to ensure that the instruments are serviced as needed so that they will perform accurately in testing procedures. Instruments must be calibrated using calibration standards whenever they are used for patient tests or whenever new lots of reagents are introduced.

Inventory-Control Manual. In order for POLs to operate smoothly, they must have an adequate supply of necessary reagents and other supplies. The **inventory-control manual** maintains records of the routine inventory of supplies on hand and orders that have been placed. It generally consists of two parts, (a) a file containing supply house addresses and orders and (b) a calendar for keeping a daily tally of supplies on hand. Chapter 3 describes how to construct the files and calendar record for this manual.

PATH OF PATIENT'S TEST—FROM START TO FINISH

The most important record in POLs is the patient's test result. It is supported by all other lab records. Figure 7.1 shows the path of the patient's test, beginning with the physician's requisition and ending with posting of the result in the patient's chart.

✦✦ *An Important Note on Filing Patient-Test Results*

Test results, when completed, are filed in the progress notes of patients' charts and highlighted to draw attention to them. Each test result should be reported with its normal range for the average, healthy individual. This way, the physician can see at a glance if a patient's test result is abnormal.

While all test results should be posted to the patient's chart as soon as possible, some test results must be called to the attention of the physician immediately. There are test results that indicate the need for prompt medical screening or treatment. Action, or panic, test values are those that call for immediate ("stat") medical attention. Not all abnormal test re-

---

✦✦✦ **Action Values** ✦✦✦

Some of the abnormal test results that should be brought to the physician's immediate attention are shown below:

- high urine protein
- high urine-glucose and blood-glucose levels
- many white blood cells, red blood cells, or bacteria in a freshly collected urine specimen
- grossly abnormal blood cells on a blood-differential slide
- pronounced anemia
- abnormal chemistries and test values indicating possible malignancy

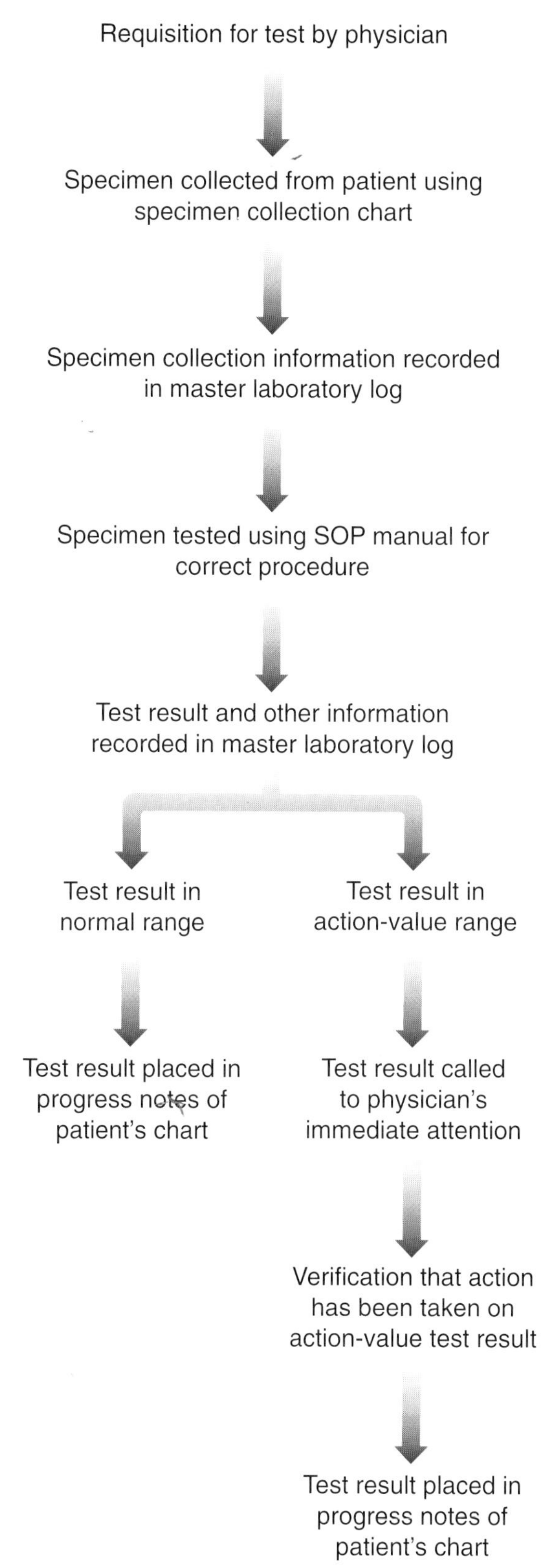

Requisition for test by physician

↓

Specimen collected from patient using specimen collection chart

↓

Specimen collection information recorded in master laboratory log

↓

Specimen tested using SOP manual for correct procedure

↓

Test result and other information recorded in master laboratory log

↓ ↓

| Test result in normal range | Test result in action-value range |

↓ ↓

| Test result placed in progress notes of patient's chart | Test result called to physician's immediate attention |

↓

Verification that action has been taken on action-value test result

↓

Test result placed in progress notes of patient's chart

Figure 7.1. The path of a patient's test.

---

sults are action values. It is up to the physician to decide for each lab test how far outside the normal range of values a test result must fall before it is considered to be an action value. A chart of action-value ranges for testing procedures carried out in the POL should be posted in an obvious place so that such test results are not overlooked.

There should be an established procedure for dealing with action values in the POL, including delegation of responsibility for reporting results. A sign-off procedure such as a written report initialed by both the responsible lab worker and the physician may be used to ensure that the physician has received the report and taken the necessary action. Only then should the action-value test result be posted in the progress notes of the patient's chart.

PROCEDURE

7.1 ◆ Using Lab Manuals and Personal Lab Journals

Goal

- After successfully completing this procedure, you will have hands-on experience using POL manuals to find information and rewriting the information in personal lab-journal format.

Completion Time

- 60 minutes

Equipment and Supplies

- POL manuals
- notebook and pen/pencil

Instructions

Read through the list of equipment and supplies that you will need and the steps of the procedure. Then complete the procedure. If your completion time is too long, spend additional time familiarizing yourself with the contents and format of the manuals.

S = Satisfactory U = Unsatisfactory	S	U
1. Assemble the needed supplies.		
2. Study the contents and format of each manual.		
3. Locate information on centrifuging urine samples.		
4. Locate information on cleaning up biohazardous spills.		

5. Locate information on collecting blood through capillary puncture.

6. Write a summary of one of the procedures that would allow you to follow the procedure correctly at a later date. Use the POL lab-journal format.

OVERALL PROCEDURAL EVALUATION

Student's Name _____

Signature of Instructor _____ **Date** _____

Comments

CHAPTER 7 REVIEW

Using Terminology

Define the following terms in the spaces provided.

1. Action value: _____

_____

2. Procedure: _____

_____

3. Manual: _____

_____

4. General-policy manual: _____

_____

5. Record: _____

_____

6. Requisition: _____

_____

7. Standard operating procedure (SOP) manual: _____

_____

8. Master laboratory log: _____

_____

Acquiring Knowledge

Answer the following questions in the spaces provided.

9. What are some advantages of computerized record keeping in POLs?

_____

_____

_____

10. Why should even experienced lab workers refer to the appropriate manual when performing lab tests?

_____

_____

11. Where are daily quality-control results recorded?

_____

_____

12. From legal, malpractice, and quality-control perspectives, why is the daily recording of the temperature controls in the POL important?

_____

_____

13. Why should oral transmission of information be avoided in the POL?

_____

_____

14. What primary purpose of the POL must all POL records support?

_____

_____

15. What information should be found in the POL's specimen-collection manual?

_____

_____

16. Which medical professional(s) can order laboratory tests for a patient?

_____

17. Describe the path of a patient's test in the POL (when results are normal)—from the doctor's requisition to recording the result in the patient's chart.

_____

_____

_____

18. List test results classified as action values in POLs.

_____

_____

_____

_____

19. Where are values for quality-control tests recorded?

_____

_____

20. How long must proficiency testing records be kept on file to satisfy legal regulations?

_____

_____

21. How is a split specimen used to check accuracy?

_____

_____

_____

22. What is the best way to prove that a POL is not negligent in a malpractice suit?

_____

_____

_____

23. Explain how the master laboratory log is used as a backup record of all POL functions.

_____

_____

_____

_____

24. How is a statute-of-limitations law related to POL records?

_____

_____

_____

_____

25. When can a patient's laboratory-test results be released to insurance companies or other individuals who request them?

_____

_____

26. Which POL manual would you look in to find information about vacation, sick leave, and hiring and firing procedures?

_____

27. Why is it crucial that POL records be protected against loss by theft, fire, and other disasters?

_____

_____

28. Who has the ultimate authority and responsibility for the policies of a POL?

_____

29. What is contained in a typical requisition form?

_____

_____

_____

30. Where are patient-test results permanently recorded?

_____

_____

31. How do quality-control records safeguard the accuracy of laboratory-test results?

_____

_____

32. What POL manual serves as a daily diary of all lab activities?

_____

33. What response should be made when an action value is obtained in patient testing? Why?

_____

_____

34. Who decides at what level of abnormality to treat patient-test results as action values?

_____

_____

35. What information does the SOP manual contain?

_____

_____

Applying Knowledge—On the Job

Answer the following questions in the spaces provided.

36. Dr. Singh is very upset. Mrs. Levy, one of his patients, just informed him that a neighbor had started a rumor that Mrs. Levy's thirteen-year-old daughter is pregnant. The neighbor had seen the thirteen-year-old's name recorded with a positive pregnancy test result in the POL's master laboratory log. The log had been left open on a table near the test-collection site where the neighbor had a blood specimen drawn. In fact, the pregnancy test report belonged to a thirty-year-old woman with the same name as the thirteen-year-old. Why should this mixup never have occurred? How could it have been prevented?

_____

_____

_____

_____

_____

37. Dr. Paro had lunch with some friends who told her that they overheard her POL staff gossiping about her patients at a local restaurant. How should Dr. Paro deal with this problem?

_____

_____

_____

_____

38. Jera has been asked to collect a fasting blood specimen from a patient named Mr. Boroughs. When she checks to be sure that he has fasted according to instructions, he tells her that he had only a doughnut for breakfast instead of his usual bacon and eggs. When Jera tries to explain that fasting means no food at all, Mr. Boroughs becomes angry and tells her that she had better take his blood now anyway because he is not going to miss any more work. What should Jera do?

_____

_____

_____

_____

39. Anne, a new worker in the POL, has been told by a coworker that she lacks seniority and has to take whatever shift the other lab workers do not want. During her job interview, Anne had been assured of fair rotation. How can she find out which is the correct policy of the POL?

_____

_____

_____

_____

40. Debbie has just completed a patient urinalysis. The urine contained many bacteria and had a high level of glucose and protein. She is not sure if she should call it to the physician's attention, because he is having a very busy morning. What do you think Debbie should do?

_____

_____

_____

_____

41. Mrs. Bond is upset because she has been asked to return to the doctor's office this morning for another blood test. The lab worker failed to draw enough blood yesterday for all of the tests that were requested. How could this problem have been avoided?

_____

_____

_____

_____

42. The POL where Tony works has been accused of reporting an erroneous positive result for a syphilis test to an insurance company. The report embarrassed the patient and caused him to lose a job. How should the POL staff determine if they were negligent?

_____

_____

_____

_____

43. The mother of a child with a birth defect believes that her doctor's office lab failed to report a positive test for protein in her urine before the child was born. The mother is suing the clinic for malpractice in causing the birth defect of her child. What evidence is needed to determine if the POL met acceptable medical standards?

_____

_____

_____

_____

UNIT

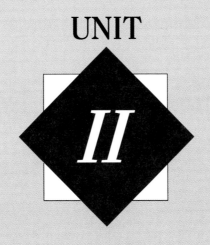

II

Urinalysis

Anatomy and Physiology of the Urinary System

COGNITIVE OBJECTIVES

After studying this chapter, you should be able to

- use each of the vocabulary terms appropriately.
- describe the structure and function of the organs of the urinary system.
- discuss the role of the kidneys in maintaining body homeostasis.
- describe the physiological basis for several diseases that involve the urinary system.
- identify the factors that affect the volume and composition of urine.
- list three reasons for performing urinalysis.
- explain why urinalysis is used frequently in POLs to diagnose disease.

PERFORMANCE OBJECTIVE

After studying this chapter, you should be able to

- develop a model that shows the path of urine formation, from arterial blood through the kidneys, ureters, and bladder, to micturition.

TERMINOLOGY

Addis count: the quantitative measurement or count of cells and casts in a twelve-hour sample of urine.

Bowman's capsule: a thin-walled, saclike structure at the closed end of a nephron, surrounding the glomerulus.

cystitis: inflammation of the urinary bladder.

diabetes insipidus: an uncommon type of diabetes, resulting from a deficiency of antidiuretic hormone, ADH. Diabetes insipidus is characterized by the output of large quantities of urine with a low specific gravity, less than 1.006.

distal convoluted tubule: the part of the coiled renal tubule that begins after the loop of Henle.

electrolyte: a substance, like an ion, that in solution conducts electricity. The kidneys regulate the concentration of electrolytes in the blood, including sodium, potassium, chloride, and bicarbonate ions.

glomerular filtrate: a plasmalike fluid formed by hydrostatic pressure when fluid from the blood passes through the thin-walled membranes of the glomerular capillaries. After traveling through the convoluted tubules, it becomes urine.

glomerulonephritis: a condition in which the glomerular capillaries are inflamed and become permeable to proteins.

glomerulus: in general, a small spherical mass. The renal glomerulus is a tangled cluster of capillaries in the renal corpuscle of the nephron.

glucosuria (glycosuria): the condition in which there is glucose in the urine.

homeostasis: an equilibrium state of the body maintained by feedback and internal regulation of body processes. Homeostasis helps keep individuals healthy by returning their physical state to normal following stress or trauma. For example, when the body is dehydrated, the kidneys decrease excretion of water by producing more concentrated urine.

kidney stone (calculus): a hard calcium stone that forms in the hollow passages of the urinary system in some individuals.

loop of Henle: a U-shaped portion of the renal tubule. It is located between the proximal and distal convoluted tubules.

micturition: also called urination; the voiding, or passing, of urine from the bladder through the urethra.

nephrology: from *nephr* meaning *kidney* and *ology* meaning *study of;* the study of the structure and function of kidneys.

nephron: the basic functional unit of the kidneys, composed of a renal corpuscle and proximal and distal convoluted renal tubules. Each kidney has over a million nephrons.

peritoneum: a membrane lining the abdominal cavity.

pH: the degree of acidity or alkalinity (basic) expressed in hydrogen ion concentration. Acids have a pH less than 7.0. Bases have a pH greater than 7.0.

proteinuria: a condition in which protein appears in the urine.

proximal convoluted tubule: the part of the coiled renal tubule closest to the glomerulus, before the loop of Henle.

renal: pertaining to the kidney.

renal artery: one of a pair of arteries that branch from the abdominal aorta and go directly to the kidneys, where they supply nutrients and bring blood to be filtered.

renal corpuscle: located at the proximal end of a convoluted tubule; a renal glomerulus enclosed in its Bowman's capsule.

renal plasma threshold: spillover point; the concentration of a substance in the blood above which the substance is not reabsorbed and remains in the urine for excretion; often used with reference to glucose.

ureteritis: inflammation of the ureters.

uria: a suffix that denotes urine or urination.

urinalysis (UA): clinical analysis of urine. Complete, or routine, urinalysis includes examination of the physical, chemical, and microscopic properties of urine.

urinary sediment: substance found in standing or centrifuged urine, including bacteria, cells, renal casts, mucus, uric acid, and salts.

• • • • • • • • • • • • • • • • •

Because urine is easily obtained and has great diagnostic value, **urinalysis,** or the clinical analysis of urine, is the most frequently performed patient test in POLs. Therefore, familiarity with the structure and function of the urinary system—the organs that produce, store, and excrete urine—is important.

THE URINARY SYSTEM

The urinary system consists of two kidneys, which form the urine, two ureters, which carry the urine from the kidneys to the bladder where the urine is stored, and the urethra, which carries the urine out of the body. These structures are shown in Figure 8.1.

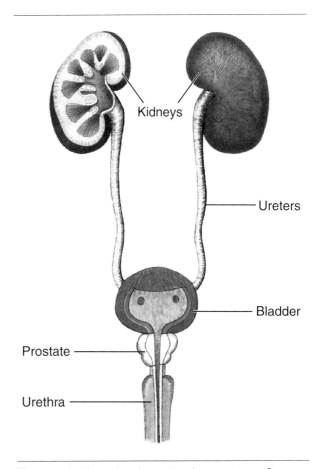

Figure 8.1. Normal male genitourinary system. Courtesy of Miles, Inc., Diagnostics Division.

◆◆ The Kidneys

The kidneys are the main organs for the removal of excretory materials from the human body. They help maintain body **homeostasis,** or equilibrium, by selectively excreting or retaining various substances according to specific body needs. The kidneys play a vital role in water, **electrolyte,** and **pH** balance. They also secrete renin, an enzyme that helps control blood pressure, and erythropoietin, a hormone that stimulates red blood-cell production by the bone marrow.

The kidneys are dark red, bean-shaped organs about the size of an adult's fist. They are located within the back wall of the abdominal cavity, just below and behind the liver. The kidneys are positioned outside the **peritoneum,** which lines the abdominal cavity, and against the deep muscles of the back on either side of the spinal column. They are held in place by connective tissue. Masses of adipose tissue, or fat, surround them and help protect them from injury.

The inner region of each kidney is called the medulla, and the outer region is the cortex. The lateral side of each kidney is convex and the medial side concave. The medial concavity leads into a hollow chamber called the **renal** sinus. The entrance to the renal sinus is called the hilum. Through the hilum passes various blood and lymphatic vessels, nerves, and the ureter. The renal pelvis is the expanded proximal end of the ureter that lies within the renal sinus.

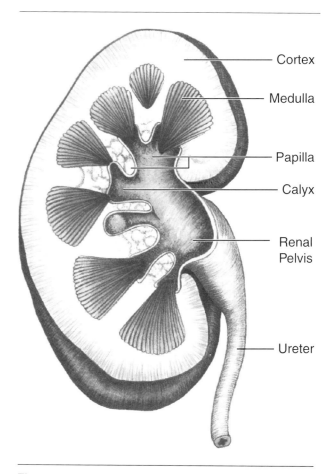

Figure 8.2. A kidney. Courtesy of Miles, Inc., Diagnostics Division.

It is divided into cuplike cavities called calyces (singular, *calyx*). See Figure 8.2.

Blood is supplied to the kidneys by the **renal arteries,** which branch from the main abdominal artery, the aorta. About 1,200 mL of blood per minute enters the renal arteries. This is about 25 percent of total cardiac output. The renal arteries enter the kidneys through the hilum and further subdivide as they pass through to the cortex, where the **nephrons** are located.

Venous blood is returned through a series of blood vessels that correspond generally to the arterial pathway. These vessels join to form the renal vein, which leaves each kidney through the hilum. The renal veins join the inferior vena cava, the principal vein of the lower part of the body.

Nephrons are the structural and functional units of the kidneys. They remove waste products from the blood and regulate water and electrolyte concentrations in blood and other body fluids. There are an astonishing one million nephrons per kidney. Not all

---

◆◆◆ Diseases of the ◆◆◆ Kidney

Patients who are tested in POLs may have several different kidney diseases and conditions with which you should be familiar:

- *nephropathy:* any disease of the kidney.

- *nephrotic syndrome:* any kidney disease showing chronic protein loss in urine.

- *nephrosis:* protein loss due to noninflammatory degeneration of the kidney.

- *nephritis:* any inflammation of the kidney.

- *nephrocystitis:* inflammation of the kidney and bladder.

- *pyelonephritis:* inflammation of the kidney and pelvis.

- *renal failure:* the kidney no longer functions.

- *renal insufficiency:* the kidney functions inadequately to maintain health.

of these nephrons are actively functioning in healthy individuals, but they can be called into action to maintain normal kidney function if an individual loses a kidney.

Each nephron (see Figure 8.3) consists of a renal corpuscle and renal tubule. The **renal corpuscle** is composed of a tangled cluster of capillaries called a **glomerulus,** which is surrounded by a thin-walled, saclike structure called the **Bowman's capsule.** The tubule leading away from the Bowman's capsule becomes highly coiled and is called the proximal convoluted tubule. The tubule then follows a straight path, forming the **loop of Henle** (descending and ascending), and finally becomes highly coiled again, at which point it is called the distal convoluted tubule.

Distal convoluted tubules merge from several nephrons and drain into a collecting tubule.

A number of collecting tubules, in turn, coalesce in the renal cortex to form a collecting duct. The collecting ducts increase in size as they join together into papillae (singular, *papilla*) and ultimately empty into calyces that drain first into the funnel-shaped renal pelvis and then through the hilum into the ureter.

❖❖ *The Ureters*

Each ureter is a tubular organ about 25 cm long that carries urine from the kidney to the urinary bladder. The wall of the ureter is muscular, and peristaltic

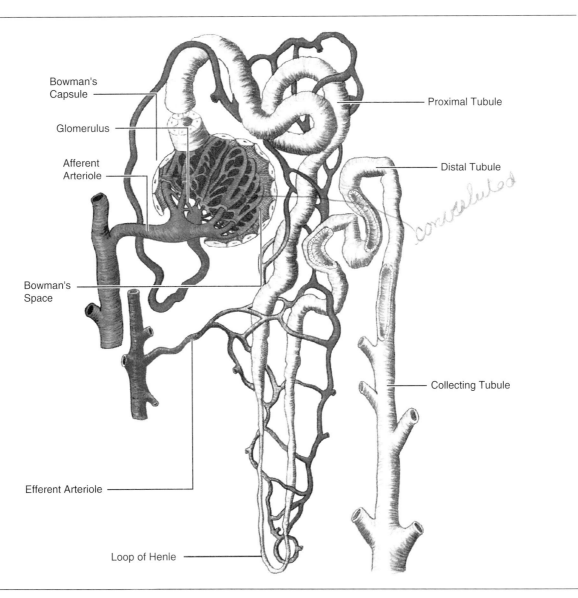

Figure 8.3. A nephron. Courtesy of Miles, Inc., Diagnostics Division.

waves originating in the renal pelvis move the urine along its length. The flaplike fold of mucous membrane covering the opening to the bladder acts like a one-way valve, allowing urine to enter the bladder but not to leave it.

◆ ◆ ◆ Kidney Stones ◆ ◆ ◆

Kidney stones, or **calculi,** sometimes form in the renal pelvis. They may be composed of uric acid or magnesium phosphate, but most often, they are composed of calcium compounds, such as calcium oxalate or calcium phosphate. If the stones pass into the ureter, they cause severe pain, typically beginning in the region of the kidney and radiating into the abdomen, pelvis, and legs. Kidney stones also may cause nausea and vomiting. The causes of kidney stone formation are diverse, including excess calcium intake, gout, and abnormal functioning of the parathyroid glands, which regulate calcium-phosphorus metabolism.

◆◆ *The Urinary Bladder*

The urinary bladder is a hollow, expandable, muscular sac located behind the pubic symphysis and below the parietal peritoneum. The walls of the empty bladder have many folds that smooth out when the bladder is filled with urine, allowing it to swell to a capacity of several hundred milliliters.

Micturition, also called urination, is the voiding, or passing, of urine from the bladder through the urethra. It is triggered by the micturition reflex center in the sacral region of the spinal cord. Although the bladder may hold as much as 600 mL, the desire to urinate usually is triggered when the bladder contains about 150 mL. Micturition is accomplished by voluntary muscle tissue surrounding the urethra.

◆ ◆ ◆ Urinary Infections ◆ ◆ ◆

Bladder infections are more common in women than in men. The urethra is shorter in women, allowing infectious agents like bacteria easier access to the bladder. Because the linings of the ureters and the bladder are continuous, infectious agents introduced to the bladder may enter the ureters. Inflammation of the bladder is called **cystitis,** and inflammation of the ureters is called **ureteritis.**

◆◆ *The Urethra*

The urethra is a tube that carries urine from the bladder to the outside of the body. In males, the urethra carries semen as well. The wall of the urethra consists of a relatively thick layer of smooth muscle lined with mucous membrane. Numerous mucous glands, called urethral glands, secrete mucus into the urethral canal.

◆ ◆

URINE FORMATION

Urine contains wastes, excess water, and excess electrolytes. It is formed in the nephrons in a three-stage process consisting of glomerular filtration, tubular reabsorption, and tubular secretion.

◆◆ *Glomerular Filtration*

The formation of urine begins when the plasma portion of the blood passes through the thin-walled membranes of the glomerular capillaries. If the entering, or afferent, arteriole is larger than the exiting, or efferent, arteriole, this will create a higher blood pressure than is found in most capillaries. The hydrostatic pressure forces water and other substances out of the blood. The resulting fluid, the **glomerular filtrate,** has about the same composition as tissue fluid elsewhere in the body. The concentrations of electrolytes, calcium, magnesium, sulfate, phosphate, glucose, urea, and uric acid, for example, are the same as in plasma. The glomerulus filtrate lacks only the larger protein molecules.

◆ ◆ ◆ Glomerulonephritis ◆ ◆ ◆

Glomerulonephritis is a condition in which the glomerular capillaries are inflamed and become permeable to protein. Because protein appears in the glomerular filtrate and is excreted in the urine, the condition also is called **proteinuria.**

The glomerular filtration rate in both kidneys in the average adult is about 125 mL per minute, or some 180,000 mL in twenty-four hours. Loss of fluid from the body in urine is typically less than 1,500 mL per day. Obviously, most of the glomerular filtrate is reabsorbed by the plasma.

◆◆ Tubular Reabsorption

Much of the glomerular filtrate is reabsorbed in the renal tubules of the nephron. As a result, the fluid leaving the renal tubules as urine has a much different composition than does the glomerular filtrate entering them via Bowman's capsule membrane. The substances that remain in the renal tubules, like urea and uric acid, tend to become more and more concentrated as water is reabsorbed from the filtrate. Fluid absorption from the renal tubules is enhanced by the permeable wall and low pressure of the surrounding capillaries.

Reabsorption of most substances, including glucose and water, occurs in the **proximal convoluted tubule.** All of the glucose in the filtrate is reabsorbed in most people. Water reabsorption depends on the rate of absorption of sodium ions—as sodium reabsorption increases or decreases, so does the absorption of water. Almost all of the sodium in the glomerular filtrate is eventually reabsorbed. (See Table 8.1.)

When the blood concentration of a substance rises, it may reach its **renal plasma threshold,** or spillover point, the concentration above which the substance is not reabsorbed and remains in the urine for excretion. The renal threshold for a substance like glucose varies from person to person.

The reabsorption of water from the tubule is regulated by antidiuretic hormone, ADH, which is produced by the hypothalamus. ADH inhibits the loss of water when there is danger of dehydration. It does this by increasing the permeability of the tubule and collecting duct, causing rapid reabsorption of water.

◆◆ Tubular Secretion

Some substances are secreted from the tubule into the urine, bypassing glomerular filtration. Penicillin and histamine, for example, are secreted into the proximal convoluted portion of the tubule, and hydrogen ions are secreted into both the proximal and **distal** segments.

TABLE 8.1	Composition of Glomerular Filtrate and Urine	
	Glomerular Filtrate	**Urine**
Glucose concentration	100 mg/100 mL (or dL)	0
Urea concentration	26 mg/100 mL (or dL)	1820 mg/100 mL (or dL)
Uric acid concentration	4 mg/100 mL (or dL)	53 mg/100 mL (or dL)

VOLUME AND COMPOSITION OF URINE

Typical urine output for the average adult is 50 to 60 mL per hour or about 1,200 to 1,500 mL per day. The exact amount depends on many factors, including fluid intake, environmental temperature, relative humidity of the surrounding air, respiratory rate, body temperature, and emotional state. An output of less than 30 mL per hour may indicate kidney failure.

The composition of urine varies considerably from time to time in the same individual because of changes in dietary intake and level of physical activity. In addition to being approximately 95 percent water, urine usually contains urea from the breakdown of amino acids and uric acid from the breakdown of nucleic acids. Urine also contains a variety of electrolytes, such as sodium, potassium, chloride, and bicarbonates. The concentration of electrolytes tends to vary directly with their concentration in the diet.

URINALYSIS

Urine may be analyzed for its physical, chemical, or microscopic properties. When all three types of analysis are made, this is referred to as complete, or routine, urinalysis (UA). On the other hand, only a few specific parameters of urine may be analyzed, such as the urine-glucose level, which is measured in routine testing for diabetes and in monitoring diabetic patients. Urinalysis is performed for three general reasons:

- Screening of large groups of people for unsuspected disorders, such as when testing urine-glucose levels in diabetes screening.

- Diagnosis of suspected disease in individual patients, such as when looking for the presence of bacteria in a suspected urinary tract infection.

- Monitoring the course of treatment to assess its effectiveness, such as when checking the effect of an antibiotic on the bacteria count in a urinary tract infection or of a particular dosage or type of insulin on the glucose level in diabetes.

Urinalysis as a Diagnostic Tool

Diagnosis of disease is the main purpose of urinalysis in POLs. Urine may be abnormal because the kidneys are malfunctioning, or it may reflect problems in metabolism affecting other organs. Urinalysis in POLs can be used to detect kidney disease and many endocrine and metabolic disorders.

Detecting Kidney Disease. Patients with diseased kidneys may have abnormal urine because substances normally filtered out of the urine by the kidneys may appear in the urine or substances normally in the urine may not be present. In either case, urinalysis may be an important diagnostic tool. Protein in the urine, for example, may be indicative of glomerulonephritis.

Detecting Changes in Endocrine and Metabolic Function. Patients with endocrine or metabolic diseases, such as diabetes mellitus, may produce abnormal amounts of metabolic products such as ketones. These metabolic products often are excreted in the urine, where they may be detected through urinalysis. Abnormally high levels of glucose in the urine, especially in a fasting patient, is a positive clinical sign of diabetes mellitus.

Historical Note

The use of urine to diagnose disease dates back thousands of years. In 400 B.C., Hippocrates discovered that changes in the color and odor of urine often occur in patients with elevated temperatures. By the Middle Ages, the significance of urine in detecting disease was so widely recognized that the urine flask came to be an accepted symbol for physicians.

In 1827, an English physician named Richard Bright described the relationship between proteinuria, protein in the urine, and kidney disease. He made urine testing a regular part of medical examinations. By the middle of the nineteenth century, medical textbooks recommended that urinalysis be performed for every patient.

In the early part of this century, the American physician Thomas Addis advanced the diagnostic use of urine when he discovered the diagnostic value of examining **urinary sediments,** substances found in standing urine. In 1920, Addis developed a method for the quantitative analysis of urinary sediments, which we now call the **Addis count.**

PROCEDURE

8.1 ◆ Urine Formation and Excretion

Goal

- After successfully completing this procedure, you will be able to demonstrate the path of urine formation and excretion and explain how urine is formed.

Completion Time

- 60 minutes

Equipment and Supplies

- paper and pencil

Instructions

Read through the list of equipment and supplies that you will need and the steps of the procedure. Be sure that you understand each step before you begin. Then complete each step correctly and in the proper order. If your completion time is too long, repeat the procedure until you increase your speed. Do this procedure with a partner or the rest of the class.

S = Satisfactory	U = Unsatisfactory	S	U
1. Collect the needed equipment and supplies.			
2. Review the description of urine formation in the text while tracing the route of urine formation and excretion in Figures 8.1, 8.2, and 8.3.			
3. In your own words, write a brief description of how urine is formed and make a simple, well-labeled drawing showing the path of urine formation and excretion.			

4. Use your drawing to demonstrate the path of urine formation and excretion to your partner or the rest of the class, while you explain the formation in your own words.

5. Clarify any questions raised or errors noted by your partner or the class.

OVERALL PROCEDURAL EVALUATION

Student's Name _____

Signature of Instructor _____ **Date** _____

Comments

Using Terminology

Label the indicated parts in the following drawings.

1.

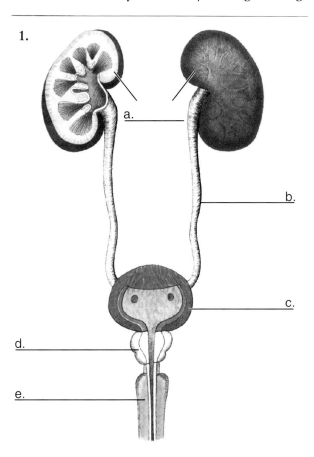

a.

b.

c.

d.

e.

2.

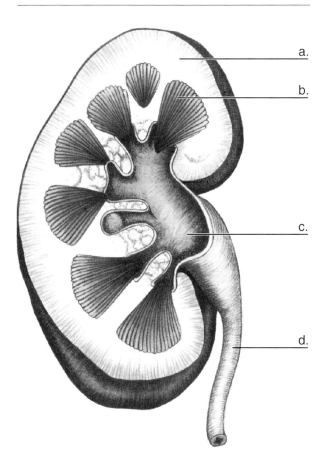

a.

b.

c.

d.

3.

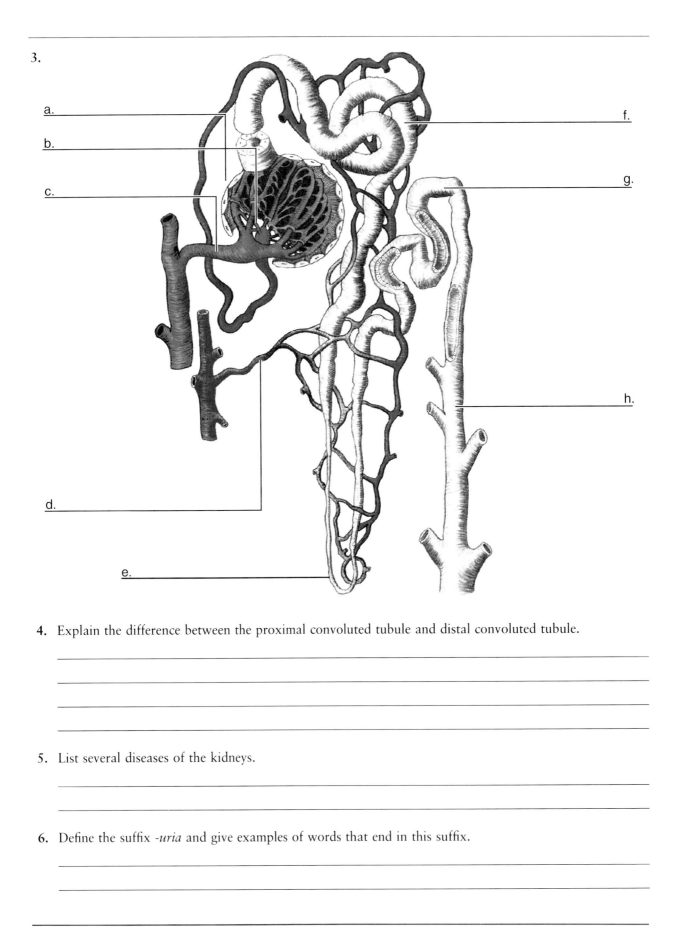

a. _____

b. _____

c. _____

d. _____

e. _____

f. _____

g. _____

h. _____

4. Explain the difference between the proximal convoluted tubule and distal convoluted tubule.

_____

_____

_____

_____

5. List several diseases of the kidneys.

_____

_____

6. Define the suffix *-uria* and give examples of words that end in this suffix.

_____

_____

7. What terms describe the passing of urine from the body?

_____

_____

8. What electrolytes are regulated by the kidneys?

_____

_____

Match the term or suffix in the right column with the appropriate definition in the left column.

_____ 9. closer

_____ 10. equilibrium

_____ 11. farther

_____ 12. inflammation

_____ 13. kidney

_____ 14. kidney stone

_____ 15. metabolic abnormality

_____ 16. study

_____ 17. urination

a. diabetes insipidus
b. distal
c. -itis
d. calculus
e. homeostasis
f. micturition
g. nephro-
h. -ology
i. proximal

Acquiring Knowledge

Answer the following questions in the spaces provided.

18. List three reasons for performing a urinalysis.

_____

_____

_____

19. Give two diagnostic purposes for urinalysis.

_____

_____

20. Who was the first physician to make urinalysis a routine part of the medical exam?

_____

21. What three types of tests are included in a complete urinalysis?

_____

_____

_____

22. How do blood vessels, nerves, and the ureter enter the kidney?

_____

_____

23. How does urine go from the kidney to the ureter?

_____

_____

24. How does blood enter and leave the glomerulus?

_____

_____

25. What are the two main parts of nephrons?

_____

_____

26. What are the primary functions of nephrons?

_____

_____

27. What roles do the nephrons play in the formation of urine?

_____

_____

_____

28. How is blood pressure related to filtration by nephrons?

_____

_____

29. Describe glomerulonephritis.

_____

_____

30. What is proteinuria?

_____

_____

31. What term denotes the presence of glucose in the urine?

_____

32. Explain the cause of diabetes insipidus.

_____

_____

33. What is the source of urea in urine?

_____

_____

34. What volume of urine output per hour is considered normal?

_____

35. Name three electrolytes found in urine.

_____

36. Who are more prone to bladder infections, men or women? Why?

_____

_____

_____

37. What is homeostasis?

_____

_____

38. What factors influence the volume of urine?

_____

_____

_____

_____

39. What is the renal plasma threshold?

_____

_____

_____

40. Describe renal failure.

_____

_____

_____

41. Rearrange the following list of urinary tract structures to show the path of urine from the blood to micturition: loop of Henle, proximal convoluted tubule, collecting duct, collecting tubule, distal convoluted tubule, urethra, ureter, urinary bladder, renal pelvis, calyx.

_____

_____

_____

_____

Applying Knowledge—On the Job

Answer the following questions in the spaces provided.

42. Why does a patient with diabetes insipidus not have to take insulin or watch his or her diet? Can you describe the urine specimen?

_____

_____

_____

43. Mrs. Kinsey just called with regard to her new prescription. The doctor said that she had a bladder infection but the pharmacist mentioned cystitis. Now, Mrs. Kinsey is worried that she either has the wrong medication or she has a cyst instead of a bladder infection. How would you straighten out this mix-up?

_____

_____

_____

_____

44. A patient has a reading of 4+ urine glucose on the test strip. The normal reading is negative. What metabolic disorder might you suspect? Why is the glucose present in the urine?

_____

_____

_____

_____

_____

45. A patient's urine has a high level of protein. What might this finding indicate?

_____

_____

9

Collection and Preservation of the Urine Specimen

COGNITIVE OBJECTIVES

After studying this chapter, you should be able to

- use each of the vocabulary terms appropriately.
- describe several different types of urine specimens and identify their diagnostic uses.
- describe the different methods of urine collection and explain why they are used.
- discuss what must be communicated to patients to assure that urine specimens are collected correctly.
- explain the role of refrigeration and preservatives in accurate urinalysis.
- list the labeling requirements for urine specimens.

PERFORMANCE OBJECTIVES

After studying this chapter, you should be able to

- give instructions and necessary supplies to patients for collection of different types of urine specimens.
- receive a urine specimen from a patient, disinfect the container, label it correctly, and refrigerate it appropriately.

TERMINOLOGY

catheterization, urinary: the process of inserting a tube through the urethra into the urinary bladder to obtain a urine specimen.

clean-catch specimen: a urine specimen collected midstream after thoroughly cleaning the surrounding area to prevent contamination of the specimen; used when urine is to be cultured.

double-voided specimens: two specimens collected within a specified time interval, usually thirty minutes, to compare the concentration of particular substances.

eight-hour specimen: also called overnight, early morning, or first morning specimen; a urine specimen collected as soon as the patient arises in the morning, consisting of urine that has collected in the bladder during the night.

glucose-tolerance test (GTT): a test of the ability to metabolize glucose, in which the patient is tested for blood and urine glucose at short intervals after consuming a known quantity of glucose in solution.

midstream urine specimen: a specimen collected after voiding the first urine in order to reduce contamination with bacteria and debris from the urethra and perineum.

perineum: the outside area of the body immediately surrounding the rectum and urethra.

postprandial specimen: an after-meal specimen; used most often to test for the presence of glucose in urine.

random specimen: a urine specimen that is taken at any time of day or night, usually during a visit to the physician's office.

timed specimens: urine specimens collected at timed intervals to diagnose diabetes or to assess the rate of renal clearance.

twenty-four hour specimen: the total urine output of a patient for a twenty-four hour period; usually collected by the patient at home and often used for quantitative analysis.

two-hour specimen: the total urine output of a patient for a two-hour period.

urinary casts: microscopic solid molds formed from protein precipitates in the renal tubules and voided in the urine.

urobilinogen: a colorless derivative of bilirubin; formed by the action of intestinal bacteria.

• • • • • • • • • • • • • • • • • • • •

The care that goes into collecting, handling, and preserving a urine specimen is the first stage of ensuring the accuracy of urinalysis. No degree of accuracy in performing subsequent tests on the urine in the lab can compensate for errors made in the process of getting the sample from the patient to the lab. Urine must be collected at the correct time, in the right way, into an appropriate container, and then labeled and preserved correctly. Only then is the analysis of the urine in the lab likely to be based on a reliable, representative specimen.

TYPES OF URINE SPECIMENS

Several different types of urine specimens are routinely collected in POLs. Random specimens are the easiest and most frequently done. Other types of specimens, such as the postprandial and double voided, are more difficult to obtain but must be performed for particular lab tests.

◆◆ *Random Specimens*

Random specimens are so named because they are collected randomly in terms of time. They may be collected at any time of the day or night. They are convenient to collect in the physician's office restroom and require only a few simple instructions to the patient. Random specimens are useful for qualitative assessment of chemical and microscopic properties of urine, but they are not useful for quantitative assessments.

◆◆ *Eight-Hour Specimens*

Also called overnight, early morning, or first morning specimens, **eight-hour specimens** are samples collected at the first urination upon arising in the morning. The concentration of urine varies during a twenty-four hour period, depending on fluid intake and activity level. Urine concentration is usually greatest in the first urination of the day, after the urine has collected undisturbed in the bladder throughout the night when there has been little, if any, fluid intake. Concentrations of bacteria in the urine also tend to be greatest at this time.

Eight-hour specimens are best for nitrite and protein tests as well as for microscopic examination of the urine. The only drawback is that particles like red and white blood cells may decompose after standing in urine throughout the night, especially if the pH of the urine is high or the specific gravity is low.

◆◆ *Timed Specimens*

Timed specimens are urine samples collected at specific intervals. Timed specimens often are collected to diagnose diabetes. They are also used in renal clearance tests, which are performed to diagnose and evaluate kidney function.

Two-Hour Postprandial Specimens. Postprandial specimens, or after-meal specimens, often are collected to assess glucose metabolism. The patient is instructed to eat a meal high in carbohydrates. Two hours later, the urine specimen is collected. Later, it is analyzed for the presence of glucose.

Specimens for Glucose-Tolerance Tests. The glucose-tolerance test (GTT) uses blood and urine levels of glucose to diagnose diabetes mellitus. The first urine specimen is collected after the patient has fasted. Then, the patient is given a known quantity of glucose in solution to drink, and urine specimens are collected one-half hour, one hour, and two hours later. Sometimes, additional samples are collected after two hours if the patient is slow to metabolize the glucose. Blood samples are taken at the same time as the urine samples.

Double-Voided Specimens. For double-voided specimens, two specimens are collected within a specified time interval, usually thirty minutes, to compare the concentration of particular substances, such as glucose. Blood samples are collected at the same time.

◆◆ *Volume Specimens*

Volume specimens are cumulative samples collected over a specified time interval—most often two or twenty-four hours. The entire volume of urine voided during the time interval is collected in one container and preserved for analysis at the end of the interval.

Two-Hour Volume Specimens. For two-hour specimens, urine is collected from the patient over a two-hour period. This type of specimen usually is used to assess the level of **urobilinogen** in the urine.

Twenty-Four Hour Volume Specimens. For **twenty-four hour specimens,** urine is collected over a twenty-four hour interval. The large volume of urine can be used for quantitative analysis of the urine, which is usually performed in a reference lab, not the POL.

A twenty-four hour specimen should be collected in the following manner:

- Empty the bladder on arising in the morning. Do not save this sample but note the exact time at which urination occurred.

- Collect all urine samples throughout the next twenty-four hours and add each to the same collection container, taking care to avoid spills or contaminating the inside of the container. Refrigerate the collection container, keep it on ice, or use a chemical preservative.

- At exactly the same time as the first day, empty the bladder completely and add this sample to the collection container.

COLLECTING THE SAMPLE

The first step in patient testing in POLs is preparation of the patient to collect the specimen.

✦✦ *The Patient's Role*

Collecting the urine specimen is usually up to the patient, who must be provided with the instructions and materials necessary to follow the collection procedure precisely. Patients who may need special assistance are the very weak, the extremely ill, the elderly, or very young children. Some patients may require urinary **catheterization,** which involves placing a tube called a catheter through the urethra into the bladder to obtain a urine specimen.

Midstream Specimens. To reduce the risk of contamination from the urethra or **perineum,** all urine specimens should be **midstream specimens.** The patient starts voiding directly into the toilet. Then, he or she should collect about half a cup or 20 mL from the middle portion of the urination into the container. The remaining portion of the urination should go into the toilet.

Clean-Catch Specimens. Clean-catch specimens are collected only after a strict cleansing procedure has been followed by the patient. This greatly minimizes the chance that the specimen will be contaminated with extraneous organisms during the collection procedure. They are required for cultures to prevent extraneous organisms from proliferating in the culture medium and making the results meaningless.

Collecting clean-catch specimens requires careful patient instructions in procedure, so it is virtually always done in the POL, not at home. Posting illus-

---

✦ ✦ ✦ Collecting Clean-Catch Specimens ✦ ✦ ✦

For males:

- Wash and dry your hands before starting.
- If uncircumcised, retract your foreskin with a towelette.
- Clean the urethral opening three times, using a fresh towelette each time in a single wipe toward the glans.
- Start urinating into toilet with the foreskin still retracted.
- Collect a midstream specimen of about 20 mL in the collection container. Do not touch the inside of the container or its lid!
- Void the rest of the urine into the toilet.
- Cap the container and take it to the lab.

For females:

- Wash and dry your hands before starting.
- Sit on the toilet seat with your legs spread apart as far as comfortable.
- If you are menstruating or have a heavy vaginal discharge, such as from a yeast infection, first insert a clean tampon.
- Spread the outer labia with your left hand (right hand if you are left handed).
- Clean both inner labia and the urethral opening, using a fresh towelette each time to wipe from front to back in a single stroke.
- Start urinating into toilet with the outer labia still spread.
- Collect a midstream specimen of about 20 mL in the collection container. Do not touch the inside of the container or its lid!
- Void the rest of the urine into the toilet.
- Cap the container and take it to the lab.

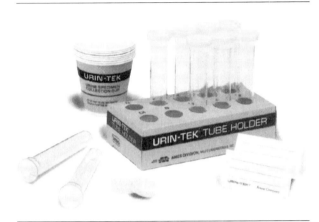

Figure 9.1. The Urin-Tek System consists of a disposable collection system that includes paper collection cups, 15 mL centrifuge tubes with snap lids, and self-adhesive identification labels. Courtesy of Miles, Inc., Diagnostics Division.

trated instructions in the POL patient bathroom is a good idea. The patient should be provided with an adequate supply of sterile towelettes saturated with cleansing solution and a sterile collection container. When the container arrives in the lab, the outside should be wiped with disinfectant before it is labeled.

❖❖ *Specimen Collection Supplies*

The preferred urine-specimen container is a paper or plastic disposable cup with a capacity of 50 to 100 mL and an opening at least 5 cm. wide. Specimen containers must always be scrupulously clean and completely dry, but they need not be sterile unless the specimen will be cultured.

Urine collection systems are available to help assure quality control in urine collection, including Urin-Tek (Miles, Inc., Diagnostics Division; see Figure 9.1) and KOVA System (ICL Scientific). The collection systems consist of a flat-bottomed paper collection cup, a nonsterile 15 mL plastic tube with a plastic cap, a self-adhesive identification label, and a disposable tube holder. The patient is instructed to void into the paper cup and then to transfer the specimen to the tube and put on the cap to avoid contamination and spillage. The patient labels the tube, reducing the risk of mislabeling in the lab. Testing can be performed directly in the tube, including centrifuging for urine sediment analysis, thereby decreasing handling and potential contamination and spillage.

Pediatric collection systems are available to collect urine specimens from infants and young children. The disposable collection apparatus consists of a plastic bag with an adhesive backing around the opening. This is attached to the child so that the urine goes directly into the bag. (See Figure 9.2.)

❖ ❖

LABELING AND PRESERVING THE SPECIMEN

It is important that the urine specimen be labeled and preserved to prevent spoilage.

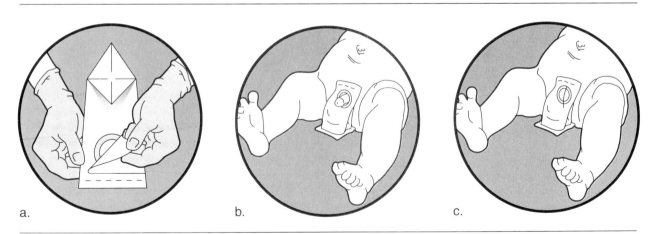

a.   b.   c.

Figure 9.2. a. A pediatric collection unit consists of a clear plastic bag with adhesive for attaching to the child. b. A male collection unit. c. A female collection unit.

❖❖ Labeling

The label should be attached to the container, not the lid, which may become separated from the specimen. The label should include:

- the patient's name
- the patient's identification number—usually the chart number
- the name of physician requesting the test
- the date of specimen collection
- the time of specimen collection

❖❖ Preserving

A fresh urine sample should be used when a routine urinalysis is performed. If the specimen cannot be analyzed within one hour of collection, it should be refrigerated at a temperature of 4 to 6 degrees Celsius. Before being analyzed, the refrigerated specimen should be returned to room temperature and mixed thoroughly. Although refrigeration is the preferred method of preservation, chemical preservatives may be used when a specimen cannot be refrigerated, such as when a patient transports a specimen from home to the POL or when the specimen is sent by mail to a reference laboratory.

Without proper preservation, decomposition and deterioration will occur. The following may characterize urine that has "gone bad":

- Glucose and ketones are reduced by bacterial consumption.
- Urea is converted to ammonia, making the urine alkaline.
- If the urine is alkaline or has low specific gravity, **urinary casts** (microscopic molds of tubules) and red blood cells decompose.
- Bilirubin is reduced due to light sensitivity.
- Urobilinogen is converted to urobilin, causing the urine to darken.
- Nitrite is produced by bacteria.
- The urine has a foul odor.

♦♦♦ Note ♦♦♦

Never discard a patient's urine sample until after the doctor sees the patient and the patient's urinalysis report. If the doctor decides that a urine culture should be done, you may have thrown out the only specimen that the patient can provide. Sometimes, physicians decide that they want a culture on a urine you might have thought was unremarkable. A second sample can be especially difficult to obtain from the pediatric patient.

❖❖ Drug Screen Urine Collections

The Drug Testing Custody and Control Form is the legal external chain of custody document used by the Department of Transportation (DOT) and industry (NON-DOT). The form identifies the urine sample and who has handled the sample from the time of collection until it is analyzed and released by the laboratory. Each company has specific forms and collection kits. These are typical collection procedure steps.

1. Verify identification. Ask for a photo I.D. (e.g., driver's license) to properly identify the donor. If a photo I.D. is not available, an agent of the company may make a positive identification. Document on the form, "I.D. made by _____." Be sure to also examine proper I.D. of the agent. If the donor's identification cannot be established, *discontinue the collection procedure.*

2. Enter the donor's social security number and any other information requested at the top of the form.

3. Secure the rest room. (Check the rest room for specimens that might have been left, that dye is present in the toilet bowl, and that faucets have been taped off with security tape.)

4. Have the donor remove outer clothing, such as a coat, sweater, or hat. These items, along with purses or parcels, are to remain outside the actual collection facility.

5. When the donor comes out of the rest room, check the time, to make certain the temperature check is done within the required four minutes. Temperature of the specimen must be between 90.5 and 99.0 degrees. If the temperature is out of range, another specimen should be collected. If any difficulty occurs in collecting a new sample, the client/employer should be contacted for further instruction regarding what course of action to take.

6. The collector is now in receipt of the sample. Continue to fill out the custody form according to instructions on the form. Have the donor sign in the appropriate section.

7. Secure the specimen in a bag and the shipping container. Be sure to include the paperwork for the testing lab. Mail copies of the paperwork to the Medical Review Officer (MRO) and the employer. Log the specimen in the Drug Screen Log and call a courier for pickup.

PROCEDURE

9.1

Collecting a Clean-Catch Specimen: Instructing the Patient

Goal

- After successfully completing this procedure, you will be able to instruct a patient in the correct procedure for collecting a clean-catch urine specimen.

Completion Time

- 10 minutes

Equipment and Supplies

- impermeable jacket, gown, or apron
- disposable latex gloves
- hand disinfectant
- surface disinfectant
- paper towels and tissues
- biohazard container
- premoistened towelettes
- tampon
- disposable, clean graduated urine containers with lids
- labels and pens

Instructions

Read through the list of equipment and supplies that you will need and the steps of the procedure. Be sure that you understand each step before you begin. Then complete each step correctly and in the proper order. If your completion time is too long, repeat the procedure until you increase your speed. For this procedure, you must work with a partner. One of you will assume the patient role, and the other will assume the role of lab technician. After working through the procedure, switch roles, and repeat the procedure.

	S	U
1. Put on a protective jacket, gown, or apron; wash your hands with disinfectant, dry them, and put on gloves.		
2. Follow the Universal Precautions.		
3. Collect and prepare the appropriate equipment.		
4. Verify identification of the patient and direct the patient to the toilet facility.		
5. Using the instructions below, explain the collection procedure to the patient. If a chart illustrating the procedure is available, use it to clarify your explanation. Ask the patient if he or she has any questions.		
6. If the patient is a male, explain the collection procedure as follows:		
a. Wash and dry your hands before starting.		
b. If uncircumcised, retract your foreskin with a towelette.		
c. Clean the urethral opening three times, using a fresh towelette each time in a single wipe toward the glans.		
d. Start urinating into the toilet with your foreskin still retracted.		
e. Collect a midstream specimen of about 20 mL in the collection container. Do not touch the inside of the container or its lid.		
f. Void the rest of the urine into the toilet.		
g. Cap the container and take it to the lab.		
7. If the patient is a female, explain the collection procedure as follows:		
a. Wash and dry your hands before starting.		

b. Sit on the toilet seat with your legs spread apart as far as comfortable.

c. If you are menstruating or have a heavy vaginal discharge, such as from a yeast infection, first insert a clean tampon.

d. Spread the outer labia with your left hand (right hand if you are left handed).

e. Clean both inner labia and the urethral opening, using a fresh towelette each time to wipe from front to back in a single stroke.

f. Start urinating into the toilet with the outer labia still spread.

g. Collect a midstream specimen of about 20 mL in the collection container. Do not touch the inside of the container or its lid.

h. Void the rest of the urine into the toilet.

i. Cap the container and take it to the lab.

8. Receive the urine specimen from the patient and tell the patient to return to the examination room.

9. Wipe the outside of the container with a tissue soaked in disinfectant and place the container on the counter.

10. Fill in the label with the patient's name, the patient's chart number, the physician's name, the date, and the time of day.

11. Attach the label to the urine container, not the lid.

12. Store the urine specimen in the refrigerator.

13. Discard disposable equipment.

S = Satisfactory	U = Unsatisfactory	S	U

14. Disinfect other equipment and return it to storage.

15. Clean the work area following the Universal Precautions.

16. Remove your jacket, gown, or apron, and gloves; wash your hands with disinfectant, and dry them.

OVERALL PROCEDURAL EVALUATION

Student's Name _____

Signature of Instructor _____ **Date** _____

Comments

CHAPTER 9 REVIEW

Using Terminology

Supply the identifying term in the space provided.

1. A urine specimen that is always collected at the clinic, never at home:

   _____

2. The process of collecting urine by inserting a tube through the urethra into the bladder:

   _____

3. The urine specimen collected as soon as the patient first arises in the morning:

   _____

4. The urine specimen from the middle part of a single urination:

   _____

5. The urine specimen taken after meals to check for glucose:

   _____

6. The urine specimen collected as needed at any time of day or night:

   _____

7. The area of the body immediately surrounding the rectum and urethra:

   _____

8. Microscopic solid molds formed from protein in the renal tubules:

   _____

9. The amount of liquid, such as water and juices, drunk by a patient:

   _____

10. The specimen collected at home by the patient over a twenty-four hour period:

    _____

11. The test that assesses the ability of the patient to metabolize glucose:

    _____

12. The urine test that requires a sterile container:

    _____

13. The disease characterized by glucose and ketones in the urine:

    _____

14. The container used to collect urine specimens from infants and young children:

    _____

15. The urine specimen that must be either refrigerated or chemically preserved from the beginning:

    _____

Acquiring Knowledge

Answer the following questions in the spaces provided.

16. At what temperature should urinalysis be performed? What should be done with refrigerated specimens?

    _____

    _____

    _____

17. How is the glucose-tolerance test used to diagnose diabetes mellitus?

    _____

    _____

    _____

18. Why is an eight-hour urine specimen best for microscopic examination and for tests of nitrite and protein? What do these tests reveal?

_____

_____

_____

19. Why are elaborate instructions given to patients for a midstream, clean-catch specimen?

_____

_____

_____

20. How soon must fresh urine be used for urinalysis without refrigeration or chemical preservation? Why?

_____

_____

_____

21. Why is a twenty-four hour urine specimen used for quantitative tests?

_____

_____

_____

22. Why is a postprandial urine specimen used for a urine-glucose test?

_____

_____

23. Describe the preferred urine-collection container.

_____

_____

24. How is urine collected from infants?

_____

_____

25. Describe how a urine container should be labeled.

_____

_____

_____

26. Why are random specimens called random? What are their advantages?

_____

_____

_____

27. Why is the middle part of a urination best for urinalysis?

_____

_____

_____

28. What special precautions should menstruating females take when collecting a urine specimen? Why?

_____

_____

_____

29. Describe a midstream, clean-catch urine specimen.

_____

_____

_____

30. Why does urine concentration vary during a twenty-four hour period?

_____

_____

31. When collecting a midstream, clean-catch sample, how should the patient handle the container?

_____

_____

32. What precautions are taken with the urine container to protect laboratory workers against disease?

_____

_____

33. Why are double-voided urine specimens collected?

_____

_____

34. When is a two-hour postprandial urine specimen collected?

_____

35. What happens to glucose, ketones, and urea in long-standing urine?

_____

36. Why should urine specimens be protected from light?

_____

_____

Applying Knowledge—On the Job

Answer the following questions in the spaces provided.

37. A twenty-month-old toddler is in the doctor's office and needs a random urine specimen. How will you collect it?

_____

_____

_____

_____

38. A female patient is referred to the laboratory for a midstream, clean-catch urine specimen. What instructions should you give the patient to ensure that the urine specimen is not contaminated?

_____

_____

_____

_____

39. Two patients with urinalysis requisition slips come to the lab where you work. A sample is collected from each and the patients leave the office. When you go to do the urinalyses, you realize that the samples are unidentified, so you don't know which sample belongs to which patient. What should you do? What are some changes that should be made in the urine-collection procedure in the lab?

_____

_____

_____

_____

40. A patient is referred to the laboratory for a two-hour postprandial urine specimen. What instructions should you give to the patient?

_____

_____

_____

_____

41. An eight-hour urine specimen collected at home is handed to you by a patient's relative. What should you do?

_____

_____

_____

_____

42. A very elderly woman comes to the laboratory with a urinalysis request. What should you do?

_____

_____

_____

43. A twenty-four hour urine specimen has been ordered for a patient. He has come to the laboratory for instructions. What instructions should you give the patient?

_____

_____

44. In the POL, when should you discard a patient's urine sample?

_____

_____

10 Physical Properties of the Urinalysis

COGNITIVE OBJECTIVES

After studying this chapter, you should be able to

- use each of the vocabulary terms appropriately.
- list the physical properties of urine.
- describe the abnormal colors of urine and explain their clinical significance.
- identify the different causes of turbidity in urine.
- identify the factors affecting the volume of urine.
- define specific gravity and explain its relationship to urine concentration.
- list and describe three methods used to measure specific gravity of urine.

PERFORMANCE OBJECTIVES

After studying this chapter, you should be able to

- measure specific gravity using a urinometer, a refractometer, and a reagent strip.
- calibrate a urinometer and a refractometer.

TERMINOLOGY

anuria: the complete absence of urine excretion.

bilirubin: a product of the breakdown of red blood cells. A high serum level of bilirubin may result in excretion through the kidneys, in addition to the usual route of excretion through the intestines.

dehydration: the loss of body water in excess of intake, resulting in a net deficiency of water in the tissues. Dehydration is caused by either decreased intake or increased loss of water

and may be due to excessive vomiting, diarrhea, sweating, or uncontrolled diabetes.

diuretic: an agent that increases the production of urine.

foam test: a test to detect the presence of bilirubin in urine that appears yellow-orange.

hematuria: the presence of erythrocytes (red blood cells) in urine. Hematuria is a serious clinical finding that may be caused by several different diseases.

hypersthenuria: the production of urine with high specific gravity. Hypersthenuria may be caused by several different diseases.

hyposthenuria: the production of urine with low specific gravity. Hyposthenuria may be caused by several different diseases.

isosthenuria: the production of urine with consistently low specific gravity regardless of fluid intake. Isosthenuria is a sign of marked impairment of renal function.

lipiduria: the presence of fat in urine.

maple-syrup urine disease: a very rare inborn error of metabolism that is fatal if not treated. The urine of patients with this disorder has a maple-syrup odor.

oliguria: the excretion of less than 400 mL of urine in twenty-four hours in adults. Oliguria is a life-threatening condition requiring immediate correction.

opalescence: the milky appearance in urine due to bacteria or lipids.

phenylketonuria (PKU): an inborn error of protein metabolism that results in mental retardation if not treated. The urine of patients with PKU often has a distinctive mousy odor.

polyuria: the excretion of excessive amounts of nearly colorless urine. Polyuria is confirmed by a twenty-four hour urine volume greater than 2,000 mL.

Pseudomonas: a genus of gram-negative, rod-shaped bacteria with many species. It is widespread and often causes opportunistic infections in humans.

refractometer: an instrument for measuring the refractive index, which is the ratio of the velocity of light in air to the velocity of light in a solution such as urine.

specific gravity (SG) of urine: the density of urine relative to the density of distilled water. The concentration of dissolved substances gives urine greater specific gravity because these substances give urine greater weight.

turbidity: cloudiness in a solution due to suspended particles, which scatter light and produce the cloudy appearance.

urinometer: an instrument for measuring specific gravity of urine. Graduations on the cylindrical stem of a weighted rod are read while the urinometer is floating in a column of urine.

urochrome: the yellow pigment that causes the characteristic yellow color of urine.

• • • • • • • • • • • • • • • • • • • •

A routine urinalysis examines the chemical, microscopic, and physical properties of urine. Physical properties include appearance (color and turbidity), odor, volume, and specific gravity. This chapter describes each of these physical properties of urine. Later chapters describe the chemical and microscopic properties of urine.

— — — — — — — — — — ◆ ◆

THE APPEARANCE OF URINE

The appearance of urine depends on its color and its **turbidity,** or cloudiness.

◆◆ *Color*

A freshly voided normal urine specimen may range in color from pale yellow to amber, depending on its concentration. The yellow color comes from the pigment **urochrome,** which is more concentrated with increased metabolism. Patients with fever, starvation, or goiter (hyperthyroidism) have more urochrome and thus, darker urine. Other factors that may affect the color of urine include food pigments and dyes, some medications, and blood contamination of the specimen. Several pathological conditions also affect urine color, so any unusual urine color should be noted in the patient's chart. Table 10.1 lists abnormal urine colors and some of their causes.

◆ ◆ ◆ **Detecting Bilirubin** ◆ ◆ ◆
in the Urine

A **foam test** is sometimes performed to determine if **bilirubin** is present in a urine specimen that appears yellow-orange. The procedure is as follows:

- Place a small volume of urine in a test tube. Cap the tube and shake it vigorously.

- If the foam on the top is white, bilirubin is absent. If the foam is orange, bilirubin is present. (*Note:* urinary analgesics, like phenazopyridine, also cause orange foam.)

◆◆ *Turbidity*

A freshly voided normal urine specimen is clear to slightly hazy. A turbid, or cloudy, urine specimen may be due to a number of nonpathological causes or to disease.

Turbidity in Healthy Urine. Healthy urine specimens may appear cloudy due to sediment that precipitates when urine drops below body temperature. Acid urines may have a white or pink haze due to urate precipitates. They can be cleared by warming the urine to 60 degrees Celsius. Alkaline urines precipitate phosphates and carbonates. They can be cleared by adding dilute acetic acid. Both acidic and alkaline urines may collect precipitates as the urine stands in the patient's bladder. Sperm and prostatic fluid may cause turbidity in specimens from males. This turbidity will not clear when the sample is acidified or heated.

Turbidity Due to Disease. Cloudy, or turbid, urine samples that are pathologically significant are caused most often by white blood cells, red blood cells, or bacteria.

TABLE 10.1 Abnormal Urine Colors and Their Causes

Color	Possible Causes Pathological	Possible Causes Nonpathological
Red or reddish brown	Hemoglobin Red blood cells Myoglobin Porphyrins	Beets, rhubarb Senna (cathartic) drugs and dyes Menstrual blood
Orange	Bile pigments	Drugs (e.g., pyridium and phenothiazine)
Yellow-orange or yellow-brown	Dehydration or fever Bilirubin Urobilin	Carrots Riboflavin Nitrofurantoin (urinary antibiotic)
Green	Biliverdin (from oxidation of bilirubin) Bacteria (especially *Pseudomonas*)	Vitamin preparations Psychoactive drugs Proprietary diuretics
Blue or blue-green	None	Proprietary diuretics Methylene (urinary germicide)
Black or brownish black	Melanin Urobilin Methemoglobins	Iron complexes Levodopa (Anti-Parkinson drug)

Leukocytes (white blood cells) may form a white cloud similar to that caused by phosphates, but it will not disappear when dilute acetic acid is added to the sample. Leukocytes, may be detected microscopically. **Hematuria,** or the presence of erythrocytes (red blood cells) in urine, may give the sample a pink or red appearance. Red blood cells in the specimen may give a "smokey" appearance. Red blood cells also may be detected microscopically.

Large numbers of bacteria may appear in the urine specimens of patients with urinary tract infections. The presence of the bacteria themselves may cause a uniform **opalescence,** or milky appearance, that is not cleared when the sample is acidified. It also remains after filtration through paper. Increased alkalinity of the urine and high phosphate concentrations also contribute to cloudiness of urine when bacteria are present.

Fat globules also cause urine to appear opalescent. The presence of fat in urine is called **lipiduria.** It may be caused by degenerative nephron tubular disease.

THE ODOR OF URINE

Normal, freshly voided urine has a faint characteristic odor due to the presence of volatile acids. The odor is more marked in concentrated urine. Certain foods, such as asparagus, may produce a harmless, but characteristic, odor in the urine.

The odor of urine usually is not considered to be of special diagnostic significance. Nonetheless, urine with an abnormal smell should be investigated more closely. Several pathological states are characterized by urine with a marked odor. Some are very distinctive.

Bacteria in urine cause an odor of ammonia because they split urea. Patients with **phenylketonuria (PKU)** produce urine with a distinctive mousy odor. Patients with **maple-syrup urine disease** produce urine that smells like maple syrup. The urine of patients with diabetes may have a sweet or fruity odor due to the presence of ketones. Malnutrition, vomiting, and diarrhea can also produce urine that smells sweet.

VOLUME OF URINE

The volume of urine produced in the healthy patient is determined by several factors, including:

- water intake
- diet, especially salt and protein intake
- drugs
- ambient temperature, humidity, and activity level, which influence the rate of sweating

---

◆◆◆ The Role of Drugs ◆◆◆ in Urine Volume

The volume of urine is increased with drugs that exert a **diuretic** effect, including:

- caffeine
- alcohol
- thiazides
- oral hypoglycemic agents

The volume of urine is decreased with drugs that cause nephrotoxicity, including:

- analgesics (e.g., salicylates)
- antimicrobial agents (e.g., neomycin, streptomycin, and penicillin).

Urinary output also varies with age and sex, as shown in Table 10.2, but average adult volume is 1500 mL/day.

Urinary output may be affected by disease, so the measurement of urine volume during a timed interval, such as twenty-four hours, may be a valuable diagnostic aid. Diseases like diabetes mellitus, diabetes insipidus, and chronic renal disorders are characterized by **polyuria,** or the excretion of excessive amounts of urine. Polyuria is confirmed by a twenty-four hour urine volume greater than 2,000 mL. **Oliguria,** which is the excretion of less than 400 mL of urine in twenty-four hours, may result from **dehydration,** shock, edema, or acute kidney disease. **Anuria,** or the complete absence of urine excretion, may be due to acute renal failure, acute glomerulonephritis, or urinary tract obstruction.

SPECIFIC GRAVITY

Specific gravity is the density of a substance relative to the density of distilled water. Assessing the **specific gravity (SG) of urine** is part of routine urinalysis. It is usually calculated as:

$$SG = \frac{\text{Weight/Volume of urine}}{\text{Weight/Volume of water}}$$

In addition to water, urine contains minerals, salts, and organic compounds, which give it a density greater than that of distilled water and a specific gravity greater than 1.000. The specific gravity of

---

TABLE 10.2 Age and Sex Variation in Urine Volume Ranges

Age Group/Sex		Normal Volume
Newborn:	1–2 days	30–60 mL/day
Infant:	3–10 days	100–300 mL/day
	60–365 days	400–500 mL/day
Child:	1–3 years	500–600 mL/day
	8–14 years	800–1,400 mL/day
Middle-aged adult:		
	Female	600–1,600 mL/day
	Male	800–1,800 mL/day
Elderly adult		250–2,400 mL/day

normal urine ranges between 1.005 and 1.030, with most samples falling between 1.010 and 1.025. The specific gravity of urine varies throughout the day. It is generally highest (greater than 1.020) in the first morning specimen.

❖❖ Causes of Abnormal Specific Gravity

Specific gravity of urine may be either abnormally low or abnormally high.

Low Specific Gravity. Production of urine with low specific gravity (**hyposthenuria**) characterizes patients with diabetes insipidus, in whom antidiuretic hormone (ADH) is lacking. Patients with glomerulonephritis and pyelonephritis also may have urine with low specific gravity because of tubular damage. The production of urine with a consistent low specific gravity (1.010), varying little from specimen to specimen regardless of fluid intake, is known as **isosthenuria.** It is a sign of marked impairment of renal function, occurring in patients with chronic renal disorders, whose kidneys are unable to concentrate or dilute urine. This urine has the same specific gravity as plasma filtrate.

High Specific Gravity. Production of urine with high specific gravity (**hypersthenuria**) occurs with diabetes mellitus, adrenal insufficiency, hepatic disease, and congestive cardiac failure. Patients who are dehydrated due to sweating, fever, vomiting, or diarrhea also may have urine with high specific gravity.

❖❖ Measuring Specific Gravity

The specific gravity of urine may be determined using a urinometer, refractometer, or reagent test strip.

The Urinometer. The **urinometer** is an instrument for measuring the specific gravity of urine. It consists of a weighted, bulb-shaped instrument with a cylindrical stem containing a scale of specific graduations (see Figure 10.1). The urinometer floats in the cylinder, which contains the urine. The depth to which the urinometer sinks in the urine indicates the specific gravity of the sample, which is read on the scale at the meniscus.

The urinometer, an adapted hydrometer, is calibrated to read 1.000 in distilled water at a specific temperature (usually 16 degrees Celsius), which is indicated on the instrument. At different temperatures, the specific gravity will vary slightly. In very

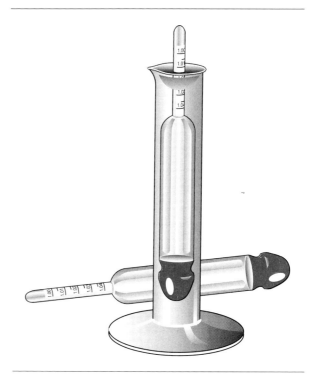

Figure 10.1. A urinometer measures the specific gravity of urine. Remember to read the lowest part of the meniscus at eye level.

precise work, a temperature correction may be required, but most often, urine at room temperature can be used. Refrigerated urine always should be allowed to come to room temperature before the specific-gravity reading is made with the urinometer. A change in specific gravity of ± 0.001 occurs for each 3 degrees Celsius change above (minus) or below (plus) the 16 degrees Celsius temperature.

The urinometer should be checked frequently to test the reliability of the instrument by placing it in distilled water, in which it should read 1.000. Another check is to use a solution of known specific gravity to test the urinometer. When 20.29 grams of potassium sulfate are dissolved in 1 liter of distilled water, the solution should have an SG of 1.015.

The Refractometer. The **refractometer** measures the refractive index, which is the ratio of the velocity of light in air to the velocity of light in a solution such as urine. The ratio varies directly with the concentration of dissolved particles in the solution because the light beam that enters the instrument is bent and slowed by the solutes in the specimen. This value is read on a scale, which is viewed through the ocular of the refractometer. It is important to read the scale of the instrument with the refractometer held toward a

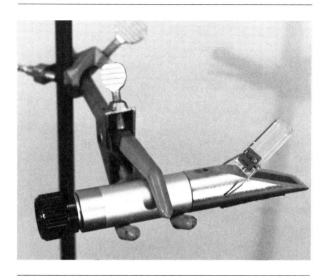

Figure 10.2. A refractometer is used for determining the specific gravity of urine. The window is open for cleaning. Photo by Mark Palko.

light source. The refractometer is accurate with samples in the temperature range of 16 to 38 degrees Celsius (see Figure 10.2).

The refractometer should be calibrated daily using distilled water and using the set screw to adjust the scale to read 1.000. The refractive index varies with but is not identical to the specific gravity of a urine sample, the refractive index usually being lower by about 0.002.

The Reagent Strip. The disposable colorimetric reagent strip that measures specific gravity of urine can be used at the same time as other routine urinalysis tests. No special equipment is required.

Urines with a high specific gravity have high ion concentrations, and urines with low specific gravity have low ion concentrations. Changes in ion concentration affect pH, causing a color change in the reagent strip. This color change is compared to color blocks on the reagent vial to measure specific gravity. The color of the reagent strip ranges from blue (SG = 1.000) to blue-green to yellow (SG = 1.030).

The chemical nature of the reagent-strip test may produce results that differ slightly from those of other methods when elevated amounts of protein and glucose are present. Highly buffered alkaline urines also may show low readings relative to other methods. A urine quality-control solution, discussed in Chapter 13, may be used to check the accuracy of the reagent strip.

Measuring the Specific Gravity of Urine

Goal

- After successfully completing this procedure, you will be able to measure specific gravity with a urinometer and a refractometer and to calibrate both instruments.

Completion Time

- 20 minutes

Equipment and Supplies

- impermeable jacket, gown, or apron
- disposable latex gloves
- hand disinfectant
- surface disinfectant
- paper towels and tissues
- biohazard container
- urine specimen
- distilled water
- urinometer and glass cylinder
- refractometer
- glass rod
- dropping pipette
- urine report form and pen

Instructions

Read through the list of equipment and supplies that you will need and the steps of the procedure. Be sure that you understand each step before you begin. Then complete each step correctly and in the proper order. If your completion time is too long, repeat the procedure until you increase your speed.

◆◆ *Part 1: Calibrating and Using a Urinometer*

S = Satisfactory	U =Unsatisfactory	S	U

1. Put on a protective jacket, gown, or apron; wash your hands with disinfectant, dry them, and put on gloves.

2. Follow the Universal Precautions.

3. Collect and prepare the appropriate equipment.

4. Verify identification of the specimen and label the container.

5. Place the clean glass cylinder on a level surface and fill it two-thirds full with distilled water at room temperature. Use enough water to float the urinometer without overflowing the cylinder.

6. Insert the urinometer into the distilled water and twirl it gently, so that the urinometer is centered and upright while floating freely.

7. If the urinometer reads 1.000, no correction factor is needed. If the urinometer does not read 1.000, the amount by which it reads over or under 1.000 is the correction factor.

8. Empty and dry the glass cylinder.

9. Allow the urine to come to room temperature.

10. Mix the urine specimen in the container by stirring it with a clean glass rod.

11. Place the clean glass cylinder on a level surface and fill it two-thirds full with urine.

12. Place the urinometer in the urine. If there is too little urine to float it, record QNS (quantity not sufficient) on the lab form.

13. Twirl the urinometer so that it remains centered and upright in the urine.

	S	U

14. Read the specific gravity at the bottom of the meniscus while viewing it from eye level.

15. Repeat steps 12–14 to obtain a second reading as a quality-control measure.

16. Record both results on the lab form.

17. Flush the urine sample down the toilet.

18. Discard disposable equipment.

19. Disinfect other equipment and return it to storage.

20. Clean the work area following the Universal Precautions.

21. Remove your jacket, gown, or apron, and gloves; wash your hands with disinfectant, and dry them.

❖❖ Part 2: Calibrating and Using a Refractometer

S = Satisfactory   U = Unsatisfactory

	S	U

1. Put on a protective jacket, gown, or apron; wash your hands with disinfectant, dry them, and put on gloves.

2. Follow the Universal Precautions.

3. Collect and prepare the appropriate equipment.

4. Verify identification of the specimen and label the container.

5. Read the refractometer manufacturer's instructions.

6. With a pipette, place a drop of distilled water on the exposed area of the refractometer prism (glass plate) and close the coverplate gently.

7. Hold the refractometer toward a light source.

8. Look through the ocular and rotate the eyepiece until the scale comes into view. Read the specific gravity at the point on the scale where the dark area meets the light area.

9. If the urinometer reads 1.000, no correction is needed. If the urinometer does not read 1.000, adjust the refractometer with a screwdriver until you obtain a reading of 1.000.

10. Wipe the prism clean with a tissue.

11. Allow the urine to come to room temperature.

12. Mix the urine specimen in the container by stirring it with a clean glass rod.

13. With a pipette, place a drop of urine on the exposed area of the prism and close the coverplate gently.

14. Hold the refractometer toward a light source.

15. Look through the ocular and rotate the eyepiece until the scale comes into view. Read the specific gravity at the point on the scale where the dark area meets the light area.

16. Record the results on the lab form.

17. Flush the urine sample down the toilet.

18. Discard disposable equipment.

19. Clean the prism with a tissue soaked in disinfectant and wipe the rest of the refractometer with disinfectant.

20. Disinfect other equipment and return all equipment to storage.

21. Clean the work area following the Universal Precautions.

22. Remove your jacket, gown, or apron, and gloves; wash your hands with disinfectant, and dry them.

OVERALL PROCEDURAL EVALUATION

Student's Name _____

Signature of Instructor _____ _____ Date _____

Comments

CHAPTER 10 REVIEW

Using Terminology

Match the term on the right with the most appropriate description on the left.

_____ 1. urine with mousy odor

_____ 2. urine with reddish color

_____ 3. urine with bluish color

_____ 4. yellow foam that persists

_____ 5. opalescence persisting with acid

_____ 6. urine with fruity odor

_____ 7. specific gravity of 1.035

a. urine bacteria

b. medication

c. diabetes mellitus

d. hematuria

e. concentrated urine

f. PKU

g. urinary bilirubin

For each of the following questions, provide the correct term in the space provided.

8. What term describes the presence of erythrocytes (red blood cells) in urine?

_____

9. What is another term for "milky" urine?

_____

10. What term refers to the complete absence of urine excretion?

_____

11. What term refers to the excretion of excessive amounts of nearly colorless urine?

_____

12. What term designates urine secretion of less than 400 mL in twenty-four hours?

_____

13. What term refers to the density of a liquid relative to the density of distilled water?

_____

14. What condition results when the body loses more water than it takes in?

_____

15. What end product of protein metabolism is secreted into the urine?

_____

16. What instrument measures specific gravity by floating in urine?

_____

17. What term describes urine with suspended matter in it?

_____

18. Name the curved surface read in a specific gravity test at the top of the urine in a cylinder. It is caused by the attraction of the liquid molecules to the wall of the container.

_____

Acquiring Knowledge

Answer the following questions in the spaces provided.

19. What properties of urine are examined in a routine urinalysis?

_____

_____

_____

20. Name five physical properties of urine.

_____

_____

_____

_____

_____

21. What visible clue may indicate that urine is concentrated?

_____

22. List two factors that may cause an orange color in urine.

_____

_____

23. List two factors that may cause a black color in urine.

_____

_____

24. What does a positive yellow foam test indicate?

_____

25. What disease may cause a sweet or fruity odor in urine?

_____

26. What odor in urine may be caused by a urinary infection?

_____

27. Name two congenital metabolic disorders that have characteristic urine odors.

_____

_____

28. List three drugs or food substances that are diuretics.

_____

_____

_____

29. Name two substances in urine that influence specific gravity.

_____

_____

30. What does a very low specific gravity that is consistent indicate?

_____

_____

31. What are some causes of high specific gravity of urine?

_____

_____

_____

_____

32. List three ways of measuring the specific gravity of urine and state how each works.

_____

_____

_____

_____

33. What is the range of specific gravity of normal urine?

_____

34. What specific gravity reading is obtained with distilled water?

_____

Applying Knowledge—On the Job

Answer the following questions in the spaces provided.

35. Assume that you are employed in a clinical laboratory and that one of your duties is performing urinalyses. The urine specimens submitted for testing have a variety of appearances. Some are clear, others are cloudy, and there are variations in color. Some also have distinctive odors. Why is it important to make note of these physical characteristics of urine?

_____

_____

_____

_____

36. A patient has just handed you a urine specimen with an intense orange-gold color. Yellow foam floats on top. What might be the cause of the abnormal appearance of the urine?

_____

_____

_____

_____

_____

37. This morning's work load includes a urine specimen of particular interest. It appears to have chalk suspended in it. What might cause this unusual appearance?

_____

_____

_____

_____

38. Among the urine specimens this morning is one with a pungent odor of ammonia. Why is it important that you call this to the physician's attention?

_____

_____

_____

_____

_____

39. Assume that you perform the urinalyses in the POL where you work. What quality control will you employ to ensure that your specific gravity readings are accurate?

_____

_____

_____

_____

_____

CHAPTER 11

Chemical Properties of the Urinalysis

COGNITIVE OBJECTIVES

After studying this chapter, you should be able to

- use each of the vocabulary terms appropriately.
- explain the general methodology of reagent-strip tests.
- describe the quality-control methods applicable to strip-test methods.
- list the reagent-strip tests usually performed in routine urinalysis and identify the pathological conditions that each can detect.
- distinguish between screening and confirmatory tests in diagnosis and describe when it is appropriate to use each type of test.
- identify the confirmatory tests commonly used to follow up reagent-strip tests for reducing sugars, ketones, protein, and bilirubin.

PERFORMANCE OBJECTIVES

After studying this chapter, you should be able to

- use reagent strips to assess the pH of a urine sample.
- evaluate a urine specimen for glucose using a reagent-strip test.
- assess urine for ketones, protein, or blood using appropriate reagent-strip test methods.
- use an ICTOTEST to confirm the bilirubin concentration in a urine specimen.
- perform a CLINITEST analysis of a urine sample to assess the presence of reducing sugars.

TERMINOLOGY

acidemia: abnormally low blood pH. The blood is more acidic than normal.

alkalemia: abnormally high blood pH. The blood is more alkaline than normal.

ascorbic acid: vitamin C.

bacteriuria: the presence of bacteria in the urine.

Bence Jones protein: an abnormal protein found in patients with multiple myeloma and other conditions. The reagent-strip test for urinary protein is not sensitive to it.

bilirubinemia: a high level of bilirubin in the blood.

bilirubinuria: the presence of bilirubin in the urine.

confirmatory test: a more precise and specific test used to confirm the results of a reagent-strip test.

galactose: a simple sugar formed from the breakdown of lactose (milk sugar).

galactosemia: the presence of galactose in the blood. Galactosemia is the condition in which galactose is not converted to glucose due to a lack of the enzyme galactase.

hemoglobinuria: the presence of hemoglobin in the urine.

jaundice: yellowing of the eyes and skin caused by excess bilirubin in the blood.

ketoacidosis: an acid condition of the body caused by excretion of ketones with basic ions in the urine.

ketone: an intermediary product of fat metabolism.

ketonuria: the presence of ketones in the urine.

lyse: to break down a formed substance, such as red blood cells.

myoglobinuria: the presence of myoglobin in the urine.

occult blood: blood that cannot be detected with the naked eye. It must be detected by chemical or microscopic analysis.

pyuria: the presence of white blood cells in the urine.

reagent-strip test: also called dry reagent test; a quick and easy way to assess urine pH and abnormal urine constituents. It uses a test strip impregnated with reagents.

reduction test: also called Benedict's test. It tests for simple sugars, such as lactose, galactose, fructose, and pentose, in the urine, not just for glucose.

renal tubular acidosis: a condition in which the renal tubules are unable to excrete hydrogen ions that increase body acidity.

reticuloendothelial cell: cell of the spleen or bone marrow in which hemoglobin from lysed red blood cells is degraded to bilirubin.

urobilinogenuria: excess urobilinogen in the urine.

• • • • • • • • • • • • • • • • •

The diagnostic information provided by chemical analysis of urine is the reason that urinalysis is the most common laboratory test performed in POLs. Urinalysis is also one of the easiest and quickest due to **reagent-strip tests.**

—————————————————— ◆ ◆

REAGENT-STRIP TESTS

The most widely used technology in POLs for performing chemical analysis of urine is the reagent-strip test. Reagent strips are popular because they are convenient, easy, disposable, and available for a variety of chemical tests, including urinary pH, glucose, ketone, protein, and blood, among others. Two types of reagent strips commonly used are Multistix from Miles, Inc., Diagnostic Division and CHEMSTRIP from Boehringer Mannheim Corporation. Some examples of reagent-strip tests are shown in Figure 11.1.

The test-strip results are qualitative in that color change indicates presence or absence of the analyte—as well as semiquantitative in that degree of

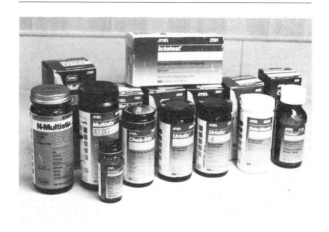

Figure 11.1. Many reagent systems for individual tests are available as convenient test strips and tablets. Reagent strips should be enclosed in the airtight, dark container supplied by the manufacturer and kept away from heat, fumes, light, and moisture.

color change indicates approximate concentration of the analyte. Test strips are used most often for initial, noninvasive screening of large numbers of patients for health problems, such as diabetes and kidney disease. Those who test positive on the reagent-strip test are followed up with **confirmatory tests,** which are more precise and specific diagnostic tools.

◆◆ *Materials and Procedure*

The reagent strip consists of a firm plastic strip to which a pad or pads are attached. Each pad contains chemical reactants for a specific analyte, such as glucose or protein. The color reaction produced on the pad is compared to a color chart provided by the

> ◆ ◆ ◆ **Using Test** ◆ ◆ ◆
> **Strips Safely**
>
> Test-strip technology advances lab safety because it requires only minute amounts of reagents. However, urine, like all biological specimens, is potentially hazardous. Urine specimens should be kept covered in their containers as much as possible. Carefully discard contaminated testing equipment and emptied, used specimen containers into the biohazardous waste container.

manufacturer. The color chart usually is placed on the label of the test-strip container. Many reagent-strip tests must be accurately timed for valid test results. The read time varies from thirty seconds to two minutes. The recommended read time for each test is printed on the manufacturer's instruction sheet inserted in the package. The general test-strip procedure is illustrated in Figure 11.2.

Reacted test strips also can be interpreted by instruments. Some labs have semiautomated bench-top analyzers that read test strips and print out the results. The saturated test strip is placed on a feed-load table and drawn into the instrument for reading. The specimen identification number and appearance can be entered and printed out along with the results of the chemical analysis. Analyzers are described in more detail in Chapter 13.

◆◆ *Quality Control*

Quality control in urinalysis begins with proper sample collection and storage. Fresh urine specimens should be tested within one hour, refrigerated specimens should be tested within eight hours. Refrigerated specimens should be brought to room temperature before testing.

Known controls should be tested each day with the reagent strips. Controls may be purchased from commercial sources. Proficiency testing using unknown positive and negative urines also may be used. The results should be recorded in the quality-control manual.

◆◆ *Storage*

Always consult the manufacturer's instructions on the package insert for proper storage of reagent strips. Generally, the test strips should be stored at room temperature in tightly closed containers that protect them from heat, light, fumes, and moisture. Care must be taken to protect the test strips from other laboratory chemicals. Even detergents may react with the strips if they are placed nearby.

◆◆◆ **Note** ◆◆◆

Always check the expiration date on reagent strips before use. If test strips change color before use, you should discard them, regardless of expiration date.

◆◆

CHEMICAL URINALYSIS

Routine urinalysis always measures pH as well as the presence of several chemicals, including glucose, ketone, protein, bilirubin, urobilinogen, and blood.

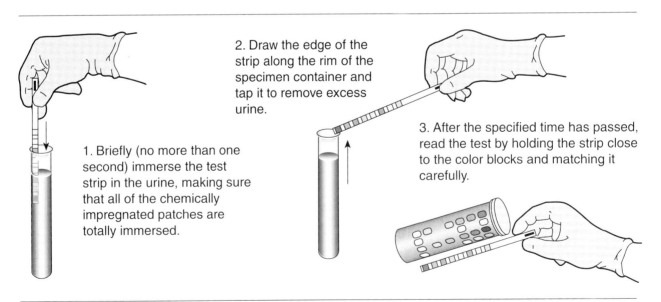

2. Draw the edge of the strip along the rim of the specimen container and tap it to remove excess urine.

1. Briefly (no more than one second) immerse the test strip in the urine, making sure that all of the chemically impregnated patches are totally immersed.

3. After the specified time has passed, read the test by holding the strip close to the color blocks and matching it carefully.

Figure 11.2. The test-strip procedure is easy. Follow the manufacturer's instructions; they will be in the format of this dip-and-read test.

Many POLs also routinely measure leukocytes and nitrite to detect bacteria in the urine. With the exception of urobilinogen, normal urines should test negative for all of these chemicals. A positive test result indicates possible pathology. Test data provide the physician with information on the patient's carbohydrate metabolism, kidney and liver function, infections of the urinary tract, and acid-base balance.

♦ ♦ ♦ Medical Terms ♦ ♦ ♦

The following terms describe abnormal urines:

- **bacteriuria:** the presence of bacteria in the urine
- **bilirubinuria:** the presence of bilirubin in the urine
- *glucosuria:* the presence of glucose in the urine
- *hematuria:* the presence of red blood cells in the urine
- **hemoglobinuria:** the presence of hemoglobin in the urine
- **ketonuria:** the presence of ketones in the urine
- *proteinuria:* the presence of proteins in the urine
- **urobilinogenuria:** excess urobilinogen in the urine

♦♦ Urinary pH

A solution's pH, or concentration of hydrogen ions, can range from 0 to 14. See Figure 11.3. A pH reading of 7 is neutral; a reading above 7 is alkaline (basic); below 7 is acidic. The lower the reading, the more acidic; the higher the reading, the more alkaline.

Acid-Base Balance. The pH of the blood and other body tissues is referred to as the body's acid–base balance. Blood pH varies between 7.35 and 7.45 in normal individuals. This balance is regulated by the kidneys and lungs, which excrete the waste products of body metabolism. The lungs excrete volatile wastes, predominantly carbon dioxide, and the kidneys excrete nonvolatile acid wastes, like uric acid. The kidneys help regulate blood pH by selectively secreting less acid when the blood is too alkaline (basic), **alkalemia,** or more acid when the blood is too acidic, **acidemia.**

Factors Affecting Urinary pH. Normal adult urine tends to be slightly acidic, at an average pH of 6.0. The normal adult range is from 4.5 to 8.0 pH. The following factors may decrease blood pH and result in urine that is more acidic:

- a high protein diet
- uncontrolled diabetes mellitus
- respiratory diseases involving carbon dioxide retention

The following factors may increase blood pH and result in urine that is more alkaline:

- diets high in vegetables, citrus fruits, or dairy products
- urinary tract infections
- bacterial contamination of the specimen
- respiratory diseases involving hyperventilation and loss of carbon dioxide
- sodium bicarbonate and potassium citrate, which are often used in conjunction with antibiotics in treating urinary tract infections

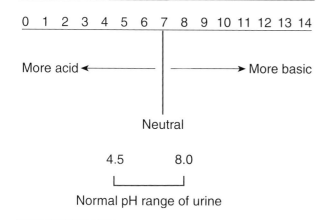

Figure 11.3. The pH scale.

♦ ♦ ♦ Renal Tubular ♦ ♦ ♦ Acidosis

Patients with **renal tubular acidosis** tend to have a neutral urine pH regardless of their body's acid level. Their renal tubules are unable to excrete hydrogen ions that increase systemic acidity.

Measuring Urinary pH. The test strip for measuring urinary pH gives colors in the range from orange through yellow and green to blue. This covers the entire urinary pH range. Protein buffers from adjacent pads on the strip should not be allowed to run over on the pH pad and alter its pH indicators.

Glucose

Healthy individuals will have a negative urine glucose test if their blood glucose levels are 110 mg/dL or less. However, if blood-glucose concentration rises as high as 180 mg/dL, which is the renal threshold for glucose, the reabsorption capacity of the renal tubules is surpassed and glucose spills over into the urine. This condition may be benign due to emotional stress or ingestion of a large meal or pathological due to diabetes mellitus.

Diabetes Mellitus. Patients with diabetes mellitus have elevated blood glucose because they are unable to produce or use insulin, the pancreatic hormone that is needed to transport glucose across cell membranes. Measuring blood and urine glucose is important for screening and monitoring these patients.

Testing for Glucose. The glucose test strip is specific for glucose. No other substance normally excreted in urine is known to give a positive result with this test. A negative result is normal. Even other sugars, including lactose, galactose, and fructose, do not give a positive result with the glucose test. However, the test may have reduced sensitivity, tending to produce false negatives, if the urine has a high specific gravity or contains a large quantity of **ascorbic acid.**

When glucose in urine reacts with the reagent on the test strip, it changes the color of the strip. The exact color change depends on the manufacturer. The Ames Reagent Strip color ranges from green to brown when glucose is present; for CHEMSTRIP, the color ranges from yellow to green.

Ketones

Glucose is the energy source usually utilized by the cells. However, when the patient's diet is inadequate in carbohydrates or the patient has a defect in carbohydrate metabolism or absorption, fat is used as the primary energy source. This results in incomplete metabolism of fatty acids and accumulation of intermediary products of fat metabolism, called **ketones.** Ketones include acetoacetic acid, acetone, and betahydroxybutyric acid.

Ketones appear in the urine before they increase significantly in the blood. When they are excreted in the urine, the condition is called ketonuria. Patients with ketonuria always excrete ketone bodies in the same proportions—20 percent acetoacetic acid, 2 percent acetone, and 78 percent betahydroxybutyric acid. Because ketones are excreted in combination with basic ions (Na, K, and Ca), ketonuria produces **ketoacidosis,** an acid condition of the body. Patients with ketoacidosis frequently have a fruity odor to their breath because acetone is highly volatile and is blown off in small amounts with air that is expelled from the lungs.

Causes of Ketonuria. The most important pathological condition that may produce ketonuria is diabetes mellitus. Ketonuria in a diabetic patient indicates the need for a change in insulin dosage or other aspect of treatment. Other conditions that may cause ketonuria include anorexia, starvation, vomiting, diarrhea, and fever.

Testing for Ketones. The ketone test strip, which is based on a nitroprusside reaction, checks for the presence of acetoacetic acid, one of the three ketone bodies. The reaction occurs in the presence of a basic buffer. A positive result is indicated by a color change from buff through lavender to maroon.

Proteins

Normally, only small amounts of protein are excreted each day in the urine, ranging up to 150 mg/day or 20 mg/dL, because most of the protein filtered out of the blood into the kidneys is reabsorbed in the tubules of the nephrons. Urine specimens normally test negative for protein. In several pathological conditions of the kidney, however, protein is detectable in the urine at relatively high concentrations, a condition called proteinuria. The degree of proteinuria is classified according to the amount of protein excreted per day.

The detection of protein in the urine is one of the most important indicators of renal disease in which there is glomerular or tubular damage. Usually, albu-

---

♦ ♦ ♦ Bence Jones Protein ♦ ♦ ♦

Another type of protein that can produce proteinuria is **Bence Jones protein,** a globulin observed in the urine of over 50 percent of patients with multiple myeloma. It is also found in the urine of patients with macroglobulinemia and malignant lymphomas. Bence Jones protein is not sensitive to the reagent-strip test for protein, which predominantly screens for albumin. It must be detected using a precipitation test or a coagulation test.

---

min is lost in greatest amounts in renal disease, making up 60 to 90 percent of protein excreted. Albumin normally makes up only about one-third of urinary protein. Other types of protein in normal urine are globulins and Tamm-Horsfall protein.

Testing for Protein. When the protein test-strip indicator, tetrabromphenol blue, is buffered at pH 3, it is yellow. If protein is added to the test-strip indicator, it changes to green and then blue, according to the concentration of protein. If no protein is present in the urine, the indicator remains yellow. The reagent area is more sensitive to albumin than to globulins or other proteins.

◆◆ *Blood*

A normal urine sample should not have any detectable blood even when the most sensitive tests are used. When urine contains blood, it may appear pink or red, but more often, blood is present in such minute quantities that it can be detected only by microscopic or chemical means. This blood, which cannot be seen by the naked eye, is called **occult blood.** Three different ways to detect blood in the urine are (1) chemically (by means of reagent strips), (2) visually (by observing the specimen), and (3) microscopically (by examining the urine under magnification).

Blood in urine may be in the form of intact red blood cells, which is referred to as hematuria. Blood may be in the form of free hemoglobin from **lysed** red blood cells that are also present, which is called hemoglobinuria. Finally, a positive test for occult blood may be detected in urine in which no red blood cells are present. This usually means that there is myoglobin in the urine. This is called **myoglobinuria.** Myoglobin is a hemoglobin-like molecule that stores oxygen in muscle tissue.

Causes of Blood in Urine. Detection of blood in urine indicates damage or disease of the kidney or urinary tract and, often, bleeding in the urinary tract. In infectious diseases like yellow fever, smallpox, and malaria, hemoglobin from lysed red blood cells is present in the urine, producing hemoglobinuria. Hemoglobinuria also occurs with renal disorders, kidney stones, and severe infections of the urinary tract. Myoglobinuria is usually a result of traumatic muscle injury. The only nonpathological reason for blood in urine is menstrual blood contamination, which can be ruled out if proper specimen-collection procedures are followed.

Testing for Blood. The reagent-strip test for blood is based on the oxidizing activity of hemoglobin, which produces spots of color change if the blood consists of intact red blood cells and a uniform color change in the presence of free hemoglobin or myoglobin. The test can detect 5 to 20 intact red blood cells per microliter or 0.015 to 0.060 mg/dL of free hemoglobin. A positive test strip for blood should be followed up with a microscopic examination of urine sediment.

◆◆ *Bilirubin*

Bilirubin is a yellow-orange bile-pigmented compound formed when red blood cells are lysed or ruptured.

The Formation and Excretion of Bilirubin. Figure 11.4 shows the process by which bilirubin normally is formed and excreted. Bilirubin forms when red blood cells reach the end of their life span, which averages 120 days. When old red cells lyse, hemoglobin is degraded to bilirubin in the **reticuloendothelial**

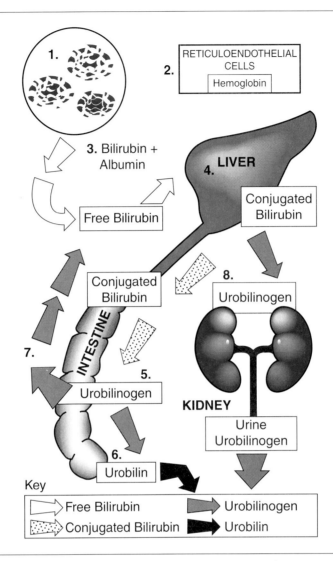

Figure 11.4. Normal bile pigment metabolism. 1. Red blood cells disintegrate from age or disease and release hemoglobin. 2. Hemoglobin enters the reticuloendothial cells of the spleen and bone marrow where it is degraded to bilirubin. 3. Bilirubin enters the circulatory system and binds with albumin to form free bilirubin (not soluble). 4. Free bilirubin enters the liver and forms conjugated bilirubin (soluble) which enters the intestine by way of the bile duct. 5. Conjugated bilirubin is converted to urobilinogen by bacterial action in the intestine. 6. Some of the urobilinogen is oxidized to the brown pigment urobilin and is excreted in the feces. 7. Much of the urobilinogen in the intestine is reabsorbed into the blood. 8. A small amount of the reabsorbed urobilinogen in the blood is filtered by the kidneys. A small amount of urine urobilinogen is normal.

cells of the spleen and bone marrow. The bilirubin then binds to albumin in the blood and is transported to the liver. This form of bilirubin, called free bilirubin, is not water soluble, so it cannot be excreted in the urine.

In the liver, Kupffer cells change free bilirubin to conjugated bilirubin, a soluble form. This is excreted into the small intestine through the bile duct and converted by bacterial action to urobilinogen, a colorless compound. Some of the urobilinogen thus formed is oxidized to brown-pigmented urobilin and excreted in the feces, where it gives color to fecal material. However, up to 50 percent of the urobilinogen formed in the intestine is reabsorbed into the blood, and a small amount of the reabsorbed urobilinogen is excreted in the urine.

When conjugated bilirubin levels are abnormally high, the conjugated bilirubin reenters the blood from the liver and a high level of bilirubin in the blood results. This condition is called **bilirubinemia.**

Excess bilirubin in the blood causes yellowing of the eyes and skin, a condition referred to as **jaundice.**

There are two types of jaundice—hemolytic and obstructive. Hemolytic jaundice is due to excess destruction of red blood cells, which may occur in several forms of anemia, infectious hepatitis, and malaria. Obstructive jaundice occurs when the liver fails to excrete bile or the bile ducts are obstructed.

Testing for Bilirubin. If blood levels of bilirubin are high, excess amounts will be excreted in the urine. Bilirubin in the urine is called *bilirubinuria*. Bilirubin in the urine can be detected only if the specimen is fresh because bilirubin decomposes rapidly in bright light. If the urine is allowed to stand, the bilirubin will be converted to biliverdin, a green compound not detected by the bilirubin reagent-strip test. The bilirubin strip test is based on the reaction of bilirubin with a diazonium salt in a strongly acid medium. This produces a color change that is proportional to the concentration of bilirubin in the sample. Normally, the amount of bilirubin in the urine is too small to be detected.

◆◆ Urobilinogen

As described, urobilinogen is a bile pigment formed directly from bilirubin by bacterial action in the intestine. Much of the urobilinogen is reabsorbed into the circulating blood, and some is filtered by the kidneys into the urine. Therefore, urine specimens normally test positive for urobilinogen.

Because urinary urobilinogen is higher whenever there is an increase in the production of bilirubin, knowing the concentration of both bile pigments, bilirubin and urobilinogen, may be more useful for diagnosis than knowing one alone. Table 11.1 gives urinary bilirubin and urobilinogen concentrations for healthy individuals and for patients with pathological liver conditions.

Testing for Urobilinogen. The test for urobilinogen on the reagent strip involves the Ehrlich aldehyde reaction, which forms a red azo dye. The test must be performed using fresh urine because urobilinogen is unstable and breaks down to urobilin on standing. The test detects urobilinogen in concentrations of at least 0.1 mg/dL. The normal urobilinogen range obtained with this method is 0.2 to 1.0 mg/dL. A concentration of 2.0 mg/dL represents the transition from normal to abnormal, indicating that the patient needs further evaluation or that the test result should be confirmed with a follow-up test.

◆◆ Nitrite

Nitrite in the urine is significant because it is an indicator of bacteriuria, or bacteria in the urine. Most of the common pathogens that cause bacteriuria (see Table 11.2) produce reductase enzymes, which reduce nitrate, from the diet, to nitrite while the urine is held in the bladder (see Figure 11.5). For the reduction reaction to occur, the bacteria must be

TABLE 11.1   Correlation of Urobilinogen and Bilirubin Tests

	In Health	In Hemolytic Disease	In Hepatic Disease	In Biliary Obstruction
Urine Urobilinogen	Normal	Increased	Increased	Low or Absent
Urine Bilirubin	Negative	Negative	Positive or Negative	Positive

Courtesy of Miles, Inc., Diagnostics Div.

TABLE 11.2 Common Causes of Bacteriuria	
Type of Pathogen	**Percent of All Urinary Tract Infections**
E. coli	72%
Klebsiella/Enterobacter	16%
Proteus	5%
Staphylococcus	5%
Pseudomonas	1%
Streptococcus faecalis*	1%

*Does not reduce nitrate to nitrite.

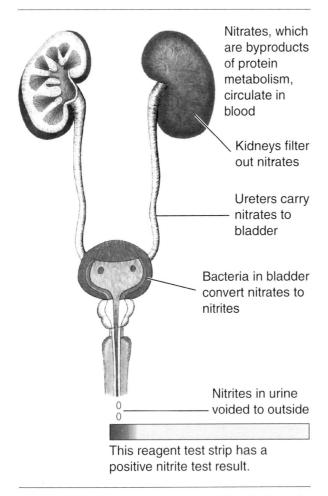

Nitrates, which are byproducts of protein metabolism, circulate in blood

Kidneys filter out nitrates

Ureters carry nitrates to bladder

Bacteria in bladder convert nitrates to nitrites

Nitrites in urine voided to outside

This reagent test strip has a positive nitrite test result.

Figure 11.5. Confirmation of bacterial infection is made using a nitrite test strip. The test is based on the ability of bacteria in the bladder to convert nitrate to nitrite.

held in the bladder for a minimum of four hours. First morning specimens are therefore the best samples to test. The urine has been held in the bladder for many hours and the number of bacteria is relatively great.

Testing for Nitrite. The nitrite test is based on the conversion of nitrate to nitrite by the action of gram-negative bacteria in the urine. The nitrite will react with the acid pH of the reagent pad to produce a pink color. A negative nitrite result does not completely rule out bacteriuria, however. The pathogen may be one that does not reduce nitrate or there may be too few organisms present to produce nitrite at a detectable level. A positive nitrite test result should be confirmed by microscopic findings of bacteria and leukocytes. Some POLs also perform cultures and smears with Gram stain.

◆◆ *Leukocytes*

The presence of significant numbers of white blood cells in the urine (**pyuria**) usually indicates bacteriuria. It is associated with lesions of the urethra, ureters, bladder, and kidneys, and with urinary tract infections.

Testing for Leukocyte Esterase. Neutrophilic leukocytes contain granules that release esterases into the urine. These esterases can be detected by chemical means using the leukocyte esterase test strip. The esterase splits an ester to form a pyrrole compound, which reacts with a diazo reagent to form a purple azo dye. The intensity of color is proportional to the amount of esterase in the urine and, indirectly, to the number of leukocytes present. The test can detect as few as 5 to 15 white blood cells per high-power microscope field. Zero to 2 cells per high-power field is normal. The leukocyte esterase test is not affected by the presence of a large number of erythrocytes or bacteria in the urine, but urinary tract antibiotics like cephalexin and tetracycline may affect the results, producing false negatives.

CONFIRMATORY TESTS

When the test results of a reagent-strip test used in routine urinalysis are questionable, an additional testing method should be used to confirm the results. Confirmatory tests generally are not used to screen patients because they are too time consuming and costly—nor should they be run on every specimen just to confirm the accuracy of test results. Their use should be confined to cases in which there is reasonable doubt about a test result, such as when a test result seems illogical in light of other medical evidence. Repeating the reagent-strip test on the same specimen or on a new specimen from the same patient may negate the need for a confirmatory test.

The four most often used confirmatory tests in POLs are those for bilirubin, protein, reducing sugars, and ketones.

ICTOTEST® for Bilirubin

The ICTOTEST® is highly sensitive, and it is convenient for qualitative determination of bilirubinuria. This test can detect bilirubin concentrations as low as 0.05 mg/dL and as high as 0.10 mg/dL. Materials needed include an ICTOTEST reagent tablet, ICTOTEST mat, dropper, and water. The reagent tablets must not be exposed to light, heat, or moisture, and they never should be used past the expiration date on the bottle. Deterioration of the tablets is indicated by a tan or brown discoloration.

Figure 11.6 illustrates the general procedure for ICTOTEST. Remember always to check the instruc-

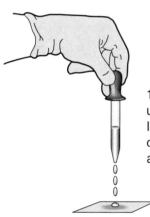

1. Place ten drops of fresh urine on one of the ICTOTEST mats. Remove one ICTOTEST reagent tablet and recap the bottle.

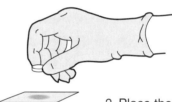

2. Place the tablet in the center of the moistened area.

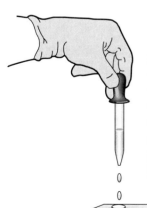

3. Place one drop of water on the tablet. Wait 5 seconds, then place a second drop of water onto the tablet, so that the water runs off the tablet onto the mat, where the reaction occurs. Time the reaction for 60 seconds.

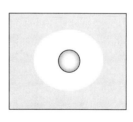

4. Observe the color of the mat around the tablet at the end of 60 seconds. Blue or purple color on the mat means the test is positive—bilirubin is present in the urine. The speed of color development and the intensity of color are proportional to the amount of bilirubin in the urine.

Figure 11.6. ICTOTEST procedure.

tions given in the manufacturer's package insert when you run the test.

◆◆ *Tests for Protein*

There are three simple yet sensitive tests for protein in the urine: the acetic acid, sulfosalicylic acid, and concentrated nitric acid tests. In all three, protein in the urine is coagulated and/or precipitated by the addition of acid or acid and heat. The acetic acid method uses acid and heat to test urine for protein. It is the most sensitive method for detecting protein at low concentrations—as low as 2 to 3 mg/dL, compared with 15 to 30 mg/dL for reagent-strip tests.

◆ ◆ ◆ Interpreting Protein Precipitation and Coagulation Test Results

The following factors will help you interpret protein precipitation and coagulation test results:

- no turbidity—negative (no protein in the urine)
- faint precipitation when viewed against a black background—a trace
- a small degree of turbidity—one plus
- moderate turbidity—two plus
- heavy turbidity—three plus
- heavy flocculation (like cotton wool)—four plus

◆◆ *CLINITEST® for Reducing Sugars*

The reagent-strip test for urinary sugar detects only glucose. A **reduction test,** also called Benedict's test, is needed to detect other simple sugars, such as lactose, galactose, fructose, and pentose. In POLs, the most frequently used reduction test is CLINITEST®.

CLINITEST is used to test for lactase deficiency and galactosemia, among other disorders of carbohydrate metabolism. A blue result is negative, and an orange-red result is positive. Always consult the color chart in the package insert. A negative result means that no sugar is present in the urine. A positive result means that some type of sugar, although not necessarily glucose, is present in the urine.

◆ ◆ ◆ Galactosemia ◆ ◆ ◆

Galactose is a simple sugar formed from the breakdown of lactose, or milk sugar. Normal individuals do not test positive for galactose in the urine because they are able to convert galactose to glucose with the enzyme galactase. People who are born without the ability to manufacture the enzyme have an inborn error of metabolism called **galactosemia,** which is characterized by the presence of detectable levels of galactose in the urine. Galactosemia can be treated by eliminating sources of both galatose and lactose from the diet. Untreated infants with this disease deteriorate rapidly, both physically and mentally, and die at an early age, literally of starvation. A patient with galactosemia tests negative for sugar with the reagent-strip tests but positive with CLINITEST.

◆◆ *ACETEST® for Ketones*

ACETEST® is a confirmatory test for ketones. Like reagent-strip tests, ACETEST is based on a nitroprusside reaction, which detects both acetone and acetoacetic acid. Materials needed include an ACETEST tablet, the ACETEST color chart, and white paper. The procedure for ACETEST is:

- Remove an ACETEST tablet from the bottle and recap the bottle.
- Place the tablet on a clean surface, preferably white paper.
- Put one drop of urine on the tablet.
- Time the reaction on the tablet for thirty seconds.
- Compare the color change on the tablet to the ACETEST color chart at thirty seconds.

◆ ◆ ◆ Testing Blood for Ketones ◆ ◆ ◆

Serum, plasma, or whole blood also can be tested for ketones by substituting one drop of the fluid in place of one drop of urine. When using serum or plasma, take the reading at two minutes after applying the specimen to the tablet. When whole blood is added, wait ten minutes before removing clotted blood from the tablet.

PROCEDURE

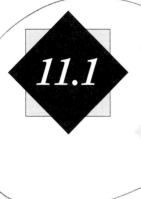

11.1 ◆ Chemical Analysis of Urine

Goal

- After successfully completing this procedure, you will be able to perform a reagent-strip test, CLINITEST, and ICTOTEST on urine.

Completion Time

- 45 minutes

Equipment and Supplies

- impermeable jacket, gown, or apron
- disposable latex gloves
- hand disinfectant
- surface disinfectant
- paper towels and tissues
- biohazard container
- fresh urine sample
- distilled water
- disposable reagent strip and color chart
- watch with second hand
- disposable pipettes
- CLINITEST tablet
- ICTOTEST tablet and mat
- small test tube (16 × 125 mm)
- test tube rack
- forceps
- glass rod
- urinalysis report form and pen

Instructions

Read through the list of equipment and supplies that you will need and the steps of the procedure. Be sure that you understand each step before you begin. Then complete each step correctly and in the proper order. If your completion time is too long, repeat the procedure until you increase your speed.

S = Satisfactory	U = Unsatisfactory	S	U

1. Put on a protective jacket, gown, or apron; wash your hands with disinfectant, dry them, and put on gloves.

2. Follow the Universal Precautions.

3. Collect and prepare appropriate equipment and supplies.

4. Verify identification of the specimen and label the container. If the specimen has been refrigerated, allow it to come to room temperature.

5. Mix the urine specimen in the container by stirring it with a clean glass rod.

6. Remove a reagent strip from the bottle and recap the bottle immediately.

7. Note the time, and then dip the reagent strip into the urine, wetting all reagent pad areas. Immerse the reagent strip no longer than one second.

8. Remove the reagent strip from the urine by drawing the edge of the strip along the rim of the specimen container to remove excess urine. Hold the strip horizontally to prevent mixing chemicals from adjacent pads.

9. At the time specified and in good light, hold the reagent strip next to the color chart on the bottle. Be careful not to let the strip touch and contaminate the chart.

10. Find the colors that match the reagent-strip pads and record the results for each test on the urinalysis report form.

S = Satisfactory	U = Unsatisfactory	S	U

11. Place a small test tube in a test tube rack and add five drops of urine and ten drops of distilled water.

12. Dispense one CLINITEST tablet into the cap of the bottle, remove it with forceps, and close the bottle tightly.

13. Add the CLINITEST tablet to the test tube. *Caution:* Heat is produced from the chemical reaction that occurs as the tablet dissolves. To avoid burns, do not touch the tube or point it toward anyone.

14. When boiling has ceased, note the time. After fifteen seconds, compare the color of the liquid in the test tube to the CLINITEST color chart.

15. Record the result on the urinalysis report form, either as negative or as a percent.

16. Place ten drops of urine on an ICTOTEST test mat.

17. Place an ICTOTEST reagent tablet on the center of the moistened area of the mat.

18. With a disposable pipette, flow two drops of distilled water over the tablet. Note the time.

19. Watch for sixty seconds. The rapidity and depth of color formation are proportional to the amount of bilirubin present. A blue to purple color indicates the presence of bilirubin. An orange to red color indicates the absence of bilirubin.

20. Record the result on the urinalysis report form.

21. Flush the remaining urine down the toilet.

S = Satisfactory	U = Unsatisfactory	S	U

22. Discard disposable equipment.

23. Disinfect other equipment and return it to storage.

24. Clean the work area following the Universal Precautions.

25. Remove your jacket, gown, or apron, and gloves; wash your hands with disinfectant, and dry them.

OVERALL PROCEDURAL EVALUATION

Student's Name _____

Signature of Instructor _____ Date _____

Comments

Using Terminology

Match the term in the right column with the appropriate definition in the left column.

_____ 1. abnormally high blood pH

_____ 2. abnormally low blood pH

_____ 3. abnormal protein

_____ 4. break down

_____ 5. insulin deficiency

_____ 6. intermediate product of fat metabolism

_____ 7. invisible and hemolyzed

_____ 8. pus in the urine

_____ 9. yellowing

a. acidemia

b. alkalemia

c. Bence Jones protein

d. diabetes mellitus

e. jaundice

f. ketone

g. lyse

h. occult blood

i. pyuria

Reagent strips are used to detect abnormal levels of each of the following. In the space provided, identify the clinical significance of each.

10. Glucose

_____

11. Ketones

_____

12. Protein

_____

13. Blood

_____

14. Bilirubin

_____

15. Urobilinogen

_____

16. Nitrite

_____

17. Leukocytes

_____

Acquiring Knowledge

Answer the following questions in the spaces provided.

18. Why is routine urinalysis the most commonly performed laboratory procedure?

19. Name the analytes included in routine urinalysis.

20. What is a screening test? When is it used?

21. What is a confirmatory test? When is it used?

22. How is the concentration of hydrogen atoms in a solution expressed?

23. How is the acid-base balance of the body measured?

24. What is the pH of acidic urine?

25. What is the pH of alkaline urine?

26. What type of sugar most often is found in urine?

27. What disease is the chief cause of glucosuria?

28. What is the role of insulin in diabetes mellitus?

29. For which kind of sugar do the reagent strips test?

_____

30. What form of energy is utilized by body cells?

_____

31. Explain the cause of ketosis (ketoacidosis).

_____

_____

32. What analyte in urine is indicative of renal disease?

_____

33. What is jaundice? What causes it?

_____

_____

_____

34. What test-strip parameter detects bacteria in a first morning specimen?

_____

35. What abnormal protein is not detected by a reagent-strip test? What does its presence mean?

_____

_____

36. What type of testing is performed with reagent strips: screening or confirmatory?

_____

Applying Knowledge—On the Job

Answer the following questions in the spaces provided.

37. You just tested Mr. Gomez's urine with a reagent strip and the pH was 4.4. What might cause Mr. Gomez to have acidic urine?

_____

_____

_____

38. Mrs. Vukovich has come to the doctor's office with a urinary tract infection. She has been prescribed sodium bicarbonate to increase urinary pH and an antibiotic. She has heard that a good home remedy is cranberry juice, supposedly because it makes the urine more acidic. Now Mrs. Vukovich is confused about the role of urinary pH in treating urinary tract infections. Set her straight.

_____

_____

_____

39. An infant's urine has been submitted to the laboratory with a request for a CLINITEST® along with routine urinalysis. Why would such a request be made?

40. In the lab where you work, several patients have tested positive for urinary protein. Classify each of the following protein levels as marked, moderate, or minimal, and list two possible causes of each:

(a) 5 grams/day:

(b) 2 grams/day:

(c) 0.2 grams/day:

41. Mrs. Jones' urine specimen tests positive for nitrite and leukocyte esterase, and is strongly alkaline (8.5). It also has an ammonia smell. What type of illness might she have?

42. Mr. Chan's reagent-strip test for protein was negative, yet the physician has ordered a precipitation test for him, which you know also screens for protein. Why did the doctor order a confirmatory test for an analyte when the screening test was negative?

43. Elaine's urine specimen appears normal, but the reagent-strip test reveals occult blood. She does not understand how blood can be present without being obvious. The doctor has asked you to explain this to her. What do you say?

44. One of the urine specimens that you analyzed today tested positive for occult blood. What is the clinical significance of this finding?

_____

_____

_____

_____

_____

45. Your student group is visiting a clinical laboratory. One of the students asks why both screening and confirmatory tests are done for a single analyte. She thinks that it might be quicker and cheaper to do just confirmatory tests in the first place and eliminate screening. Explain to her why the laboratory uses screening tests in addition to confirmatory tests.

_____

_____

_____

_____

_____

46. You are employed in a clinical laboratory where you perform a urinalysis that tests positive for bilirubin. Why should this finding lead you to treat the urine specimen with special caution?

_____

_____

_____

47. As the clinical worker in charge of the urinalysis section, how will you maintain quality control of urine testing?

_____

_____

_____

48. Jerry is having a busy day in the laboratory. He dips reagent strips into several different urine specimens at the same time and attempts to read several reagent strips simultaneously. What problem do you see in this scenario?

_____

_____

_____

_____

CHAPTER 12

Microscopic Properties of the Urinalysis

COGNITIVE OBJECTIVES

After studying this chapter, you should be able to

- use each of the vocabulary terms appropriately.

- explain the relationship between a microscopic examination of urine and the diagnosis and treatment of patients.

- describe how to differentiate among the various elements found in urine under microscopic examination.

- identify the normal and pathological ranges of particular elements in urinary sediment.

- discuss the significance of abnormally high amounts of particular elements found in urinary sediment.

- outline the technical procedure for obtaining precise and reproducible microscopic examinations of urine.

- identify the tissue origins of the various elements found in urine under the microscope.

PERFORMANCE OBJECTIVES

After studying this chapter, you should be able to

- demonstrate how to prepare a urine specimen for microscopic examination of sediment.

- identify and count casts, cellular elements, and crystals in a urine-sediment slide.

TERMINOLOGY

balanitis: inflammation of the glans penis, most often due to *Trichomonas vaginalis*, herpes, or *Chlamydia trachomatis*.

crenated: shrunken; usually used to refer to shrunken red blood cells, which appear small and scalloped around the edges.

cylindruria: the condition characterized by large numbers of casts in the urine.

desquamation: the shedding of layers of cells or skin.

erythrocyte: a red blood cell.

fatty cast: renal cast that contains fat droplets because of chronic renal disease.

granular cast: fine- or coarse-grained dark renal cast that has degenerated from a hyaline or waxy cast. An increase in the number of granular casts may indicate pyelonephritis.

hyaline cast: the most common type of renal cast. Hyaline casts are colorless, homogeneous, and semitransparent. An increase in the number of hyaline casts indicates damage to the glomerular capillary membrane, permitting leakage of protein.

hypertonic urine: urine with a specific gravity of 1.030 or greater (concentrated).

hypotonic urine: urine with a specific gravity of 1.003 or less (diluted).

leukocyte: a white blood cell.

lymphocyte: a nongranular white blood cell with a single nucleus.

neutrophil: the most commonly found type of white blood cell in urine sediment; so named because it stains with neutral dyes.

phase microscopy: the type of microscopy in which differences in the refractive index are translated into difference in brightness; used to view unstained specimens.

prostatitis: inflammation of the prostate.

renal cast: the tube-shaped element in urine sediment, formed in the tubules of the kidney by the deposition of protein.

spermatozoan (sperm): the male gamete that fertilizes the female egg. As seen in urine, it has an expanded head and a long whiplike tail and appears black.

supravital stain: dye added to cells while they are living.

urine sediment: the solid material that settles to the bottom of urine when it stands or is centrifuged.

waxy cast: the renal cast that is yellowish, with irregular broken ends.

● ● ● ● ● ● ● ● ● ● ● ● ● ● ● ● ●

Microscopic examination of urine sediment is considered to be the most valuable diagnostic technique in urinalysis. **Urine sediment,** which is the solid material that settles to the bottom when it stands or is centrifuged, contains all of the insoluble materials in urine, including **erythrocytes, leukocytes,** casts, crystals, bacteria, fungi, parasites, mucous threads, and, in males, **sperm.** Next to actual biopsies of kidney tissue, microscopic findings are the clearest indicators of intrinsic renal disease. In fact, urine-sediment analysis is sometimes referred to as "liquid biopsy" for this reason.

━━━━━━━━━━━━━━━━━━━━━ ◆ ◆

THE CONVENTIONAL METHOD OF MICROSCOPIC ANALYSIS

This section outlines the method of preparing and examining urine sediment that is most widely used in POLs today.

◆◆ *Preparation of the Specimen*

Most urine specimens are centrifuged before microscopic examination of sediment to concentrate the formed elements. (See Figure 12.1 for a centrifuge.) The specimen used for centrifugation must be fresh and thoroughly mixed (see Figure 12.2). About 10 to 15 mL of urine are poured into a disposable centrifuge tube and centrifuged for five minutes at 1,500 to 2,000 rpm. After centrifuging, the supernatant, the

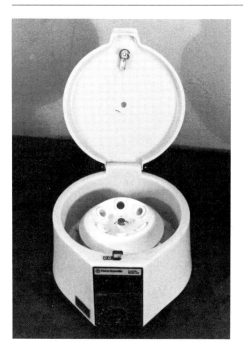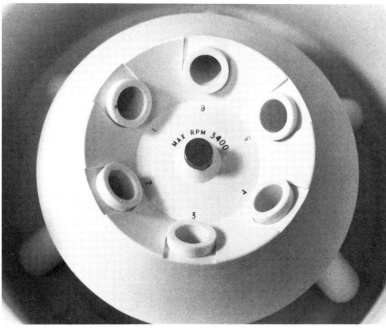

Figure 12.1. a. The six-tube capacity of this centrifuge is typical of those found in POLs. b. The centrifuge must be balanced to avoid breaking the tubes. When centrifuging two tubes, place them opposite each other—in slots 1 and 4 or 2 and 5, for example. Place three tubes in alternate slots. Photos by Mark Palko.

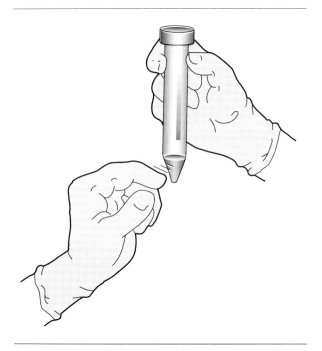

Figure 12.2. To mix the contents of the centrifuge tube, hold the top of the tube with the thumb and index finger of one hand and flick the bottom of the tube sharply several times with the index finger of the other hand.

fluid that floats on top, is poured off without disturbing the sediment. The amount of urine left with the sediment may vary from a few drops to one milliliter.

The sediment is resuspended in the remaining urine and a drop is placed on a microscope glass slide and covered with a 22 mm-square plastic coverslip. The coverslip assures that the slide has a uniform thickness, helps keep the specimen still, and protects the microscope objective from contamination with specimen material (see Figure 12.3). To prevent the formation of bubbles when placing the coverslip on the drop of urine, let one edge of the coverslip touch the liquid first and then let the rest drop into place. If liquid runs out from under the coverslip or allows it to float, you have used too large a drop.

Staining. Sediment may be stained to improve refraction and to clarify the image at lower light intensities. Add one or two drops of stain to the sediment in the centrifuge tube and thoroughly mix it before placing the sediment on the microscope slide. Avoid overstaining.

A number of different stains may be used for urine sediment. A toluidine blue stain is used to stain cells and casts. Sternheimer-Malbin (S-M) stain is most helpful in the identification of nucleated elements as well as casts, but some staining solutions require filtration before using because they form sediments that interfere with viewing.

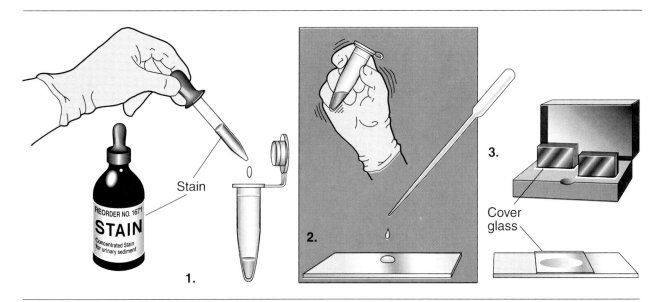

Figure 12.3. To stain urine sediment, follow these steps: 1. Add one drop of stain to approximately 1/2 mL of centrifuged urine sediment and mix together by shaking the tube. 2. Place one drop of stained urine sediment on the slide. 3. Place coverslip over drop on the slide, and then view the slide in the microscope and count formed elements in the sediment.

A stabilized modification of S-M stain, which does not require filtration, is SEDI-STAIN®, produced by Clay-Adams. SEDI-STAIN contains both crystal violet and safranine dyes, which are taken up in varying proportions depending on the chemical and physical properties of formed elements in the sediment. The results vary from pale pink to dark purple.

◆◆ Scanning the Slide

After the slide is coverslipped, it is placed on the microscope stage for examination. Under low-power (10X) magnification and subdued light (with the condenser lowered and/or the iris diaphragm partly closed), the entire slide is systematically scanned around all four sides of the coverslip. The fine focus adjustment knob should be used as needed to sharpen the image. This initial scan is necessary to locate the fields in which most of the formed elements are present.

◆◆ Counting Formed Elements

Ten to fifteen of the fields containing formed elements should be examined using high-power (45X) magnification and higher light intensity (with the condenser raised and/or the iris diaphragm opened). Under high power, the number of erythrocytes, leukocytes, and epithelial cells in the selected fields are counted and then the average number of each type of cell per field is calculated. The result is reported as the number per HPF, or high-power field. Casts should be identified as to type under high-power magnification and then counted in ten to fifteen fields using low-power magnification. The result is averaged and reported as the number per LPF, or low-power field.

Other elements observed in the slide may include crystals, bacteria, fungi, parasites, and sperm. These should be reported but not counted. Artifacts, extraneous materials, such as hair, clothing fibers, and talcum powder, that are not part of the urine or urinary tract, often are misinterpreted. It is common to misinterpret clothing fibers as mucous threads, for example. Take care to distinguish artifacts from any sediment elements that are to be identified and counted.

Phase microscopy, in which differences in refractive index are translated into differences in brightness, is used in some POLs to detect translucent elements in urine sediment. It is especially useful for detailing the outline of hyaline casts, mucous threads, and bacteria. Specimens are generally unstained.

◆◆

CASTS AND THEIR CLINICAL SIGNIFICANCE

Renal casts (see Figure 12.4) are cylindrical bodies with parallel sides of varying diameter that form in the renal tubules and wash into the urine. The matrix of the cast is glycoprotein (Tamm-Horsfall mucoprotein), produced by renal epithelial cells lining the ascending limb of the loop of Henle and the distal convoluted tubule.

The reference value for the number of casts in a normal urine specimen is 0 to 1 per LPF. An increased number of casts in the urine, which is called **cylindruria,** may be due to several factors, including:

- a decreased rate of tubular flow
- an increased acidity of urine
- a decreased volume of urine with increased protein or salt concentration

The significance of an increased number of casts depends on their type.

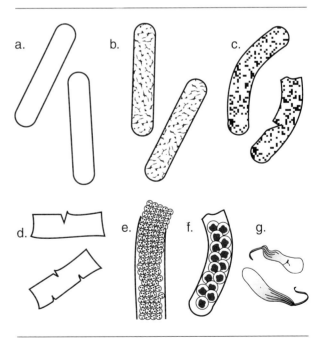

Figure 12.4. Renal casts seen during a urinalysis include a. hyaline cast, b. fine granular cast, c. coarse granular cast, d. waxy cast with sheen, e. red blood-cell cast, f. white blood-cell cast, and g. cylindroid cast.

♦♦ *Hyaline Casts*

Hyaline casts, which are colorless, homogeneous, and semitransparent, are the most common type of cast. An increase in their number indicates damage to the glomerular capillary membrane, permitting leakage of protein. This damage may be transient, resulting from fever, dehydration, emotional stress, strenuous exercise, or the effect of posture (orthostatic, lordotic), or permanent due to kidney disease. Hyaline casts usually dissolve in alkaline urine.

♦♦ *Granular Casts*

Granular casts are casts that show the degree of degeneration that has occurred in the cellular inclusions. They may be fine or coarse grained. While an occasional granular cast is considered to be normal, any increase in number may indicate pyelonephritis.

♦♦ *Waxy and Fatty Casts*

Casts may be **waxy** and yellowish, with irregular, broken ends, or they may be **fatty,** that is, containing fat droplets. Waxy casts form in the collecting tubules when the urine flow through them is reduced. Both waxy and fatty casts may be associated with the tubular inflammation and degeneration characteristic of chronic renal disease.

♦♦ *Red Blood-Cell Casts*

Red blood-cell casts indicate renal bleeding due to acute inflammatory or vascular disorders of the glomerulus. These casts should always be regarded as pathological. They may be the only symptom of acute glomerulonephritis, renal infarction, collagen disease, and kidney involvement in subacute bacterial endocarditis. Figure 12.5 shows the formation of a red blood-cell cast.

♦♦ *White Blood-Cell Casts*

White blood-cell casts may be observed in the urine of patients with acute glomerulonephritis, nephrotic syndrome, or pyelonephritis. They are especially important in diagnosing pyelonephritis because this disease may remain completely asymptomatic while progressively destroying renal tissue. Figure 12.6 shows formation of a white blood-cell cast.

♦♦ *Epithelial Cell Casts*

Epithelial cell casts are formed when epithelial cells are shed from the renal tubules and fused together. An increase in their number often indicates damage to the renal tubule epithelium, which may occur with nephrosis, eclampsia, amyloidosis, or toxic poisoning.

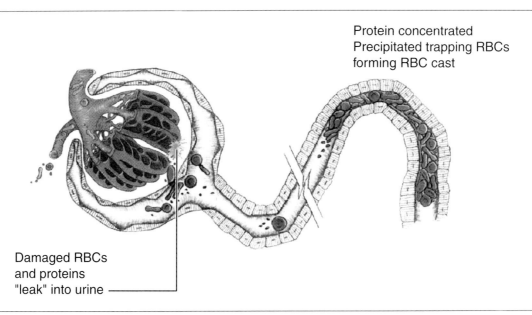

Protein concentrated
Precipitated trapping RBCs
forming RBC cast

Damaged RBCs
and proteins
"leak" into urine

Figure 12.5. Formation of a typical red blood-cell cast. Courtesy of Miles, Inc., Diagnostics Division.

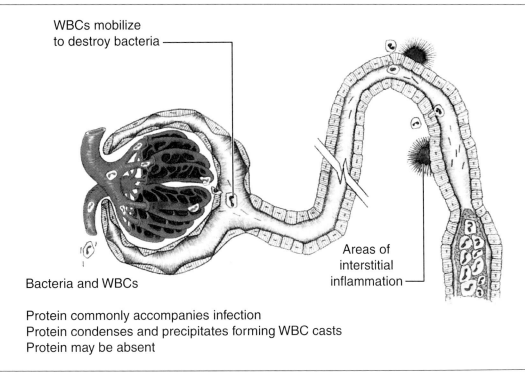

WBCs mobilize
to destroy bacteria

Bacteria and WBCs

Areas of
interstitial
inflammation

Protein commonly accompanies infection
Protein condenses and precipitates forming WBC casts
Protein may be absent

Figure 12.6. Formation of a typical white blood-cell cast. Courtesy of Miles, Inc., Diagnostics Division.

CELLULAR ELEMENTS AND THEIR CLINICAL SIGNIFICANCE

Three types of cells normally are found in urinary sediment—red blood cells, white blood cells, and epithelial cells. They are illustrated in Figure 12.7.

✦✦ Red Blood Cells

When viewed with high-power magnification, unstained red blood cells look like pale green discs of slightly varying size. In **hypotonic urine,** red blood cells tend to **lyse,** and in **hypertonic urine,** they may shrink and become **crenated** (shrunken and notched or scalloped around the edges).

Normal concentrations of red blood cells on a urine sediment slide are one or two per HPF. More than three red blood cells per HPF are considered abnormal, unless due to contamination of the specimen by menstrual blood. Blood in the urine may result from a variety of renal or systemic diseases. When an increase in red blood cells in urine is found in conjunction with red blood-cell casts, it can be assumed that the bleeding is renal in origin. An in-crease in red blood cells in the urine without casts indicates an extrarenal source (see Table 12.1).

✦✦ White Blood Cells

When viewed under high-power magnification, white blood cells in urine look like round granular bodies, about twice as large as red blood cells. The type of white blood cell most often observed is the segmented **neutrophil,** so named because it stains with neutral dyes.

In normal urine sediment, only zero to two white blood cells per HPF are observed. Increased numbers of leukocytes in the urine are usually indicative of disease, although a temporary increase may follow strenuous exercise. Diseases associated with increased white blood cells in urine include calculi, cystitis, **prostatitis,** urethritis, and **balanitis.** The presence of more than fifty leukocytes per HPF or of clumps of leukocytes is strongly suggestive of acute urinary tract infection. Gross pyuria may reflect the rupture of a renal or urinary tract abscess. When increased numbers of leukocytes are found together with leukocyte casts or mixed leukocyte-epithelial cell casts, they are most likely renal in origin, indicating renal disease, such as glomerulonephritis, lu-

ATLAS OF URINE SEDIMENT

Cells in urine

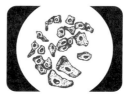

Epithelial renal tubular

Epithelial transitional

Epithelial squamous

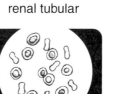

Red blood cells

Renal tubular and white blood cells

White blood cells

Crystals found in acid urine

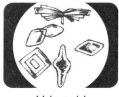

Uric acid

Tyrosine

Cystine crystals

Leucine

Crystals found in acid, neutral, and alkaline urine

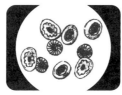

Calcium oxalate

Hippuric acid

Crystals found in alkaline urine

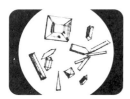
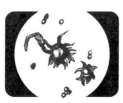

Triple phosphate

Ammonium urates

Casts in urine

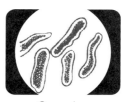

Hyaline

Granular

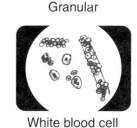

Red blood cell

White blood cell

Bacteria, fungi, parasites in urine

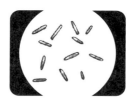
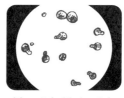

Bacteria

Yeast (with buds)

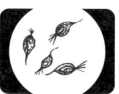

Trichomonas vaginalis

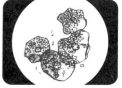
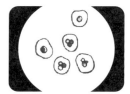
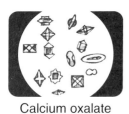
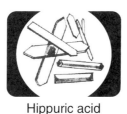

Figure 12.7. Urine sediment. Courtesy of Miles, Inc., Diagnostics Division.

TABLE 12.1 Pathological Conditions Producing Hematuria

Renal Diseases	Lower Urinary Tract Diseases
Glomerulonephritis	Acute and chronic infection
Lupus nephritis	Calculus (stone)
Calculus	Tumor
Tumor	Stricture (narrowing)
Acute infection	**Extrarenal Diseases**
Tuberculosis	Acute appendicitis
Renal vein thrombosis	Diverticulitis
Renal trauma	Tumors of the colon, rectum, pelvis
Polycystic kidney	**Drug Toxicity**
Malignant nephrosclerosis	Salicylates (aspirin)
Infarction	Anticoagulants

pus nephritis, or pyelonephritis. Large numbers of mononucleated white cells, or **lymphocytes,** in the urine of a patient who has undergone kidney transplant surgery may be an early sign of tissue rejection.

Supravital stains, such as those used to color living cells that have not been fixed or chemically treated, usually are helpful in delineating the nuclear structure of leukocytes in urine sediment. However, in dilute, or hypotonic, urine, neutrophils swell and are poorly stained with supravital stains. Then, they are called glitter cells because their cytoplasmic granules exhibit Brownian movement, causing refraction. Leukocytes are rapidly lysed in hypotonic or alkaline urine; it is estimated that half are lost after urine stands at room temperature for two to three hours, underscoring the need to use fresh urine specimens in microscopic analysis.

✦✦ Epithelial Cells

Normal urine sediment may have an occasional epithelial cell or clump of epithelial cells because the renal tubules and their epithelium are always being renewed. However, renal epithelial cells which **desquamate,** or shed, at an excessive rate are indicative of disease damage to the renal tubular epithelium.

Renal epithelial cells are round, slightly larger than

white blood cells, and have a single large nucleus. As the name implies, renal epithelial cells originate in the kidneys. Bladder epithelial cells are larger than renal cells but smaller than squamous epithelial cells. They originate in the bladder.

Squamous epithelial cells are large flat cells with a single small nucleus. They are often present in urine and originate in the urethra, vulva, or vagina. Their presence has little significance except when in sheets. If sheets of squamous cells are present, they should be reported as "sheets of squamous epithelial cells."

✦✦ Fungi and Parasites

The type of fungus most commonly seen in the urine sediment is yeast. They are sometimes confused with red blood cells. However, a close examination of yeast will reveal them to be more ovoid than round. They are colorless and vary in size, and they frequently may show budding.

Trichomonas vaginalis is the parasite most frequently seen in urine. A unicellular organism with anterior flagellae, the parasites may resemble flattened, ovoid epithelial cells, but are usually recognized by their swimming motions. Both yeast and Trichomonas are most commonly seen in the urines of females.

CRYSTALS IN URINE SEDIMENT

Crystals commonly seen in normal urine sediment include phosphates, urates, and oxalates. Most are of limited clinical significance. A few crystals are clinically significant, however, so it is important to be able to recognize and distinguish urinary sediment crystals. The most important factor in identifying crystals is the pH value of the urine.

CONFIRMATION OF MICROSCOPIC EXAMINATION

The results of microscopic examination of urinary sediment always should be verified against other results for the same sample. For example, if the microscopic examination reveals red blood cells, then the reagent-strip test for blood in the urine should be positive; or if the microscopic examination reveals white blood cells and bacteria, then reagent-strip tests for leukocyte esterase and nitrite should be positive. Whenever there is disagreement among tests for the same sample, results should be held until retesting the same sample or a new sample produces confirmatory results.

STANDARDIZATION

Despite its great diagnostic value, microscopic examination of urine sediment is considered to be the most imprecise and inaccurate part of routine urinalysis. There are several reasons, including:

- Patient variation in concentration of urine.
- Variation in sample preparation. Samples may or may not be centrifuged, varying amounts of specimen may be centrifuged, time and speed of centrifuging may vary, and varying amounts of sample may be left in the centrifuge tube for resuspension after decantation.
- Variation in the power of the microscopic field under which the sediment is examined.
- Lack of reference standards for urine sediments.

Standardization can help make microscopic examination of urine sediment more reliable for diagnosing and monitoring patients. Two methods of prepar-

---

◆ ◆ ◆ Crystals Found ◆ ◆ ◆ in Urine

Normal Acid Urine (pH = 5–6)

- *Amorphous urates:* yellow-red granular precipitate that is soluble with heat and/or sodium hydroxide.
- *Sodium acid urates:* brown spheres that revert to uric acid plates on acidification with acetic acid.
- *Uric acid:* yellow or red-brown, irregularly shaped rhomboids that are soluble in sodium hydroxide when heated to 60 degrees Celsius.
- *Calcium oxalate:* refractile, octahedral envelopes with very small to large crystals that are soluble in strong hydrochloric acid.

Normal Alkaline Urine (pH = 7 or greater)

- *Amorphous phosphates:* fine, colorless, granular precipitate that is soluble in acetic acid.
- *Triple phosphates:* colorless, three- to six-sided prisms, occasionally fern-leaf shaped, that are soluble in acids.
- *Ammonium biurates:* yellow-brown, thorny spheres that are soluble in acetic acid.
- *Calcium phosphate:* colorless, stellate, or rosette formation of individual crystals, shaped like slender prisms, which are readily soluble in acetic acid or ammonium carbonate solution.
- *Calcium carbonate:* tiny colorless spheres or dumbbell shapes that are soluble in acetic acid and give off carbon dioxide gas.

Abnormal Urine

- *Cystine:* colorless, refractile, hexagonal plates, found in congenital cystinosis, cystinuria, and cystine calculi.
- *Tyrosine:* usually yellow, silky, fine needles arranged in sheaves or clumps, occasionally found (along with leucine crystals) in severe liver disease.
- *Leucine:* yellow, oily-appearing spheres with radial, concentric markings, occasionally found, along with tyrosine crystals, in severe liver disease.
- *Sulfonamides:* yellow-brown, asymmetrical, striated sheaves, or radially striated rounds, formed from sulfa drugs (not often seen with newer, more soluble sulfa drugs).
- *Renografin:* clear, colorless, flat rhombic plates, intersecting at 80 degrees, found briefly after urinary tract radiographs.
- *Ampicillin:* long, fine, colorless crystals, formed at high dosages of the antibiotic ampicillin.

ing urine sediments for examination have been developed to improve standardization—the KOVA system and the volume quantitative method.

◆◆ KOVA® System

The KOVA® System (ICL Scientific) is a standardized slide procedure that is more reproducible than are conventional methods. The system includes a graduated centrifuge tube (12 mL), transfer pipette, supravital staining system, and clear plastic microscopic slide with four individual covered examination chambers, each holding a fixed amount of liquid.

◆◆ Volume Quantitative Method

The volume quantitative method is very time consuming and provides a level of accuracy not normally required in POLs. This method is based on the measurement of the total volume of the specimen, which may be a single random specimen or a twenty-four hour volume specimen. The sample is mixed thoroughly and a measured amount is centrifuged for five minutes at 2,000 rpm. The supernatant is decanted and the sediment is resuspended in exactly one mL of urine. A hemacytometer counting chamber is flooded, and the formed elements present are counted. Based on the total volume of the specimen, the number of formed elements in the entire sample is calculated.

◆◆ CenSlide® 1500 Urinalysis System

The CenSlide Urinalysis System (International Remote Imaging System, Inc.) is a unique system for performing a standardized urine microscopic analysis. The system includes a CenSlide 1500 Centrifuge, CenSlide tubes, CenSlide Holder, and Stak-Rak®. (See Figures 12.8 and 12.9.)

The CenSlide tube is labeled with the appropriate patient information. Urine is measured to the fill line, and the cap is pushed down until it clicks. The centrifuge is microprocessor-controlled to spin the tube for 60 seconds. The urine sediment is then redistributed evenly across the viewing area of the CenSlide tube.

The CenSlide tube is inserted directly into the CenSlide Holder, which is located on the microscope stage. Each tube viewing area is exactly the same for each sample; there is no transferring of sample to a slide. This system reduces exposure to biohazardous material at the same time that it helps laboratories control inherent variations in conventional microscopic analysis of urine sediment. The 60-second centrifugation time is an 80 percent reduction from traditional methods.

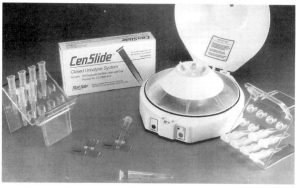

Figure 12.8. The CenSlide 1500 Centrifuge with Stak-Raks®. (Photo courtesy StatSpin, Inc., an IRIS Company.)

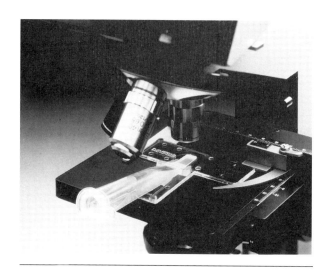

Figure 12.9. The CenSlide Holder mounted to the microscope. A mechanical stage holds a CenSlide tube ready for viewing. (Photo courtesy StatSpin, Inc., an IRIS Company.)

12.1 A Urine Microscopic Examination

Goal

- After successfully completing this procedure, you will be able to prepare a urine microscopic examination, examine the elements present, and report the results.

Completion Time

- 40 minutes

Equipment and Supplies

- impermeable jacket, gown, or apron
- disposable latex gloves
- hand disinfectant
- biohazard container
- surface disinfectant
- paper towels and tissues
- centrifuge
- four 10 mL centrifuge tubes
- microscope
- glass slides and 22 mm plastic or glass coverslips
- glass marking pen
- tissues
- disposable pipettes
- urine specimen
- Sternheimer-Malbin stain
- laboratory requisition form and pen

Instructions

Read through the list of equipment and supplies that you will need and the steps of the procedure. Be sure that you understand each step before you begin. Then complete each step correctly and in the proper order. If your completion time is too long, repeat the procedure until you increase your speed.

❖❖ Part 1

1. Put on a protective jacket, gown, or apron; wash your hands with disinfectant, dry them, and put on gloves.

2. Follow the Universal Precautions.

3. Collect and prepare the needed equipment and supplies.

4. Verify identification of the specimen and preserve the identity with a glass marking pen.

5. Mix the urine specimen well by stirring it with a pipette.

6. Pour a 10 mL sample of recently mixed urine into a clean conical 10 mL centrifuge tube. It must be graduated at the 1 mL and 10 mL marks.

7. Centrifuge at 2,000 rpm for five minutes to concentrate the urine sediment. The sediment contains the formed elements.

8. Decant the urine into another tube, reserving 1.0 mL for mixing with the sediment. The decanted urine may be used for confirmatory chemical tests for analytes such as protein.

❖❖ Part 2

9. If more than 1 mL of urine remains, recentrifuge the specimen. If less than 1 mL remains, add back supernatant urine to make the volume exactly 1 mL. The volume for suspension of sediment should remain the same from one specimen to another. Results are more reproducible if the amount of liquid urine remains constant.

10. Resuspend the sediment in the remaining liquid urine by agitating the tube.

11. If available, add one drop of Sternheimer-Malbin stain to the resuspended sediment. Allow time to stain.

12. Prepare a wet mount preparation by placing a drop of sediment onto a glass slide. Cover it with a 22 mm plastic or glass coverslip.

13. Using very reduced lighting and low-power magnification (10X objective), scan the entire area covered by the coverslip. Record the presence of all formed elements: casts, epithelial cells, red blood cells, white blood cells, crystals, mucus, sperm, contaminants, and urinary or vaginal parasites.

14. Note the number of casts in ten to fifteen LPH fields. Identify the cellular structure of casts present by going back and forth from LPF to HPF.

15. Turn to the high-power (45X) objective and observe ten to twelve representative fields. It will be necessary to increase the amount of light.

16. Identify and enumerate the following significant formed elements which are reported per high field: white blood cells, red blood cells, small crystals. Note the presence of yeast, bacteria, and spermatozoa.

◆◆ *Part 3*

17. Repeat steps 12–16 using an unstained sample of urine sediment if instructed to do so.

18. Dispose of biohazardous waste and contaminated disposable items.

19. Disinfect and return other equipment to proper storage areas.

20. Clean the work area following the Universal Precautions.

21. Complete the necessary information on the laboratory requisition form and route it to the proper place.

	S	U
22. Remove your jacket, gown, or apron, and your gloves; wash your hands with disinfectant, and dry them.		

OVERALL PROCEDURAL EVALUATION

Student's Name _____

Signature of Instructor _____ Date _____

Comments

PROCEDURE

12.2 Using the KOVA Method for a Urine Microscopic Examination

Goal

- After successfully completing this procedure, you will be able to prepare a urine microscopic examination using the KOVA method to examine the elements present and report the results.

Completion Time

- 30 minutes

Equipment and Supplies

- impermeable jacket, gown, or apron
- disposable latex gloves
- hand disinfectant
- biohazard container
- surface disinfectant
- centrifuge
- microscope
- KOVA microscope slides
- tissues and paper towels
- KOVA pipette
- urine specimen
- KOVA KUP and 2 KOVA tubes with KOVA KAPS
- glass-marking pen
- KOVA rack
- KOVA stain
- laboratory requisition form

Instructions

Read through the list of equipment and supplies that you will need and the steps of the procedure. Be sure that you understand each step before you begin. Then complete each step correctly and in the proper order. If your completion time is too long, repeat the procedure until you increase your speed.

❖❖ *Part 1*

1. Put on a protective jacket, gown, or apron; wash your hands with disinfectant, dry them, and put on gloves.

2. Follow the Universal Precautions.

3. Collect and prepare the appropriate equipment.

4. Label the KOVA tube and give it to the patient along with a tube cap and KOVA collection cup.

5. Have the patient collect the urine specimen in the KOVA KUP.

6. Verify identification of the specimen and preserve the identity with a glass-marking pen.

7. Tranfer the urine to the KOVA tube, filling it to the 12 mL mark.

8. Secure the KOVA KAP on the KOVA tube and place in KOVA rack for transportation.

9. Centrifuge the 12 mL of urine at 1,500 rpm for five minutes.

10. Insert the KOVA pipette into the centrifuge tube. Push the pipette to the bottom of the tube until it sits firmly.

11. Hold the pipette in position and decant 11 mL from the centrifuge tube into another tube.

12. Withdraw the pipette from the tube.

◆◆ *Part 2*

13. Add one drop of KOVA stain to 1 mL of urine sediment.

14. Return the pipette to the KOVA tube.

15. Use the pipette as a squeeze dropper to mix the sediment and stain together.

16. Squeeze the pipette, thus drawing up a small sample of sediment into the pipette.

17. Lay the KOVA slide flat with the covered chambers (half moon) on the upper surface.

18. Transfer the specimen to the KOVA slide by placing a drop of sediment on the open recessed area immediately adjacent to the covered chamber.

19. Tilt the KOVA slide on its edge to allow sediment to flow down into the chambers.

20. Remove any excess specimen in the open area by inverting the slide and tapping the open area on a paper towel.

21. Let the specimen stand for one minute to allow the constituents of the specimen to settle.

◆◆ *Part 3*

22. Read slide under the low-power objective and the high-power objective as instructed for the conventional method.

23. Using very reduced lighting and low-power magnification, scan the entire area covered by the coverslip. Record the presence of all formed elements: casts, epithelial cells, red blood cells, white blood cells, crystals, mucus, contaminants, and urinary or vaginal parasites.

	S	U

24. Note the number of casts in ten to fifteen LPH fields. Identify the cellular structure of casts present by going back and forth from LPF to HPF.

25. Turn to the high-power objective and observe ten to twelve representative fields. It will be necessary to increase the amount of light.

26. Identify and enumerate the following significant formed elements that are reported per high-power field: red blood cells, white blood cells, small crystals. Note the presence of yeast, bacteria, and spermatozoa.

27. Report your findings as instructed.

28. Dispose of biohazardous waste and soiled disposable equipment into proper waste receptacles.

29. Disinfect and return other equipment to proper storage area.

30. Clean the work area following the Universal Precautions.

31. Complete the necessary information on the laboratory requisition form and route it to the proper place.

32. Remove your jacket, gown, or apron, and your gloves; wash your hands with disinfectant, and dry them.

OVERALL PROCEDURAL EVALUATION

Student's Name _____

Signature of Instructor _____ **Date** _____

Comments

CHAPTER 12 REVIEW

Using Terminology

Match the term in the right column with the appropriate definition or description in the left column.

_____ 1. aspirin

_____ 2. blood in urine

_____ 3. floats on top

_____ 4. narrowing

_____ 5. nontissue contaminant

_____ 6. shedding

_____ 7. stone

_____ 8. urine crystal

_____ 9. has a flagellae

a. artifact
b. calcium oxalate
c. calculus
d. desquamation
e. hematuria
f. salicylate
g. Trichomonas vaginalis
h. stricture
i. supernatant

Write a short definition of each term in the space provided.

10. Lymphocyte: _____

_____

11. Renal cast: _____

_____

12. Cylindruria: _____

_____

13. Crenated: _____

_____

14. Phase microscopy: _____

_____

15. Urine sediment: _____

_____

Acquiring Knowledge

Answer the following questions in the spaces provided.

16. Why is microscopic examination of urine sediment considered to be the most difficult part of urinalysis to perform accurately and consistently?

_____

_____

_____

_____

17. Why is microscopic analysis of urine sediment so useful diagnostically?

_____

_____

_____

18. Why is urinary sediment analysis sometimes referred to as "liquid biopsy"?

_____

_____

_____

19. Describe how urine is decanted after centrifuging.

_____

_____

20. Why are urine specimens centrifuged before microscopic examination?

_____

_____

21. Under what magnification and lighting is the examination of urine sediment begun?

_____

_____

22. What type of magnification and lighting is used first when urine is examined for casts?

_____

_____

23. What magnification is used to identify red blood cells, white blood cells, casts, and epithelial cells?

_____

_____

24. How are the numbers of red blood cells, white blood cells, and epithelial cells reported?

_____

_____

25. What elements besides cells and casts may be observed in urine sediment?

_____

_____

26. How many casts are likely to be found in a normal urine specimen?

_____

27. What may cause an abnormal increase in the number of casts?

_____

_____

_____

28. What is the source of bleeding when both red blood-cell casts and an increased number of red blood cells are found in urine?

_____

_____

29. What is the source of bleeding when large numbers of red blood cells occur in urine without either casts or proteinuria?

_____

_____

30. What happens to red blood cells in hypotonic (dilute) urine?

_____

_____

31. What happens to red blood cells in hypertonic (concentrated) urine?

_____

_____

32. What is the clinical significance of pyuria?

_____

_____

33. What microscopic finding is indicative of an acute urinary tract infection?

_____

_____

34. What type of white blood cell is seen most often in the urine? Where does it get its name?

_____

_____

_____

35. What is the origin when many white blood cells and white blood-cell casts occur together in urine?

_____

_____

36. When are epithelial cells clinically significant in urine sediment?

_____

_____

37. If microscopic examination of urine sediment shows many red blood cells, what should chemical analysis show?

_____

_____

38. What medications may produce crystals in the urine?

_____

39. How are red blood cells distinguished from white blood cells in microscopic analysis of urine sediment?

_____

_____

40. How are casts formed?

_____

_____

_____

41. Describe the differences between hyaline casts and granular casts.

_____

_____

_____

_____

_____

42. What are some abnormal conditions that a microscopic examination of urine sediment might reveal?

_____

_____

_____

_____

Applying Knowledge—On the Job

Answer the following questions in the spaces provided.

43. If several normal urines were examined microscopically in a day's work in the POL, what might they contain?

_____

_____

_____

_____

44. What is wrong with this scenario? A microscopic analysis of urine sediment revealed many white blood cells and bacteria. Chemical analysis of the same sample was negative for leukocyte esterase and nitrite.

_____

_____

_____

_____

45. A laboratory worker reported large numbers of red blood cells in the microscopic urine sediment with a negative occult blood from the reagent-strip test. Do you think this is a correct report? How would you check the accuracy of the report?

_____

_____

_____

_____

13 Automated Urine Chemistry Instrumentation and Quality Control

COGNITIVE OBJECTIVES

After studying this chapter, you should be able to

- use each of the vocabulary terms appropriately.
- discuss the advantages of automated urinalysis.
- describe how to use and maintain the Clinitek 100 Urine Chemistry Analyzer.
- list several commercial sources for urine control specimens.
- explain how quality control is maintained in urinalysis through the use of control samples and proficiency testing.

PERFORMANCE OBJECTIVE

After studying this chapter, you should be able to

- perform routine urinalysis using a urine chemistry analyzer.

TERMINOLOGY

Clinitek 100: a urine chemistry analyzer designed for POLs. It reads urine chemistry reagent strips.

strip table: the part of the Clinitek 100 Urine Chemistry Analyzer that holds the reagent strip after the strip is immersed in urine. The strip table is automatically drawn into the instrument, where it is read.

urine control: a pretested specimen, the result and value of which are known and can be used to test the variability of the POL's procedures, reagents, and equipment in performing urinalysis.

Until recently, chemical analysis of urine specimens was done manually. Increasingly, urinalysis, like other laboratory procedures, is becoming automated.

THE NEED FOR AUTOMATION

Lab worker variability and error can lead to loss of accuracy, precision, and reproducibility in routine urinalysis. The use of automation reduces variability and error and increases standardization. Specific advantages of automated urinalysis include the following:

- Instruments eliminate the variation in reading reagent strips that is due to individual differences in visual acuity and color blindness and also to differences in quality and quantity of light illuminating the reagent strip during the reading.
- Instruments eliminate timing errors in reading results. They are programmed to read each test at the optimal time.
- Instruments go through an automatic calibration cycle at each start-up. No extra calibration procedure is required.
- Specimen identification and test results are printed by the instrument, eliminating the possibility of transcription error.

CLINITEK® 100

The Ames **Clinitek**® 100 Urine Chemistry Analyzer produced by Miles, Inc., Diagnostic Division, is a urinalysis instrument designed especially for use in POLs. It is user-friendly and very flexible. The Clinitek 100 uses either Multistix 10 SG Reagent Strips or Ames Reagent Strips. The instrument utilizes reflectance photometry in which reflected light is measured to assess the urine chemistry values of the sample. See Chapter 21 for more information and illustration of reflectance photometry. All testing is completed within one minute, including the leukocyte esterase test that takes two minutes manually, thus reducing testing time by half. Up to one hundred specimen results can be stored in the memory bank of the instrument. The results also are displayed on the instrument's screen and printed by its thermal printer. In addition, the Clinitek 100 can be interfaced with a computer printer. Figure 13.1 illustrates the Clinitek 100.

◆◆ *Using the Clinitek 100*

Urinalysis is performed on the Clinitek 100 by first immersing a reagent strip in a urine specimen. The instrument is keyed to start, and the strip is laid on the **strip table**. About ten seconds after the start key is pressed, the strip table is automatically drawn into the instrument and the specimen is read. Physical characteristics, such as color and clarity, of the sample and the identification number of the patient can be entered in and printed out before, during, or after the test is complete. As soon as the test is complete,

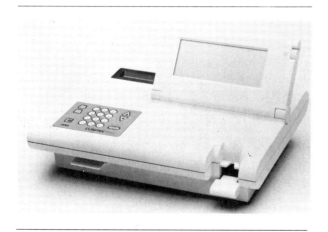

Figure 13.1. Clinitek® 100 Urine Chemistry Analyzer. Courtesy of Miles, Inc., Diagnostics Division.

the results are displayed on the screen and printed by the thermal printer. Through choice of software, results can be reported either semiquantitatively (+ system) or quantitatively (mg/dL). Abnormal results have an asterisk printed by the test name.

◆◆ *Calibration and Quality Control*

The Clinitek 100 has a calibration disk on the strip table. When turned on, the instrument automatically goes through a calibration cycle and no extra calibration procedure is required. Quality-control checks are performed daily by running a known-value urine control specimen, using the regular testing procedure. The sample is identified as a urine control specimen, and the results of the control-sample test are recorded in the control record. The results also are compared with the expected values for that control specimen. If the results fall outside the range of expected values, the instrument needs servicing, which must be done at the factory. The manufacturer will provide a temporary replacement to POLs.

◆◆ *Maintenance*

The only maintenance recommended for Clinitek 100 is routine cleaning of the strip table, which can be removed and washed with mild soap and rinsed with warm water. The platform of the strip table can be disinfected with a 5 percent bleach solution.

QUALITY CONTROL IN URINALYSIS

There are two essential aspects of quality control in routine urinalysis—daily testing of known-value control specimens and routine proficiency testing of unknown samples. Both are mandated by CLIA 1988, the federal law that governs certification and inspection of POLs.

◆◆ *Urine Controls*

Urine controls are known-value control specimens that are used to test the variability of the procedures, reagents, and equipment in performing urinalysis. They should be used to check all previously opened bottles of reagent strips as well as each new bottle of strips. New lab workers also should run controls to check on the precision and accuracy of their performance. Results of control testing should be considered acceptable if the correct result is obtained 95 percent of the time.

Urine controls always must be reconstituted with the appropriate diluting agent and exactly in accordance with the manufacturer's directions, which are included on the package insert. Each time a reagent strip is dipped into a control sample, some of the reagents from the strip leach out of the pads and contaminate the sample. It is important, therefore, that controls be used only the specified number of times recommended by the manufacturer.

Some manufacturers give expected values for only one brand of reagent strip, while others give expected values for several different reagents and procedures. A few list expected values for specific automated urine chemistry analyzers, like Clinitek 100. Urine controls usually can be purchased with two levels of control for each parameter—a negative, or normal, level and a positive, or abnormal, level. Table 13.1 lists several different urine quality controls and their manufacturers.

❖❖ *Proficiency Testing*

While daily testing of known-value controls is a good way to monitor day-to-day variability of test results within POLs, it does not assess how closely a particular POL's procedures match the results of other labs. Proficiency testing is required for this.

In a proficiency-testing program, control samples with unknown values are received by mail, analyzed, and the results returned to the proficiency-testing center. A report is received back indicating how closely the POL's results were to those of other participating labs using the same testing method. If the results of one POL are significantly different from those of other labs, this difference suggests a problem with the procedure, sample, reagent, or instrumentation. Most proficiency-testing reports include suggestions for identifying and correcting problem results. CLIA 1988 mandates the degree of accuracy that must be achieved in proficiency testing.

TABLE 13.1 Urine Quality Control Samples

Brand Name	Manufacturer
Lyphochek®	Biorad Laboratories 3700 East Miralome Avenue Anaheim, CA 92806 1-800-854-6737
KOVA-Trol®	Hycor BioMedical 7272 Chapman Garden Grove, CA 92641 1-800-382-2527
CHEK-STIX®	Miles, Inc. Diagnostic Division P.O. Box 70 Elkhart, IN 46515 1-800-348-8100
Urine Dipstick Control Kit™	Quantimetrix Corporation 4955 West 145th Street Hawthorne, CA 90250 1-800-624-8380
Count-10™	V-Tech, Inc. 270 East Bonita Pomona, CA 91767 1-800-762-7809

PROCEDURE

13.1

Urine Quality-Control Procedure

Goal

- After successfully completing this procedure, you will be able to perform urine quality-control procedures using CHEK-STIX control strips.

Completion Time

- 45 minutes

Equipment and Supplies

- impermeable jacket, gown, or apron
- disposable latex gloves
- hand disinfectant
- surface disinfectant
- paper towels and tissues
- biohazard container
- CHEK-STIX control strip
- disposable reagent strip with color chart
- distilled water
- small test tube (16 × 100 mm) and cap
- watch with second hand
- urinalysis-control report form and pen

Instructions

Read through the list of equipment and supplies that you will need and the steps of the procedure. Be sure that you understand each step before you begin. Then complete each step correctly and in the proper order. If your completion time is too long, repeat the procedure until you increase your speed.

S = Satisfactory U = Unsatisfactory	S	U
1. Put on a protective jacket, gown, or apron; wash your hands with disinfectant, dry them, and put on gloves.		

2. Follow the Universal Precautions.

3. Collect and prepare appropriate equipment.

4. Place 12 mL of distilled water in a small test tube.

5. Remove a CHEK-STIX control strip from the bottle and immediately recap the bottle.

6. Place the strip in the test tube and cap the tube tightly.

7. Gently invert the test tube back and forth for two minutes.

8. Let the tube stand at room temperature for thirty minutes.

9. Invert the test tube once more and remove and discard the CHEK-STIX strip.
   Note: The resulting reconstituted control should be used with no more than twelve reagent strips.

10. Remove a reagent strip from the bottle and recap the bottle immediately.

11. Note the time, and then dip the reagent strip into the urine, wetting all reagent pad areas. Immerse the reagent strip no longer than one second.

12. Remove the reagent strip from the urine by drawing the edge of the strip along the rim of the specimen container to remove excess urine. Hold the strip horizontally to prevent mixing chemicals from adjacent pads.

13. At the time specified and in good light, hold the reagent strip next to the color chart on the reagent strip bottle (be careful not to let the strip touch and contaminate the chart).

14. Find the colors that match the reagent strip pads and record the results for each test on the urinalysis-control report form.

15. Discard disposable supplies into proper waste container.

16. Disinfect other equipment and return it to storage.

17. Clean the work area following the Universal Precautions.

18. Remove your jacket, gown, or apron, and gloves; wash your hands with disinfectant, and dry them.

OVERALL PROCEDURAL EVALUATION

Student's Name _____

Signature of Instructor _____ Date _____

Comments

CHAPTER 13 REVIEW

Using Terminology

Match the term in the right column with the appropriate definition or description in the left column.

_____ 1. holds reagent strip for reading

_____ 2. known-value specimen

_____ 3. urine chemistry analyzer

a. Clinitek 100
b. strip table
c. urine control

Acquiring Knowledge

Answer the following questions in the spaces provided.

4. What sources of variation do urine chemistry analyzers eliminate?

5. What other advantages are associated with automated urinalysis?

6. Describe the capabilities of the Clinitek 100 Urine Chemistry Analyzer.

7. Describe briefly how the Clinitek 100 is used.

8. What is the difference between semiquantitative and quantitative results?

9. What differences among individuals may cause great variation in their interpretation of reagent strips?

10. How are precision and accuracy affected by variation among workers in the interpretation of reagent strips?

11. How does the Clinitek 100 calibrate itself? How are quality-control tests performed?

12. What two factors in laboratory work produce reliable test results?

_____

13. What is the best way to assure reliability in laboratory testing?

_____

14. How are urine controls prepared for testing?

_____

_____

15. Why can each urine-control sample be used only a limited number of times?

_____

_____

_____

16. What maintenance does the Clinitek 100 require?

_____

_____

_____

17. How does the Clinitek 100 analyzer mark abnormal test results?

_____

18. How is proficiency testing used to maintain quality control in routine urinalysis?

_____

_____

_____

19. What does it mean when proficiency-test results of one POL are significantly different from those of other labs?

_____

_____

_____

20. What are some specific uses of urine controls?

_____

_____

_____

_____

Applying Knowledge—On the Job

Answer the following questions in the spaces provided.

21. Your laboratory has just purchased a urine chemistry analyzer. What are some things you can do to familiarize yourself with the instrument and how it works? What should you do if you run into problems using it?

_____

_____

_____

_____

_____

22. Clarisse has just gotten the printout from the new urine chemistry analyzer for the first batch of samples that she is testing using the new instrument. She cannot find anything on the printout about color or clarity of the samples and fears that the instrument is malfunctioning. What do you think might be the problem?

_____

_____

_____

23. Jason has just one more urine sample to analyze before he is done with work for the day. There are no more reagent strips in the box, so he has to open a new one. The urine control has already been used the specified number of times. Jason decides just to test the urine sample and forgo quality control this one time. What should Jason have done? Why?

_____

_____

_____

_____

UNIT

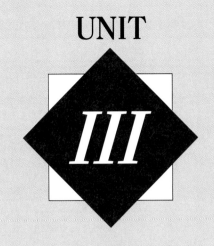

Hematology

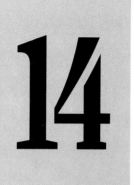

Blood Collection: Methods, Preparation, and Transport

COGNITIVE OBJECTIVES

After studying this chapter, you should be able to

- use each of the vocabulary terms appropriately.
- describe the composition of blood and list its functions.
- distinguish among whole blood, plasma, and serum.
- identify the advantages of the capillary puncture and venipuncture methods of blood drawing.
- discuss when it is best to use the vacutainer and syringe methods of venipuncture.
- list several adverse reactions to blood drawing and describe how to respond to each.
- describe how to centrifuge and store blood samples.

PERFORMANCE OBJECTIVES

After studying this chapter, you should be able to

- draw a blood sample by capillary puncture.
- collect blood by venipuncture using both the vacutainer and syringe methods.

TERMINOLOGY

antecubital: in the inner arm at the bend of the elbow; the most common site for venipuncture.

anticoagulant: an agent that prevents the clotting of blood, such as oxalate, citrate, EDTA, or heparin.

Autolet®: a semiautomatic device with a disposable lancet for capillary puncture.

blood chemistry: the quantitative analysis of the chemical composition of blood.

capillary: a small blood vessel that connects arterioles and venules.

capillary puncture: the puncture of a capillary for the purpose of drawing blood.

cyanotic: blue appearance due to deficiency of oxygen in the blood.

edematous: swollen, due to excess tissue fluid.

hematology: the study of blood cells, blood-forming tissues, and coagulation factors.

hematoma: a subcutaneous mass of blood at a venipuncture site.

hemoconcentration: the concentration of red blood cells due to decreased plasma volume.

hemoglobin (Hgb): the oxygen-carrying molecule of red blood cells.

hemolysis: the breakdown of red blood cells, with the release of hemoglobin into the plasma or serum. Hemolyzed specimens cannot be used for laboratory tests.

icteric: jaundiced; characterized by a high level of bilirubin. Icteric serum and plasma look dark yellow or greenish.

lipemic: having an abnormally high level of fat.

median cephalic vein: one of the major veins of the inner arm. It is used frequently in venipuncture.

median cubital vein: a short vein of the inner arm

just below the elbow. It is used frequently in venipuncture.

microtainer: a blood-collection system used with capillary puncture.

phlebotomy: blood collection by venipuncture.

plasma: the pale yellowish liquid part of whole blood.

platelet: a small round or oval disk in the blood that assists in blood clotting.

serum: the liquid portion of blood remaining after whole blood clots.

serum separator gel: a material added to whole blood to speed clotting. It is used in the preparation of serum.

syringe: an instrument with a needle used for drawing blood from a vein.

tourniquet: a constrictor band used to distend veins to facilitate venipuncture.

vacutainer: a vacuum tube system for drawing blood by venipuncture. It allows multiple samples to be drawn with a single puncture.

venipuncture: the puncture of a vein for therapeutic purposes or for drawing blood.

● ● ● ● ● ● ● ● ● ● ● ● ● ● ● ●

Blood analysis is an important means of diagnosing disease and monitoring patient treatment. It is performed frequently in POLs, so lab workers must know how to collect and handle blood samples properly. Proper technique in blood collection and handling, in turn, requires knowledge of the composition and function of blood.

━━━━━━━━━━━━━━━━━━━━ ◆ ◆

BLOOD COMPOSITION AND FUNCTIONS

Blood is a body tissue made up of plasma and blood cells. **Plasma** is a pale yellowish liquid part of whole blood. Plasma is composed of water, proteins, carbohydrates, lipids, electrolytes, enzymes, vitamins, trace metals, and coagulation factors, which help form blood clots and stop bleeding. Plasma also contains hormones at very low but measurable levels. The blood cells suspended in the plasma include leukocytes, also called white blood cells, erythrocytes, also called red blood cells, and thrombolytes, also called **platelets,** which are involved in clot formation.

Blood performs several functions crucial for life, including transportation of nutrients and oxygen to the cells and removal of waste products from the cells. Blood combats infections and also produces antibodies used by the immune system to defend against foreign antigens.

━━━━━━━━━━━━━━━━━━━━ ◆ ◆

THE ANALYSIS OF BLOOD

In POLs, the analysis of blood usually consists of three components: hematology, serology, and blood chemistry. **Hematology** is the study of blood cells, blood-cell forming tissues, and coagulation factors. Plasma without the protein fibrinogen, which is one of the coagulation factors, is called **serum.** Serum is the liquid portion that remains after whole blood clots. Serology is the study of blood serum. It is concerned primarily with antigen-antibody reactions. **Blood chemistry** is the quantitative analysis of the chemical composition of blood. It measures blood levels of carbohydrates, lipids, proteins, gases such as oxygen and carbon dioxide, electrolytes, hormones, and enzymes.

━━━━━━━━━━━━━━━━━━━━ ◆ ◆

BLOOD-COLLECTION METHODS

Blood samples can be collected by two different methods—**capillary puncture** or **venipuncture.** The method selected depends on the type of test that will be performed as well as the age and condition of the patient. Capillary puncture is the method of choice if only a small quantity of blood is needed. It is also the only method suitable for infants, and it may be preferable for elderly patients. Venipuncture has the advantage of drawing a larger quantity of blood, which may be required for some procedures or if a test must be repeated. Unlike capillary samples, venipuncture samples can be stored for later processing and testing. Although capillary and venous blood are not identical—capillary blood is more like arterial blood—they are close enough to be used interchangeably in most cases.

Both blood-collection methods should be described in detail in the SOP manual of your POL. In addition, blood-collection procedures may be outlined on a wall chart posted by the blood-drawing station. For all blood-collection procedures, the patient should be seated in a blood-collection chair. A blood-collection chair makes venipuncture easier to

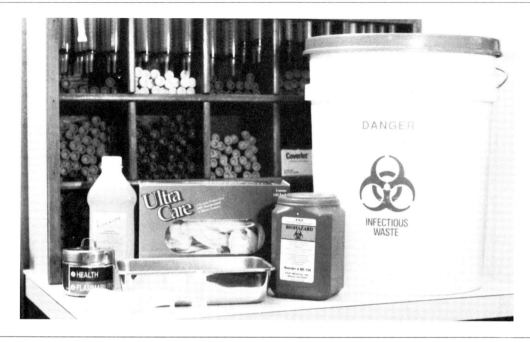

Figure 14.1. A blood-collection station containing supplies. Note the sharps container for biohazardous waste and the disposable latex gloves. Photo by Mark Palko.

perform and more comfortable for the patient. The best type of chair has two armrests, allowing blood to be drawn from either arm. The armrests should adjust to different angles. Using an armrest prevents the patient's elbow from bending back and flattening the vein. Drawers under the armrests keep blood-drawing supplies readily available. Figure 14.1 shows other blood-collection supplies.

◆◆ *Capillary Puncture*

Capillaries are small blood vessels that connect arterioles and venules. As Figure 14.2 shows, sites used to collect capillary blood include fingers, toes, heels, and earlobes. The capillaries are close to the surface of the skin in the fingers and ear lobes. Moist heat on the foot, or massage, increases circulation at the site, making it easier to collect the sample. Areas that are **edematous,** swollen, or **cyanotic,** bluish, should be avoided because blood at these sites may be atypical.

When a finger site is used, the ring finger or middle finger on the left hand in right-handed patients, on the right hand in left-handed patients, should be used. Callouses should be avoided because they are difficult to puncture. The puncture site should be at the tip of and slightly to the side of the finger to cause the least amount of discomfort over the next few

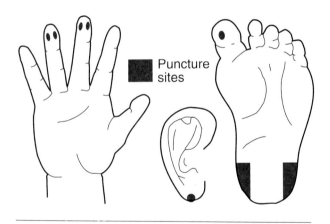

Figure 14.2. Sites for a capillary puncture.

days. In small infants, the fingers are too small to be used for capillary blood collection. The puncture site should be on the side of the heel to avoid hitting the calcaneus, the heel bone (see Figure 14.3).

How It Is Done. Swab the site with alcohol to disinfect it. Allow the alcohol to dry. Residual alcohol will cause stinging and **hemolysis.** Make a puncture about 2 to 3 mm deep with a hand-held blood lancet or with a semiautomatic device, such as an **Autolet®,** which has a disposable lancet. Because capillary blood usually clots quickly, you should have all of the

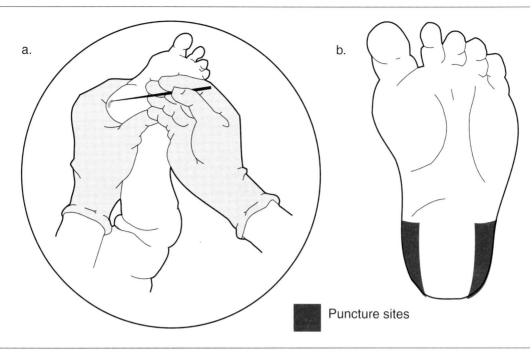

Figure 14.3. An infant capillary puncture. a. Collection of a hematocrit from an infant using the heel as the site of the capillary puncture. Stroke the foot and then warm it before puncture to increase circulation. b. The capillary puncture site in infants should be the sides of the heel to avoid the calcaneus (heel bone). The puncture should not be too deep.

Puncture sites

necessary equipment and supplies at hand before the puncture is made. If the blood is not drawn fast enough to prevent clots from forming, discard the whole sample, because the consistency of the remaining blood is altered. Avoid squeezing the puncture to encourage blood flow. This can produce excess tissue fluid that dilutes the sample. Squeezing also can cause hemolysis (see Figure 14.4).

When the Patient Is a Child. You should be especially patient when collecting a blood specimen from an infant or a child. Assistance is required, preferably from a parent, who can make the child feel more secure. Infants must be held to prevent them from squirming and possibly rolling off the examination table while you are taking the sample. Tell older children that their finger will be stuck, that the stick will hurt a little, and that it is all right to cry. Also tell children that the blood is needed to help the doctor find out what is making them sick. Ask the child to try to hold still so the blood collection will be over more quickly and praise the child for any effort to cooperate.

Particularly useful with infants and children, as well as with geriatric, cancer, and burn patients, is the **Microtainer** capillary whole-blood collector,

> ### ◆ ◆ ◆ Hemolysis ◆ ◆ ◆
>
> Hemolysis releases red-pigmented **hemoglobin (Hgb)**, the oxygen-carrying molecule of red blood cells. The released hemoglobin interferes with the optical reading of chemistry tests. Because hemolysis changes the composition of the plasma or serum, it also prevents accurate results for many other tests, including the complete blood count, hemoglobin determination, hematocrit, and tests for potassium, magnesium, lactic dehydrogenase, and aspartate aminotransferase. For this reason, hemolyzed blood samples generally are discarded. Clearly, then, you should avoid anything that may cause hemolysis of the sample.

shown in Figure 14.5. A widemouthed collector encourages capillary blood to flow quickly and freely into the tube. After collecting the sample to the fill line, remove the collector and seal the tube with a color-coded plug, which permits it to be centrifuged. The color coding indicates whether or not the tube contains an **anticoagulant** to prevent clotting.

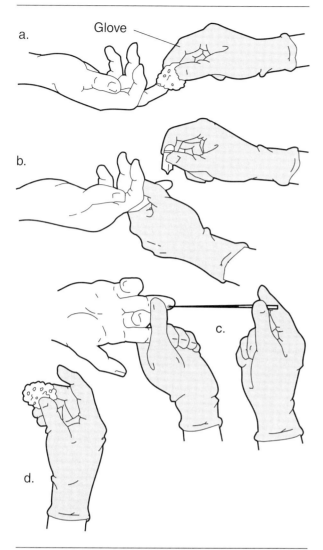

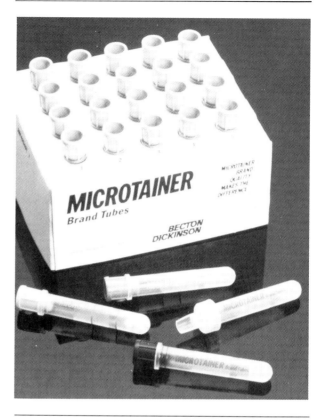

Figure 14.5. Microtainer tubes allow collection of whole blood, serum, or plasma specimens from capillary punctures for use in microchemistry and hematology procedures. Photo courtesy of Fisher Scientific.

Figure 14.4. After collecting supplies for a capillary puncture: a. apply antiseptic to puncture site to disinfect the skin; b. puncture the skin using either an automatic lance or a manual lance; c. collect specimens; d. give the patient a sterile gauze pad or a cotton ball to help control further bleeding.

◆◆ *Venipuncture*

Blood collected by the venipuncture method, also called **phlebotomy,** is taken directly from a vein, most commonly in the **antecubital** area of the arm, that is, the inner arm at the bend of the elbow. The veins used most often are the **median cephalic vein** and the **median cubital vein.** Other sites sometimes used are the lower forearm, the back of the hand, and the wrist. Occasionally, a vein in the foot or ankle may be used.

Venipuncture Tourniquets. A venipuncture **tourniquet** should be used around the upper arm to pool the blood in the veins by preventing its return. The volume of blood pooling in the veins is greater if the patient opens and closes the fist several times. Unlike a blood-pressure cuff, the venipuncture tourniquet should not be applied so tightly that arterial blood flow is cut off. Never leave a tourniquet on longer than two minutes before drawing blood. This can result in **hemoconcentration,** the concentration of red blood cells. Stopping venous blood flow for more than three minutes will increase the cholesterol value by 5 percent compared to a one-minute stoppage. If it is necessary to wait longer than two minutes after putting on the tourniquet, remove the tourniquet and reapply it when ready.

Two types of tourniquets are available. One type has a velcro closing and is available in both child and adult sizes. Although easy to use, velcro-type tourniquets have the serious disadvantage of not being easily disinfected and cleaned because of the velcro material. The other type is a soft, pliable rubber strip,

1 inch × 15 inches, that you simply tie around the arm (see Figure 14.6); one size fits all. Never use rubber tubing as a makeshift tourniquet. It can cut into the arm when applied tightly. Disinfect tourniquets frequently with 70 percent alcohol.

◆ ◆ ◆ Note ◆ ◆ ◆

Release the tourniquet before removing the needle from the vein. Many laboratory workers prefer to release the tourniquet as soon as the blood begins to flow into the syringe or vacutainer.

Which Method to Use. A venipuncture sample can be collected by either **vacutainer** or **syringe**. Both work on the same principle. A vacuum in the tube or syringe pulls the blood out of the vein in which a needle has been inserted. In the case of the vacutainer, the amount of vacuum is predetermined, and a precise amount of blood is collected if the fill line of the tube is reached. The tube is then ready for processing. In the case of the syringe, the plunger of the syringe is withdrawn manually, thus creating a vacuum. The contents of the syringe then must be injected into stoppered tubes before processing.

The vacutainer method usually is preferred because it reduces handling of the blood sample. The syringe, however, is easier to maneuver and requires less cooperation from the patient. The syringe method is preferable when performing venipuncture on children and elderly patients. The intravenous pressure of elderly patients may be so low that the negative pressure in the vacutainer collapses the vein. With the syringe method, the amount of negative pressure created by pulling the plunger of the syringe can be controlled.

Types of Blood-Collection Tubes. If the sample required is whole blood or plasma, an anticoagulant must be added to the blood right after it is collected to prevent coagulation. Anticoagulants used include oxalate, citrate, and EDTA (ethylenediamine tetraacetate), which prevent coagulation by removing calcium ions that are needed for clot formation. Heparin also is used. It prevents coagulation by antagonizing thrombin and thromboplastin, blood components essential in the clotting process.

Venipuncture tubes to which anticoagulant has been added are color coded gray, blue, lavender, or green, depending on which of these four anticoagulants has been added. They are used for whole-blood and plasma samples. Tubes that are red or red/black contain no anticoagulant and are used for serum samples. Blood collection tubes vary in size from 2 to 15 mL. See Table 14.1 for the color codes.

How It Is Done. Always precede venipuncture by explaining the procedure and attempting to reassure the patient. The procedure will go much more easily and quickly if the patient is relaxed and comfortable.

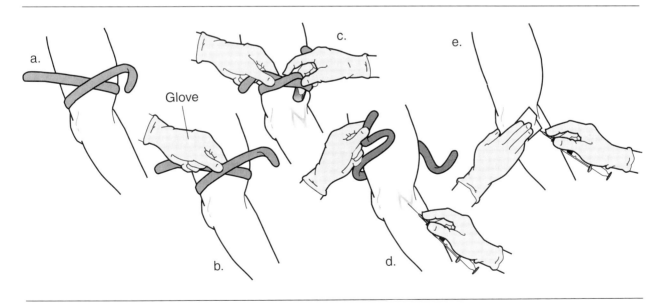

Figure 14.6. To use a tourniquet of flat rubber tubing, follow this procedure: a. and b. Crisscross the tubing snuggly around the arm. c. Make a tuck in the tubing. d. Find the vein and make the venipuncture. Remove the tourniquet by pulling on one end; it will come apart. e. Withdraw the needle and syringe, applying pressure with a gauze square.

Also, make sure that the patient has followed any pretest instructions, such as fasting or abstinence from medication.

Thoroughly examine the vein before sticking the patient. Feel the vein to be sure that it is surrounded by tissue. If it is, it will be easier to puncture. Though easy to find, prominent veins are not necessarily the most suitable. They may have small lumens and roll because they are attached superficially. Sometimes, you can anchor a rolling vein by pressing down on it, holding the thumb and index finger 2 to 5 cm apart. Release the pressure before drawing the blood.

There are several ways to make a vein more prominent for venipuncture, including hanging the arm down at the side for two to three minutes, massaging the vein toward the trunk of the body, and lightly slapping the site to be punctured. Do not attempt venipuncture if you are uncertain of the exact loca-

tion of the vein, and never probe with the needle to find a vein. This is very painful. It is better to try again with another puncture. If the second puncture also fails, seek the help of the physician or someone more experienced at drawing blood.

Figure 14.7 shows the procedures for vacutainer and syringe venipunctures. For the vacutainer method, you insert one end of a double-pointed needle into the vein with the opposite end in a collection tube that has had a predetermined amount of air removed from it. This allows only the proper amount of blood to enter the tube, which is set into a plastic holder. Allow tubes containing anticoagulant to fill until the vacuum is exhausted and the blood flow ceases. This will ensure the correct ratio of anticoagulant to blood.

TABLE 14.1 The Color Codes of Blood-Collection Tubes

Color of Tube Stopper	Laboratory Use	Additive
Gray	Glucose test	Oxalate and fluoride
Blue	Coagulation studies	Citrate
Lavender	Hematology testing	EDTA
Green	Plasma determinations in chemistry	Heparin
Red	Serum testing	None
Red/black or Red	Serum determinations; speeds clot formation	Serum separator gel

Figure 14.7. The procedures for venipuncture. a. Apply a tourniquet and palpate the arm to locate a prominent vein. b. Release the tourniquet to allow a fresh flow of blood. c. Reapply the tourniquet. (It may be necessary to relocate the selected venipuncture site by palpation.) d. Disinfect the venipuncture site, usually with 70 percent isopropyl alcohol on a gauze pad or a cotton ball. e. Enter the vein with bevel of the needle upward and at about a 15 degree angle. f. Puncture the vein using a *syringe*. g. Withdraw blood using the syringe method. h. Puncture the vein using a *vacutainer*. i. Engage the vacuum tube by forcing the covered needle through the rubber stopper of the tube. j. Release the tourniquet *before* withdrawing the needle. k. Cover the needle with a clean gauze pad and withdraw the needle quickly. l. Apply pressure over the puncture site. Have the patient continue to apply pressure for three to five minutes, keeping the arm straight. Put a bandage over the site if the patient wishes.

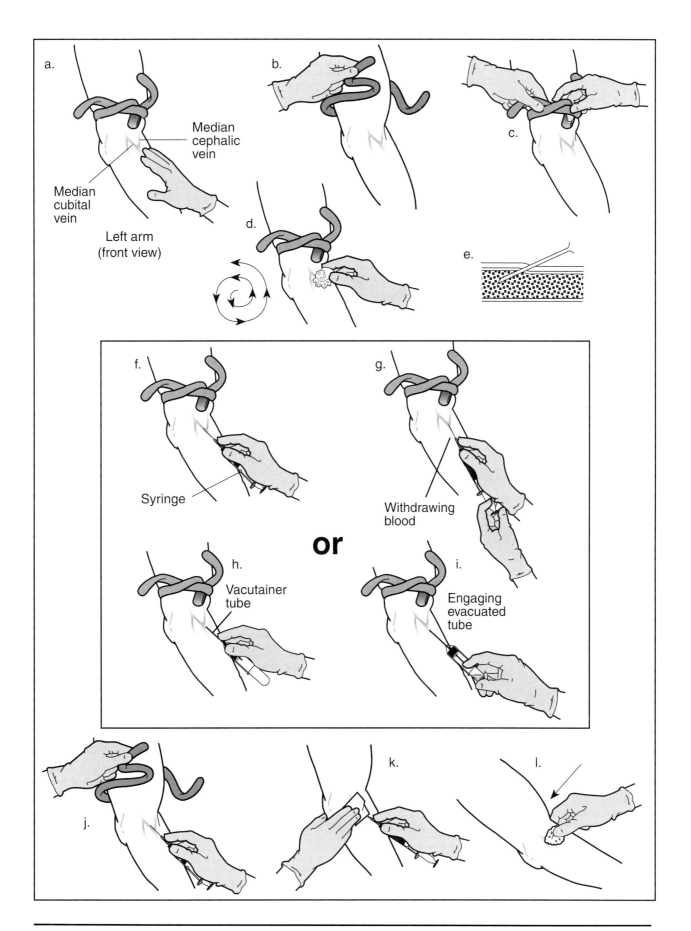

a.

Median cephalic vein

Median cubital vein

Left arm (front view)

b.

c.

d.

e.

f.

Syringe

g.

Withdrawing blood

or

h.

Vacutainer tube

i.

Engaging evacuated tube

j.

k.

l.

When the tube is filled, remove it from the holder and replace it with a new tube while the needle is still in the vein. In this way, you may collect several samples with only one venipuncture. If blood flow is poor, there may be a problem with the vacuum. You should try another tube. If blood flow slows before all of the samples are collected, move the needle slightly backward or forward in the vein, being very careful not to push the needle out the other side of the vein.

For the syringe method of venipuncture, draw blood from a vein with a sterile needle and syringe.

Withdraw the plunger manually to collect the blood. After completing the venipuncture, puncture the stoppers of the vacuum tube with the syringe needle and the vacuum will draw the correct amount of blood into the tubes. Never fill tubes by removing the stoppers. They will no longer be sterile nor will they have the correct vacuum.

Collect tubes without anticoagulant first, then those that have anticoagulant. After filling the latter tubes with blood, invert them eight to ten times to mix the additive through the blood sample. Avoid shaking the tubes because this can hemolyze the blood cells. Label blood specimens with indelible ink when you collect them. Include on the label the date, the time if relevant (for example, glucose-tolerance test samples), and the patient's name and chart number.

When the Patient Is a Child. When performing venipuncture on a child, explain the procedure as well as possible, given the child's age. Also give reassurance and praise. It may be necessary for an assistant to hold the child's arm to stabilize it or even to wrap a bed sheet around the child to prevent movement, with only the arm that is to have the venipuncture exposed. Syringes are easier to use than are vacutainers when working with children. Use a tuberculin syringe or a 3 mL syringe with a 21 to 23 gauge needle.

TABLE 14.2 How to Respond When an Adverse Reaction Occurs

Adverse Reaction	Response
Fainting	Lower the patient's head and arms below the patient's knees; loosen tight clothing; check and record the pulse, blood pressure, and respiration rate. Alert the physician if the patient fails to respond.
Nausea	Tell the patient to take deep breaths and to lower the head. Make the patient comfortable and place a cold cloth on the patient's forehead. Give the patient a basin, tissues, and a glass of water if vomiting occurs. Alert the physician to the patient's condition.
Excessive bleeding	If bleeding continues after the venipuncture, keep pressure over the venipuncture site with a clean gauze pad, changing pads as needed. Alert the physician if bleeding continues past five minutes.
Convulsions	Alert the physician immediately. Do not restrain the convulsing patient except to prevent self-injury. Do not insert anything into the patient's mouth except a soft padded tongue depressor to prevent choking, if needed.
Hematomas	These are usually harmless, but they may alarm the patient. They are less likely if the tourniquet is removed before the needle is withdrawn and if pressure is applied to the puncture site until bleeding has stopped.

Butterfly-Winged Collection Set. An alternate method for drawing blood from a child or infant is to use the Butterfly-Winged Collection Set. This is a device used by the phlebotomist to collect blood samples from pediatric, elderly, neonate, and severely traumatized patients. The butterfly-winged device consists of a needle with plastic wings, plastic tubing and adapter. The easy-to-grasp, flexible wing design allows an entry angle almost parallel to the vein. The needles are extremely short, three-fourths of an inch, and thin gauge to minimize trauma. The adapter attaches directly to evacuated collection tubes, which eliminates messy transfers.

The Appearance of the Blood. Normal venous blood in the collection tube is thick, dull, and dark wine red. In the lab report, note any blood sample that shows marked deviation from normal appearance. For example, if blood is bright red and less viscous, the patient may have anemia.

Adverse Reactions. Drawing blood occasionally triggers adverse reactions in patients who are frightened or weak. Typical adverse reactions include fainting, nausea, vomiting, excessive bleeding, convulsions, and **hematomas,** which are subcutaneous masses of blood. If a patient shows signs of distress, notify the physician immediately and administer appropriate first aid treatment (see Table 14.2). Also make a written report of the incident.

Injectable Training Arm. The Lifeform Injectable Training Arm Simulator (see Figure 14.8) has an internal vascular structure that simulates the large veins of the arm, wrist, and hand. The training arm is useful for practicing venipuncture, especially the vacutainer method. Steadying the plastic holder of the vacutainer while forcing the needle through the rubber stopper of the collection tube takes practice. Practice with the training arm gives trainees the experience and confidence needed to reassure patients.

◆ ◆

HANDLING AND PREPARING BLOOD SAMPLES

Blood samples require proper handling and preparation to ensure lab worker safety and accurate patient-test results.

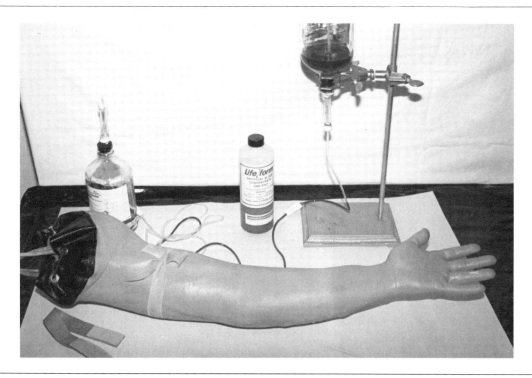

Figure 14.8. Students can perform simulated venipunctures on a practice arm before doing real venipunctures. Photo by Tommy Mumert.

⁘ Lab Worker Safety

As always when working with body fluids, you should assume that all blood is contaminated and should follow the Universal Precautions. Disinfect all work surfaces and equipment and dispose of samples and used supplies appropriately.

⁘ Preserving Sample Integrity

Blood specimens must be handled appropriately to prevent hemolysis and other decomposition. When handling blood specimens, you should always:

- keep the specimen tube in a vertical position and handle it carefully to reduce the risk of spillage, agitation, and hemolysis.
- try not to dislodge clots that stick to the top of the collecting tube. This can cause hemolysis.
- avoid exposing the specimen to light, which decomposes bilirubin and other analytes. Cover clear containers with foil or use amber-colored containers.
- refrigerate specimens at 2 to 8 degrees Celsius if they are to be kept for more than one hour before use.

⁘ Clot Formation in Serum Samples

When a test requires a serum sample, the blood must be allowed to stand until a clot forms. Only then can it be centrifuged. If the collection tube has a red and black mottled stopper, **serum separator gel** has been added to the tube to speed clot formation, and the sample needs to stand at room temperature for five to fifteen minutes. If the collection tube has a red stopper, no serum separator gel has been added, and the sample needs to stand for twenty to thirty minutes at room temperature or for thirty to sixty minutes in the refrigerator.

⁘ Centrifuging Blood Samples

Most centrifuge manufacturers recommend centrifuging blood samples for five to fifteen minutes at 1,000 to 1,200 g, but you always should check the manufacturers' recommendations. Balance sample tubes before starting the centrifuge by placing tubes of equal weight opposite each other. The centrifuge lid must remain down until all spinning has stopped. Never try to stop the centrifuge by opening the lid

and slowing it. This may cause spattering and mixing of tube contents. Clean the centrifuge and disinfect it with a 10 percent bleach solution on a regular basis as well as immediately after spills.

⁘ **Note** ◆ ◆ ◆

Do not recentrifuge blood specimens. This can lead to inaccurate test results.

⁘ Decanting and Storing Blood Samples

After centrifuging, serum samples that contain separator gel have a gel barrier between the blood cells at the bottom of the tube and the serum at the top. The serum can be stored in the refrigerator on the gel barrier for up to forty-eight hours with the tube stoppered. In samples without separator gel, plasma or serum should be pipetted into appropriately labeled tubes within one hour of centrifuging. Take care to avoid pipetting blood cells from the bottom of the tube.

After decanting, keep the tubes stoppered to reduce the risk of evaporation, spillage, and contamination. Use the samples for testing within five hours at room temperature or within forty-eight hours if they are refrigerated in a sealed container. If specimens must be kept longer than forty-eight hours, they should be frozen at −20 degrees Celsius in a freezer that does not have a self-defrost cycle.

The normal appearance of serum or plasma is a clear, straw-colored liquid. If a sample has an abnormal appearance, note this on the lab report. **Lipemic** serum and plasma, for example, appear milky and turbid because they contain a high level of lipids. **Icteric** (jaundiced) serum and plasma look dark yellow or greenish because of a high level of bilirubin. The high level of bilirubin may be due to hepatitis. Icteric samples may be very contagious, so you should handle them with great care.

⁘ Referral Laboratory Samples

Blood, serum, and plasma samples sent to a referral laboratory must be processed, labeled, and transported according to that laboratory's protocol. Referral laboratories frequently furnish collection containers and special handling instructions for such specimens.

PROCEDURE

14.1 ◆

Blood Drawing by Capillary Puncture and Venipuncture Methods

Goal

- After successfully completing this procedure, you will be able to draw blood by capillary puncture and venipuncture methods, the latter using both syringe and vacutainer procedures.

Completion Time

- 3 minutes for Part 1
- 5 minutes for Part 2
- 5 minutes for Part 3

◆◆ *Part 1: The Capillary Puncture Method*

Equipment and Supplies

- impermeable jacket, gown, or apron
- disposable latex gloves
- hand disinfectant
- surface disinfectant
- paper towels and tissues
- biohazard container
- sharps container
- cotton balls and 70 percent isopropyl alcohol or ethyl alcohol swabs
- sterile gauze pads
- Autolet with disposable lancet or manual blood lancet
- capillary tubes and test tube
- Seal-Ease or other clay sealer for capillary tube
- test tube

Instructions

Read through the list of equipment and supplies that you will need and the steps of the procedure. Be sure that you understand each step before you begin. Then complete each step correctly and in the proper order. If your completion time is too long, repeat the procedure until you increase your speed.

S = Satisfactory	U = Unsatisfactory	S	U

1. Put on the jacket, gown, or apron; wash your hands with disinfectant, dry them, and put on gloves.

2. Follow the Universal Precautions.

3. Collect and prepare the appropriate equipment.

4. Verify identification of the patient.

5. Explain the capillary blood-collection procedure to the patient and encourage the patient to relax the arm in order to increase blood flow into the hand.

6. Select an appropriate finger site and clean it with alcohol. Rubbing will improve circulation.

7. Dry the site thoroughly with a gauze pad to remove any residual alcohol.

8. Hold the patient's finger in one hand and apply gentle pressure.

9. Quickly puncture the site with the lancet.

10. Wipe off the first drop of blood with a dry gauze pad. This drop may contain tissue fluid that will dilute the sample.

11. Collect the specimen in the capillary tube. Gently massaging the finger may increase blood flow, but avoid squeezing.

12. Place a dry gauze pad over the puncture site and ask the patient to hold it on with light pressure to stop the bleeding.

13. Seal the capillary tube and place it in a test tube labeled with the patient's name and identification number, the date, and the time.

14. Ask the patient to return to the examination room.

	S	U
15. Discard disposable equipment and supplies.		
16. Disinfect other equipment and return it to storage.		
17. Clean the work area following the Universal Precautions.		
18. Remove your gloves and apron; wash your hands with disinfectant, and dry them.		

✦✦ *Part 2: The Venipuncture Method Using a Vacutainer*

◆ Equipment and Supplies

- impermeable jacket, gown, or apron
- disposable latex gloves
- hand disinfectant
- surface disinfectant
- paper towels and tissues
- biohazard container
- sharps container
- cotton balls and 70 percent isopropyl alcohol or ethyl alcohol swabs
- sterile gauze pads
- venipuncture tourniquet
- evacuated tube holder
- evacuated tubes with rubber stoppers
- sterile, disposable double-pointed needle (20 to 22 gauge, 1 to 1.5 inches long)
- bandage

◆ Instructions

Read through the list of equipment and supplies that you will need and the steps of the procedure. Be sure that you understand each step before you begin. Then complete each step correctly and in the proper order. If your completion time is too long, repeat the procedure until you increase your speed.

S = Satisfactory	U = Unsatisfactory	S	U

1. Wash your hands with disinfectant, dry them, and put on gloves and apron.

2. Follow the Universal Precautions.

3. Collect and prepare the appropriate equipment.

4. Verify identification of the patient.

5. Explain the venipuncture blood-collection procedure to the patient and encourage the patient to relax.

6. Remove the cover from the short end of the needle, screw the short end into the barrel of the plastic holder and tighten it firmly. Do not remove the cover from the long end of the needle because it must remain sterile.

7. Place the evacuated tube in the plastic holder until the short end of the needle touches the rubber stopper. Do not push the needle into the rubber stopper yet.

8. Place the tourniquet around the patient's arm above the elbow. If you cannot feel a pulse at the wrist, loosen the tourniquet.

9. Have the patient open and close the fist several times to increase the volume of blood in the veins.

10. Select a suitable vein by inspection and palpation. Determine the direction that the vein is running and its depth.

11. Clean the site with alcohol, starting at the center and moving in a circular path toward the outside, using as many cotton balls or swabs as needed.

12. Remove any residual alcohol with a gauze pad.

13. Tell the patient to make a tight fist and to hold the arm straight, resting it on the armrest of the blood-collection chair or on a table or counter for support.

14. Now remove the cover from the long needle. Grasp the vacutainer plastic holder with your right hand if you are right-handed, or with your left hand if you are left-handed, and place your index finger on the hub of the needle to guide it.

15. Grasp the patient's forearm with your other hand about 2 cm below the area to be punctured and hold the skin taut with your thumb and forefinger.

16. Hold the needle at a 15 degree angle to the vein with the bevel facing up. Insert the needle through the skin immediately adjacent to the vein to be punctured.

17. After you have penetrated the skin, hold the vacutainer holder still and push the tube all the way in to engage the vacuum.

18. Move the needle parallel to the vein, guiding it into the lumen of the vein. As the needle enters the vein, you will feel a slight "give" and see blood begin to flow into the vacutainer tube.

19. Release the tourniquet and tell the patient to open the hand.

20. After sufficient blood has filled the tube, you may collect other tubes by simply changing tubes. Do not remove the needle from the vein until you have collected all samples.

21. Cover the puncture site with a gauze pad and remove the needle quickly.

22. Have the patient press the gauze pad over the wound with the other hand for three to five minutes, keeping the arm straight.

23. Remove the tube from the vacutainer plastic holder. Gently invert the tube several times if it contains anticoagulant.

24. Label the tube with the patient's name and identification number, the date, and the time.

25. Check the puncture site to see if the bleeding has stopped. If so, apply a bandage and tell the patient to leave it on for an hour.

26. Ask the patient to return to the examination room.

27. Using safety precautions, remove the needle from the plastic holder and discard it directly into the sharps container. Do not recap the needle first.

28. Discard disposable equipment and supplies.

29. Disinfect other equipment and return it to storage.

30. Clean the work area following the Universal Precautions.

31. Remove your gloves and apron; wash your hands with disinfectant, and dry them.

◆◆ *Part 3: The Venipuncture Method Using a Syringe*

◆ Equipment and Supplies

- impermeable jacket, gown, or apron
- disposable latex gloves
- hand disinfectant
- surface disinfectant
- paper towels and tissues
- biohazard container
- sharps container
- cotton balls and 70 percent isopropyl alcohol or ethyl alcohol swabs
- sterile gauze pads
- venipuncture tourniquet
- evacuated tube with rubber stopper
- sterile, disposable syringe
- sterile needle (20 to 22 gauge, 1 to 1.5 inches long)
- bandage

◆ Instructions

Read through the list of equipment and supplies that you will need and the steps of the procedure. Be sure that you understand each step before you begin. Then complete each step correctly and in the proper order. If your completion time is too long, repeat the procedure until you increase your speed.

S = Satisfactory U = Unsatisfactory	S	U
1. Wash your hands with disinfectant, dry them, and put on gloves and apron.		
2. Follow the Universal Precautions.		
3. Collect and prepare the appropriate equipment.		
4. Verify identification of the patient.		
5. Explain the venipuncture blood-collection procedure to the patient and encourage the patient to relax.		
6. Remove the disposable syringe from the wrapper. If the needle is a separate unit, remove its wrapper but leave on the plastic sheath so that the needle will remain sterile.		
7. Place the tourniquet around the patient's arm above the elbow. If you cannot feel a pulse at the wrist, loosen the tourniquet.		
8. Have the patient open and close the fist several times to increase the volume of blood in the veins.		
9. Select a suitable vein by inspection and palpation. Determine the direction that the vein is running and its depth.		
10. Clean the site with alcohol, starting at the center and moving in a circular path toward the outside, using as many cotton balls or swabs as needed.		
11. Remove any residual alcohol with a gauze pad.		

12. Tell the patient to make a tight fist and to hold the arm straight, resting it on the armrest of the blood-collection chair or on a table or counter for support.

13. Grasp the syringe with your right hand if you are right-handed, or with your left hand if you are left-handed, and place your index finger on the hub of the needle to guide it.

14. Grasp the patient's forearm with your other hand about 2 cm below the area to be punctured and hold the skin taut with your thumb and forefinger.

15. Hold the needle at a 15 degree angle to the vein with the bevel facing up. Insert the needle through the skin immediately adjacent to the vein to be punctured.

16. Move the needle parallel to the vein, guiding it into the lumen of the vein. As the needle enters the vein, you will feel a slight "give."

17. Pull back on the plunger of the syringe to create a vacuum. You will see blood begin to flow into the syringe.

18. Release the tourniquet and tell the patient to open the hand. Draw the amount of blood required by your instructor.

19. Cover the site with a gauze pad and remove the needle quickly.

20. Have the patient press the gauze pad over the wound with the other hand for three to five minutes, keeping the arm straight.

21. Transfer the blood from the syringe to the tube, taking care not to puncture yourself when you push the needle through the rubber stopper. Gently invert the tube several times if it contains anticoagulant.

22. Label the tube with the patient's name and identification number, the date, and the time.

23. Check the puncture site to see if the bleeding has stopped. If so, apply a bandage and tell the patient to leave it on for an hour.

24. Ask the patient to return to the examination room.

25. Discard the syringe and needle directly into the sharps container. Do not recap the needle first.

26. Discard disposable equipment and supplies.

27. Disinfect other equipment and return it to storage.

28. Clean the work area following the Universal Precautions.

29. Remove your jacket, gown, or apron, and your gloves; wash your hands with disinfectant, and dry them.

OVERALL PROCEDURAL EVALUATION

Student's Name _____

Signature of Instructor _____ Date _____

Comments

Using Terminology

Define the following terms in the spaces provided.

1. Anticoagulant: _____

   _____

2. Antecubital: _____

   _____

3. Capillary: _____

   _____

4. Hematology: _____

   _____

5. Hematoma: _____

   _____

6. Autolet: _____

   _____

7. Blood chemistry: _____

   _____

8. Plasma: _____

   _____

9. Hemoglobin (Hgb): _____

   _____

10. Infant capillary puncture site: _____

    _____

11. Capillary puncture: _____

    _____

12. Hemoconcentration: _____

    _____

13. Venipuncture: _____

    _____

Match the term in the right column with the appropriate definition or description in the left column.

_____ 14. the breakdown of red blood cells

_____ 15. capillary blood collector

_____ 16. EDTA

_____ 17. having a high fat level

_____ 18. involved in clotting

_____ 19. jaundiced

_____ 20. the liquid part of clotted blood

_____ 21. used for venipuncture

a. anticoagulant
b. hemolysis
c. icteric
d. lipemic
e. platelet
f. serum
g. microtainer
h. vacutainer

Acquiring Knowledge

Answer the following questions in the spaces provided.

22. What are capillaries?

_____

_____

_____

_____

23. How is a capillary puncture made?

_____

_____

_____

24. How should needles, lancets, and syringes be disposed of?

_____

25. Why is a tourniquet used in venipuncture?

_____

_____

26. What does the color coding on the stoppers of blood-collection tubes mean?

_____

_____

_____

27. What is the role of separator gel in blood processing in POLs?

_____

_____

_____

28. How are cells (leukocytes, platelets, and erythrocytes) separated from the liquid portion of blood?

_____

29. What is the preferred site for venipuncture?

_____

30. Where can you obtain information about how to process and transport patient specimens for a referral laboratory?

_____

31. How are serum and plasma similar? How are they different?

_____

_____

_____

32. At what point during blood collection should a specimen be labeled? Why?

_____

_____

33. What are the advantages of a blood-collection chair?

_____

_____

_____

34. Where should you place a venipuncture tourniquet? How long should you leave it on?

_____

_____

_____

35. When should you use a syringe for venipuncture? Why?

_____

_____

_____

36. Why is heparin added to some blood samples?

_____

_____

37. Why should you select a finger that is not calloused for a capillary puncture?

_____

_____

38. Why should you not squeeze a finger-stick site?

_____

_____

_____

39. What information should you include on a blood-specimen label?

_____

_____

_____

40. When performing a venipuncture, when should you release the tourniquet? Why?

_____

_____

_____

41. Why are the Universal Precautions important in blood collection?

_____

_____

_____

42. Why does hemolysis ruin a blood sample?

_____

_____

_____

43. What adverse patient reactions to venipuncture require immediate attention?

_____

_____

_____

Applying Knowledge—On the Job

Answer the following questions in the spaces provided.

44. Assume that you are employed by a POL as a phlebotomist. An elderly patient has returned after a recent phlebotomy with a large bruise at the puncture site. She is very alarmed. Explain to her why a hematoma may occur after a venipuncture. What steps should have been taken to minimize the chance of a hematoma?

_____

_____

_____

_____

45. Your first phlebotomy patient on the first day of your first job has a chronic disease requiring frequent drawing of blood by venipuncture. What should you do first? Why?

_____

_____

_____

_____

46. You have just completed a venipuncture. The patient begins to jerk uncontrollably. He appears to be having a seizure. What do you do?

_____

_____

_____

_____

47. You are requested to obtain a small amount of blood from an infant. What blood-drawing method should you use? Where and how should you make the puncture? What precautions should you take for the child's safety?

_____

_____

_____

_____

_____

_____

CHAPTER 15

Hemoglobin and Hematocrit: Manual Procedures

COGNITIVE OBJECTIVES

After studying this chapter, you should be able to

- use each of the vocabulary terms appropriately.
- list the blood tests performed as part of the complete blood count.
- describe the structure, synthesis, and functions of normal hemoglobin.
- identify three types of abnormal hemoglobin and describe the health problems caused by sickle-cell hemoglobin.
- explain how the specific gravity of blood provides an indirect assessment of hemoglobin concentration.
- distinguish between hemoglobin concentration and hematocrit and give normal values for each.
- explain how hemoglobin concentration and hematocrit values are used to assess the health of patients.

PERFORMANCE OBJECTIVES

After studying this chapter, you should be able to

- use the Unopette system for the cyanmethemoglobin test to measure the hemoglobin concentration of a blood specimen.
- perform a microhematocrit by the manual method from a whole-blood specimen.

TERMINOLOGY

adult hemoglobin: hemoglobin A.

anemia: the condition in which there is a deficiency in the amount of hemoglobin in the blood, thus reducing the oxygen-carrying capacity of the blood.

arthralgia: joint pain.

buffy coat: the 0.5 to 1.0 mm thick, whitish-tan layer of white blood cells and platelets that forms between the packed red blood cells and plasma when whole blood is centrifuged.

carotenemia: the presence of carotene in the blood.

complete blood count (CBC): a battery of hematological tests often requisitioned in POLs. It includes hemoglobin concentration, hematocrit, red and white blood-cell counts, differential white blood-cell count, and sometimes erythrocyte indices.

Drabkin's reagent: a solution of potassium ferricyanide and sodium cyanide that is used to convert hemoglobin to cyanmethemoglobin in tests of hemoglobin concentration.

erythropoiesis: the formation of red blood cells.

erythropoietin: the kidney hormone that triggers red blood-cell formation. It is produced whenever hemoglobin concentration or oxygen saturation declines.

fetal hemoglobin: hemoglobin F.

hematocrit (Hct or "crit"): the volume of red blood cells packed by centrifugation in a given volume of blood. It is given as a percent.

hematological test: a blood test, including hematocrit, hemoglobin concentration, and red and white blood-cell counts, among others.

hemoglobin A: the normal adult hemoglobin. It develops by six months of age to replace hemo-globin F, or fetal hemoglobin.

hemoglobin C: an abnormal hemoglobin that is rel-atively common in African-Americans. It causes chronic hemolytic anemia, splenomeg-aly, arthralgia, and abdominal pain.

hemoglobin E: an abnormal hemoglobin that is prevalent in India, Southeast Asia, and South-east Asian refugees in the United States. It causes a mild form of hemolytic anemia.

hemoglobin F: fetal hemoglobin. This hemoglobin is found in fetuses and infants until six months of age. It is replaced by hemoglobin A, or adult hemoglobin.

hemoglobin S: sickle-cell hemoglobin.

hemoglobin S-C disease: the disease in individuals heterozygous for hemoglobin S and C. The symptoms, which usually appear after age 40, include hematuria and pain in the bones, joints, abdomen, and chest.

hemoglobinopathy: any disease caused by abnormal hemoglobin.

hemolytic anemia: the anemia that is due to the breakdown of red blood cells.

heterozygous: pertaining to the inheritance of differ-ent forms of a gene from each parent.

homozygous: pertaining to the inheritance of the same form of a gene from each parent.

hyperbilirubinemia: the presence of a high level of bilirubin in the blood.

hypochromic: low in hemoglobin.

iron-deficiency anemia: the anemia resulting from lack of available iron in the body.

leukemia: a disease characterized by unrestrained production of white blood cells.

lipemia: the presence of an abnormal amount of fat in the blood.

microhematocrit: a method of determining the he-matocrit. It uses just two or three drops of blood collected in a capillary tube.

Sahli pipette: a glass pipette that dispenses 20 μL, or 0.02 mL.

sickle-cell anemia: a life-threatening disease that oc-curs in individuals homozygous for the sickle-cell hemoglobin gene.

sickle-cell hemoglobin: the most common type of ab-normal hemoglobin in the United States. It is found primarily in African-Americans. Sickle-cell hemoglobin is so named because it causes

red blood cells to become sickle shaped under conditions of low oxygen tension, thus pro-ducing sickle-cell anemia.

splenomegaly: the enlargement of the spleen. Spleno-megaly is due to abnormal hemoglobin, among other possible causes.

stromatolytic agent: a compound that helps break down the spongy protoplasmic framework of cells such as red blood cells.

• • • • • • • • • • • • • • • • •

After urinalysis, tests on blood, or **hematological tests,** are the most frequently performed tests in POLs. Hematological tests provide valuable informa-tion about many aspects of the body in both normal and disease states.

_____ ◆ ◆

HEMATOLOGICAL PROCEDURES

The hematological requisition seen most often in POLs is the **complete blood count, CBC.** A CBC usu-ally includes the following hematological tests, which are described in this and subsequent chapters:

- _hemoglobin concentration:_ the weight of hemo-globin in grams per deciliter of whole blood.

- _hematocrit:_ the volume (percent) of red blood cells packed by centrifugation in a given volume of blood.

- _white blood-cell count:_ the number of white blood cells per cubic millimeter of blood (see Chapter 16).

- _differential white blood-cell count:_ the percent of each type of white blood cell seen on a stained blood smear (see Chapter 17).

- _red blood-cell count:_ the number of red blood cells per cubic millimeter of blood (see Chapter 16).

Note: Erythrocyte indices, described in Chapter 18, are sometimes included in the CBC.

While all of the preceding tests can be performed manually, increasingly they are performed with au-tomated hematology analyzers, which use mod-ifications of the manual methods. To improve your understanding of the automated procedures that you will most likely use on the job, this chap-ter and the next two chapters describe the manual methods.

HEMOGLOBIN

Some of the most frequently requisitioned hematological tests in POLs determine the amount of hemoglobin in the blood. To understand the tests and to know how to interpret the results, you should know more about this important blood protein.

◆◆ Normal Structure, Synthesis, and Function

Hemoglobin is the major component of red blood cells, comprising about 85 percent of their dry weight. Each hemoglobin molecule consists of four polypeptide chains, called globin chains, with a heme molecule attached to each chain, as Figure 15.1 shows. One oxygen molecule (O_2) can attach to each heme molecule. The central ion of each heme molecule is an iron atom, so synthesis of each heme portion of the hemoglobin molecule requires iron. The source is dietary iron, which is absorbed in the duodenum of the small intestine.

Hemoglobin is produced by the endoplasmic reticula of red blood cells in the early stages of **erythropoiesis,** the formation of red blood cells. Figure 15.2 illustrates erythropoiesis. When new red blood cells are released from bone marrow into the circulating blood, hemoglobin molecules are present and functioning.

The primary role of hemoglobin in the blood is to transport oxygen from the lungs to the cells. About 95 percent of the oxygen in the body is transported by the hemoglobin molecule. The remaining 5 percent is dissolved in the plasma. Oxygen binds to the iron in the hemoglobin molecule, forming the molecule oxyhemoglobin, $HgbO_2$.

A deficiency in circulating hemoglobin produces a condition called **anemia.** Anemia will result if any of the following occur:

- a reduction in the number of circulating red blood cells.
- a decrease in the amount of hemoglobin per red blood cell.
- a defect in the hemoglobin molecule.

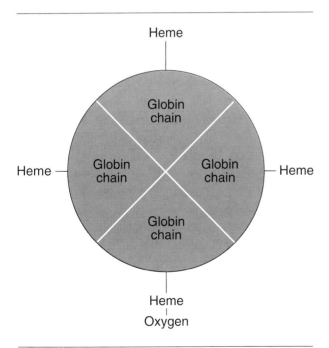

Figure 15.1. Normal hemoglobin molecule with an oxygen molecule attached to one heme molecule.

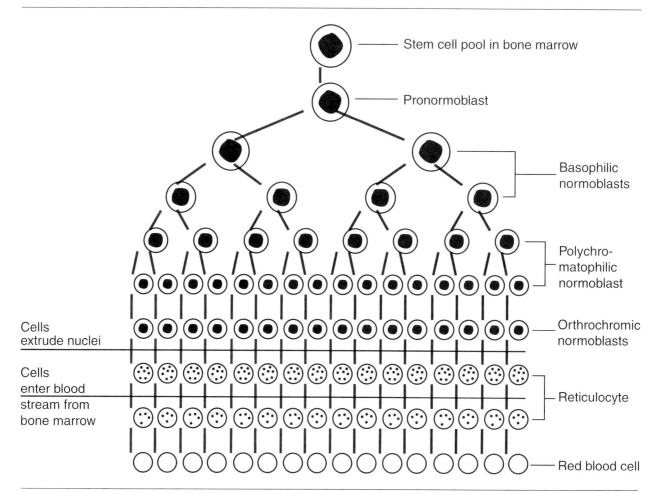

Figure 15.2. The stages of red blood-cell formation, beginning in the bone marrow. The maturation time and life span for erythropoiesis are as follows: development from pronormoblast to release of reticulocyte from bone marrow = 72 hours; final development of reticulocyte in blood stream = 1–2 days; life span of mature, circulating red blood cell = 120 days.

Anemia is not a disease in itself; it is a sign of underlying disease, just as an inflamed throat or a fever may be a sign of underlying viral infection. One cause of anemia is lack of available iron in the body. The amount of iron required varies from about 0.5 mg per day for adult males to 2 mg per day for menstruating females. Without adequate iron, hemoglobin production is hampered, and red blood cells have a lower than normal concentration of hemoglobin. The result is **iron-deficiency anemia.** It is usually treated with iron supplements.

Regardless of the cause, all patients with serious anemia are likely to be weak, easily fatigued, and prone to fainting because of reduced oxygen transport. They may be pale and have low blood pressure because of reduced blood volume. They may have heart palpitations or even congestive heart failure because of increased cardiac output.

•• *Abnormal Hemoglobins*

There are a number of relatively common forms of abnormal hemoglobin, including hemoglobins S, C, and E. All are controlled by codominant genes. Individuals who inherit two copies of one of these abnormal hemoglobin genes are said to be **homozygous.** They have only abnormal hemoglobin and suffer from **hemoglobinopathy,** or disease caused by abnormal hemoglobin. Invariably, they are anemic to some degree. Individuals with one abnormal gene and one normal gene are said to be **heterozygous.** They have enough normal hemoglobin to function without disease, but they are carriers of the abnormal gene, which they may pass on to their children.

Abnormal hemoglobins are most common in the parts of the world where the blood-borne disease malaria is prevalent. Heterozygous individuals tend to be partially resistant to malaria without suffering the harmful effects of abnormal hemoglobin. An increase in the frequency of these abnormal genes occurs in tropical Africa and Southeast Asia. This situation explains why, in the U.S. population, African-Americans and Southeast Asian refugees are at relatively high risk for hemoglobinopathies.

♦ ♦ ♦ Screening for ♦ ♦ ♦ Abnormal Hemoglobin

Most screening for abnormal hemoglobin is postponed until after six months of age because fetuses and young infants have a different form of hemoglobin than do older children and adults. It is called **fetal hemoglobin**, or **hemoglobin F**. It differs in structure from normal **adult hemoglobin**, called **hemoglobin A**.

Sickle-Cell Hemoglobin. Sickle-cell hemoglobin, or **hemoglobin S**, is the most common type of abnormal hemoglobin seen in the United States, occurring mainly in African-Americans. Individuals homozygous for the gene for hemoglobin S have the life-threatening disease **sickle-cell anemia**. Hemoglobin S causes red blood cells to become sickle, or crescent, shaped when oxygen is taken up from the red blood cells by the surrounding tissues. This shape leads to obstruction of smaller blood vessels and destruction of the red blood cells by the body's own immune response. Severe **hemolytic anemia** results, that is, anemia due to the breakdown of red blood cells. Numerous other problems also result, including hyperplasia of bone marrow, impaired mental function, poor physical development, and damage to the heart, brain, joints, lungs, and kidneys.

Other Abnormal Hemoglobins. Another type of abnormal hemoglobin relatively common in African-Americans is **hemoglobin C**, which causes chronic hemolytic anemia, **splenomegaly**—an enlarged spleen, **arthralgia**—joint pains, and abdominal pain. **Hemoglobin E** is prevalent in India and Southeast Asia, and in Southeast Asian refugees in the United States. It causes a mild form of hemolytic anemia.

Some people inherit two different forms of abnormal hemoglobin, hemoglobin S and hemoglobin C. This combination produces **hemoglobin S-C disease**. The symptoms, which are not life threatening, include hematuria—blood in the urine—and pain in the bones, joints, abdomen, and chest. Symptoms may not appear until the patient is in middle age.

♦♦ Measuring Hemoglobin Concentration

The hemoglobin concentration, g/dL, of whole blood is measured routinely as part of the complete blood count. Hemoglobin concentration alone may be measured if the doctor suspects that a patient is anemic. The most common test to measure hemoglobin concentration is the cyanmethemoglobin test. There is also a specific-gravity test that provides an estimate of hemoglobin concentration.

The Specific-Gravity Test. The specific gravity of blood provides an estimate of hemoglobin concentration because the specific gravity of blood is largely determined by the amount of hemoglobin that it contains. The specific-gravity test commonly is used to screen patients in public health agencies and blood banks.

The specific-gravity test determines if a single drop of a patient's blood is dense enough to fall in a copper sulfate solution of known density. The test result is normal when the drop of blood falls through the copper sulfate solution without hesitating or rising, indicating that the blood has at least as great a density as the solution. Two different copper sulfate solutions are used. One solution, which is used for testing samples from females, has the same density as blood with 37 percent red cells—the normal value for females. The other solution, which has the same density as blood with 40 percent red blood cells—the normal value for males—is used for testing samples from males.

The Cyanmethemoglobin Test. The concentration of hemoglobin in the blood is assessed most often in POLs with the cyanmethemoglobin test. It replaces earlier methods, which were less objective and less precise.

♦ ♦ ♦ Historical Note ♦ ♦ ♦

In the 1930s and 1940s, hemoglobin concentration was estimated by matching untreated blood samples to a color scale such as the Tallqvist and Dare methods. Another method, the Sahli-Hellige and Haden-Hausser method, used 1 percent hydrochloric acid solution to convert hemoglobin to hematin. Then, a hemoglobinometer was used to match the sample with a color standard. A later method converted hemoglobin to oxyhemoglobin by adding ammonium hydroxide. The resulting solution was read with a photoelectric colorimeter.

In the cyanmethemoglobin test, hemoglobin first is converted to cyanmethemoglobin by the addition of **Drabkin's reagent,** a solution of potassium ferricyanide and sodium cyanide. A blood-to-reagent ratio of 1:250 is made by adding 0.02 mL of blood in a **Sahli pipette** to 5.0 mL of reagent. The diluted sample is stable for twenty-four hours at either room temperature or 4 degrees Celsius, but it must be protected from light to prevent fading of the color. The sample must stand at room temperature for at least ten minutes so that the Drabkin's reagent can lyse the red blood cells and release the hemoglobin.

♦ ♦ ♦ Danger! ♦ ♦ ♦

Drabkin's solution is poisonous. Use it with caution.

The solution is read photometrically using a spectrophotometer at a wavelength of 540 nm. If the solution is cloudy, due, for example, to precipitation of globulins or the presence of nonhemolyzed red cells, it should be centrifuged before spectrophotometric analysis. Otherwise, the reading will be too high. Also, the spectrophotometer cell must be clean and free of fingerprints to avoid falsely high readings.

The absorbance value of the patient sample is compared with that of a standard of known hemoglobin concentration. The following formula is used to calculate the hemoglobin concentration of the patient sample:

$$C_u = \frac{A_u}{A_s} \times C_s$$

where,

C_u = unknown concentration of the patient sample

A_u = absorbance of the patient sample

C_s = concentration of the standard

A_s = absorbance of the standard

Absorbance values for patient samples also can be located on a graph constructed from a set of hemoglobin standard solutions. The corresponding hemoglobin concentration can be read from the abscissa, or horizontal axis, of the graph. Control samples of known hemoglobin concentration should be measured each day to verify that the graph is correct.

Be aware that a number of blood conditions can cause falsely high hemoglobin readings. They include:

- **hyperbilirubinemia:** the presence of a high level of bilirubin in the blood
- **lipemia:** the presence of an abnormal amount of fat in the blood
- **leukemia:** a disease characterized by unrestrained production of white blood cells
- **carotenemia:** the presence of carotene in the blood

A high bilirubin value in neonatal jaundice, for example, can cause up to a 20 percent increase in the test result compared with the true value.

♦ ♦ ♦ Note ♦ ♦ ♦

Unopette systems are now used in all manual procedures in POLs for hemoglobin and blood-cell counts. They have totally replaced pipettes because they are more accurate and eliminate the need for a suction apparatus to make the dilution.

Unopette System. The Unopette system for the cyanmethemoglobin test uses a premeasured amount—

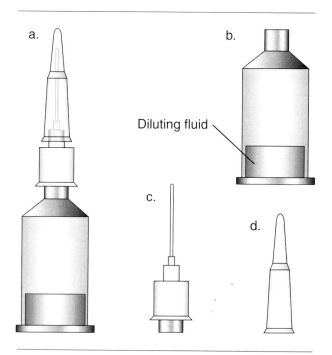

Figure 15.3. A Unopette disposable blood-diluting unit. a. A complete assembled unit. b. The reservoir with premeasured diluting fluid, sealed with a diaphragm. c. The capillary pipette with an overflow chamber and capacity marking. d. A pipette shield. Courtesy of Becton Dickinson VACUTAINER Systems.

TABLE 15.1 Normal Values for Hemoglobin Concentration

Age/Sex Group	Normal Hgb Concentration (g/dL)
Adult males	14 to 18
Adult females	12 to 16
Newborns	17 to 23
Three-month-olds	9 to 14
Ten-year-olds	12 to 14.5

4.98 mL—of modified Drabkin's reagent, called Uno-heme, in a disposable prefilled reservoir, as Figure 15.3 shows. The Unopette system also contains a 20 μL capillary pipette for collecting the blood sample and a pipette shield. The premeasured units of reagent and blood produce the same ratio of blood to reagent as does the standard method—1:250.

The Unopette system is available with a modified Uno-heme solution for use when the red blood cells in the patient sample are **hypochromic**—low in hemoglobin—or contain abnormal hemoglobin. The modified reagent contains a **stromatolytic agent** that helps break down the spongy protoplasmic framework of the red blood cells, which will not hemolyze completely with standard Drabkin's reagent.

The Normal Values for Hemoglobin Concentration. The normal values for hemoglobin concentration vary by age and sex. See Table 15.1.

♦ ♦

THE HEMATOCRIT

The **hematocrit** (Hct or "crit") is a simple yet reliable test to measure the percent volume of red blood cells per volume of whole blood. Given as a percent, it is often used as an indirect measure of hemoglobin. In POLs, a **microhematocrit** method is used because it requires only two or three drops of blood. There is also a macrohematocrit method, which requires one milliliter of blood.

♦♦ *Cellular Layers*

To measure the volume of red blood cells, you first must separate them from other blood components by high-speed centrifugation. During centrifugation, the

red blood cells are packed at the bottom of the tube, as Figure 15.4 shows. On top of the red blood cells are white blood cells and platelets, which form a 0.5 to 1.0 mm thick, whitish-tan layer called the **buffy coat.** Finally, plasma is at the top of the tube.

♦♦ *The Microhematocrit Method*

Figure 15.5 illustrates the microhematocrit method. Either capillary puncture or venipuncture can be used to obtain microhematocrit blood samples. Duplicate samples always should be run as a quality-control measure, and the results should be averaged. The two test results should agree within 2 percentage points.

Heparinized capillary tubes should be used when

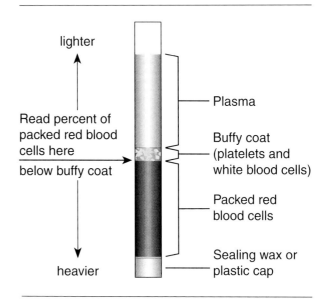

lighter

Read percent of packed red blood cells here below buffy coat

heavier

Plasma

Buffy coat (platelets and white blood cells)

Packed red blood cells

Sealing wax or plastic cap

Figure 15.4. The layers of centrifuged blood.

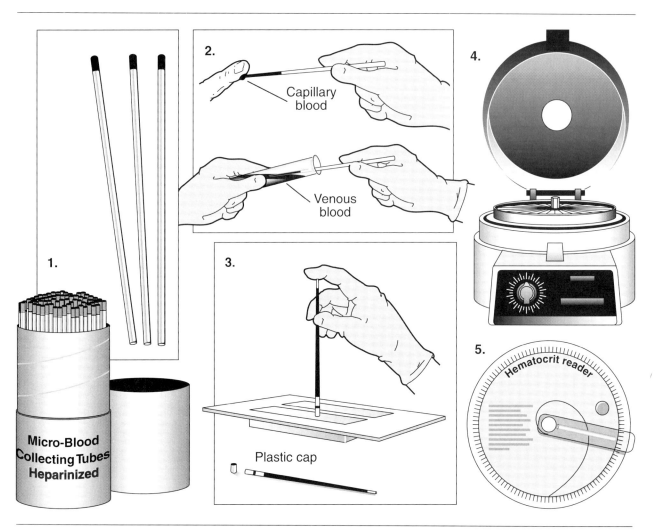

Figure 15.5. The microhematocrit method: 1. Collect the necessary supplies. Use heparinized capillary tubes for a capillary collection and nonheparinized tubes for venipuncture. 2. Collect the blood sample by either capillary puncture or venipuncture. 3. Seal the end of the capillary tube with clay or a plastic cap. 4. Place the samples in a microhematocrit centrifuge. Fasten both the inner and outer covers securely, and centrifuge the samples for the specified time. 5. Read the percent of red cells on the hematocrit reader and record the results.

collecting capillary blood samples. They are filled about three-fourths full. If venous blood is used, it should be collected in an EDTA anticoagulant tube, lavender stopper. The blood is transferred to nonheparinized plain capillary tubes, which are filled about three-fourths full. The clean end of the tube is sealed with clay or a plastic cap. A gloved index finger should be placed over the open end to prevent blood from flowing into the sealing material. The seal must be complete or the test will give erroneously low results because red blood cells will be lost from the tube when it spins.

The tubes are placed in the microhematocrit cen-

trifuge with the sealed ends against the rubber gasket and the open ends pointing toward the center. The second tube is positioned opposite the first for balance. The cover is put on the centrifuge, and the centrifuge is spun according to the manufacturer's instructions—usually for three to five minutes. Some microhematocrit centrifuges have both an inside cover plus an outer lid, and others have only the outer lid cover. Centrifuging for too short a time produces falsely high readings because plasma is trapped among the red blood cells. This is especially likely in patients with hypochromic anemias and sickle-cell anemia.

As soon as the centrifuge stops spinning, the tubes are removed to prevent settling. The volume of packed red blood cells is compared to the total volume—the packed cells plus plasma. The buffy coat, the area of white blood cells and platelets, should be excluded from the reading. The hematocrit will be elevated if the buffy coat is included as part of the packed red blood-cell volume. Some microhematocrit centrifuges have a separate reader (see Figure 15.6). Others have a built-in reader (see Figure 15.7), which allows medical assistants to determine the results while the tube is still in the centrifuge.

Quality control in hematocrit testing involves centrifuging control samples and comparing the results to the values given by the manufacturer of the controls. These usually are printed on the control bottle.

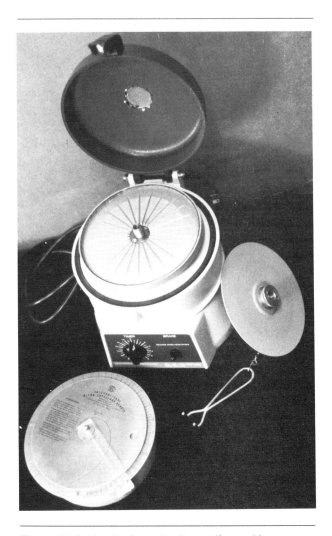

Figure 15.6. A microhematocrit centrifuge with a separate reader. Photo by Mark Palko.

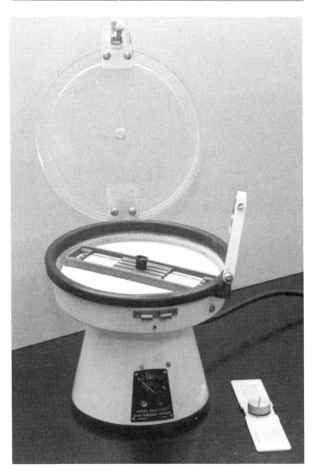

Figure 15.7. A microhematocrit centrifuge with a built-in hematocrit reader. Photo by Tommy Mumert.

❖❖ *Normal Values for the Hematocrit*

Normal values for the hematocrit vary by age and sex. See Table 15.2.

❖❖ *Interpreting Hematocrit Values*

If the hematocrit is low, the number or volume of circulating red blood cells is low. In either case, the amount of circulating hemoglobin is less than normal, and anemia results.

An elevated hematocrit can be caused by both normal physiological processes and disease states. For example, dehydration can cause an increase in hematocrit due to the decrease of body fluid, which affects the plasma level. The resulting hematocrit appears to have a greater number of RBCs but, in fact, the RBC

TABLE 15.2 Normal Values for the Hematocrit

Age/Sex Group	Normal Hct Value (%)
Adult males	42 to 52
Adult females	36 to 46
Newborns	50 to 62
One-year-olds	31 to 39

level is essentially the same as it was prior to the dehydration. Polycythemia vera, a chronic, usually fatal disease of the bone marrow, also can cause an increase in the hematocrit value. Iron deficiency ane-mias have a pattern of hematocrits that are higher than expected for the low hemoglobin reading. This is because the red blood cells lack hemoglobin due to the lack of dietary iron.

PROCEDURE

15.1 ◆ Measuring Hemoglobin Concentration and Performing a Microhematocrit by Manual Methods

Goal
- After successfully completing this procedure, you will be able to perform Unopette cyanmethemoglobin tests and manual microhematocrits on whole-blood specimens.

Completion Time
- 20 minutes for Part 1
- 8 minutes for Part 2

Equipment and Supplies
- disposable latex gloves
- apron
- hand disinfectant
- surface disinfectant
- paper towels and tissues
- biohazard container
- hemoglobin standard
- EDTA-anticoagulated blood specimens
- capillary tubes (nonheparinized)
- sealing clay or plastic caps
- microhematocrit centrifuge and reader
- distilled water sample
- 3 Unopette systems
- paper and pencil
- 3 spectrophotometer cuvettes
- spectrophotometer

Instructions
Read through the list of equipment and supplies that you will need and the steps of the procedure. Be sure that you understand each step before you begin. Then complete each step correctly and in the proper order. If your completion time is too long, repeat the procedure until you increase your speed.

◆◆ *Part 1: A Unopette Cyanmethemoglobin Test*

S = Satisfactory	U = Unsatisfactory	S	U

1. Wash your hands with disinfectant, dry them, and put on gloves and an apron.

2. Follow the Universal Precautions.

3. Collect and prepare the appropriate equipment.

4. a. Label three Unopette reservoirs containing Uno-heme reagent as follows: *B* for blank, *S* for standard, and *U* for unknown.

   b. Label 3 cuvettes.

5. Place the Unopette reservoir on a flat surface and, grasping the reservoir in one hand, take the pipette assembly in the other hand and push the tip of the pipette shield firmly through the diaphragm in the neck of the reservoir.

6. Remove the pipette and then remove the shield from the pipette assembly with a twist.

7. Add samples of 20 μL to each of the reservoirs (distilled water to reservoir B, hemoglobin standard to reservoir S, and whole blood to reservoir U.) Follow this procedure for each Unopette reservoir:

   a. Holding the pipette almost horizontally to ensure complete filling, touch the tip of the pipette to the well-mixed sample and let the pipette fill by capillary action. Filling is complete and will stop automatically when the solution reaches the end of the capillary bore in the neck of the pipette.

   b. Wipe any excess from the outside of the capillary pipette, making certain that none of the sample is removed from the capillary bore.

   c. Squeeze the reservoir slightly to force out some air, but do not expel any liquid. Maintain pressure on the reservoir.

d. Cover the opening of the overflow chamber of the pipette with your index finger and seat the pipette securely in the reservoir neck.

e. Release pressure on the reservoir, as you remove your finger from the pipette opening. Negative pressure will draw the sample into the diluent.

f. Squeeze the reservoir gently two or three times to rinse the capillary bore, forcing diluent up into but not out of the overflow chamber, releasing the pressure each time to return the mixture to the reservoir.

g. Place your index finger over the upper opening and gently invert the reservoir several times to thoroughly mix the sample with diluent.

h. Let the reservoirs stand at room temperature for ten minutes.

8. Transfer the contents of each reservoir to appropriately labeled cuvettes. *Note:* all solutions must be transferred to a cuvette before reading in the spectrophotometer.

a. Convert the reservoir to a dropper assembly by withdrawing the pipette and reseating it securely in the reverse position.

b. Place the capillary tip into the appropriately labeled cuvette and squeeze the reservoir to expel the entire contents.

9. Set the wavelength on the spectrophotometer to 540 nm or use a filter photometer with the appropriate filter.

10. Wipe the outside of the cuvettes before placing them in the spectrophotometer.

11. Check the zero stability of the instrument using distilled water.

12. Place the cuvette labeled B in the instrument and set the instrument at zero absorbance.

13. Measure the absorbance of the standard and the unknown against the blank set at zero absorbance and record the result.

14. Substitute in the formula and solve for C_u:

$$C_u = \frac{A_u}{A_s} \times C_s$$

where,

C_u = concentration of the unknown sample

A_u = absorbance of the unknown sample

A_s = absorbance of the standard

C_s = concentration of the standard

15. Record the result as the patient's hemoglobin concentration in grams per deciliter.

16. Discard disposable equipment, specimens, and used supplies in the biohazard container.

17. Disinfect other equipment and return it to storage.

18. Clean the work area following the Universal Precautions.

19. Remove your gloves and apron, wash your hands with disinfectant, and dry them.

❖❖ *Part 2: The Hematocrit*

S=Satisfactory   U=Unsatisfactory   S   U

1. Wash your hands with disinfectant, dry them, and put on gloves and apron.

2. Follow the Universal Precautions.

	S	U

3. Collect and prepare the appropriate equipment.

4. Mix a stoppered tube of EDTA-coagulated blood with a mechanical mixer or by gently rocking the tube back and forth about twenty times.

5. Remove the cap from the tube of blood, and, using a tissue or cap cover, take care to avoid spattering or contaminating your hands with blood.

6. Tilting the tube so that the blood is near the opening, insert a plain capillary tube (nonheparinized) into the blood and allow it to fill two-thirds full by capillary action or to the fill line if the tube is precalibrated.

7. Remove the tube from the blood and wipe the outside of the tube with a tissue to remove excess blood.

8. Insert the clean end of the capillary tube into a tray of sealing clay and seal the tube. The clay surface in the tube should be level. Alternately, place a plastic cap on the clean end of the tube.

9. Repeat steps 6–8 for a second capillary tube of blood.

10. Align the tubes with a number on the tray of sealing clay and write the same number on the patient requisition (or student report).

11. Transfer the capillary tubes to the same number on the microhematocrit centrifuge, placing the two tubes opposite each other for balance. The sealed ends should be against the outside rubber gasket of the centrifuge.

12. Screw on the inner lid securely and clamp down the outer lid tightly.

13. Centrifuge for the length of time recommended by the centrifuge manufacturer.

14. Allow the centrifuge to come to a complete stop before unlocking the lids.

	S	U
15. If the centrifuge requires calibrated tubes, position them as directed by the manufacturer and read the enclosed scale. If any type of capillary tubes can be used, remove the tubes carefully to preserve their identity and place them in the hematocrit reader, first matching the total volume of the capillary tube to the 100 percent volume reading on the scale.		
16. Average the two readings and report this value as the patient's hematocrit. (If the readings do not agree within 2 percent, repeat the procedure.)		
17. Discard disposable equipment, specimens, and used supplies in the biohazardous waste container.		
18. Disinfect other equipment and return it to storage.		
19. Clean the work area following the Universal Precautions.		
20. Remove your gloves and apron; wash your hands with disinfectant, and dry them.		

OVERALL PROCEDURAL EVALUATION

Student's Name _____

Signature of Instructor _____ Date _____

Comments

Using Terminology

Match the term in the right column with the appropriate definition or description in the left column.

_____ 1. a blood test measured in g/dL

_____ 2. converts hemoglobin to cyanmethemoglobin

_____ 3. a disease caused by abnormal hemoglobin

_____ 4. having two copies of the same gene

_____ 5. measures blood for a hemoglobin test

_____ 6. an oxygen-carrying molecule

_____ 7. a red blood cell

_____ 8. red blood-cell formation

_____ 9. the volume of packed red blood cells

a. Drabkin's reagent
b. erythrocyte
c. erythropoiesis
d. hematocrit
e. hemoglobin test
f. hemoglobin
g. hemoglobinopathy
h. homozygous
i. Sahli pipette

Define the following terms in the spaces provided.

10. Buffy coat: _____

_____

11. Stromatolytic agent: _____

_____

12. Microhematocrit: _____

_____

13. Hemoglobin C: _____

_____

14. Hemoglobin S: _____

_____

15. Hemolytic anemia: _____

_____

16. Hemoglobin E: _____

_____

17. Complete blood count (CBC): _____

_____

18. Erythropoietin: _____

_____

Acquiring Knowledge

Answer the following questions in the spaces provided.

19. Describe the functions of hemoglobin.

_____

_____

20. List the hemoglobin concentration and hematocrit values for normal adult males, adult females, and newborns.

_____

_____

21. What is needed to perform the cyanmethemoglobin test?

_____

22. Explain how red blood-cell formation is regulated.

_____

_____

23. How is hematocrit expressed?

_____

24. What tests usually are included in a complete blood count?

_____

_____

_____

_____

25. What disease causes a low hemoglobin concentration and a normal hematocrit? Why?

_____

_____

26. Explain how to calculate a patient's hemoglobin concentration using values for a known standard.

_____

_____

_____

27. Describe the structure of the hemoglobin molecule.

_____

_____

28. At what age would a person have a normal hematocrit reading of 60 percent? of 50 percent?

_____

29. Explain how the specific-gravity test for hemoglobin is performed.

_____

_____

30. Why are two different copper sulfate solutions required for the specific-gravity test?

_____

_____

31. Explain the principle underlying the cyanmethemoglobin test.

_____

_____

_____

_____

32. What essential element of hemoglobin must be furnished in the diet? What pathological condition results if the diet is deficient in this element?

_____

33. What are hemoglobinopathies?

_____

34. What is the most common abnormal hemoglobin in the U.S. population? What group is most often affected? Why?

_____

_____

_____

_____

35. How did sickle-cell hemoglobin acquire its name?

_____

_____

36. How do sickle-cell hemoglobin homozygous individuals differ from heterozygous individuals?

_____

_____

_____

37. What disease do physicians suspect when they order only a hemoglobin and a hematocrit?

_____

38. What is the age of a patient who has a normal hemoglobin concentration of 20 g/dL?

_____

39. Name four conditions that could cause a falsely high hemoglobin reading.

_____

_____

Applying Knowledge—On the Job

Answer the following questions in the spaces provided.

40. In the lab where Sonja works, an African-American husband and wife recently had their blood tested and were surprised to learn that each is heterozygous for sickle-cell hemoglobin. Because neither ever has had any symptoms of sickle-cell anemia nor known any close relatives to have sickle-cell anemia, they cannot understand how they could have a child with this life-threatening disease. What is the explanation for this?

_____

_____

_____

_____

_____

_____

_____

_____

41. As part of a routine complete blood count, a 35-year-old female patient's hematocrit was determined to be 38 percent and her hemoglobin concentration was measured at 10 g/dL. What diagnosis is likely? Why?

_____

_____

_____

_____

42. An apparently healthy male patient, age 44, has a hemoglobin concentration of 28 g/dL. Why should you suspect that this reading is incorrect? What might be the cause?

_____

_____

_____

43. Josh and Mark just started working in the same lab together, and they are having an argument about how to read hematocrits. Josh says that you should not include the "white part," while Mark says everything but the "watery part" should be included. Who is right? Why?

_____

_____

_____

44. When Alberto centrifuged two capillary tubes of blood from the same newborn patient for a hematocrit reading, one tube gave a result of 50 percent and the other gave a result of 56 percent. Should Alberto consider these results close enough to be in agreement? Why or why not?

_____

_____

_____

_____

16 White Blood-Cell Count and Red Blood-Cell Count: Manual Hematological Procedures

COGNITIVE OBJECTIVES

After studying this chapter, you should be able to

- use each vocabulary term appropriately.
- list normal values for white and red blood-cell counts by age and sex.
- identify the ranges of abnormally low and high white and red blood-cell counts and name at least one cause of each condition.
- explain the components of the white and red blood-cell count formulas.
- discuss how the presence of nucleated red blood cells affects the white blood-cell count and how to correct for this bias.
- describe how to clean pipettes and other equipment after performing a blood count.
- identify several sources of potential error in performing white blood-cell and red blood-cell counts.

PERFORMANCE OBJECTIVES

After studying this chapter, you should be able to

- perform a manual white blood-cell count with a Unopette kit (or a Thoma pipette) and a hemacytometer and use the result to calculate the number of white blood cells per cubic millimeter.
- perform a manual red blood-cell count with a Unopette kit (or a Thoma pipette) and a hemacytometer and use the result to calculate the number of red blood cells per cubic millimeter.

TERMINOLOGY

absolute polycythemia: erythrocytosis; an increase in the number of red blood cells because of increased red blood-cell production.

Adams suction apparatus: a device for suctioning fluids into a pipette to prevent accidental ingestion of the fluids. It has an airtight rubber gasket and a stainless steel barrel with a thumbscrew at the end to control the suction.

agglutination: a clumping together, as of red blood cells.

anoxia: a deficiency of oxygen.

aplastic anemia: anemia caused by deficient red blood-cell production, due to disorders of the bone marrow.

balanced leukocytosis: an elevation in all types of white blood cells, usually due to hemoconcentration.

diurnal: by day. In the context of this chapter, diurnal refers to normal variation in the white blood-cell count throughout the course of the day.

epinephrine: adrenaline; an adrenal gland hormone that stimulates the sympathetic nervous system.

erythremia: polycythemia vera.

erythrocyte count: red blood-cell count.

erythrocytosis: absolute polycythemia.

isotonic: having the same osmotic pressure. An isotonic solution with the same osmotic pressure as red blood cells is used to prepare blood for red blood-cell counts.

leukocyte count: white blood-cell count.

leukocytosis: an abnormally high white blood-cell count.

leukopenia: an abnormally low white blood-cell count, usually below 4,500/mm³.

neoplasm: an abnormal growth of tissue, such as a tumor.

nucleated red blood cell (nuRBC): a red blood cell that contains a nucleus. It resembles a white blood cell under low-power magnification and may inflate the white blood-cell count.

pernicious anemia: a potentially fatal form of anemia that may be due to deficiency or malabsorption of vitamin B_{12}. Pernicious anemia is associated with an abnormally low white blood-cell count.

polycythemia: an increase above normal in the number of red blood cells in circulation.

polycythemia vera: erythremia; a chronic, usually fatal disease of the bone marrow that results in greatly elevated red blood-cell counts.

pseudoagglutination: the clumping together of red blood cells as in the formation of rouleaux but differing from true agglutination in that the clumped cells can be dispersed by shaking.

red blood-cell (RBC) count: erythrocyte count; the number of red blood cells per cubic millimeter of blood; performed manually by counting red blood cells under high-power magnification on a hemacytometer. Whole blood is diluted with an isotonic solution that prevents lysing of red blood cells.

relative polycythemia: an increase in red blood cells relative to plasma volume. It occurs due to dehydration.

reticulocyte: an immature red blood cell, which retains traces of endoplasmic reticula.

rouleau: a clump of red blood cells that appear to be stacked like a roll of coins.

Thoma red blood-cell pipette: a micropipette used to dilute blood for red blood-cell counts.

Thoma white blood-cell pipette: a micropipette used to dilute blood for white blood-cell counts.

white blood-cell (WBC) count: leukocyte count; the number of white blood cells per cubic millimeter of blood; counted manually under low-power magnification on a hemacytometer. Whole blood is diluted with a solution that lyses red blood cells.

• • • • • • • • • • • • • • • • • • • •

Both white and red blood cells frequently are counted in POLs to diagnose patient conditions, follow the progress of disease, or monitor patient treatment. In this chapter, you will learn how to count white and red blood cells and how to interpret the results.

THE WHITE BLOOD-CELL COUNT

The **white blood-cell (WBC) count,** or **leukocyte count,** is one of the tests included in a complete blood count. The WBC count measures the total number of white blood cells per cubic millimeter of whole blood. The chief functions of white blood cells are to fight infection and to provide immunity, so the WBC count is performed most often to diagnose infection in the body.

◆◆ Normal Values for the WBC Count

Normal values for the WBC count vary by age (see Table 16.1). In general, the count declines as individuals get older. In healthy individuals, the WBC count varies throughout the day, that is, **diurnally.** It is lowest in the morning and gradually rises by about 2,000 cells/mm³ through midafternoon, when it peaks. The WBC count also rises with meals, strenuous exercise, stress, exposure to temperature extremes such as cold baths, and during pregnancy. The WBC count decreases when an individual is at rest.

◆◆ Abnormal Values for the WBC Count

A WBC count may reveal either more or fewer white blood cells than normal due to a variety of pathological conditions (see Figure 16.1).

Abnormally High WBC Count. Leukocytosis refers to an abnormally high WBC count. Pathological conditions that may cause leukocytosis include, most commonly, bacterial infections and leukemia. Other causes include acute hemorrhage, sudden hemolysis of red blood cells, growing malignant **neoplasms** of the gastrointestinal tract or liver, epileptic seizures, **epinephrine** or adrenaline injections, pain, and **anoxia,** a deficiency of oxygen. The anoxia caused by

TABLE 16.1 Variation in WBC Count by Age	
Age Group	**WBC Count (cells/mm³)**
Newborns	9,000 to 30,000
One-year-olds	8,000 to 14,000
Adults	4,500 to 12,000

cigarette smoking, for example, increases the WBC count by as much as 30 percent.

Most often, only one or a few types of white blood cells occur in high numbers. It is rare to see an elevation in all types of white blood cells, which is called **balanced leukocytosis.** This elevation occurs primarily in cases of acute hemoconcentration, in which there is a decrease in plasma volume due, for example, to dehydration.

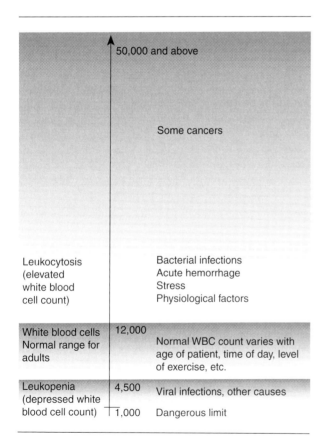

Figure 16.1. Normal and abnormal variation in the WBC count.

Abnormally Low WBC Count. Leukopenia refers to an abnormally low WBC count, usually below 4,500 cells/mm³. Conditions that may produce leukopenia include viral infections, such as flu and measles, and exposure to radiation, lead, and mercury. Patients with **pernicious anemia,** a potentially fatal form of anemia that may be due to deficiency or malabsorption of vitamin B_{12}, also have an abnormally low WBC count. In pernicious anemia, the WBC count usually is in the range of 3,000 to 4,000 cells/mm³ and may fall below 2,000 cells/mm³. A WBC count of 1,000/mm³ or lower is considered to be dangerously low.

❖❖ A Manual WBC Count

For a manual WBC count, a sample of whole blood is diluted in a micropipette with a solution that hemolyzes the red blood cells, leaving only the white blood cells intact. The solution used to lyse the red blood cells is either 1 percent hydrochloric acid or 3 percent acetic acid. After mixing, the diluted specimen is introduced into a hemacytometer counting chamber and the white blood cells are systematically counted under low-power magnification.

Figure 16.2 illustrates Thoma pipettes and the Unopette system. However, all manual hematology counts that are now performed in POLs utilize the Unopette system.

Diluting the Sample. Thoma white blood-cell pipettes are used for diluting and mixing the blood sample. The pipettes are available with calibrations at 0.5, 1.0, and 11.0 marks for the WBC count, and at 0.5, 1.0, and 101 marks for the RBC count. For a WBC count, blood is drawn to the 0.5 or 1.0 mark and then diluting solution is added to the 11.0 mark. For very high WBC counts, over 50,000 cells/mm³, a red blood-cell pipette is used, blood is drawn to the

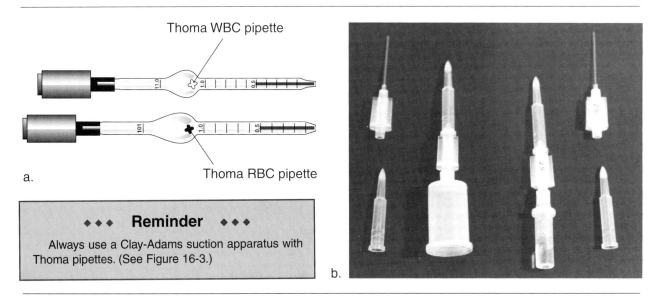

Thoma WBC pipette

a.

Thoma RBC pipette

b.

Figure 16.2. These instruments are used to obtain samples for red blood cells and white blood cells. a. The traditional Thoma pipettes are still used in many training programs. b. The Unopette systems are shown in the photo, with the red blood-cell equipment on the left and the white blood-cell equipment on the right. Photo by Mark Palko.

1.0 mark, and then diluting solution is added to the 101 mark.

Draw the blood sample exactly to the mark. If too much is drawn in, remove the excess by touching the tip of the pipette to a nonabsorbent surface, such as a gloved index finger. Never use a tissue or other absorbent material. It will wick away fluid and increase the blood count. Wipe any excess blood from the sides of the pipette with a tissue before you place it in the container of diluting solution.

To avoid ingesting blood or diluting solution when filling the pipette, always use a suction device, such as the **Adams suction apparatus** (see Figure 16.3). This suction apparatus consists of an airtight rubber gasket and a stainless steel barrel with a thumbscrew at

♦♦♦ **Thoma Blood-Cell** ♦♦♦
Pipettes

Thoma blood-cell pipettes are no longer used in POLs to perform blood-cell counts. They are used in sperm count determinations. Thoma blood-cell pipettes are explained in this chapter because they are still used in many laboratory teaching settings. Thoma pipettes provide an opportunity for students to observe how the change in the ratio of blood sample to diluting fluid will affect the results of the blood-cell count. This variation in the ratio of blood to diluting fluid also is used in automated hematology instruments. These are explained in Chapter 18. The hemacytometer is used in the same manner to perform a blood-cell count with both the Unopette system and the blood-cell pipette. It is also used when performing a sperm count.

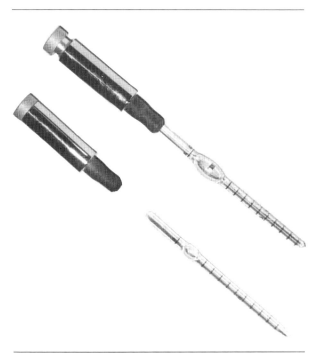

Figure 16.3. The Adams suction apparatus with white blood-cell and red blood-cell pipettes. The suction device eliminates the need for mouth pipetting. Photo by Tommy Mumert.

the end. Insert the pipette into the hole in the gasket. Then, screw out the thumbscrew to draw the liquid into the pipette and screw it in to force the liquid out again.

Mixing the Sample. After filling the pipette with blood and diluting solution, mix the sample into a homogenous solution with a mechanical shaker, like the one in Figure 16.4, or by hand using a figure-eight motion, as in Figure 16.5. When mixing by hand, hold the pipette horizontally and cover both ends with your finger and thumb to prevent leakage. Mix the sample for at least one minute, preferably two minutes.

Charging the Hemacytometer. Before charging the hemacytometer, be sure that the counting chamber and coverslip are free of dust and grease. Always expel the first three drops from the pipette to get rid of any diluting solution remaining in the stem (see Figure 16.6). The sample counted must contain just the mixture from the bulb of the pipette. With the coverslip positioned over both sides of the counting chamber, let the sample from the pipette flow evenly under the coverslip, avoiding the depressed area, or moat, around the platform. Most hemacytometers have a *V*-shaped trough to help in the filling process. If the chamber is overflooded or if air bubbles form, clean the counting chamber, dry it, and refill it. After

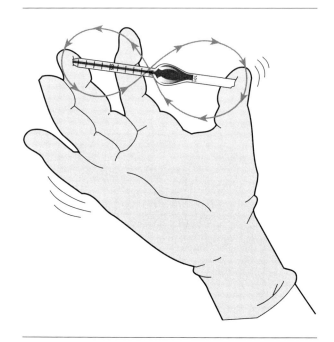

Figure 16.5. Mixing a blood-cell pipette by hand using a figure-eight motion.

flooding one side of the chamber, repeat the process on the other side. Then allow the filled chambers to stand two minutes before counting to let the cells settle and stabilize.

Counting the Sample. As Figure 16.7 shows, count the cells in the four corner squares, first on one side of the counting chamber and then on the other side. Use the average of the two sides in the WBC count formula. Each corner square measures 1 mm × 1 mm and is divided into sixteen smaller squares.

Under low-power magnification, begin the count in the upper left corner and move through the sixteen small squares systematically (see Figure 16.8). Move horizontally across each row, starting at the top, and then go to the next adjacent row and repeat. Count the cells touching the border lines on just two sides of the corner square, omitting from the count cells that touch the border lines of the other two sides (see Figure 16.9).

After counting all the cells in the upper left corner square in this way, repeat the process for the remaining three corner squares. If the counts for the four corner squares differ from one another by more than ten cells, discard the count, clean the counting chamber, refill it, and start the counting process over again. Such an uneven distribution of cells usually is caused by a dirty hemacytometer or coverslip.

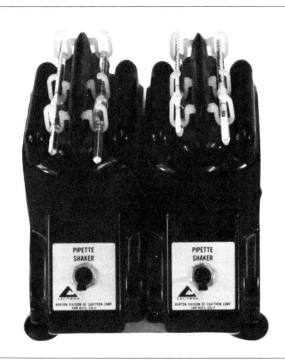

Figure 16.4. A mechanical blood-cell pipette shaker.

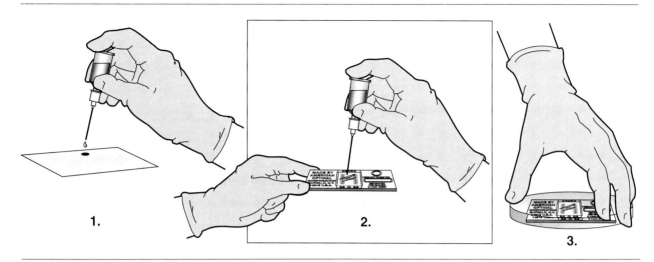

Figure 16.6. Charging a hemacytometer. 1. Expel two or three drops of fluid from the Unopette pipette or blood-cell pipette onto an absorbent tissue. 2. Let the fluid from the pipette fill the space between the coverslip and the hemacytometer. 3. Let the filled hemacytometer stand for two minutes before counting.

When Nucleated Red Blood Cells Are Present. Nucleated red blood cells, **nuRBC**, resemble white blood cells when viewed under low-power magnification. Very few nucleated red blood cells normally are present in circulating blood, but they may reach significant numbers in cases of hemorrhage. Because nucleated red blood cells are not lysed by hydrochloric acid or acetic acid, they may remain intact in the sample and inflate the WBC count. Nucleated red blood cells must be distinguished from white blood cells under high-power (100X) magnification on a stained blood smear, and their number per 100 white

Figure 16.7. The ruled areas of a hemacytometer. Count the four corner squares labeled *W* for a WBC count under the 10X objective. Count the five areas labeled *R* for an RBC count under the 45X objective.

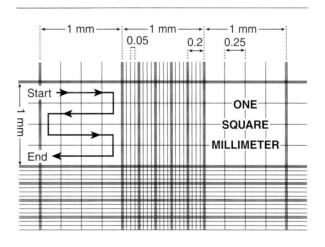

Figure 16.8. Counting the sixteen small squares in each corner square. The direction followed in a WBC count through the sixteen small squares must be consistent on each large square to prevent overlooking cells in the count.

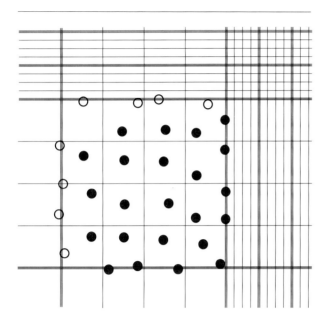

○ **Skip** these cells in the white blood cell count

● Count these cells in the white blood cell count

Figure 16.9. Count the cells that touch the borderlines on two sides of the corner square. Leave uncounted the cells that touch the borderlines of the other two sides of the square.

blood cells must be noted on the lab report. See Chapter 17. Their number per one hundred white cells is used to correct the overall WBC count, as described below.

Using a Unopette Kit. The principle underlying the Unopette kit for performing a manual WBC count is the same as that just described for the Thoma diluting pipette. Whole blood is added to a hemolyzing solution, mixed, and counted in a hemacytometer. The Unopette kit contains a prefilled disposable reservoir of 3 percent acetic acid as the diluting solution, a capillary pipette for measuring and mixing, and a pipette shield. A reservoir containing 0.475 mL of diluting solution is used with a 25 μL pipette of blood to yield a dilution of 1:20. A reservoir containing 1.98 mL of diluting solution is used with a 20 μL pipette of blood to yield a dilution of 1:100. The latter should be used when the WBC count is high.

After mixing blood and diluting fluid in the reservoir, let the sample stand at least ten minutes for the red blood cells to hemolyze before charging the hemacytometer and counting the white blood cells. The sample may stand up to three hours at room temperature. (A Unopette kit was shown in Figure 15.3.)

⁙ Calculating the WBC Count

The following formula is used to calculate the number of white blood cells per cubic millimeter of blood in the sample:

$$\text{WBC/mm}^3 = \frac{\text{Average number} \times \text{Dilution} \times \text{Depth}}{\text{Area counted}}$$

Components of the WBC Count Formula. The number of cells counted in the WBC count formula is the average of the cells counted on both sides of the hemacytometer counting chamber, as described. The dilution factor is the ratio of blood to the total volume of blood plus diluting solution. The total volume of the mixed solution in the bulb of the white blood-cell pipette is always ten units. The diluting fluid present in the stem of the pipette is not included as part of the total volume. If blood is drawn to the 0.5 mark, the dilution is $\frac{0.5}{10}$, or 1:20. If blood is drawn to the 1.0 mark, the dilution is $\frac{1.0}{10}$, or 1:10. If a red blood-cell pipette is used and blood drawn to the 1.0 mark, the dilution is 1:100 because red blood-cell pipette bulbs contain one hundred units of volume. The value substituted into the formula for the dilution factor is 20, 10, or 100, respectively.

The depth factor in the formula is a constant, 10. It represents the depth of fluid between the counting chamber platform and the coverslip. The actual distance always is 0.1 mm, but the constant 10 is used so that the answer gives the number of cells present in 1 mm of depth (0.1 mm × 10 = 1.0 mm). The area counted is most often the four corners of the hemacytometer counting chamber, which cover a total of 4 mm². If the total area on each side of the counting chamber is counted instead of just the four corners, the area counted is 9 mm². The total area may be counted when the WBC count is low.

Whenever the dilution is 1:20 and just the four corners are counted, so the counting area is 4 mm², you can use this shorthand formula for calculating the WBC count:

$$\text{WBC/mm}^3 = \text{No. of cells counted} \times 50$$

because,

$$\frac{\text{Dilution factor} \times \text{Depth factor}}{\text{Area counted}}$$

$$= \frac{(20 \times 10)}{4} = \frac{200}{4} = 50.$$

Using the Formula: A Worked Example. Assume that you have counted 28, 32, 33, and 26 white blood cells in the four corners of one side of the counting chamber and 31, 32, 25, and 33 white blood cells in the four corners of the other side. The total cells counted on the two sides are 119 and 121, for an average of 120 cells counted. Use your calculator to verify this. Also assume that blood was drawn to the 0.5 mark on the white blood-cell pipette, so the dilution is 1:20. Depth and area are the constants 10 and 4, respectively. Substituting into the formula, you get:

$$\text{WBC/mm}^3 = \frac{120 \times 20 \times 10}{4} = 6,000$$

Correction for Nucleated Red Blood Cells. When significant numbers of nucleated red blood cells are present in a sample, the WBC count will be inflated unless their number per 100 white blood cells is known and used to correct the WBC count. The following two formulas are used:

- WBC/mm^3 (corrected) $= \text{WBC/mm}^3 - \text{nuRBC/mm}^3$
- $\text{nuRBC/mm}^3 = \dfrac{\text{nuRBC}}{100 + \text{No. nuRBC}} \times \text{WBC/mm}^3$

Consider the following example. Assume that the WBC count is 11,000 and a blood smear under high-power magnification shows 10 nucleated red blood cells per 100 white blood cells. The number of nucleated red blood cells/mm^3 is calculated as:

$$\text{nuRBC/mm}^3 = \frac{10}{(100 + 10)} \times 11,000 = 1,000$$

The corrected WBC count is then:

$$\text{WBC/mm}^3 \text{ (corrected)} = 11,000 - 1,000$$
$$= 10,000$$

THE RED BLOOD-CELL COUNT

The **red blood-cell (RBC) count,** or **erythrocyte count,** is another test included in the complete blood count. The RBC count determines the number of red blood cells per cubic millimeter of blood. Both mature red blood cells and immature red blood cells, called **reticulocytes,** are included in the count. The chief role of red blood cells is to transport oxygen to the tissues. A deficiency of red blood cells produces anemia, and diagnosing anemia is the most common reason for performing an RBC count. Normal values for an RBC count vary by age and sex (see Table 16.2).

TABLE 16.2 Normal Values for the RBC Count

Age/Sex Group	RBC Count (millions/mm³)
Newborns	5.0 to 6.5
One-year-olds	4.0 to 5.0
Adult females	4.0 to 5.5
Adult males	4.5 to 6.0

❖❖ Abnormal Values for the RBC Count

An RBC count may reveal either more red blood cells or fewer red blood cells than normal due to a variety of pathological conditions (see Figure 16.10). Both conditions are stressful for the body.

An Abnormally High RBC Count. Polycythemia is an increase above normal in the number of red blood cells in circulation. There are two ways this may come about—through a decrease in blood fluid or through an increase in red blood-cell production.

Relative polycythemia is the increase in red blood cells relative to plasma volume, which occurs with dehydration. This can be caused by a decrease in fluid intake or by loss of body fluids due to diarrhea or vomiting.

Absolute polycythemia, also known as **erythrocytosis,** is an increase in red blood-cell production for any of a variety of reasons, including:

- low oxygen tension in the blood due to high altitude or pulmonary diseases like emphysema
- slowing of the circulation due to heart disease
- defects in the hemoglobin molecule

Polycythemia vera, also known as **erythremia,** is a type of absolute polycythemia in which RBC counts may be as high as 7 to 10 million cells/mm^3. It is due to an unknown disorder of the bone marrow and usually is fatal.

An Abnormally Low RBC Count. A low RBC count means that there are fewer than normal red blood cells per given volume of blood. With fewer red blood cells, there is less hemoglobin, and anemia results. Causes of abnormally low RBC counts include some therapeutic drugs and bone marrow disorders that reduce red blood-cell production. The latter produce **aplastic anemia.**

◆◆◆ Drugs and Anemia ◆◆◆

Many different drugs may reduce red blood-cell production or cause hemolysis of red blood cells, leading to a low RBC count. If your patient has a low RBC count, find out if it may be due to a drug such as the following:

- antineoplastic drugs, such as azathioprine
- analgesics, such as aspirin
- antimicrobials, such as penicillin
- anticonvulsants, such as primidone
- antimalarials, such as primaquine
- heavy metals, such as gold compounds
- oral hypoglycemics, such as tolbutamide
- psychotropics, such as chlorpromazine
- diuretics, such as acetazolamide
- antihistamines, such as chlorpheniramine

❖❖ A Manual RBC Count

Performing a manual RBC count is very similar to performing a manual WBC count. A sample of whole blood is diluted in a micropipette, mixed, and introduced into a hemacytometer for counting. For RBC counts, however, the diluting solution is an **isotonic** solution, not an acid. The isotonic solution prevents hemolysis of the red blood cells because it has the same osmotic pressure as the red blood cells. Also for RBC counts, high-power magnification is used instead of low-power magnification for counting the cells.

Diluting the Sample. Use **Thoma red blood-cell pipettes,** with calibrations at 0.5, 1.0, and 101 marks, for diluting and mixing the blood sample for the RBC count. Draw blood to the 0.5 mark (see Figure 16.11) or the 1.0 mark, and then add diluting solution to the 101 mark. Use the 1.0 mark for blood from patients with severe anemia. The measurements must be pre-

Increased RBC count → Pathological conditions with high RBC count

— Erythemia
— Polycythemia
— Erythrocytosis

6.0 million/cmm^3

Normal RBC count in healthy individuals

4.0 million/cmm^3

Decreased RBC count → Pathological conditions with low RBC count → Anemia (loss of oxygen-carrying capacity of blood)

Figure 16.10. Normal and abnormal variation in the RBC count.

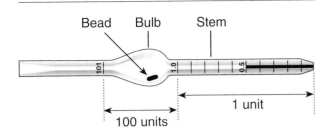

Figure 16.11. A Thoma red blood-cell pipette, showing blood drawn to the 0.5 mark.

cise, and you must remove any excess blood before adding diluting solution. As always, use a suction device, such as the Adams suction apparatus for filling the pipettes.

The diluting solution used may be normal saline solution, which is 0.85 percent sodium chloride in water, Hayem and Gower solution, or Gower solution. Because the bulb of the red blood-cell pipette contains 100 units, the dilution is 1:200 when the pipette is filled to the 0.5 mark ($\frac{0.5}{100}$) and 1:100 when the pipette is filled to the 1.0 mark ($\frac{1.0}{100}$).

Mixing the Sample. Mix the diluted sample in the pipette for approximately three minutes before performing the RBC count. Mixing may be done with a mechanical shaker or by hand using a figure-eight motion. When mixing by hand, do not forget to hold the pipette horizontally and to cover both ends with your finger and thumb to prevent spills.

Charging the Hemacytometer. Charge the hemacytometer the same way as for a WBC count. Be sure that the counting chamber and coverslip are clean, and discard the first two or three drops from the pipette so that only the mixture from the bulb of the pipette enters the counting chamber. Let the sample flow evenly under the coverslip. If any sample flows into the moat or if air bubbles form, clean the counting chamber and start over again. After filling both sides of the counting chamber, let the sample stand for three minutes before performing the count.

If the blood sample is too cold, it may cause **agglutination**, or clumping, of red blood cells on the hemacytometer. If you observe agglutination, dilute another specimen and warm it to body temperature before charging the hemacytometer. If warming does not eliminate the agglutination, it may be due to the presence of paraprotein in the sample, which is an indicator of multiple myeloma or other immunoglobulin disorder. Paraprotein produces **pseudoagglutination** of red blood cells, with the formation of

rouleaux, clumps of red blood cells that appear to be stacked like rolls of coins. In pseudoagglutination, the red blood cells can be dispersed by shaking the sample.

Counting the Sample. It is at this stage of the procedure that the RBC count differs most from the WBC count. The RBC counting area on the hemacytometer is the 1 mm² square area located in the center of the counting chamber (see Figure 16.12). The five smaller squares labeled R in the figure are included in the count, making up a total of $\frac{1}{5}$ mm². Follow the same procedure that you used for the WBC count to systematically count the sixteen smaller squares within each of the five squares labeled R:

- Begin counting in the upper left corner of each square and move horizontally across the row.
- After finishing one row, go on to the adjacent one until each row of the square has been counted.
- Count the cells that touch the border lines on just two sides of each square.

RBC counts are made under high-power magnification using the 45X objective (40X or 43X on some microscopes). First locate the field under low-power magnification and then change to high-power magnification following the procedure outlined in Chap-

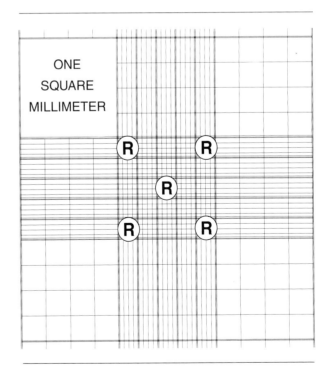

Figure 16.12. The area of the hemacytometer counted in an RBC count.

ter 2. If there is a difference greater than twenty-five cells among any of the five larger squares, discard the count, clean and refill the counting chamber, and start the counting process over again. Count cells on both sides of the counting chamber in this way and average the counts for the two sides.

Using a Unopette Kit. The Unopette kit for performing manual RBCs is very similar to that described for WBC counts. The red blood-cell Unopette kit contains a disposable reservoir prefilled with 1.99 mL of saline solution containing sodium azide, a 10 μL capillary pipette, and a pipette shield. The dilution always is 1:200. After blood and diluting fluid are mixed in the Unopette reservoir, the sample can be kept at room temperature for about six hours, although it is best to use the sample immediately.

♦ ♦ ♦ Watch Out ♦ ♦ ♦
for Hydrazoic Acid!

The diluent used in the Unopette prefilled reservoir contains sodium azide. Under acidic conditions, sodium azide may produce hydrazoic acid, which is extremely toxic. Take great care to avoid contact with this compound. When discarding used diluent into the sink, dilute it with running water to avoid damage to the sink and pipes.

♦♦ *Calculating the RBC Count*

The following formula is used to calculate the number of red blood cells per cubic millimeter of blood:

RBC/mm^3 = No. of cells counted ×

Dilution factor × Depth factor × Area counted

Components of the RBC Count Formula. The components of the RBC count formula that differ from the WBC count formula are the area counted and the dilution factor. In the RBC count, the area counted is just $\frac{1}{5}$ mm^2. The value 5 is substituted into the formula in order to get the number of red blood cells in 1 mm^3 of blood. The dilution factor for the RBC count depends on how much blood was added to the red blood-cell pipette. The dilution usually is 1:200, so the dilution factor is 200. The depth factor is the same as for the WBC count—the constant 10. Whenever the dilution is 1:200, you can use this

shorthand formula for calculating the RBC count:

RBC/mm^3 = No. of cells counted × 10,000

because dilution factor × depth factor × area counted = 200 × 10 × 5 = 10,000.

Using the Formula: A Worked Example. Assume that you have counted 101, 92, 112, 95, and 104 red blood cells in the five squares on one side of the counting chamber and 99, 98, 100, 102, and 97 red blood cells in the five squares on the other side. The total cells counted on the two sides are 504 and 496, for an average of 500 cells counted. Verify this on your calculator. Also assume that blood was drawn to the 0.5 mark on the red blood-cell pipette, so the dilution is 1:200. Substituting into the formula, you get:

RBC/mm^3 = 500 × 200 × 10 × 5 = 5,000,000

♦ ♦

CLEANING UP

Follow this procedure for cleaning up after both WBC and RBC counts.

♦♦ *Pipettes*

Never let undiluted blood samples dry in pipettes. Instead, always draw water or diluting solution into pipettes and clean them immediately or soak them for later cleaning. Clean WBC and RBC pipettes in a microliter-pipette washer, like the one shown in Figure 16.13, which can clean up to eighteen pipettes per operation.

To use the pipette washer, first fill the chamber with low-sudsing detergent and water for cleaning the pipettes. See Figure 16.14. Use tap or distilled water in the chamber for rinsing. The detergent solution and rinse water are pulled through the inserted pipettes with an aspirator pump connected to the faucet. Disinfectant also can be aspirated through the pipettes. Aspirate both the detergent solution and rinse water for several minutes for thorough cleaning and rinsing. Use distilled or deionized water for the final rinse. After rinsing, remove excess water with the aspirator pump and dry the pipettes in a drying oven to remove any remaining water and destroy any pathogens that may be present. Excess water also can be removed using acetone, but this requires a hood and great care because acetone is highly flammable and extremely toxic.

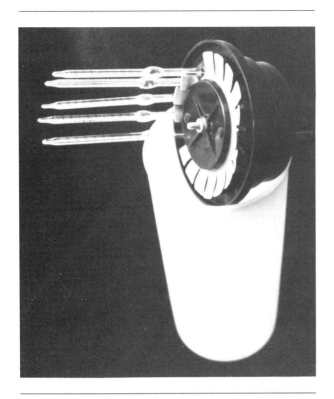

Figure 16.13. A pipette washer. Photo by Mark Palko.

✦✦ *Other Equipment*

Clean the pipette suction device with soap and water and disinfect it with a 10 percent bleach solu-

tion if it becomes contaminated. Always clean the hemacytometer and coverslip thoroughly after the count is complete. Store both under a glass cover when they are not in use. Even a very small scratch can cause serious damage to these precision instruments.

TRACKING ERRORS

Errors may occur in performing WBC and RBC counts for several reasons. Following is a list of some of the most common sources of error to help you resolve problems in performing blood counts:

- chipped pipette tips, which may cause inaccurate dilutions
- moist or dirty pipettes, which may contaminate the sample
- contaminated diluting fluid (if in doubt, filter it)
- too much time elapsed between drawing the sample and performing the procedure
- too much time elapsed between diluting the sample and charging the hemacytometer
- misinterpretation of the counting area on the hemacytometer

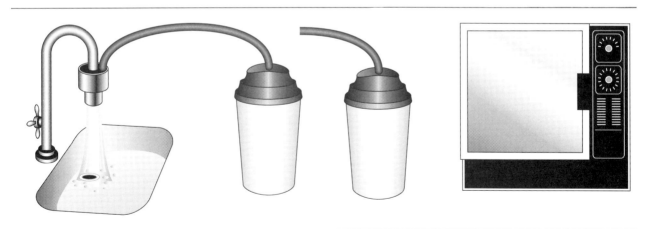

Figure 16.14. The cleaning procedure for white blood-cell and red blood-cell pipettes. First fill the pipette washer with a detergent solution. Use tap water for rinsing. Use distilled water for final rinsing. After removing excess water with the aspirator pump, place the pipettes in a drying oven.

PROCEDURE

16.1 Determining a WBC Count by the Manual Method

Goal

- After successfully completing this procedure, you will be able to dilute a blood sample in a Thoma pipette or Unopette kit, charge a hemacytometer, count white blood cells under low-power magnification, and calculate the WBC count.

Completion Time

- 30 minutes

Equipment and Supplies

- disposable latex gloves
- apron
- hand disinfectant
- surface disinfectant
- paper towels and tissues
- biohazard container
- mechanical blood mixer (optional)
- automatic pipetting device
- Thoma white blood-cell pipette (or a Unopette kit)
- EDTA-anticoagulated blood
- white blood-cell diluting solution
- pipette shaker (optional)
- test tube rack
- glass-marking pen
- Neubauer ruled hemacytometer and coverslip
- lens paper
- 70 percent alcohol
- microscope
- hand tally counter
- pipette washer
- paper and pencil

Instructions

Read through the list of equipment and supplies that you will need and the steps of the procedure. Be sure that you understand each step before you begin. Then complete each step correctly and in the proper order. If your completion time is too long, repeat the procedure until you increase your speed.

S = Satisfactory U = Unsatisfactory	S	U
1. Wash your hands with disinfectant, dry them, and put on gloves and an apron.		
2. Follow the Universal Precautions.		
3. Collect and prepare the appropriate equipment.		
4. Mix the blood sample gently by hand or with a mechanical blood mixer.		

5. Two alternate methods of dilution:
   a. Attach the pipetting suction device to the Thoma white blood-cell pipette.
   b. Use a WBC Unopette kit per manufacturer's instructions on package insert.		

6. Holding the pipette nearly horizontally in your dominant hand between your thumb and index finger and the tube of blood in your other hand, tilt the tube slightly and insert the pipette tip into the blood.		
7. Using the pipetting suction device, draw blood up to the 0.5 mark of the pipette but not past the mark, taking care to avoid air bubbles.		
8. Clean the outside of the pipette with a soft tissue, avoiding the tip so that you do not siphon any blood out of the pipette by accident.		
9. Holding the pipette almost vertically to prevent air bubbles from collecting, insert the tip of the pipette into the diluting solution and aspirate fluid to the 11.0 mark, taking care not to drop any blood into the diluting solution.		
10. Hold your gloved finger over the pipette tip to prevent loss of fluid and remove the pipette suction device from the other end of the pipette.		
11. Label the pipette with the marking pen.		

12. After cleaning the hemacytometer and coverslip with 70 percent alcohol and drying them thoroughly with lens paper, align the coverslip on the hemacytometer.

13. Mix the diluted blood sample in the pipette for two minutes using either the manual figure-eight method or a mechanical pipette mixer.

14. Placing the tip of your index finger over the stem of the Thoma pipette to control the flow of fluid, expel the first three drops of fluid from the tip of the pipette by holding it vertically above a tissue.

15. Touch the pipette tip to the edge of the counting chamber and coverslip.

16. By gently releasing your fingertip, allow the fluid to flow into one side of the hemacytometer and to fill the ruled area by capillary action. Do not overfill. Only about three-fourths of a drop is needed.

17. Fill the other side of the hemacytometer in the same way.

18. Allow the hemacytometer to sit undisturbed for two minutes to allow the cells to settle, and place the pipette in disinfectant to soak for later cleaning.

19. Place the low-power (10X) objective of the microscope in the viewing position.

20. Place the filled hemacytometer on the lowered stage of the microscope, centered over the opening in the stage, and secure it with the clamps.

21. Adjust the light for comfortable viewing by narrowing the diaphragm and lowering the condenser.

22. Raise the microscope stage carefully while watching from the side until the hemacytometer is near but not touching the 10X objective.

23. Looking through the ocular of the microscope, focus with the coarse-focus adjustment knob until the squares of the hemacytometer come into view.

24. Refocus with the fine-focus adjustment knob and light until you see the cells clearly.

25. Inspect the field of vision to see if the white blood cells appear to be evenly distributed over the field. If so, proceed to the next step. If the cells are not evenly distributed, go back to step 12 to clean and refill the hemacytometer.

26. Count the white blood cells in the four corners of the ruled area, pressing the button of the hand tally each time that you count a cell, following the counting rules described in the text. Do not forget that you should count the cells on only two sides of each square.

27. When you have finished counting each corner square, record the number of cells counted, reset the tally to zero, and proceed to the next corner square until you have counted all four corner squares. If the counts differ by more than ten cells, go back to step 12 and clean and recharge the hemacytometer again.

28. Total the number of cells counted in all four corner squares.

29. Count the white blood cells on the other side of the hemacytometer in the same way.

30. Average the counts from the two sides.

31. Substitute the average number of cells counted into the WBC count formula given in the text and calculate the WBC count.

32. Record the results as the number of white blood cells/mm^3.

33. Discard disposable equipment.

34. Clean and disinfect the automatic pipetting device and the hemacytometer and coverslip and return them to storage.

S = Satisfactory	U = Unsatisfactory	S	U
35. Clean the pipette in the pipette washer and then place it in the drying oven.			
36. Clean the work area following the Universal Precautions.			
37. Remove your gloves and apron; wash your hands with disinfectant, and dry them.			

OVERALL PROCEDURAL EVALUATION

Student's Name _____

Signature of Instructor _____ Date _____

Comments

PROCEDURE

16.2 ◆ Determining an RBC Count by the Manual Method

Goal

- After successfully completing this procedure, you will be able to dilute a blood sample in a Thoma pipette or Unopette kit, charge a hemacytometer, count red blood cells under high-power magnification, and calculate the RBC count.

Equipment and Supplies

- disposable latex gloves
- apron
- hand disinfectant
- surface disinfectant
- paper towels and tissues
- biohazard container
- mechanical blood mixer (optional)
- automatic pipetting device
- Thoma red blood-cell pipette (or a Unopette kit)
- EDTA-anticoagulated blood
- Hayem normal saline solution
- pipette shaker (optional)
- test tube rack
- glass-marking pen
- Neubauer ruled hemacytometer and coverslip
- lens paper
- 70 percent alcohol
- microscope
- hand tally counter
- pipette washer
- paper and pencil

Instructions

Read through the list of equipment and supplies that you will need and the steps of the procedure. Be sure that you understand each step before you begin. Then complete each step correctly and in the proper order. If your completion time is too long, repeat the procedure until you increase your speed.

S = Satisfactory	U = Unsatisfactory	S	U

1. Wash your hands with disinfectant, dry them, and put on gloves and an apron.

2. Follow the Universal Precautions.

3. Collect and prepare the appropriate equipment.

4. Mix the blood sample gently by hand or with a mechanical blood mixer.

5. Two alternate methods of dilution:
   a. Attach the pipetting device to the Thoma red blood-cell pipette.
   b. Use an RBC Unopette kit per manufacturer's instructions on package insert.

6. Holding the pipette nearly horizontally in your dominant hand between your thumb and index finger and the tube of blood in your other hand, tilt the tube slightly and insert the pipette tip into the blood.

7. Using the pipetting device, draw blood up to the 0.5 mark of the pipette but not past the mark, taking care to avoid air bubbles.

8. Clean the outside of the pipette with a soft tissue, avoiding the tip so that you do not siphon away blood out of the pipette by accident.

9. Holding the pipette almost vertically to prevent air bubbles from collecting, insert the tip of the pipette into the diluting solution and aspirate fluid to the 101 mark, taking care not to drop any blood into the diluting solution.

10. Hold your gloved finger over the pipette tip to prevent loss of fluid and remove the pipetting device from the other end of the pipette.

11. Label the pipette with the marking pen.

12. After cleaning the hemacytometer and coverslip with 70 percent alcohol and drying them thoroughly with lens paper, align the coverslip on the hemacytometer.

13. Mix the diluted blood sample in the pipette for two to three minutes using either the manual figure-eight method or a mechanical pipette mixer.

14. Placing the tip of your index finger over the stem of the Thoma pipette to control the flow of fluid, expel the first three drops of fluid from the tip of the pipette by holding it vertically above a tissue.

15. Touch the pipette tip to the edge of the counting chamber and coverslip.

16. By gently releasing your fingertip, allow the fluid to flow into one side of the hemacytometer and to fill the ruled area by capillary action. Do not overfill. Only about three-fourths of a drop is needed.

17. Fill the other side of the hemacytometer in the same way.

18. Allow the hemacytometer to sit undisturbed for two minutes to allow the cells to settle, and place the pipette in disinfectant to soak for later cleaning.

19. Place the low-power (10X) objective of the microscope in the viewing position.

20. Place the filled hemacytometer on the lowered stage of the microscope, centered over the opening in the stage, and secure it with the clamps.

21. Raise the stage carefully while watching from the side.

22. Focus and center the large center square of the counting area under the low-power objective by simultaneously turning the coarse-focus adjustment knob and moving the mechanical stage.

23. Switch to the high-power (45X) objective and focus with the fine-focus adjustment knob.

24. Adjust the light source until the cells are easy to see.

25. Inspect the field of vision to see if the red blood cells appear to be evenly distributed over the field. If so, proceed to the next step. If the cells are not evenly distributed, go back to step 12 to clean and refill the hemacytometer.

26. Pressing the button of the hand tally each time that you count a cell, count the red blood cells in the five smaller squares (the four corners and one center square) within the large center square. Follow the counting rules described in the text and do not forget to count the cells on only two sides of each square.

27. When you have finished counting each of the five small squares, record the number of cells counted, reset the tally to zero, and proceed to the next square until you have counted all five squares. If the counts differ by more than twenty-five cells, go back to step 12 and clean and recharge the hemacytometer again.

28. Total the number of cells counted in all five squares.

29. Count the red blood cells on the other side of the hemacytometer in the same way.

30. Average the counts from the two sides.

31. Substitute the average number of cells counted into the RBC count formula given in the text and calculate the RBC count.

32. Record the results as the number of red blood cells/mm^3.

33. Discard disposable equipment.

34. Clean and disinfect the automatic pipetting device and the hemacytometer and coverslip and return them to storage.

35. Clean the pipette in the pipette washer and then place it in the drying oven.

36. Clean the work area following the Universal Precautions.

37. Remove your gloves and apron; wash your hands with disinfectant, and dry them.

OVERALL PROCEDURAL EVALUATION

Student's Name _____

Signature of Instructor _____ **Date** _____

Comments

CHAPTER 16 REVIEW

Using Terminology

Define the following terms in the spaces provided.

1. Agglutination: _____

   _____

2. Isotonic: _____

   _____

3. Leukocytosis: _____

   _____

4. Leukopenia: _____

   _____

5. Polycythemia: _____

   _____

6. Reticulocyte: _____

   _____

7. Erythrocytosis: _____

   _____

8. Pseudoagglutination: _____

_____

9. Nucleated red blood cell (nuRBC): _____

_____

10. Rouleau: _____

_____

Match the term in the right column with the appropriate definition or description in the left column.

_____ 11. adrenaline

_____ 12. bone marrow disorder

_____ 13. daily variation

_____ 14. lack of oxygen

_____ 15. polycythemia vera

_____ 16. WBC count

_____ 17. result of dehydration

_____ 18. tumor

_____ 19. vitamin B$_{12}$ deficiency

_____ 20. RBC count

a. anoxia

b. aplastic anemia

c. diurnal

d. epinephrine

e. erythemia

f. erythrocyte count

g. leukocyte count

h. neoplasm

i. pernicious anemia

j. relative polycythemia

Acquiring Knowledge

Answer the following questions in the spaces provided.

21. What functions do white blood cells serve in the body?

_____

_____

22. What does the WBC count measure? What is the most common reason it is performed?

_____

_____

23. How does the normal WBC count for newborns differ from that of adults?

_____

_____

_____

24. What are some causes of normal and abnormal variation in the WBC count?

_____

_____

_____

_____

_____

_____

25. When performing a WBC count, why must you add acid to the blood before counting the white cells?

_____

_____

26. Why is an Adams suction apparatus used when performing blood counts? How does it work?

_____

_____

_____

_____

27. Why are the first three drops of fluid from the pipette always discarded when doing a blood count?

_____

_____

28. Describe the area of the hemacytometer that is counted when performing a WBC count. What is the total area counted?

_____

29. How does the presence of nucleated red blood cells affect the WBC count? Why? What must be done to correct for this?

_____

_____

_____

30. Why is the depth factor in the WBC count formula 10 when the sample in the hemacytometer is only 0.1 mm deep?

_____

_____

31. Explain why the dilution is 1:20 in a white blood-cell pipette in which blood is drawn to the 0.5 mark and diluting fluid is drawn to the 11.0 mark.

_____

_____

32. What types of cells are included in an RBC count?

_____

33. How does the RBC count of the normal woman compare with that of the normal man?

_____

_____

34. List some of the causes of normal and abnormal variation in the RBC count.

_____

_____

_____

_____

_____

_____

35. When performing an RBC count, why must saline or a similar solution be added to the blood before the count is made?

_____

_____

36. Describe the area of the hemacytometer that is counted when performing an RBC count. What is the total area counted?

_____

_____

_____

37. What may cause agglutination and pseudoagglutination of red blood cells on the hemacytometer? How can you tell which has occurred? What should you do with an agglutinated sample?

_____

_____

_____

_____

38. When counting red or white blood cells, what is the rule for counting cells that fall on the borderlines between squares?

_____

_____

39. What is the most common reason for performing an RBC count?

_____

Applying Knowledge—On the Job

Answer the following questions in the spaces provided.

40. If a patient is taking the drug primidone, how may his or her RBC count be affected? Why?

_____

_____

41. Mrs. Potts just had a urinalysis and a complete blood count as part of a routine physical exam. Her WBC count was 16,000 and the urinalysis revealed a small amount of blood in her urine. What diagnosis do you think the doctor will make? Why?

_____

_____

_____

_____

_____

42. Assume that your coworker in the lab performs an RBC count and siphons blood into the pipette by mouth with a rubber tube. She passes the 0.5 mark and uses a tissue to drain out the excess blood. She then tosses the tissue into an unlabeled wastebasket and the rubber tube onto the countertop. What errors did your coworker make? What should your coworker have done instead?

_____

_____

_____

_____

_____

_____

_____

43. In the POL where you work, you are responsible for doing blood counts. How would you respond to each of the following situations and why?
   a. In the first square you count on the hemacytometer, there are 30 white blood cells and in the second there are 45.

   _____

   _____

   b. There appears to be an air bubble under one corner of the hemacytometer coverslip.

   _____

   _____

   c. The red blood cells appear to be clumped together in bunches on the hemacytometer.

   _____

   _____

d. A blood sample was left at room temperature overnight because it was overlooked the day before, and the doctor wants to know what happened to the blood count that she ordered.

44. It was nearing the end of Brad's shift, and he had just one more blood count to perform for the day. As soon as he flooded the hemacytometer, he focused the microscope and began counting red blood cells. To save time, he counted cells on only one side of the counting chamber. What errors did Brad make? What should he have done instead?

45. Assume that you are performing an RBC count in the POL where you work. In preparing the sample, you draw blood to the 0.5 mark of the red blood-cell pipette and diluting fluid to the 101 mark. You count the red blood cells under high-power magnification and come up with these tallies for the five squares on one side of the hemacytometer counting chamber: 100, 99, 103, 94, and 105. For the other side of the counting chamber the numbers are: 103, 105, 98, 97, and 101. Calculate the patient's RBC count, showing all of the steps.

46. Before performing an RBC count for a patient, you notice on her chart that she is taking an anticonvulsant drug for epilepsy and a diuretic for high blood pressure. How will these medications affect her RBC count?

47. You have just performed a WBC count, which turned out to be 990/mm^3. What should you do?

17 *Differential White Blood-Cell Count: Manual Procedure*

COGNITIVE OBJECTIVES

After studying this chapter, you should be able to

- use each vocabulary term appropriately.
- list several potential reasons for examining a blood smear under 100X objective magnification (oil immersion).
- describe the relative sizes and numbers of the formed elements in blood.
- identify the regions of a properly prepared blood smear and explain why the body of the smear is the region examined under the microscope.
- describe differences among the five types of white blood cells and list their identifying features on a differential blood smear.
- define the normal range of adult values for differential white blood-cell counts and list several causes of abnormal values.
- discuss the relationship between staining and identification of formed elements in the blood.

PERFORMANCE OBJECTIVES

After studying this chapter, you should be able to

- diagnose staining errors from the appearance of a differential blood-smear slide.
- correctly prepare a differential blood-smear slide.
- stain a differential blood-smear slide using the quick-stain method.
- perform a differential white blood-cell count.
- examine and describe the morphology and hemo-

globin concentration of red blood cells on a differential blood-smear slide.
- estimate the number of platelets on a differential blood-smear slide.

TERMINOLOGY

agranulocytes: the third of white blood cells, including both monocytes and lymphocytes, that have few, if any, visible granules.

agranulocytosis: an acute disorder characterized by severe sore throat, fever, complete exhaustion, and an extreme reduction in the number of neutrophils.

anisocytosis: the excessive variation in the size of cells, especially red blood cells.

basophil: the least common type of granular white blood cell, containing large cytoplasmic granules that stain blue-black with alkaline dyes.

brucellosis: a bacterial disease primarily of cattle, which leads to an increase in lymphocytes and a decrease in neutrophils.

cell counter: a manual counter for differential white blood-cell counts with keys for each type of white cell.

chronic granulocytic leukemia: a type of chronic leukemia caused by a chromosomal abnormality, leading to an overproduction of basophils in the bone marrow.

differential white blood-cell count: differential or "diff"; a determination of the percent of each type of white blood cells out of a total of 100 white blood cells observed under magnification by the oil immersion objective (100X) on a stained blood smear.

endocarditis: the inflammation of the lining of the heart. Endocarditis may be associated with an increase in the number of monocytes.

eosin: a red-orange acidic dye used to stain blood smears for microscopic examination.

eosinophil: a granular white blood cell with a bilobed nucleus and cytoplasmic granules that stain brilliant red with eosin dye. Increased numbers of eosinophils are associated with allergies and internal parasitic infections.

granulocyte: a polymorphonuclear white blood cell that contains granules in its cytoplasm. This class includes neutrophils, eosinophils, and basophils.

hyperchromic: having excess hemoglobin; refers to red blood cells with excess hemoglobin.

hypersegmented: having a nucleus with more than five segments, or lobes; used to describe certain neutrophils.

hypochromic: having too little hemoglobin; refers to red blood cells.

infectious lymphocytosis: a rare disorder, probably of viral origin, that leads to an increase in the number of small lymphocytes.

infectious mononucleosis: an acute infectious disease in which lymphocytes are both more numerous and larger than normal and often contain vacuoles, causing them to resemble monocytes—hence the name of the disease.

lymphocyte: the most common of all white blood cells in children; typically small and round with a nonsegmented nucleus and no cytoplasmic granules.

lymphocytic leukemia: predominantly a children's disease, in which the blood-forming tissues produce an excessive number of lymphocytes.

macrocyte: a red blood cell that is unusually large (greater than 12 microns in diameter).

megakaryocyte: a large bone marrow cell with large or multiple nuclei. Megakaryocytes give rise to platelets, which are cytoplasmic fragments of megakaryocytes.

methylene blue: a blue alkaline dye used to stain blood smears for microscopic examination.

microcyte: a red blood cell that is unusually small (less than 6 microns in diameter).

monocyte: the largest type of cell in the blood; an agranulocyte that has gray-blue cytoplasm with the appearance of ground glass.

monocytic leukemia: a form of acute leukemia in which abnormal monocytes proliferate and invade the blood, bone marrow, and other tissues.

mononuclear: having an undivided nucleus, such as lymphocytes and monocytes.

neutropenia: a decrease below normal in the number of neutrophils in the blood, due to certain drugs, some acute infections, radiation, or certain diseases of the spleen or bone marrow.

neutrophil: the most common type of white blood cell; a granulocyte with a multilobed nucleus and cytoplasm filled with fine pink granules.

normochromic: normal in color; used to describe red blood cells that have the normal amount of hemoglobin.

normocyte: an average-sized red blood cell, about 7.5 micrometers (μm) in diameter.

poikilocytosis: a condition in which many red blood cells have abnormal shapes.

polychromatic stain: a stain containing dyes of two or more colors, such as Wright's stain, which contains methylene blue and eosin.

polymorphonuclear: having a multilobed nucleus; used to describe cells such as granulocytes.

pyogenic: pus producing; includes organisms such as staphylococcus and streptococcus.

quick-stain method: a method of staining blood smears, in which the smear is dipped sequentially in fixative, acidic stain, and alkaline stain; also called the three-step method.

vacuole: a clear space in cell cytoplasm that is filled with fluid or air.

Wright's stain: a polychromatic stain for fixing and staining blood smears. It contains eosin and methylene blue dyes in a methyl alcohol solution.

• • • • • • • • • • • • • • • • • • •

Stained blood smears are examined under the highest power of magnification as part of the complete blood count. The main purpose is to count the different types of white blood cells. Another reason for examining blood smears under the highest power of magnification is to identify abnormalities in white blood cells and in the other formed elements in the blood—the red blood cells and platelets. Microscopic examination of a blood smear also can provide an estimate of WBC and RBC counts, platelet count, and the hematocrit.

♦ ♦

AN OVERVIEW OF THE FORMED ELEMENTS IN THE BLOOD

The most numerous formed elements in the blood observed on a differential slide are red blood cells. Each cubic millimeter of blood in the normal adult averages 5,000,000 red blood cells. Red blood cells have no nuclei and are smaller than the average white blood cells. The average life span of mature red blood cells is just 120 days, and new red blood cells are constantly being produced in the bone marrow to replace those that are worn out. Old red blood cells are removed from circulation by the spleen.

Unlike red blood cells, white blood cells are nucleated. They also are highly differentiated for their specialized functions, and they are larger than red blood cells. Normal adult blood has an average of 7,000 white blood cells per cubic millimeter. Figure 17.1 shows types of blood cells found on a normal peripheral blood smear for an individual.

White blood cells fall into two general classes. One class is called **granulocytes** because they have granules in their cytoplasm that are visible after staining. Granulocytes also are called **polymorphonuclear** leukocytes because of their multilobed nuclei. There are three types of granulocytes—**neutrophils, eosinophils,** and **basophils,** with neutrophils being by far the most common. The average life span of granulocytes is about nine to ten days.

The other class of white blood cells is called **agranulocytes** because they have few, if any, visible granules after staining. There are two types—**monocytes** and **lymphocytes.** Monocytes are the largest cells in the blood, but they are relatively few in number. Lymphocytes, which are responsible for the formation of antibodies and cell-mediated immunity, are further subdivided by size into small and large lymphocytes. Small lymphocytes are just a little larger than red blood cells and make up the majority of lymphocytes. Next to neutrophils, they are the most common white blood cells. In children, lymphocytes are the most common white blood cells observed on a stained blood smear.

Platelets are the smallest formed elements in blood, being less than half as big as red blood cells.

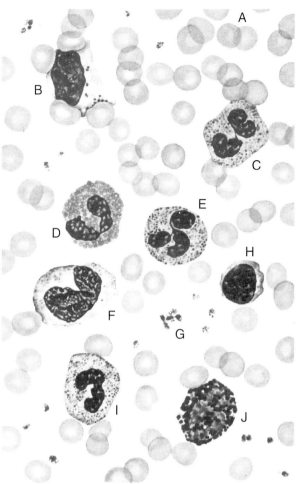

Figure 17.1. Cell types found in smears of peripheral blood from normal individuals. a. Erythrocytes. b. Large lymphocyte with azurophilic granules and deeply indented by adjacent erythrocytes. c. Neutrophilic segmented. d. Eosinophil. e. Neutrophilic segmented. f. Monocyte with blue-gray cytoplasm, coarse linear chromatin, and blunt pseudopods. g. Thrombocytes. h. Lymphocyte. i. Neutrophilic band. j. Basophil. (*Note:* Arrangement is arbitrary, and the number of leukocytes in relation to erythrocytes and thrombocytes is greater than would occur in actual microscopic field.) Reproduction of pictures from *The Morphology of Human Blood Cells* has been granted with approval of Abbott Laboratories; all rights reserved by Abbott Laboratories.

They are called platelets because of their platelike flatness. They also are called thrombocytes for their role in clot, or thrombus, formation. Platelets are not cells but fragments of the cytoplasm of large cells called **megakaryocytes,** which remain in the bone marrow. Platelets average some 250,000 per cubic millimeter of blood, making them more numerous than white blood cells but less numerous than red blood cells. Their average life span in the circulating blood is eight to ten days.

PREPARING AND STAINING BLOOD SMEARS

Blood smears are examined under the oil-immersion, 100X, objective of the microscope. Correct preparation and staining of the smear are crucial first steps in obtaining accurate results.

◆◆ *Preparing the Smear*

The most common method of preparing a blood smear is the two-slide method. A glass slide, called the spreader, is used to spread a drop of whole blood on another glass slide, which holds the smear. Both slides must be free of dust, dirt, and oil, and they should be handled only by their edges to avoid smudges. Blood smears are made in duplicate, so the second one can be referred to if the need arises.

◆◆◆ Note ◆◆◆

Blood used for a smear can be collected by either venipuncture or capillary puncture. A tube containing EDTA anticoagulant must be used for collecting the sample unless the smear is made before the blood has time to clot.

Figure 17.2 illustrates how to make a blood smear. Place the smear slide on a flat surface, and hold the spreader slide in the dominant hand. Place a single drop of blood about half an inch from the end of the smear slide—the right end for right-handed people, the left end for left-handed people. The drop of blood should be small, about twice the size of a pin head. Hold the spreader slide at a 35 to 40 degree angle and place it to the left of the drop of blood, or to the right for left-handed people. Back the spreader slide into the drop of blood until blood covers about three-fourths of its width. Then, push the spreader slide in the opposite direction in a quick, steady movement, reducing the angle as you go across the slide. Avoid jerky movements and pressure on the spreader slide.

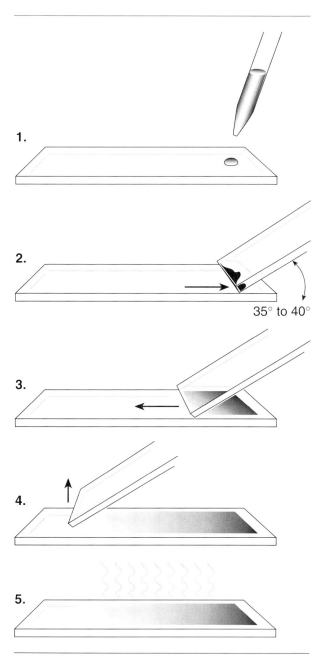

Figure 17.2. Making a peripheral blood smear. 1. Place a small drop of blood toward one end of the slide. 2. Place a new glass slide over the first slide and pull it backward into the drop of blood. 3. Push the upper slide across the bottom slide with a quick, even motion. 4. Pull the upper slide up and away. 5. Allow the smear to air dry. Do not blow on it.

Air dry the blood smear as quickly as possible to avoid contraction artifacts of the cells. To hasten drying, wave the slide in the air or place it in front of an electric fan. Never blow on the slide. Exhaled water droplets may make holes in the smear.

After preparing and drying the slide, label it with a pencil on the end where the blood drop was placed. The label should include the patient's name, the date, and the doctor's name. If you cannot stain the slide immediately, preserve the cellular components by immersing the slide in methyl alcohol for thirty to sixty seconds and air drying again.

Preparing a blood smear is a skill that takes practice to perfect. If correctly done, a blood smear covers about two-thirds the length of the slide and coats the slide smoothly without grainy streaks or ridges. A correctly prepared smear has three different regions, as Figure 17.3 illustrates:

- *The heel:* the thick end of the smear, where the drop of blood was placed, which contains stacked red blood cells
- *The feathered edge:* the end opposite the heel,

which is the thinnest area of the smear, with spaces between the red blood cells

- *The body:* the middle region of the slide, where the red blood cells barely touch one another and do not overlap.

Only the body of the blood smear is examined under the oil-immersion objective of the microscope. The cells are easiest to examine in this region because they are numerous yet arranged in a single layer, with minimal distortion from adjacent cells. Figure 17.4 shows a correct smear and some that would be difficult to read.

♦♦ *Staining the Smear*

Before the slide is examined under the microscope, the smear must be stained. Staining heightens the contrast among the different types of cells and other structures and therefore differentiates them.

In today's POLs, a **polychromatic stain,** also known as Romanowsky stain, is used most often. Polychromatic stains are multicolored, containing both an alkaline dye, such as **methylene blue,** and an acidic dye, such as **eosin,** which is red-orange. Acidic structures in the blood, such as cell nuclei, appear blue after staining because they attract alkaline, or basic, dye. That is why they are called basophilic. Alkaline structures in the blood, such as cytoplasm, attract acidic dye, hence the name eosinophilic, or acidophilic. Structures that attract neutral dyes are termed neutrophilic. Both normal and abnormal formed elements in the blood are differentiated by their staining affinities.

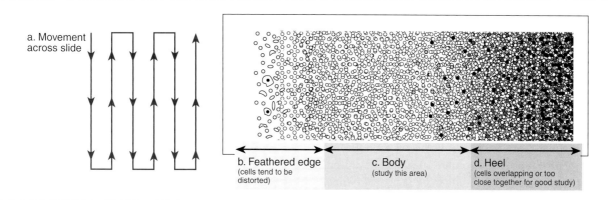

Figure 17.3. Representation of a correctly stained blood smear. a. A serpentine (snakelike) counting pattern across the slide ensures thorough, nonrepetitive coverage. b. Inspect the feather edge when studying abnormal lymphocytes. c. The body of the slide reveals the most cell morphology of both red and white blood cells. Observe the numbers of platelets in this area. d. The heel end of the smear shows stacked red blood cells.

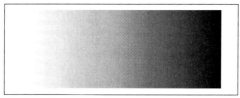

a. Ideal blood smear changes evenly from a thick area to a very thin area when spread from right to left.

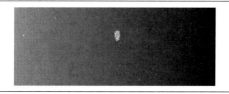

b. This smear has a thick, even layer of blood that does not permit viewing the individual cells' structures.

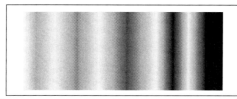

c. This smear was made with uneven pressure, so it does not permit accurate counts.

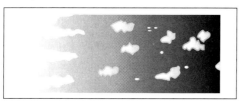

d. The slide this smear was made on was not clean; it probably had minute oil droplets on the surface.

Figure 17.4. Correct and incorrect types of slides.

Wright's Stain. **Wright's stain** is one of the most widely used polychromatic stains in POLs. It is a solution of methyl alcohol, eosin, and a complex mixture of thiazines, including methyl blue. Because it contains methyl alcohol, Wright's solution both stains and fixes the smear in one operation.

To stain a slide with Wright's stain, place the air-dried slide on a rack, blood side up, and cover it with Wright's stain. Let the slide stand for two minutes and then cover it with an equal amount of buffer solution. Mix the stain and buffer by gently blowing on the mixture. Let the slide stand again, this time for two and one-half to five minutes. A green metallic scum should appear on the surface of the mixture, and the margins should show a reddish tint. Wash the slide with distilled water, first gently, then more vig-

orously, using an overhead water bottle until all traces of excess stain are removed. Remove excess water by tilting the slide. Then leave the slide to dry in a tilted position.

An incorrectly prepared or incorrectly stained slide has a telltale appearance. Use the following guide to assess your technique:

- If a slide appears too blue or too dark:
  The smear may be too thick.
  The stain may have been left on too long.
  The stain may have been washed off inadequately.
  The stain or buffer may be too alkaline.

- If a slide appears too pink or too light:
  The staining time may have been too short.
  The stain may have been washed too long or too vigorously.
  The stain or buffer may be too acidic.

- If a slide has precipitate on the blood film:
  The slide may be dirty.
  The slide may have dried during staining.
  The stain may have been washed off inadequately.
  The stain may have been filtered inadequately.

The Quick-Stain Method. The **quick-stain method,** also called the three-step method, is used widely in POLs because it is quicker and easier to use than is Wright's stain. The quick-stain method uses the same dyes as Wright's stain, but the two dyes, methylene blue and eosin, are in separate aqueous (water) solutions. Because the dyes are applied separately, there is more control over staining time with each dye (see Figure 17.5).

First, dip the air-dried, blood-smear slide in a fixative solution five times, allowing one second for each dip. Wick away excess fixative from the slide by touching the edge of the slide to a paper towel. Next, dip the slide three to five times, allowing one second for each dip, in the eosin staining solution. Allow excess stain to drain away, but do not dry the slide.

♦ ♦ ♦ Caution! ♦ ♦ ♦

The fixative solution used in the quick-stain method contains methyl alcohol in greater than 99 percent concentration. This solution can be fatal or cause blindness if ingested. Be certain that all supplies are closed tightly after use because evaporation can distort results and can cause chemical changes.

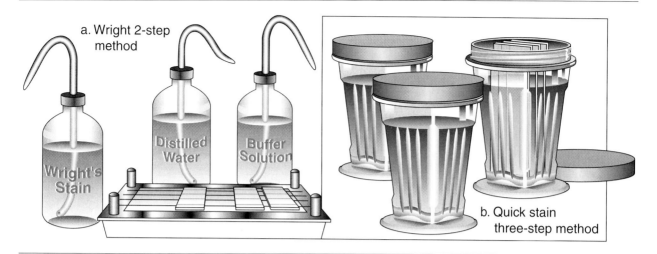

Figure 17.5. Two methods for staining blood smears. Both use a timed exposure to the stains. a. The Wright's-stain method utilizes a rack, where the stains are added to the blood smear. b. With the quick-stain method, the smear is immersed in three solutions.

Finally, dip the slide three to five times in the methylene blue staining solution, again allowing one second for each dip and allowing the excess stain to drain. Follow this by a rinse with distilled or deionized water and air drying.

If a pale stain is desired, dip the slide just three times in each dye solution. Red tone may be intensified by increasing the number of dips in the first, acidic, stain solution. Blue tone may be intensified by increasing the number of dips in the second, alkaline, stain solution.

◆◆

DIFFERENTIATING AND COUNTING WHITE BLOOD CELLS

The **differential white blood-cell count**, also known as the differential or "diff," determines the percent of each type of white blood cell in a stained blood smear out of a total of at least 100 white blood cells. The white cells also are examined for abnormal morphology. The differential white blood-cell count assists in the diagnosis and treatment of many diseases.

◆◆ *Differentiating White Blood Cells by Type*

To perform a differential white blood-cell count, you must be able to distinguish the different types of

white cells in a stained blood smear. A good blood-cell atlas, such as Abbott Laboratories' *The Morphology of Human Blood Cells*, is indispensable for this purpose.

Features that must be examined to differentiate the various types of white blood cells include:

- the size of the cell
- the nuclear characteristics, such as shape, size, structure, and color
- the cytoplasmic characteristics, such as amount, color, and types of inclusions

Figure 17.6 shows characteristics of white blood cells.

Neutrophils. The neutrophil, also called a "seg" for segmented nucleus or "poly" for polymorphonuclear, is a granulocyte ranging from 10 to 15 micrometers in diameter. The nuclei of neutrophils usually have three to five lobes, each connected by an invisible, threadlike membrane. The arrangement of the lobes may resemble the letters *E*, *S*, or *Z*. The nuclear material is coarse and condensed, and it stains deeply with blue.

The cytoplasm of neutrophils is abundant and either colorless or stained light pink. Neutrophils are so named because the fine granules that fill their cytoplasm are stained by neutral stains. With Wright's stain they appear pink or lilac.

Band neutrophils, or "bands," are an immature form of neutrophil. They have the same diameter as the mature form, but the lobes of the nuclei are still connected by a wide strip of membrane that is clearly

	Segmented neutrophil	Neutrophilic band (stab)	Eosinophil	Basophil	Lymphocyte	Monocyte
Cell size	10 – 15 µm	10 – 15 µm	10 – 15 µm	10 – 15 µm	6 – 15 µm	14 – 20 µm
Nucleus shape	2–5 lobes connected by slender filaments	sausage or band shaped	bilobed	segmented	usually round (oval)	round or kidney-shaped
structure	coarse, condensed	course	course	difficult to see; obscured by cytoplasmic granules	lumpy or clumped; smudged (smoothly stained)	folded, convoluted, may be deeply indented
Cytoplasm amount	abundant	abundant	abundant	abundant	scant	abundant
color	pink to colorless or bright pink	pink to tan	pink to tan	pink to tan	clear to medium blue	opaque, blue-gray
inclusions	small purple, lilac granules	small lilac granules; fine pale blue or pink granules	course, red or orange granules	course, large blue-black granules	occasional granules, red-purple	fine stain or ground-glass appearance, evenly cytoplasmic distributed; lilac granules

Figure 17.6. White blood cells (leukocytes) are identified by the individual characteristics of their nucleus and cytoplasm and according to size and color.

visible. The coarse-appearing nucleus is shaped like a link sausage or a band, and it stains deep purple-blue. The cytoplasm of band neutrophils is abundant and contains fine pale blue or pink granules.

Eosinophils. Eosinophil granulocytes have about the same diameter as neutrophils—10 to 15 micrometers —but the nucleus has just two lobes and

stains less deeply. The cytoplasm has a faint sky-blue tinge or is colorless. The most distinguishing features of eosinophils are the large, coarse, spherical granules in the cytoplasm. These granules are uniform in size, they usually are evenly distributed, and they fill the cell without overlying the nucleus. The granules stain bright red with the acidic dye, eosin.

Basophils. Basophils average 10 micrometers in diameter. Like other polymorphonuclear leukocytes, they have a nucleus with lobes. Their distinguishing features are the large, irregularly shaped cytoplasmic granules, which stain blue-black with Wright's stain. In fact, the nucleus often is obscured by the cytoplasmic granules.

Lymphocytes. Lymphocytes are **mononuclear,** or single-nucleus, cells without visible cytoplasmic granules. Small lymphocytes range from 6 to 12 micrometers in diameter, being only slightly larger than red blood cells. Large lymphocytes range from 12 to 15 microns in diameter, comparable in size to granulo-

---

**♦ ♦ ♦   Is It a Neutrophil   ♦ ♦ ♦
or a Basophil?**

Neutrophils sometimes have large, darkly stained granules that resemble basophilic granules. When in doubt, it is usually safe to assume the cell is a neutrophil because basophils are far less numerous and are seldom seen on a blood differential slide. (Basophils average one-half percent or less of the total leukocytes.)

cytes. Large lymphocytes are more common in the blood of children and generally are less mature cells, although size is not a reliable criterion for the age of lymphocytes. Small lymphocytes have less cytoplasm, perhaps because they shed cytoplasm as they supply antibodies. In any event, the size of lymphocytes usually is not relevant in diagnosis or treatment.

In the blood stream, lymphocytes are actively motile cells with irregular shapes. When a smear is prepared, the lymphocytes are exposed to air, chilled, brought into contact with glass surfaces, and dried. These disturbances give lymphocytes the spherical shape that they take on in a differential smear.

Lymphocytes have a single, sharply defined nucleus that contains heavy blocks of chromatin and stains a coarse dark blue or blue-black. The nucleus occupies a major portion of the cell in small lymphocytes, which may appear to have just a narrow rim of cytoplasm around it. The nucleus usually is round, but it may have an indentation at one side caused by the pressure of neighboring cells.

The cytoplasm of lymphocytes usually contains few granules, if any, and it stains a pale blue. However, about one-third of large lymphocytes have cytoplasmic granules that are large, round, and stain red-purple. The granules are larger than the granules of neutrophils.

Monocytes. Monocytes are the largest cells normally found in circulating blood. They have a diameter of 14 to 20 micrometers, making them two to three times the size of the typical red blood cell. The nuclei of monocytes usually are round or kidney shaped, but they may be deeply indented or folded. Some monocytes have nuclei with superimposed lobes that look like convolutions of the brain.

The cytoplasm of monocytes is abundant. It stains gray-blue with Wright's stain and has a finely granular appearance, like ground glass. The cytoplasm also may contain fine lilac granules that are smaller and less distinct than are the granules of neutrophils.

Cytoplasmic **vacuoles** are common in monocytes, and they may contain phagocytized red blood cells, leukocytes, cell fragments, or bacteria.

Figure 17.7 shows the sequence of origin and maturation of myelocytic white blood cells. The stages of progressive maturation start with the myeloblast and end with the segmented cells. Only band and segmented forms of the cell on stained smears are considered to be normal. Classify any form of the cell that is younger than the band as an abnormal cell and refer it to the laboratory director for identification.

♦♦ *Counting White Blood Cells*

The only area counted in a differential blood cell count is the middle portion of the slide, called the body, where the red blood cells are just one layer thick. First, locate the body of the smear under the low-power, 10X, objective. This also is a good time to identify cells that appear abnormal for closer examination under the oil-immersion objective. After locating the body of the slide under the low-power objective, perform the count using the oil-immersion objective. The light must be bright enough for the colors and small structures to be readily distinguishable.

Follow a definite pattern when counting cells on the slide, like the serpentine pattern shown in Figure 17.3, to avoid the possibility of counting the same area of the slide twice. A manual **cell counter**, such as those shown in Figure 17.8, is used to tally the dif-

---

♦ ♦ ♦ **Is It a Lymphocyte** ♦ ♦ ♦
or a Monocyte?

If you are having difficulty distinguishing monocytes and large lymphocytes from each other on differential smears, look closely at the chromatin. In lymphocytes, the chromatin is all in a clump. In monocytes, light spaces between the chromatin strands give the chromatin a coarse, linear appearance.

♦ ♦ ♦ **Estimating the** ♦ ♦ ♦
WBC Count

You can estimate the total WBC count by counting the white blood cells in one field in the body portion of a blood smear under the low-power objective and then multiplying the count by 500. This method is less accurate than the one described in Chapter 16, but it is useful as a check on the WBC count using the preferred method.

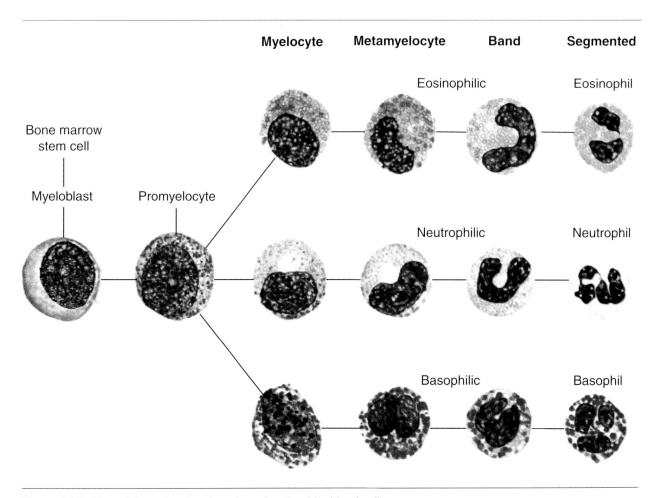

Myelocyte	Metamyelocyte	Band	Segmented

Figure 17.7. The origin and maturation of myelocytic white blood cells.

ferent types of white blood cells observed. Counters vary, but most can count up to six different types of cells per operation. When a total of 100 cells has been counted, the counter rings or locks. The counter can be reset if more than 100 cells are to be counted. The more cells counted, the greater the accuracy of the count. Error is on the order of ± 10 percent when 100 cells are counted and ± 7 percent when 200 cells are counted.

Express the number of each type of white blood cell as a percentage of the total number of white blood cells counted. Table 17.1 gives normal adult values for each type of white cell.

◆◆ *Abnormal Values for the Differential White Blood-Cell Count*

A rise or fall in the number of white blood cells occurs in many pathological conditions. It usually leads to a change in the proportion of the various types of white blood cells. Changes in the proportions of the various types may be important in diagnosis.

An Increase in the Number of White Blood Cells. An increase in the number of white blood cells usually is due to an increase in the number of granulocytes, especially neutrophils. Increased numbers of neutrophils, in turn, are most often associated with infection by **pyogenic,** or pus-producing, organisms, such as streptococcus, staphylococcus, gonococcus,

---

◆ ◆ ◆ **Hypersegmentation** ◆ ◆ ◆

When neutrophils have nuclei with six or more lobes, they are said to be **hypersegmented.** Hypersegmentation may indicate anemia, vitamin B_{12} deficiency, or folic acid deficiency. It is usually the last sign of the disease to disappear after therapy.

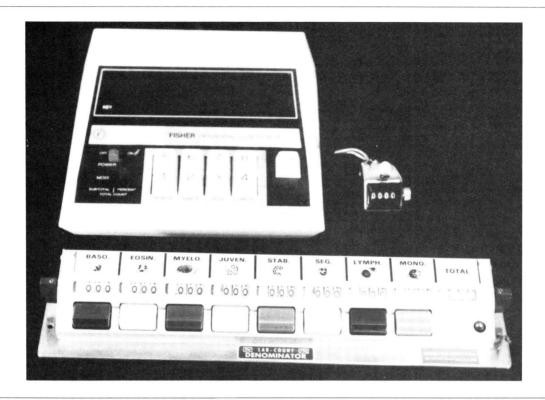

Figure 17.8. Cell counters make counting and classifying cells easier. The two differential white blood-cell counters have keys labeled for each cell type. The small hand-held tally is for total RBC and WBC counts. Photo by Mark Palko.

pneumococcus, or meningococcus, which cause appendicitis, pneumonia, and other acute infections.

An increase in the number of neutrophils is always accompanied by an increase in the "band" neutrophils, the immature form of a neutrophil. This increase in band forms is referred to as a "shift to the left" (Figure 17.7).

An increase in the percent of eosinophils is found in association with allergic reactions, such as hay fever, and skin disorders, such as eczema. Parasitic infestations, such as trichinosis and tapeworm, also may be associated with elevated numbers of eosinophils. If basophils are elevated, the patient may have **chronic granulocytic leukemia.**

TABLE 17.1 Normal Differential White Blood-Cell Values in Adults

Type of WBC	Percent of Total WBCs Counted
Neutrophil ("poly")	54 to 62
Neutrophil ("band")	3 to 5
Eosinophil	1 to 3
Basophil	0 to 1
Lymphocyte	25 to 33
Monocyte	3 to 7

An increase in the number of small lymphocytes is associated with whooping cough, tuberculosis, **brucellosis**—a bacterial disease primarily of cattle—and **infectious lymphocytosis**, a rare disorder that is probably of viral origin. In **infectious mononucleosis**, lymphocytes are both more numerous and larger than normal, and they often contain vacuoles, causing them to resemble monocytes—hence the name of the disease. A very high lymphocyte count also may indicate **lymphocytic leukemia**, predominantly a children's disease, in which there is excessive production of lymphocytes by the blood-forming tissues.

An increase in monocytes may be found in tuberculosis and acute **monocytic leukemia**. The latter is a form of acute leukemia in which abnormal monocytes proliferate and invade the blood, bone marrow, and other tissues. **Endocarditis**, inflammation of the lining of the heart, and ulcerative colitis also may be associated with an increased number of monocytes.

A Decrease in the Number of White Blood Cells.
A decreased WBC count usually is due to **neutropenia**, or a decrease below normal in the number of neutrophils. Of itself, neutropenia causes no symptoms, but it may lead to frequent and severe bacterial infections. An extreme reduction in the number of neutrophils or even their complete disappearance from the blood is called **agranulocytosis**. It is an acute disorder characterized by severe sore throat, fever, and complete exhaustion.

A number of pharmaceutical drugs may cause neutropenia in sensitive people. These include pain relievers, antihistamines, tranquilizers, anticonvulsants, antimicrobial agents, sulfonamide derivatives, and antithyroid drugs. Neutropenia also is associated with some acute infections (such as typhoid fever, brucellosis, and measles), exposure to radiation, and certain diseases involving the spleen or bone marrow (such as aplastic anemia).

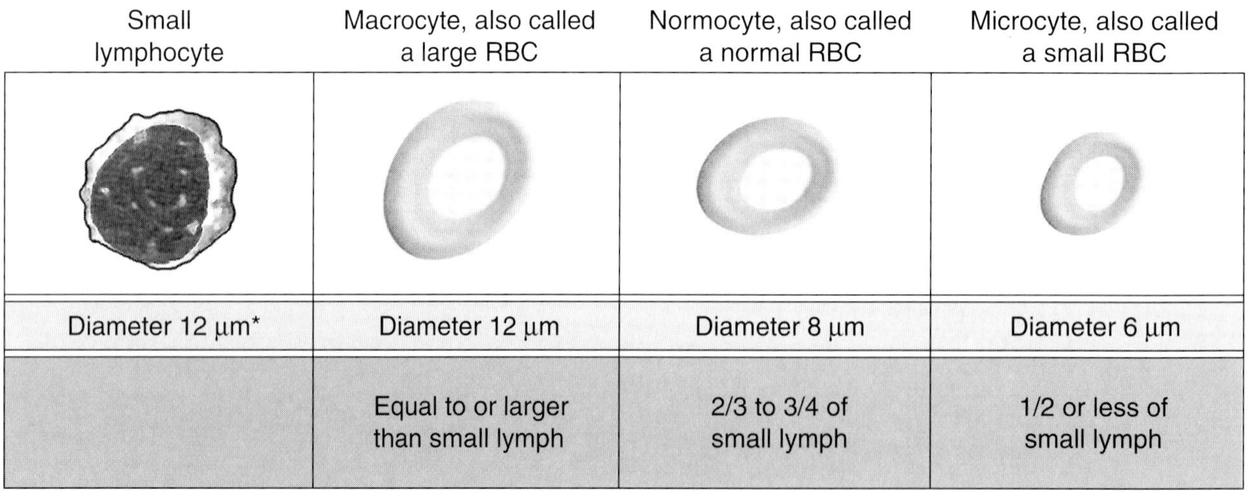

Small lymphocyte	Macrocyte, also called a large RBC	Normocyte, also called a normal RBC	Microcyte, also called a small RBC
Diameter 12 μm*	Diameter 12 μm	Diameter 8 μm	Diameter 6 μm
	Equal to or larger than small lymph	2/3 to 3/4 of small lymph	1/2 or less of small lymph

* μm = a measure of the metric system
μm = micrometer
μm = 1/millionth of a meter
μm = 1/1000 of a millimeter

μm = .001 millimeter
μm = 10^{-3} mm
μm = micron

(all of the above are ways of expressing the same measurement)

Figure 17.9. Use small lymphocytes as a standard of reference to estimate the size of red blood cells on a stained differential blood smear.

EXAMINING RED BLOOD CELLS

Red blood cells are easy to identify under the oil-immersion objective of the microscope. They stain light red or pinkish tan with Wright's stain and have no nuclei. They are examined under the oil-immersion objective for their size, shape, and hemoglobin content.

Red blood cells normally range from 6 to 8 micrometers in diameter. Small lymphocytes are used as a point of reference to judge the size of red blood cells on the slide, as Figure 17.9 shows. A normal-sized red blood cell, a **normocyte,** has about two-thirds to three-fourths the diameter of a small lymphocyte. Small red blood cells, called **microcytes,** are half or less the diameter of small lymphocytes. They are common in patients with iron-deficiency anemia. Large red blood cells, called **macrocytes,** are equal to or larger than small lymphocytes. They are found in patients with vitamin B_{12} deficiency or folic acid deficiency. Occasional small or large red blood cells may be observed in normal individuals. A great deal of variation observed in the size of the red blood cells is referred to as **anisocytosis.**

+ + + **What Is in a Shape?** + + +

Red blood cells develop in the bone marrow, where they contain a nucleus and have a spherical shape. Before a red blood cell is released into the circulating blood, it extrudes the nucleus, which causes the cell to collapse on both sides, giving it the biconcave disk shape that characterizes circulating red blood cells. This shape has more surface area per volume than does the spherical shape. The relatively greater surface area helps the hemoglobin in the cell function more effectively in transporting oxygen.

Normal red blood cells appear as circular, homogeneous disks that are concave on both sides (see Figure 17.10). Occasional abnormally shaped cells are observed in normal individuals. The condition in which many red blood cells have abnormal shapes is

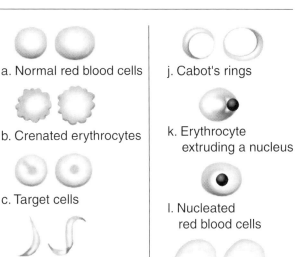

a. Normal red blood cells

b. Crenated erythrocytes

c. Target cells

d. Sickle cells

e. Oval, elliptical cells

f. Spherocytes (spherical erythrocytes)

g. Hypochromic cells

h. Reticulocytes

i. Howell-Jolly bodies

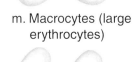

j. Cabot's rings

k. Erythrocyte extruding a nucleus

l. Nucleated red blood cells

m. Macrocytes (large erythrocytes)

n. Microcytes (small erythrocytes)

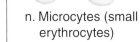

o. Pear shape cell (tear drop)

p. Helmet cell

q. Erthrocyte with HgbC

Figure 17.10. Types of red blood cells seen on stained blood smears.

poikilocytosis. Other abnormal cells may take on sickle, helmet, target, or pear shapes. Sickle-shaped red blood cells are due to the presence of hemoglobin S in the cells, as Chapter 15 describes.

Nucleated red blood cells, which are difficult to distinguish from white blood cells under low-power magnification, are easy to identify under the oil-immersion (100X) objective on a stained blood smear. Nucleated red blood cells have the color and appearance of large erythrocytes containing a dense nucleus (see Figure 17.11).

The hemoglobin content of red blood cells is indicated by the depth of staining of the cells. The more hemoglobin present, the darker the stain. Red blood cells with normal hemoglobin content are **normochromic.** Red blood cells with excess hemoglobin are **hyperchromic.** Red blood cells with too little hemoglobin are **hypochromic.** Hypochromic red blood cells may indicate a deficiency of iron, vitamin B$_{12}$, or folic acid.

Another indicator of hypochromia is the size of the pale area in the center of the cell. Normal red blood cells have a central pale area, measuring about one-third the diameter of the cell, where the hemoglobin concentration is low. Hypochromic cells have larger pale areas, measuring about two-thirds the diameter of the cell. Borderline hypochromic cells have pale

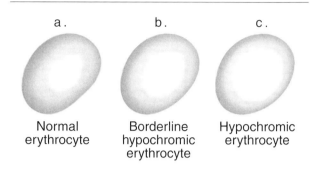

a.   b.   c.

Normal erythrocyte   Borderline hypochromic erythrocyte   Hypochromic erythrocyte

Figure 17.12. Normal and hypochromic cells. The amount of hemoglobin present in red blood cells is estimated according to the intensity of color. a. A normal erythrocyte shows a thick outer ring of darker color, approximately two-thirds the diameter of the cell, denoting hemoglobin. b. A borderline hypochromic cell has a smaller outer ring of darker color, approximately one-half the diameter of the cell. c. A hypochromic cell has only a thin ring of dark color, about one-third the diameter of the cell.

areas over about half the cell diameter (see Figure 17.12).

COUNTING PLATELETS

Normal platelets, illustrated in Figure 17.13, vary in diameter from 1 to 4 microns. They may have round, oval, spindle, or disk shapes. Platelets usually

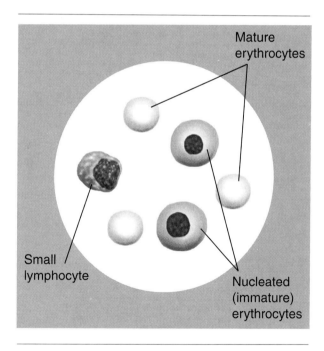

Mature erythrocytes

Small lymphocyte

Nucleated (immature) erythrocytes

Figure 17.11. Nucleated red blood cells. Viewed under the oil-immersion (100X) objective of a stained smear, they have the distinctive coloring and appearance of large erythrocytes containing a dense nucleus.

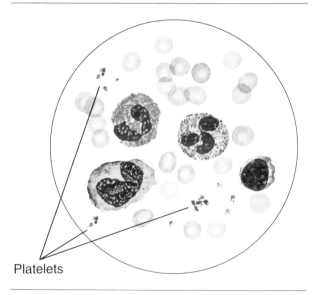

Platelets

Figure 17.13. The appearance of platelets with erythrocytes and white blood-cell types on a stained blood-cell differential smear.

have multiple tentacle-like protrusions, but some have smooth margins. The cytoplasm fragments of platelets stain light blue and contain variable numbers of small blue granules. The granules usually aggregate in the center of the cytoplasm, with the marginal zone being nongranular.

On a slide, platelets tend to adhere to each other. Both individual and clumps of platelets are more numerous at the feather end of the blood smear. In the body portion of the smear, the number of platelets per oil-immersion field normally varies from five to twenty, with about one platelet for every ten to thirty red blood cells.

Estimate the platelets per cubic millimeter by counting the number of platelets in a few oil-immersion fields and multiplying the average by 20,000. For example, if you counted 10 platelets in one field, 20 in the next, and 15 in the next, for an average of 15 per high-power field, the platelet count would be 15 × 20,000, or 300,000 per cubic millimeter.

The normal range for the platelet count is 140,000 to 400,000 per cubic millimeter. A reduced platelet count occurs in acute bacterial infections, immunological disorders, certain hemorrhagic diseases, and anemias. An increased platelet count occurs after surgery, especially splenectomy, following violent exercise, and in inflammatory disorders.

PROCEDURE

17.1

Preparing and Staining a Blood Smear and Examining Formed Elements Under High-Power Magnification

Goal

- After successfully completing this procedure, you will be able to correctly prepare and quick stain a blood-differential slide, examine the slide under the microscope, perform a differential white blood-cell count, note blood-cell morphology, and estimate the number of platelets.

Completion Time

- 40 minutes

Equipment and Supplies

- disposable latex gloves
- goggles and apron
- hand disinfectant
- surface disinfectant
- paper towels and tissues
- biohazard container
- 70 percent alcohol
- EDTA-anticoagulated blood
- clean glass slides
- capillary tube
- fixative and the two staining solutions of Hema 3® (Curtin Matheson Scientific Company)
- Coplin jars or staining dishes
- microscope
- immersion oil
- lens paper
- differential cell counter or notepad and pencil

Instructions

Read through the list of equipment and supplies that you will need and the steps of the procedure. Be sure that you understand each step before you begin. Then complete each step correctly and in the proper order. If your completion time is too long, repeat the procedure until you increase your speed.

S = Satisfactory U = Unsatisfactory	S	U
1. Put on a protective jacket, gown, or apron; wash your hands with disinfectant, dry them, and put on gloves.		
2. Follow the Universal Precautions.		
3. Collect and prepare the appropriate equipment.		
4. If slides are not precleaned, wash them, wipe them with 70 percent alcohol, and dry them.		
5. Mix the blood specimen thoroughly but gently.		
6. Lay a clean glass slide on the table or counter, holding it only by the edges with your nondominant hand.		
7. Dispense a small drop of blood with a capillary tube onto the slide about one-half inch from the end (the right end if you are right-handed, the left end if you are left-handed).		
8. Holding another clean slide, the spreader slide, in your dominant hand, place it at a 35 to 40 degree angle in front of the drop of blood. Pull the slide back into the drop of blood.		
9. Push the spreader slide forward with a smooth quick motion, maintaining the angle and allowing the blood to spread about three-quarters the width of the other slide. Continue holding the other slide with the nondominant hand to prevent it from moving.		
10. Gently but rapidly wave the slide to air dry.		
11. Stand the slide with the thick end down to allow complete drying.		

12. Label the slide with the patient's name, the date, and the doctor on the thick end with a graphite pencil.

13. Repeat steps 6–12 until you obtain two satisfactory slides.

14. Following the manufacturer's instructions, transfer each of the three Hema 3 solutions into a Coplin jar or staining dish.

15. Dip one of the air-dried blood-smear slides into the Hema 3 fixative solution for one second. Allow any excess fixative to drain, but do not dry the slide.

16. Dip the slide three to five times (one second for each dip) into Hema 3 solution (eosin) # 1. Allow any excess to drain, but do not dry the slide.

17. Dip the slide three to five times (one second for each dip) into Hema 3 solution (methylene blue) # 2. Allow the slide to drain, but do not dry the slide.

18. Rinse the slide with deionized water.

19. Allow the slide to air dry by standing it on its end.

20. Wipe the back of the slide with a tissue to remove excess stain.

21. Repeat steps 15–20 with the other air-dried blood-smear slide.

22. Clean the lenses of the microscope with lens paper.

23. Place one of the stained slides, stain side up, on the mechanical stage and secure the slide.

24. Focus with the 10X objective, adjusting the light as needed.

25. Scan the slide to find the body region of the slide; that is, find the area where the cells barely touch one another.

26. While scanning, observe the smear for any abnormal appearing cells. Large abnormal cells tend to congregate in the feather edge. If abnormal cells are present, ask your instructor to examine them.

27. Rotate the nosepiece so that the 45X objective is in place, and bring the cells into clear focus with the fine-focus adjustment knob. Adjust the light to a comfortable level.

28. Rotate the 45X objective out of place so that oil does not touch it. Place a drop of immersion oil on the slide and carefully rotate the oil-immersion (100X) objective into place while watching from the side of the microscope.

29. Adjust the fine-focus adjustment knob until you focus the details of the cells clearly. Adjust the lighting to the correct level. If you lose the focus, return to 10X and begin the focusing process again.

30. Check the quality of staining on the slide, using the following criteria:
    a. red blood cells—pinkish tan
    b. nuclei of lymphocytes—purple
    c. platelets—purple
    d. eosinophil granules—red

31. Repeat steps 22–30 with the other slide and select the best slide for further analysis in the remaining steps of the procedure.

32. Scan the selected slide systematically as Figure 17.3 shows. Count 100 consecutive white blood cells and record the types of cells observed with a differential cell counter, if available, or with a notepad and pencil. Also record any unusual findings or questionable cells.

33. Again using the systematic movement, examine the appearance of red blood cells in at least ten fields, noting:
    a. color—normochromic or hypochromic
    b. size—normocytic, microcytic, or macrocytic
    c. shape—description of any abnormal shapes present
    d. inclusions—description of any inclusions present

S = Satisfactory	U = Unsatisfactory	S	U

34. Systematically observe the platelets in at least ten fields, noting:
    a. if they are clumped or single
    b. the approximate number in each field (5 to 15 per field = adequate; fewer than 4 per field = decreased; more than 15 per field = increased)

35. Rotate the 10X objective into place and remove the slide from the microscope stage.

36. Clean all lenses beginning with 10X and finishing with the 100X objective gently with lens paper to remove any debris or oil. Clean the microscope stage and condenser, if needed, with lens paper.

37. Discard disposable supplies and equipment.

38. Disinfect other equipment and return it to storage.

39. Clean the work area following the Universal Precautions.

40. Remove your jacket, gown, or apron, and gloves; wash your hands with disinfectant, and dry them.

OVERALL PROCEDURAL EVALUATION

Student's Name _____

Signature of Instructor _____ Date _____

Comments

Using Terminology

Write a brief definition of each of the following terms in the spaces provided.

1. Anisocytosis: _____

_____

2. Eosin: _____

_____

3. Hypersegmented: _____

_____

4. Infectious mononucleosis: _____

_____

5. Megakaryocyte: _____

_____

6. Methylene blue: _____

_____

7. Neutropenia: _____

_____

8. Poikilocytosis: _____

_____

9. Polychromatic stain: _____

_____

10. Polymorphonuclear: _____

_____

11. Quick-stain method: _____

_____

12. Wright's stain: _____

_____

13. Monocytic leukemia: _____

_____

14. Lymphocytic leukemia: _____

    _____

15. Endocarditis: _____

    _____

Compare and contrast each of the following sets of terms by listing their similarities and differences in the spaces provided.

16. Granulocyte, agranulocyte _____

    _____

    _____

    _____

17. Neutrophil, eosinophil, basophil _____

    _____

    _____

    _____

    _____

18. Normochromic, hyperchromic, hypochromic _____

    _____

    _____

    _____

19. Lymphocyte, monocyte _____

    _____

20. Macrocyte, microcyte _____

    _____

Acquiring Knowledge

Answer the following questions in the spaces provided.

21. How do red blood cells differ from most other cells?

    _____

22. How many formed elements of each type normally are found in one cubic millimeter of blood? What are the size relationships among the different types of formed elements?

    _____

    _____

    _____

23. Which type of leukocyte normally is the most numerous in adults? the least numerous?

    _____

24. How should a blood-smear slide be dried? Why should you never blow on a smear to dry it?

_____

_____

25. Why is it important that a blood smear not be too thick or too thin? How is thickness of the smear related to the manner in which the spreader slide is held?

_____

_____

_____

_____

_____

26. Describe the characteristics of a properly prepared blood-smear slide.

_____

_____

27. What region of a blood-smear slide is examined under the microscope in a differential count? Why?

_____

_____

28. Why are cell nuclei called basophilic and why is cell cytoplasm called acidophilic or eosinophilic?

_____

_____

29. What may cause a stained blood smear to appear too blue? too pink?

_____

_____

_____

_____

30. What are the advantages of quick stain over Wright's stain?

_____

_____

_____

31. Explain the relationship between staining and the identification of formed elements in the blood.

_____

_____

32. What features must be examined to differentiate among the various types of white blood cells?

_____

_____

33. How can you tell if an agranulocyte is a lymphocyte or a monocyte?

_____

_____

_____

_____

_____

34. Explain how white blood cells are counted on a differential blood-smear slide.

_____

_____

_____

_____

_____

35. What are some causes of an abnormally high or low neutrophil count in a differential blood smear?

_____

_____

_____

_____

36. What disorders may lead to an increase in the number of small lymphocytes?

_____

_____

37. Which features of red blood cells are examined in a differential blood-smear slide?

_____

_____

38. Explain how hemoglobin concentration can be assessed from examination of a differential blood-smear slide.

_____

_____

_____

39. What is the physiological relevance of the shape of normal red blood cells?

_____

_____

_____

40. What are the origin and function of platelets?

_____

_____

41. How are platelets counted on a differential blood-smear slide?

_____

_____

_____

42. What factors may lead to a reduced platelet count? an increased platelet count?

_____

_____

Applying Knowledge—On the Job

Answer the following questions in the spaces provided.

43. Assume that you have been instructed by your lab supervisor to help a new lab worker identify stained white blood cells in a differential blood-smear slide. What characteristics of stained white cells would you point out as most useful in distinguishing the different types?

_____

_____

_____

44. Assume that you just got a platelet count of 30,000 using the automated hematology machine in your POL. How can you confirm the low platelet count by examining the patient's stained blood-smear slide?

_____

_____

45. You have a stained differential blood-smear slide for a nine-month-old infant, showing small red cells with very little color. The pale center is larger than in a normal red cell. What condition does this child have? What is the child's hemoglobin concentration likely to be?

_____

_____

46. Assume the lab director in your POL has given you a blood-smear slide and asked you to perform a differential white blood-cell count. The smear has no feather edge, and when you scan it under low power you find that the cells are very crowded. What has caused the smear to be this way? What should you do about it?

_____

_____

47. A patient's differential blood-smear slide, which was stained using the quick-stain method, is too dark for good viewing. What is the problem and how can it be corrected?

_____

_____

_____

48. A differential blood-smear slide that you are examining has dark blue and purple sediment scattered over it, which interferes with a clear view of the formed elements. What is the problem and how can it be corrected?

_____

_____

_____

18 Automated Hematology and Quality Control

COGNITIVE OBJECTIVES

After studying this chapter, you should be able to

- use each of the vocabulary terms appropriately.
- explain the principle behind the operation of electrical impedance cell counters.
- describe how to use an electrical impedance cell counter.
- discuss why electrical impedance cell counters require two different sample dilutions.
- list the tests that can be performed with electrical impedance cell counters.
- explain the principle behind the operation of electron-optical cell counters.
- describe how the QBC (quantitative buffy coat) instrument works.
- discuss the differences and similarities between controls and calibrators used for automated hematology instruments.

PERFORMANCE OBJECTIVES

After studying this chapter, you should be able to

- decide whether a particular POL would benefit from the use of automated hematology instruments.
- make a list of factors to consider in choosing an automated hematology instrument for a particular POL.

TERMINOLOGY

aperture: an opening, as in the probe of an electrical impedance or electron-optical cell counter, through which blood cells and other formed elements in diluting solution pass in single file.

cyanmethemoglobin: a very stable cyanide and hemoglobin compound that results when a solution of potassium ferrocyanide and potassium cyanide is added to blood, lysing the red blood cells and releasing their hemoglobin content.

dilution #1: the 1:250 sample dilution that is used with electrical impedance cell counters for WBC counts and hemoglobin determinations. It is made by adding 40 μL of blood to 10 mL of isotonic saline solution.

dilution #2: the 1:62,500 sample dilution that is used with electrical impedance cell counters for RBC and platelet counts. It is made by adding 40 μL of dilution #1 to 10 mL of isotonic saline solution.

electrical impedance cell counter: an automated hematology instrument, such as the Danam and Cell Dyn instruments, that analyzes formed elements in the blood on the basis of their impedance of an electrical current.

electrical impedance method: the method of studying the formed elements in the blood that depends on their resistance to the flow of an electrical current.

electron-optical cell counter: the automated hematology instrument that analyzes formed elements in the blood on the basis of their interruption of a beam of light from a laser lamp.

hematology calibrator: a hematology control that is certified to be highly stable over its entire life; used to set the electronics of automated hematology instruments.

hematology control: an artificial blood, containing both human and animal cells, that is used to check the stability of electronic settings of automated hematology instruments.

light-beam method: the method of studying formed elements in the blood that depends on their interruption of a beam of light from a laser lamp.

photomultiplier tube (PMT): an electron multiplier in which electrons released by photoelectric emission are multiplied in successive stages by dynodes that produce secondary emission; used to detect reduction in intensity of the light beam from an electron-optical cell counter.

QBC (quantitative buffy coat) calibration check tube: the tube used with a QBC instrument to perform a daily quality-control check. It gives a set of expected values and acceptable deviation values for each parameter.

QBC (quantitative buffy coat) instrument: an automated hematology instrument that centrifuges nondiluted blood samples and estimates blood parameters such as hemoglobin, hematocrit, platelet counts, and WBC counts, on the basis of differences in density and fluorescence.

● ● ● ● ● ● ● ● ● ● ● ● ● ● ● ● ●

Automated hematology instruments have become widely used in POLs because of the greater accuracy and speed of automated methods over manual methods. Automation is especially useful in POLs that perform more than ten blood counts a day.

———————————————————— ◆ ◆

AN OVERVIEW OF AUTOMATED HEMATOLOGY INSTRUMENTS

While automated hematology instruments differ in the specific tests that they can perform, all have the

---

◆ ◆ ◆ **Tests Performed With** ◆ ◆ ◆
Automated Hematology Instruments

The range of tests performed with automated hematology instruments includes the following:

- WBC count
- RBC count
- platelet count
- hematocrit
- hemoglobin
- mean cell volume (MCV)
- mean cell hemoglobin concentration (MCHC)
- mean cell hemoglobin (MCH)
- granulocyte count (neutrophils, eosinophils, basophils)
- percentage of granulocytes
- nongranulocyte count (lymphocytes and monocytes)
- percentage of nongranulocytes
- mid-range cell count (monocytes and band granulocytes)
- percentage of mid-range cells
- lymphocyte count
- percentage of lymphocytes
- red blood-cell distribution width (RDW)

---

main purposes of differentiating and counting formed elements in the blood and determining hemoglobin concentration.

Automated hematology instruments differ in their degree of automation. Some require the operator to make dilutions of the blood samples and to add lysing reagents, while others are completely automated, requiring only introduction of well-mixed EDTA blood samples. The instrument then pierces the rubber stoppers in the tubes, makes the appropriate dilutions, performs the selected test(s), cleans the instrument, and reports the results. Many automated hematology instruments print out complete results, and most can be programmed to flag abnormal results.

Automated hematology instruments also differ in the underlying methods that they use to differentiate and count formed elements in the blood. One type of instrument uses a diluted sample, distinguishing and counting formed elements with an electric current or a beam of light. The other type of instrument uses an undiluted sample, separating formed elements by centrifugation.

The type of instrument best suited for a particular POL depends on several considerations, including:

- the hematological tests most commonly performed
- the degree of automation required
- the cost of instrument and maintenance
- the amount of laboratory space available
- the number of staff

HEMATOLOGY INSTRUMENTS REQUIRING DILUTED SAMPLES

Instruments using diluted samples may use an electrical current or a beam of light to differentiate and count formed elements in the blood.

❖❖ Instruments Using Electrical Impedance

The automated hematology instruments used most commonly in POLs count particulate matter in blood by counting electrical impulses generated when blood cells impede an electrical current. This is called the **electrical impedance method,** and the instruments are called **electrical impedance cell counters.** Figure 18.1 shows two of them.

As Figure 18.2 shows, a known volume of diluted blood is drawn through a small (100 μm) **aperture,** or opening, in the probe of the electrical impedance counter. A constant current is passed across the aperture from one side to the other. When a cell passes through the aperture, it causes a change in resistance, which in turn causes a voltage pulse, which is read on a voltage meter.

The size of the pulse is proportional to the size of the cell passing through the aperture. The larger the cell, the greater the pulse. Pulse magnitude can be used to measure cell volume as well as to differentiate types of cells by size. Figure 18.3 shows how cells of two different sizes generate pulses of different magnitudes. If the pulses labeled *a* and *c* were produced by platelets, those labeled *b* and *d* would have been produced by red blood cells, which are considerably larger. See also Table 18.1.

Because blood cells are so highly concentrated, it is necessary to dilute the blood sample before counting cells using this type of instrument. Dilution ensures that the cells can be conducted in single file past the counting point. The greater the dilution, the better the separation of cells and the less likely that more than one cell will pass the counting point simultaneously and bias the count.

The more concentrated the cells, the more dilute the blood sample must be. Because red blood cells

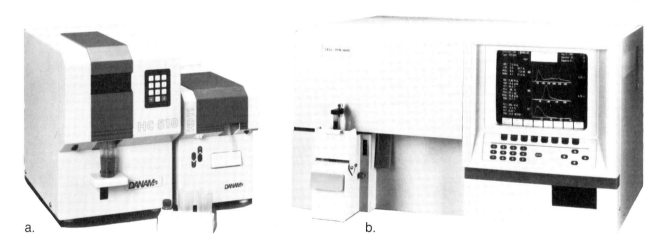

a.   b.

Figure 18.1. a. A Danam HC-510 hematology unit with diluter. This semiautomated instrument performs five hematology parameters: WBC count, RBC count, hemoglobin, hematocrit, and mean cell volume. Photo courtesy of Danam Electronics, Inc. b. The CELL-DYN 1600 is a fully automatic/self-cleaning hematology instrument that performs sixteen hematology parameters, including mean cell volume, mean cell hemoglobin concentration, mean cell hemoglobin, and a three-part WBC differential. It punctures the blood tube automatically, eliminating contact with the blood, and performs quality-control and data-management functions. Photo courtesy of Abbott Laboratories.

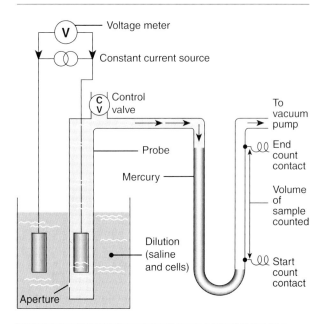

Figure 18.2. A schematic of an electrical impedance counter. Courtesy of Danam Electronics, Inc.

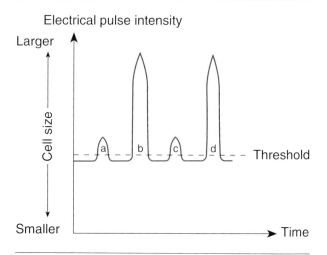

Figure 18.3. Electrical pulses from cells of different sizes.

and platelets are much more numerous than are white blood cells, counting them requires a more dilute sample. Two dilutions are therefore used. **Dilution #1,** which is used for counting white blood cells and determining hemoglobin, is 1:250. It is made by adding 40 μL of blood to 10 mL of diluent. Verify on your calculator that this produces the desired dilution of 1:250. **Dilution #2,** which is used to count red blood cells and platelets, is 1:62,500. It is made by further diluting 40 μL of Dilution #1 with another 10 mL of diluent. Verify that this produces a dilution of 1:62,500.

The diluent, a 0.85 percent saline solution, is isotonic with blood cells, thus preventing any alteration in cell size through the transfer of water in or out of the cells. Dilutions are made in plastic cuvettes be-

cause platelets tend to stick to glass. Most companies produce plastic cuvettes with antistatic treatment to prevent them from attracting dust.

The dilution can be made either manually or with an automated diluter. If the procedure is done manually, the blood sample is collected in a 40 μL calibrated capillary pipette from a finger stick, and the filled pipette is dispensed immediately into the 10 mL of diluent. Speed is essential to prevent the formation of fibrin clots and platelet aggregates.

For WBC counts and hemoglobin determinations, a lysing reagent must be added to the blood sample to

---

◆ ◆ ◆ **Danger—Poison!** ◆ ◆ ◆

Remember that the lysing reagent used to rupture red blood cells is a poisonous cyanide compound. Use it with caution.

TABLE 18.1 Normal Sizes of Blood Cells by Type	
Type of Cell	**Range in Volume (in cubic microns)**
White Blood Cells	120 to 1,000
Red Blood Cells	85 to 95
Platelets	3 to 30

rupture the red blood cells and release their hemo-globin content. A solution of potassium ferrocyanide and potassium cyanide is used most commonly. In about thirty seconds, this solution breaks down the red blood cells and converts the hemoglobin to the very stable compound, **cyanmethemoglobin.**

WBC Counts. WBC counts are performed using Di-lution #1 (1:250) with lysing reagent added. Differ-ential white blood-cell counts can be performed using differences in pulse amplitude to distinguish among the different types of white blood cells on the basis of cell size. Some instruments perform a two-part dif-ferential, giving the numbers and percents of granu-locytes and lymphocytes. Other instruments perform a three-part differential, giving the numbers and per-cents of granulocytes, lymphocytes, and midrange cells (monocytes and band neutrophils, eosinophils, and basophils).

RBC and Platelet Counts. RBC counts are per-formed using Dilution #2 (1:62,500). Diluted sam-ples are not lysed and contain intact red blood cells as well as platelets and white blood cells. As a conse-quence, some white blood cells are included in the counts. These are usually ignored because the normal concentration of white blood cells is so much lower than is the concentration of red blood cells. In cases of elevated WBC counts, however, the RBC count should be corrected by subtracting the WBC count. Platelets are much smaller than are red blood cells, so they can be distinguished from red blood cells and counted at the same time as the red blood cells.

Hematocrits. Hematocrits, or the percent of whole blood volume that is composed of red blood cells, can be calculated using an electrical impedance counter. Volumes of the red blood cells detected are added, and their sum is multiplied by a calibration constant. This method provides an accurate value for the he-matocrit.

Hemoglobin Determinations. Hemoglobin deter-minations made with an electrical impedance counter use a colorimetric method. Red blood cells are lysed to form the stable cyanmethemoglobin compound. This compound absorbs green light of wavelength 540 nm in a logarithmic ratio to the concentration of hemoglobin present. As Figure 18.4 shows, the amount of light transmitted through the solution is measured with a photodetector. This is compared with the amount of light transmitted through a ref-erence solution. Most electrical impedance counters do a reference zero check before each hemoglobin measurement.

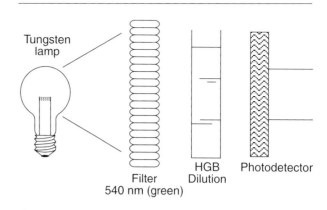

Figure 18.4. The hemoglobin colorimetric measurement method. Courtesy of Danam Electronics, Inc.

This same method of hemoglobin determination is used with automated hematology instruments that work on a light-scattering principle. These are de-scribed next.

❖❖ Instruments Using Light Scattering

Some automated hematology instruments count particulate matter in blood by counting light-scatter-ing events. This is called the **light-beam method,** and the instruments are called **electron-optical cell counters.** Electron-optical cell counters are not used commonly in POLs. They are designed to handle large volumes of blood samples, and the start-up and shut-down processes are not as easy as those with hematology instruments used more commonly in POLs.

As with electrical impedance counters, electron-optical counters use blood samples diluted in an ac-curate known ratio. An isotonic saline solution is used to avoid changes in cell size. Again, dilution ensures cell separation so that the cells can be con-ducted in single file past the counting point. The elec-tron-optical counter uses sample dilutions that are much lower than those used for the electrical imped-ance method. This makes it possible to count a larger number of cells in a given volume of diluted sample. Figure 18.5 shows how an electron-optical counter works.

Electron-optical cell counters use a laser lamp, which has an extremely sharp focus of discrete, monochromatic light. This allows the beam to be fo-cused to a point that approaches the total diameter of the aperture through which the cells pass. The inten-sity of the beam is a known, specific value at this

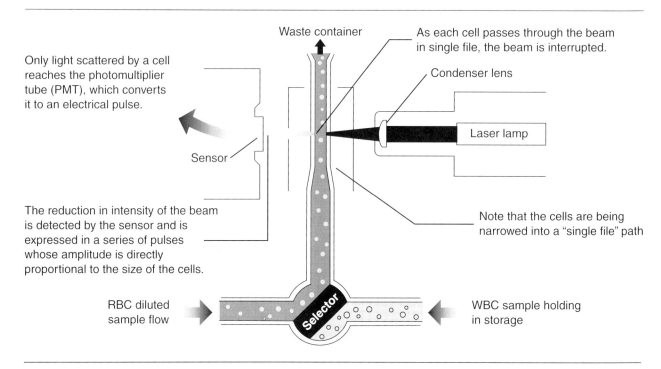

Only light scattered by a cell reaches the photomultiplier tube (PMT), which converts it to an electrical pulse.

Waste container

As each cell passes through the beam in single file, the beam is interrupted.

Condenser lens

Laser lamp

Sensor

The reduction in intensity of the beam is detected by the sensor and is expressed in a series of pulses whose amplitude is directly proportional to the size of the cells.

Note that the cells are being narrowed into a "single file" path

RBC diluted sample flow

Selector

WBC sample holding in storage

Figure 18.5. The flow of cells in an electron-optical cell counter.

point. As each blood cell in the flow cell passes through the beam, it interrupts the beam and reduces the intensity of the beam by a degree proportional to the size of the cell. This reduction in intensity is detected by the sensor, a **photomultiplier tube (PMT)**, and is expressed in a series of pulses, with an amplitude that is directly proportional to cell size.

Electron-optical cell counters can be changed by the selector for either WBC or RBC counts. The instruments also can calculate the hematocrit at the same time it is performing an RBC count, using information on the number and size of the red blood cells.

HEMATOLOGY INSTRUMENT REQUIRING UNDILUTED SAMPLES

The **QBC (quantitative buffy coat) instrument,** shown in Figure 18.6a, is an automated hematology instrument that uses an undiluted blood sample. The QBC instrument is a centrifugal system that can be used to perform the following hematology parameters:

- hemoglobin
- hematocrit
- platelet count
- total WBC count
- total granulocyte count
- percent granulocytes
- total lymphocyte/monocyte count
- percent lymphocytes/monocytes
- mean cell hemoglobin concentration (MCHC)

In the QBC instrument, a sample of whole blood, which is collected either by finger puncture or venipuncture, is drawn into a very precise capillary tube.

A special capillary cap is placed on the end of the

♦ ♦ ♦ **Note** ♦ ♦ ♦

The QBC instrument does not perform an RBC count. It cannot be used to calculate mean cell volume (MCV) or the mean cell hemoglobin (MCH), two of the red blood-cell indices described in the next chapter. The QBC instrument does calculate a mean cell hemoglobin concentration (MCHC).

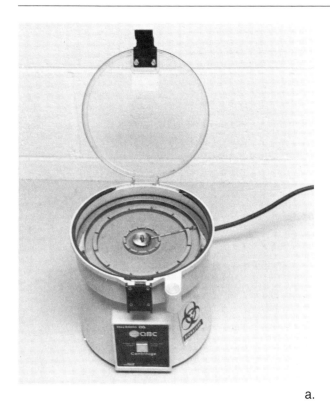

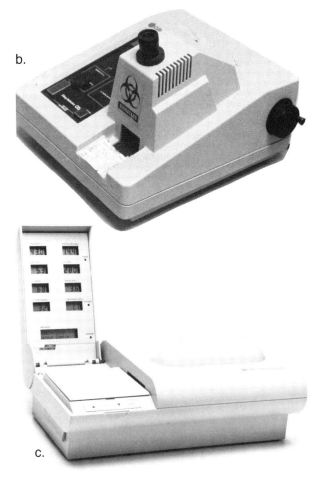

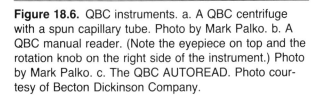

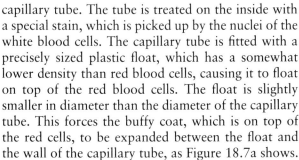

Figure 18.6. QBC instruments. a. A QBC centrifuge with a spun capillary tube. Photo by Mark Palko. b. A QBC manual reader. (Note the eyepiece on top and the rotation knob on the right side of the instrument.) Photo by Mark Palko. c. The QBC AUTOREAD. Photo courtesy of Becton Dickinson Company.

capillary tube. The tube is treated on the inside with a special stain, which is picked up by the nuclei of the white blood cells. The capillary tube is fitted with a precisely sized plastic float, which has a somewhat lower density than red blood cells, causing it to float on top of the red blood cells. The float is slightly smaller in diameter than the diameter of the capillary tube. This forces the buffy coat, which is on top of the red cells, to be expanded between the float and the wall of the capillary tube, as Figure 18.7a shows.

First, blood is centrifuged in the capillary tube for five minutes at 12,000 rpms. Then the capillary tube is placed in a reader that contains a fluorescent microscope and a micrometer. In the older QBC instruments, the tube is moved manually, by turning the transport knob to advance the tube in the reader. In an automated reader (QBC Autoread or QBC Hemascan), it is moved automatically until it comes to a distinct interface in the buffy column. Chemical and physical differences among the cells cause them to

fluoresce different colors. The different layers of the buffy coat represent different types of white cells and platelets in the column, as Figure 18.7b shows.

Hemoglobin concentration is indicated by the height of the plastic float in the red blood-cell column. Red blood cells that contain large amounts of hemoglobin are more dense and cause the float to ride high. Red blood cells that are low in hemoglobin have a lower density, causing the float to sink in the column when it is centrifuged.

♦ ♦

QUALITY CONTROL

As is true with all other instruments used in POLs, automated hematology instruments require a good system of quality control to test their accuracy and precision. Quality control must be an ongoing process and not just part of the initial installation. Qual-

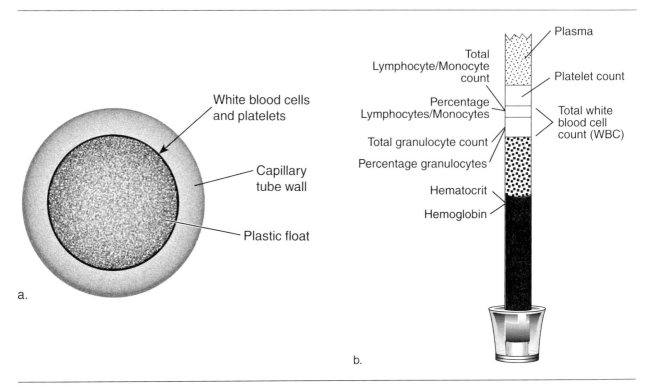

Figure 18.7. a. A cross-section of a capillary tube in the buffy coat area. Expansion of the buffy coat (platelets and white blood cells) is seen between the plastic float and the capillary tube wall. b. A spun capillary tube. Centrifugation of the tube separates the formed elements of the blood into distinct layers. Courtesy of Becton Dickinson Primary Care Diagnostics.

ity-control testing involves the use of controls and calibrators to test the accuracy and precision of the instrument, the procedure, and the operator. Some automated hematology instruments store test results in their computers and provide a monthly printout that can be mailed to the manufacturer of the controls and calibrators to verify the accuracy of the instrument. Required reagents also must be checked daily for quality.

Some POLs use split samples in their quality-control program. Part of a sample is analyzed in the POL, and part is sent to an outside reference laboratory for comparison. Split-specimen testing is useful for detecting inaccurate or imprecise test results caused by improper calibrations, mechanical problems, and operator errors.

◆◆ *Controls*

A **hematology control** is an artificial blood that is used to check the stability of electronic settings of automated hematology instruments. Most hematology controls include both human and animal cells. Human red blood cells are used, but instead of human leukocytes, bird red blood cells are substituted. They have the same volume as human leukocytes but are more stable. Bird RBCs have nuclei and are very similar in size to human WBCs, and they have very long life spans. Swine platelets are also used in hematology controls.

Hematology controls normally are available in three levels—abnormal low values, normal values, and abnormal high values. The manufacturers provide the expected values and the allowable deviation for each level of the control for a given instrument using the stated reagent systems. Thus, the values stated for one instrument will not be the same as those for a different instrument. Most manufacturers also list expected values for manual determinations.

Controls for a test must be run before you perform that test on a patient's specimen. CLIA 1988 requires performing two levels of controls. Controls are usually performed at the beginning of each workday or whenever an instrument has been shut down for four hours or more. CLIA 1988 also requires POLs with extended hours to run controls at eight-hour intervals. Quality-control checks on the QBC instrument are performed daily using a **QBC calibration check tube.** This gives a set of expected values and acceptable deviations for each parameter.

❖❖ *Calibrators*

A **hematology calibrator** normally is a control that is certified to be highly stable over its entire life. Calibrators are used to set the electronics of the instrument, while controls are used to check the stability of

---

❖ ❖ ❖ Caution—Biohazard! ❖ ❖ ❖

Because hematology controls and calibrators contain human blood, you must handle them with the same caution as with other blood samples.

---

these settings. Calibrators are specially prepared for specific instruments, as listed on the insert sheet that comes with each set of calibrators, and they must be used with the reagent system on which the expected values have been determined.

Automated electronic hematology instruments should be calibrated as scheduled by the manufacturer or whenever controls give erroneous results. CLIA 1988 requires calibration of automated hematology instruments at three-month intervals and that the POL enroll in a proficiency testing program for the automated hematology instrument.

❖❖ *Reagents*

In addition to checking the instrument daily with controls, it is also necessary to check all reagents. For example, a background check must be run on the isotonic diluent each day to be sure that yeast or mold is not growing in the solution. Yeast and mold would be counted as blood cells and would give falsely high readings.

CHAPTER 18 REVIEW

Using Terminology

Define the following terms in the spaces provided.

1. Cyanmethemoglobin: _____

   _____

2. Electrical impedance method: _____

   _____

3. Electron-optical cell counter: _____

   _____

4. Hematology calibrator: _____

   _____

5. Photomultiplier tube (PMT): _____

   _____

6. QBC (quantitative buffy coat) instrument: _____

   _____

7. Aperture: _____

_____

8. Dilution #1: _____

_____

9. Electrical impedance cell counter: _____

_____

10. Light-beam method: _____

_____

Acquiring Knowledge

Answer the following questions in the spaces provided.

11. What are the main advantages of using automated hematology instruments over using manual methods?

_____

_____

12. What are the main purposes of automated hematology instruments?

_____

_____

13. What are some of the specific functions that automated hematology instruments perform?

_____

_____

_____

_____

14. List several factors that should be considered when selecting an automated hematology instrument for a particular POL.

_____

_____

_____

15. Briefly state how an electrical impedance cell counter works.

_____

_____

16. How does the electrical impedance cell counter differentiate cells on the basis of size?

_____

_____

17. Why is it necessary to dilute blood samples when performing tests with some automated hematology instruments?

_____

_____

_____

_____

18. Describe how to make Dilution #1 and Dilution #2 for use with electrical impedance cell counters.

_____

_____

_____

_____

19. Explain why two different dilutions are necessary when using electrical impedance cell counters. When is each dilution used?

_____

_____

_____

_____

20. What diluent is used to dilute samples for testing with electrical impedance cell counters? Why is this diluent used?

_____

_____

21. Why must a lysing agent be added to the blood sample for WBC counts and hemoglobin determinations when using an electrical impedance cell counter? What lysing agent is used?

_____

_____

_____

22. What method is used to determine hemoglobin concentration with an automated cell counter? How does it work?

_____

_____

_____

23. Why are electron-optical cell counters not used commonly in POLs?

_____

_____

24. Briefly state how an electron-optical cell counter works.

_____

_____

25. How are different types of blood cells distinguished with a QBC instrument?

_____

_____

26. Describe how hemoglobin concentration is estimated with a QBC instrument.

_____

_____

_____

27. What is the role of quality control in the use of automated hematology instruments? What are some ways in which quality control is achieved?

_____

_____

_____

_____

28. What are hematology controls? Why are they used?

_____

_____

_____

_____

29. List the hematology parameters that can be estimated with a QBC instrument.

_____

_____

_____

_____

Applying Knowledge—On the Job

Answer the following questions in the spaces provided.

30. A coworker in your POL is setting up the QBC instrument to run several tests on a patient's blood sample. The tests requisitioned include a differential white blood-cell count and a red blood cell count. What problem will your coworker run into if he tries to run these tests on the QBC instrument? What should he do instead?

_____

_____

_____

31. One of the patients in the clinic where you work has acute leukemia with a WBC count of 100,000/mm³. How will this affect the RBC count? What can you do to correct it?

_____

_____

_____

_____

_____

32. The physician whom you work for has ordered a manual differential white blood-cell count in addition to the one furnished by the QBC instrument. What additional information can be obtained from a manual differential?

_____

_____

_____

_____

33. One of your duties in the POL is to operate an automated hematology instrument. What precautions should you take when handling the artificial blood used as a control?

_____

_____

34. The laboratory where you are employed is required to calculate erythrocyte indices. What type of automated hematology instrument should be purchased for this purpose? Why?

_____

_____

19

Advanced Hematology Procedures

COGNITIVE OBJECTIVES

After studying this chapter, you should be able to

- use each of the vocabulary terms appropriately.
- define the three erythrocyte indices and explain what high and low values for each index mean.
- list potential sources of error in performing platelet counts.
- identify the three stages of erythrocyte sedimentation.
- discuss the pros and cons of the Wintrobe and Westergren methods for measuring the erythrocyte sedimentation rate.
- list potential sources of error in measuring the erythrocyte sedimentation rate.
- discuss the factors that influence the erythrocyte sedimentation rate.
- explain how the erythrocyte sedimentation rate is used as a diagnostic tool.
- list potential sources of error in performing reticulocyte counts.
- explain why the reticulocyte count is a valuable indicator of erythropoiesis.
- describe the clinical applications of the reticulocyte count.

PERFORMANCE OBJECTIVES

After studying this chapter, you should be able to

- calculate and interpret erythrocyte indices.
- count platelets using direct and indirect methods.
- calculate the platelet count.

- use Wintrobe and Westergren methods to measure erythrocyte sedimentation rates.
- prepare a smear and count reticulocytes.
- calculate the percent and absolute number of reticulocytes.

TERMINOLOGY

erythrocyte indices: three indicators of the size or hemoglobin content of the red blood cells that are used in the diagnosis of anemia. They include the mean cell volume (MCV), the mean cell hemoglobin (MCH), and the mean cell hemoglobin concentration (MCHC).

erythrocyte sedimentation rate (ESR or sed rate): the rate at which red blood cells settle out of plasma when placed in a vertical tube.

mean cell hemoglobin (MCH): the average weight of hemoglobin in red blood cells in a sample (also called mean corpuscular hemoglobin).

mean cell hemoglobin concentration (MCHC): the average concentration of hemoglobin in a given volume of packed red blood cells in a sample (also called mean corpuscular hemoglobin concentration).

mean cell volume (MCV): the average volume of a red blood cell in a sample (also called mean corpuscular volume).

reticulocytopenia: the lowering of the number of circulating reticulocytes; usually found in patients with pernicious anemia, aplastic anemia, or bone marrow failure.

spherocytosis: a condition in which red blood cells assume a spherical shape.

supravital stain: a stain that stains only living cells, not dried blood smears.

• • • • • • • • • • • • • • • • •

This chapter describes the following advanced hematology indices and procedures that may be performed in POLs:

- erythrocyte indices
- platelet counts
- the erythrocyte sedimentation rate
- reticulocyte counts

———————————— ◆ ◆

ERYTHROCYTE INDICES

Three **erythrocyte indices** were introduced by Dr. Maxwell Wintrobe:

- the mean cell volume (MCV)
- the mean cell hemoglobin (MCH)
- the mean cell hemoglobin concentration (MCHC)

The indices are indicators of the size and hemoglobin content of the average red blood cell in a given sample of blood. They are used primarily for diagnosing anemia.

◆◆ *Calculating the Indices*

Each index is calculated from two of the following three blood parameters: RBC count, hemoglobin, and hematocrit. The validity of the indices depends on the accuracy of these three blood parameters. For this reason, the indices became a routine part of the complete blood count only when automated methods increased the accuracy of the RBC count. Even with automated methods, the validity of the erythrocyte indices always should be checked against the appearance of the red blood cells on a stained differential blood-smear slide.

Erythrocyte indices are expressed in very small units, some of which were defined in Chapter 4. See Table 19.1.

The Mean Cell Volume. Mean cell volume (MCV) is the average volume of a red blood cell in the sample. It is expressed in femtoliters (fL) or their equivalent, cubic micrometers (μm^3), and reported to the nearest whole number.

MCV is calculated from the RBC count and the hematocrit (Hct), using the formula:

$$MCV = \frac{Hct\ (\%) \times 10}{RBC\ (millions)}$$

The Mean Cell Hemoglobin Concentration. The **mean cell hemoglobin concentration (MCHC)** is the average concentration of hemoglobin in a given volume of packed red blood cells in the sample. It is expressed in percent (%), or grams per deciliter (g/dL), and reported to the nearest tenth. The ratio of the weight of hemoglobin to the volume of red blood cells, the MCHC is calculated from the hemoglobin concentration (Hgb) and hematocrit (Hct) using the formula:

$$MCHC = \frac{Hgb\ (g/dL) \times 100}{Hct\ (\%)}$$

The Mean Cell Hemoglobin. The **mean cell hemoglobin (MCH)** is the average weight of hemoglobin in a red blood cell in the sample. It is expressed in pi-

▼▼

TABLE 19.1 A Review of Metric Units

Unit	Symbol	Equivalent
Deciliter	dL	0.1 liters
Femtoliter	fL	10^{-15} liters
Micrometer	μm	10^{-6} meters
Picogram	pg	10^{-12} grams
Micromicrogram	$\mu\mu$g	10^{-12} grams

▲▲

cograms (pg) or micromicrograms (μμg) and is reported to the nearest tenth.

MCH is directly proportional to the amount of hemoglobin and size of the red blood cell. It is calculated from the hemoglobin concentration (Hgb) and the RBC count using the formula:

$$MCH = \frac{Hgb \ (g/dL) \times 10}{RBC \ (millions)}$$

❖❖ Interpreting the Indices

In healthy adults, the erythrocyte indices show little variation from the normal ranges (see Table 19.2). A deviation of more than one unit from the normal range usually indicates some type of anemia.

The Mean Cell Volume. The MCV indicates the size of the red blood cells. Cells in the normal range of 82 to 102 fL are considered normocytic. Cells with MCV less than 80 fL are considered microcytic. Those over 102 fL are considered macrocytic. The greater the deviation of MCV from the normal range, the more the cells differ from normal size.

MCV is higher than normal in anemia caused by vitamin B_{12} deficiency and in pernicious anemia. These conditions are referred to as macrocytic anemias. In macrocytosis with many oval macrocytes, MCV is usually in the range of 120 to 140 fL. MCV is decreased in iron-deficiency anemia, which is characteristically microcytic.

The Mean Cell Hemoglobin Concentration. The MCHC indicates whether the red blood cells are normochromic, meaning that they have normal color and hemoglobin content, or hypochromic, meaning that they are pale and low in hemoglobin. MCHC values below 32 percent indicate hypochromia, which is associated with iron-deficiency anemia. In macrocytic anemias, MCHC is normal or slightly reduced. MCHC values above 38 percent only occur with **spherocytosis,** a condition in which erythrocytes assume a spheroid shape. It is characteristic of certain hemolytic anemias.

❖❖❖ Interpretation Tips ❖❖❖

- When the MCHC is above 40 percent and other blood parameters are normal, the automated hematology instrument should be checked for malfunction.
- When all three indices are markedly elevated, the cause may be autoagglutination of the red blood cells or rouleau formation. Figure 19.1 illustrates roleaux.

The Mean Cell Hemoglobin. The MCH indicates the weight of hemoglobin in the average red blood cell. Elevated MCH values are present in macrocytic anemia. The cells contain more hemoglobin because they are large, although the concentration of hemoglobin per unit volume of the cell (MCHC) may be normal or even slightly reduced. Lower than normal MCH values are found in microcytic anemia, unless the red blood cells also are spherocytic. MCH also is lower than normal in normocytic cells that are hypochromic. If the cells are both microcytic and hypochromic, the MCH value is even lower.

TABLE 19.2   Normal Adult Values for Erythrocyte Indices

Index	Normal Adult* Range
MCV	82 to 102 fL or μm^3
MCH	27.0 to 33.0 pg or μμg
MCHC	33.0 to 38.0 % or g/dL

*MCV and MCH values are higher at birth and lower at one year of age than they are in adulthood. Both rise to adult values by puberty.

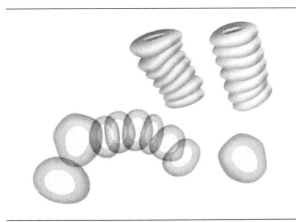

Figure 19.1. Erythrocytes in rouleau formation resemble a stack of coins. Because they fit together in less space, rouleau cells have a higher sedimentation rate than do normal cells. Rouleau formation results from pathologic changes in the blood.

⁕ Calculating Erythrocyte Indices: Two Worked Examples

The following two worked examples show how to calculate and interpret the erythrocyte indices. See Table 19.3 for patient data.

Patient A:

$$MCV = \frac{Hct\ (\%) \times 10}{RBC\ (million)} = \frac{24 \times 10}{4.2} = 57\ fL$$

$$MCH = \frac{Hgb\ (g/dL) \times 10}{RBC\ (million)} = \frac{6.5 \times 10}{4.2}$$

$$= 15.5\ pg$$

$$MCHC = \frac{Hgb\ (g/dL) \times 100}{Hct\ (\%)} = \frac{6.5 \times 100}{24}$$

$$= 27.1\ g/dL$$

Compared with normal values, Patient A has low values for all three indices. This means that the patient's red blood cells are both microcytic and hypochromic, which is characteristic of iron-deficiency anemia.

Patient B:

$$MCV = \frac{Hct\ (\%) \times 10}{RBC\ (million)} = \frac{27 \times 10}{2.2} = 123\ fL$$

$$MCH = \frac{Hgb\ (g/dL) \times 10}{RBC\ (million)} = \frac{9.0 \times 10}{2.2}$$

$$= 40.9\ pg$$

$$MCHC = \frac{Hgb\ (g/dL) \times 100}{Hct\ (\%)} = \frac{9.0 \times 100}{27}$$

$$= 33.3\ g/dL$$

Compared with normal values, Patient B has elevated MCV and MCH values but a normal MCHC value. This means that the patient has macrocytic normochromic red blood cells, which are characteristic of pernicious anemia.

PLATELET COUNTS

Platelets can be counted directly using a Thoma pipette or the Unopette system and a hemacytometer or with an automated hematology instrument. They are counted indirectly using a stained blood-smear slide and an oil-immersion objective.

⁕ The Direct Method

The direct method of counting platelets is a modification of the method of Brecker and Cronkie and similar to the direct method of counting blood cells that was described in Chapter 16. The blood sample

TABLE 19.3 Patient Data			
Patient	**RBC (millions/mm³)**	**Hgb (g/dL)**	**Hct (%)**
Patient A	4.2	6.5	24
Patient B	2.2	9.0	27

is diluted in a Thoma pipette with a hemolytic reagent, and the platelets are counted using a Neubauer hemacytometer and a phase contrast or bright-light microscope.

Diluting the Sample. Attach an Adams suction apparatus to a Thoma white blood-cell pipette, and draw a sample of EDTA-anticoagulated venous blood to the 0.5 mark. After cleaning the outside of the pipette, draw a fresh solution of filtered 1 percent ammonium oxalate solution (the hemolytic reagent) to the 11.0 mark, producing a dilution of 1:20.

♦ ♦ ♦ Note ♦ ♦ ♦

Capillary blood may be used instead of venous blood for a platelet count. Be aware, however, that blood collected by capillary puncture usually is lower in platelets than is blood collected by venipuncture. Because the function of platelets is to adhere to wounds and skin punctures, there is inevitably a loss of platelets during the collection process.

If you use a Thoma red blood-cell pipette instead of a white blood-cell pipette, you can draw blood to either the 0.5 mark or the 1 mark, and you draw diluting solution to the 101 mark. If you draw blood to the 0.5 mark, the dilution is 1:200. This dilution is recommended if the platelet count is high. If you draw blood to the 1.0 mark, the dilution is 1:100.

Charging the Hemacytometer. Mix the diluted sample on a mechanical shaker for two minutes, and expel the first two or three drops of liquid from the pipette to ensure that the sample used to charge the hemacytometer comes only from the bulb of the pipette. Then charge both sides of the counting chamber of the hemacytometer, following the procedure described in Chapter 16. Place the charged hemacytometer in a covered petri dish that is lined with a disk of moist filter paper to prevent evaporation of the sample. Allow the sample to stand for twenty minutes so that the platelets can settle out.

Counting the Platelets. The area of the hemacytometer counted is the central ruled area of 1 square millimeter. If you use a light microscope, the condenser must be well down to view the platelets, which appear as small refractile bodies under the high-

power objective. White blood cells in the sample are unaffected by the lysing reagent and are readily visible. However, because they are much larger than platelets, they are unlikely to be confused with them during the count.

Using a Unopette Kit. This method is a variation of the one just described. The Unopette kit contains a 20-μL capillary pipette and a prefilled reservoir containing 1.98 mL of reagent, giving a dilution of 1:100. Blood collected by venipuncture using EDTA anticoagulents should be used for the test, if possible. The reagent is ammonium oxalate to which Sorensen's phosphate buffer has been added to maintain the pH. The preservative, Thimerosol, has been added to the reagent as well, to act as an antibacterial agent. The reagent can be stored until the expiration date if it is kept below 30 degrees Celsius and away from sunlight. Discard it if it appears cloudy.

♦ ♦ ♦ Caution! ♦ ♦ ♦

The preservative Thimerosol may cause skin irritation. Use it with caution.

In the Unopette method, first puncture the diaphragm of the reservoir with the protective shield on the capillary pipette (see Figure 19.2). Then fill the capillary pipette with whole blood and transfer it to the reservoir. Let stand at least ten minutes to allow RBCs to completely lyse. The erythrocytes are lysed, leaving intact the platelets, white blood cells, and reticulocytes. Mix the diluted sample thoroughly by inverting the reservoir to resuspend the cells. Then, charge the hemacytometer and allow it to stand for ten minutes for the platelets to settle. Count all smaller squares in the large central one-square millimeter on the hemacytometer.

Count the platelets using bright-light or phase microscopy. Under the 45X objective, the platelets appear oval or round and frequently have one or more branches. With a bright-light microscope, they are easy to identify by their pink or purple sheen.

Calculating the Platelet Count. Use the number of platelets observed to calculate the platelet count using the standard formula for hemacytometer counts:

Platelet count = No. of platelets counted × Dilution
× Depth factor × Area counted

where,

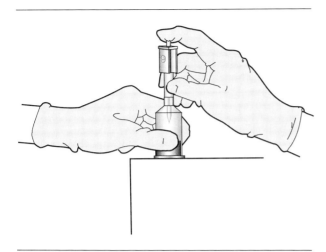

Figure 19.2. The Unopette system for counting platelets requires puncturing the diaphragm of the reservoir, which contains Thimerosol, with the pipette. To do so, place the reservoir on a flat surface. Grasp it with one hand. With the other hand, push the tip of the pipette shield firmly through the diaphragm in the neck of the reservoir. Then remove it. (Remove the shield from the pipette assembly with a quick twist.) Courtesy of Becton Dickinson VACUTAINER Systems.

Dilution = 20, 100, or 200,

depending on dilution ratio

Depth factor = the constant 10

Area counted = 1 mm^3

Assume, for example, that a red blood-cell pipette or a Unopette kit is used to dilute a blood sample to a dilution of 1:100 and that you counted 160 platelets in the central counting area of the hemacytometer. Then:

Platelet count = 160 × 100 × 10 × 1

= 160,000 platelets/mm^3

Whenever the dilution is 1:100, you may use this shorthand formula:

Platelet count = No. of platelets counted × 1,000

Sources of Error. There are several potential sources of error in performing manual platelet counts using the direct method. Take care to avoid these causes of false test results:

- improper dilution of the sample
- contaminated or cloudy reagent

- clots in the blood sample or clumping of platelets (unlikely with the use of EDTA anticoagulant)
- overfilling or underfilling the hemacytometer
- the inclusion of red blood cells or dust particles in the count
- incorrect calculations

To reduce errors in reporting the platelet count, always check it against an estimate of the platelet count made from examination of a stained blood-smear slide. The direct count and the estimate from the slide should agree. The slide also has the advantage of showing morphological characteristics of individual platelets.

✦✦ *The Indirect Method*

The indirect method for counting platelets determines the number of platelets per 1,000 red blood cells on a stained blood-smear slide using an oil-immersion objective and then multiplies that number by the RBC count.

To perform a platelet count using the indirect method, follow this procedure:

- Make a blood-smear slide using either venous blood collected in an EDTA tube or blood from a freely flowing capillary puncture.
- Allow the slide to air dry and stain it with Wright's stain or quick stain.
- Using the oil-immersion objective, count the number of platelets per 1,000 red blood cells.
- Perform an RBC count on an EDTA-anticoagulated blood sample.
- Calculate the platelet count using the formula:

$$\text{Platelet count} = \frac{P \times RBC}{1,000}$$

where,

P = number of platelets counted per 1,000 red blood cells
RBC = RBC count

Assume, for example, that 60 platelets per 1,000 red blood cells were counted on a stained blood-smear slide. For the same sample, the RBC count was found to be 5,000,000 per cubic millimeter. Then:

$$\text{Platelet count} = \frac{60 \times 5,000,000}{1,000}$$

$$= 300,000 \text{ platelets/mm}^3$$

THE ERYTHROCYTE SEDIMENTATION RATE (ESR)

The **erythrocyte sedimentation rate** (**ESR** or **sed rate**) is the rate at which red blood cells settle out of plasma when placed in a vertical tube. The ESR is calculated by measuring the distance the red blood cells travel through the plasma during a given interval of time.

❖❖ *Stages of Erythrocyte Sedimentation*

Three stages can be observed in the fall of red blood cells through the plasma column when an ESR test is performed:

- *Initial period of aggregation:* the first ten minutes, during which rouleaux form and relatively slow sedimentation of red cells occurs.
- *Period of rapid settling:* the next half hour to two hours (depending on the length of the tube), during which sedimentation occurs at a fairly constant rate.
- *Third stage:* the final stage, during which sedimentation slows as the sedimented red blood cells are packed at the bottom of the column.

The second stage, the period of rapid settling, is the most significant for the ESR.

❖❖ *Methods Used to Measure the ESR*

Two different methods are used to measure the ESR—the Wintrobe method and the Westergren method. Both methods use blood samples collected by venipuncture in EDTA tubes.

**❖❖❖ Blood Sample ❖❖❖
Storage**

The ESR test must be set up within two hours for blood left at room temperature. The sample can be refrigerated at 4 degrees Celsius up to a maximum time of twelve hours before testing. Refrigerated blood must always be brought to room temperature before testing.

The Wintrobe Method. Fill a Wintrobe sedimentation/hematocrit tube with 1 milliliter of blood, using a long-stemmed Pasteur pipette. No air bubbles should enter the blood. The meniscus should be on the 100 mm mark of the right-hand scale of the tube (or the zero mark of the left-hand scale, which reads from top to bottom). Figure 19.3 shows an ESR rack and Wintrobe sedimentation tubes.

Place the filled tube in the ESR rack on a level surface to ensure that the tube is exactly vertical. Note the time, and after exactly one hour, read the ESR as the length of the plasma column above the red cells that have settled at the bottom of the tube. Report the ESR in millimeters per hour. Figure 19.4 illustrates the Wintrobe procedure.

The Westergren Method. Mix trisodium citrate anticoagulant with the blood sample in a ratio of four volumes of blood to one volume of anticoagulant. Draw the blood-citrate mixture up to the zero mark of a Westergren ESR tube, which is graduated from 0 to 200 millimeters and has a bore of 2.55 millimeters.

Place the filled tube in its rack on a level surface at room temperature, and note the time. In exactly one hour, read the distance from the plasma meniscus to the top of the column of sedimented red cells. Report the ESR in millimeters per hour. Figure 19.5 shows the Westergren system.

Using a Sediplast Westergren System. As Figure 19.6 illustrates, a disposable Westergren system uses

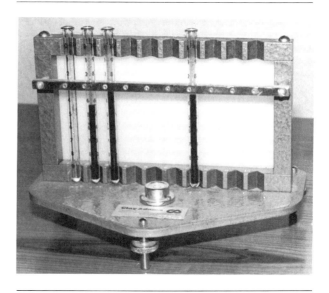

Figure 19.3. A Wintrobe sedimentation rack. The tube on the left is empty. The other tubes show sedimentation of erythrocytes. Photo by Tommy Mumert.

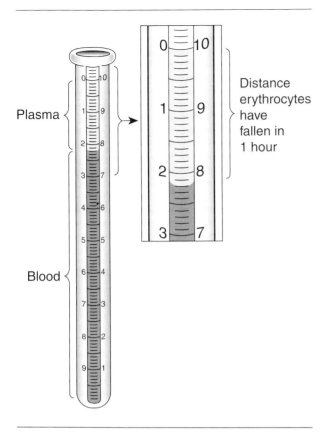

Figure 19.4. In this example of erythrocyte sedimentation, the reading at the bottom of the meniscus after one hour is 22 millimeters.

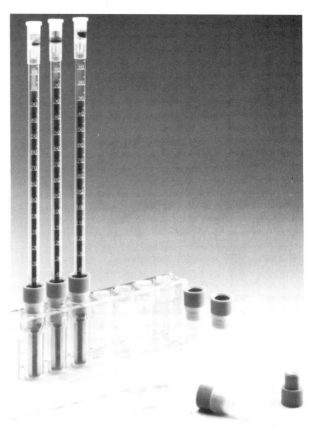

Figure 19.5. The SEDIPLAST ESR System for the Westergren erythrocyte sedimentation rate is a completely closed system that protects against risks associated with blood handling. Photo courtesy of POLYMEDCO, Inc.

> ◆ ◆ ◆ **Technique Tip** ◆ ◆ ◆
>
> Insert the autozero Westergren tube into the Sedivial with a slight, gentle twisting motion. The tube must completely touch the bottom of the Sedivial to ensure proper results.

vial. After one hour at room temperature, read the distance between the top of the plasma and the top of the sedimented red blood cells directly from the vertical scale on the tube. Report the result in millimeters per hour.

a disposable tube, called the autozero Westergren tube, for the ESR reading. The tube is inserted in a vial, called the Sedivial, which contains the diluted blood sample. Blood rises in the tube to the zero mark, and the excess blood flows into a reservoir compartment.

The Sedivial can be purchased prefilled with diluent, which is 3.8 percent sodium citrate. Use a Pasteur pipette to fill the Sedivial to the fill line with blood (about 0.8 mL are needed). Thoroughly mix the blood and diluent by replacing the cap and gently inverting. Blood and diluent are automatically added to the pipette tube when it is inserted into the Sedi-

> ◆ ◆ ◆ **For Safety's Sake** ◆ ◆ ◆
>
> The Sediplast Westergren ESR kit has the following safety features:
>
> • The autozero Westergren tube has a vented cap that prevents squirting of the blood sample from the top of the tube, thus reducing the risk of accidental exposure to biohazardous materials.
>
> • The entire Sediplast system is disposable, thus reducing the need for cleaning and handling of biohazardous materials.

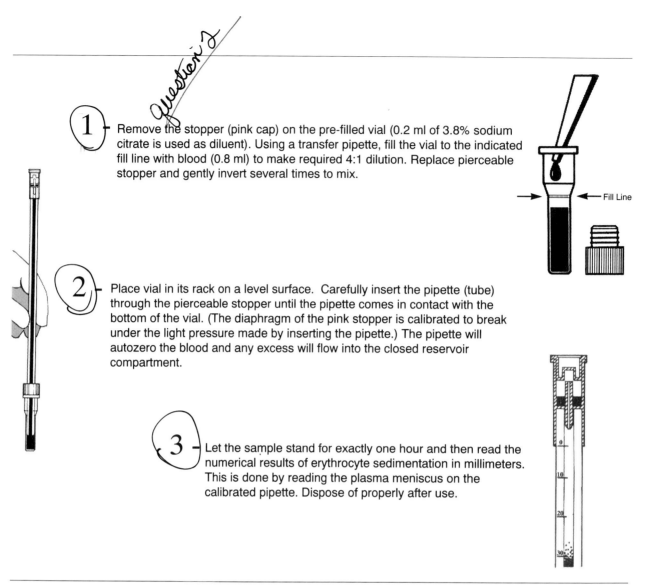

1 Remove the stopper (pink cap) on the pre-filled vial (0.2 ml of 3.8% sodium citrate is used as diluent). Using a transfer pipette, fill the vial to the indicated fill line with blood (0.8 ml) to make required 4:1 dilution. Replace pierceable stopper and gently invert several times to mix.

Fill Line

2 Place vial in its rack on a level surface. Carefully insert the pipette (tube) through the pierceable stopper until the pipette comes in contact with the bottom of the vial. (The diaphragm of the pink stopper is calibrated to break under the light pressure made by inserting the pipette.) The pipette will autozero the blood and any excess will flow into the closed reservoir compartment.

3 Let the sample stand for exactly one hour and then read the numerical results of erythrocyte sedimentation in millimeters. This is done by reading the plasma meniscus on the calibrated pipette. Dispose of properly after use.

Figure 19.6. This package insert from the SEDIPLAST ESR System explains how to use the Westergren procedure. Courtesy of POLYMEDCO, Inc.

Comparison of the Wintrobe and Westergren Methods. The Wintrobe method requires a small volume of blood without dilution. The Westergren method requires a smaller sample of blood and dilution with a reagent. Diluting the sample is a potential source of error in the Westergren method.

The undiluted blood sample in the Wintrobe test has the added advantage of being reusable for additional tests. The Wintrobe tube can be centrifuged and the hematocrit can be read directly off the tube using the right-hand bottom-to-top scale. Blood-chemistry tests can be performed on the plasma in the tube, and smears can be made of the buffy coat.

On the other hand, dilution of the blood sample in the Westergren method has the advantage of elimi-

nating the need to correct for anemia or polycythemia. While correction for these conditions can be made with the Wintrobe method based on the hematocrit, attempted corrections are not always reliable.

The Westergren method is more sensitive for the serial study of chronic diseases, such as tuberculosis, rheumatic carditis, and rheumatoid arthritis. The Wintrobe method provides a less sensitive index of systemic disease activity because of the shorter column and choice of anticoagulant.

In terms of safety, the Sediplast Westergren system is the method of choice. It is entirely disposable, and the sample is enclosed in an inverted tube. Both reduce the risk of biohazard contamination. However, even with the Wintrobe system, contamination with extraneous blood is negligible if disposable Wintrobe tubes are used to reduce handling and cleaning and disposable safety test tube cap covers (like the ones shown in Figure 1.8) are used to protect against aerosol contamination and spattering.

Sources of Error in ESR Testing. There are several potential sources of error in ESR testing. Whenever you perform an ESR test, avoid the following pitfalls:

- *Tilting:* tilting the ESR tube even slightly away from vertical accelerates the ESR; an angle of 3 degrees from vertical may accelerate the ESR by as much as 30 percent.

- *Vibrations:* vibrations to the tube, such as those caused by nearby centrifuges, increase the ESR.

- *Temperature:* deviation of room temperature from a constant 20 to 25 degrees Celsius, or placement of the ESR rack in a draft or sunlight may affect the ESR.

- *Heparin used as anticoagulant:* heparin alters the charge on the red blood cells and changes the ESR.

- *Testing time:* blood that has stood longer than two hours at room temperature after being drawn may have a falsely low ESR because the red blood cells have become spherical and less inclined to form rouleaux.

- *Reading time:* the ESR may be decreased if reading time is less than one hour and increased if reading time is over one hour.

- *Clots or air bubbles:* clots and air bubbles in the sample interfere with sedimentation of cells and affect the ESR.

** *Normal Values for the ESR*

Normal values for the ESR vary with age, sex, and test method. See Table 19.4.

** *Factors Influencing the ESR*

The speed at which red blood cells settle in the column of plasma is influenced by two general categories of factors—red blood-cell factors and plasma factors.

Red Blood-Cell Factors. Red blood cells settle in plasma because they are more dense than is the plasma; that is, they have more weight, or mass, per unit of volume. The rate at which the red blood cells settle is directly proportional to their density. If they clump together in aggregates, such as rouleaux, they tend to settle faster, leading to a higher sedimentation rate.

Countering the tendency of red blood cells to settle in the plasma column is their buoyancy, which is their tendency to float because of the upward force exerted by the plasma. The buoyancy of the red blood cells is directly proportional to their surface area-to-volume ratio—the greater their surface area relative to their volume, the more buoyant they are and the slower the rate at which they settle. Large cells have a smaller surface area in relation to volume than do small cells. Therefore, macrocytes have a relatively high sedimentation rate, and microcytes have a relatively low one.

Red blood cells in rouleau formation have a decreased surface area-to-volume ratio relative to individual red blood cells, another reason for their

TABLE 19.4 Normal Reference Values for the ESR

Method	Sex	Age	ESR (mm/hr)
Wintrobe	Males	Adult	0 to 7
	Females	Adult	0 to 15
Westergren	Males	<50	0 to 15
	Males	>50	0 to 20
	Females	<50	0 to 20
	Females	>50	0 to 30

greater sedimentation rate. Because red blood cells with abnormal shapes are less likely to form rouleaux, they have a slower than normal sedimentation rate.

Red blood-cell concentration also affects the rate at which the cells settle. Decreased red blood-cell concentration, as in some anemias, reduces the erythrocyte-to-plasma ratio, thus favoring rouleau formation. An elevated rate of sedimentation results. Increased red blood-cell concentration, as in polycythemia, has the opposite effect and results in a lowered sedimentation rate.

Plasma Factors. Three proteins in the plasma affect the rate at which red blood cells settle—fibrinogen, globulin, and albumin. Increases in the levels of fibrinogen and globulin decrease the negative charge on the surface of the red blood cells. As a consequence, the red blood cells repel each other less, promoting the formation of rouleaux and a faster rate of sedimentation. Increases in the level of albumin, on the other hand, retard the rate of sedimentation of the red blood cells.

◆◆ *ESR as a Diagnostic Tool*

Many disease processes and some normal physiological states result in an elevation of the ESR, and a few diseases lead to a decrease. As a result, the ESR is used worldwide as an index of the presence of active diseases of many different types, especially inflammatory disorders.

The ESR is elevated in patients with tissue breakdown, such as occurs in acute infectious diseases. In most acute infections, globulins and fibrinogen are increased, while albumin is somewhat reduced. This combination increases the rate at which red blood cells settle. The ESR is particularly useful as an indicator of the presence of obscure active infections, such as tuberculosis, subacute bacterial endocarditis, and systemic lupus erythematosus. The ESR may remain elevated for some time after recovery from infectious disease.

In nephrosis, a disease of the kidney, and cirrhosis, a disease of the liver, globulins are increased and albumin is decreased, resulting in an elevated sedimentation rate. The ESR also is increased in patients with nephritis and acute attacks of gout as well as heavy metal poisoning. Although the ESR is not elevated in malignancy, it is generally rapid when metastases, or the breakdown and inflammation of tumors, occur. The ESR increases after the twelfth week of pregnancy and following abortion at any time.

The ESR is slower than normal in patients with hemolytic jaundice and sickle-cell anemia due to changes in shape of the red blood cells that reduce rouleau formation.

RETICULOCYTE COUNTS

Reticulocytes are immature red blood cells that are present in small numbers in circulating blood. They are counted in POLs as a valuable index of red blood-cell production.

◆◆ *Background*

Erythropoiesis, or red blood-cell production, was described in Chapter 15, and the reticulocyte stage of red blood-cell development was described in Chapter 16. This section reviews and expands upon that material to illustrate why the number of circulating reticulocytes can be used as an index of erythropoiesis.

Erythropoiesis. The major factor that controls the rate of erythropoiesis is the oxygen content of the blood. Low blood oxygen stimulates production of the kidney hormone, erythropoietin, which acts directly on the bone marrow to increase red blood-cell production. Low blood oxygen may be due to several conditions, including anemia, cardiovascular disease, and low atmospheric oxygen, which is due, for example, to high altitude.

Erythropoiesis occurs in several stages, as Figure 15.2 showed. Stem cells in the bone marrow first differentiate into pronormoblasts, which mature into basophilic normoblasts. Polychromatophilic normoblasts, the last stage capable of mitosis, develop into orthochromic normoblasts, also known as nucleated red blood cells, which are seen occasionally on blood smears. Orthochromic normoblasts, in turn, extrude their nuclei, giving rise to reticulocytes. Each pronormoblast gives rise to sixteen reticulocytes, and the entire process takes three to five days.

Reticulocytes. After their formation from normoblasts, reticulocytes normally remain in the bone marrow for one day before being sent out into the circulating blood. There they remain as reticulocytes for another one to two days before developing into mature red blood cells. Reticulocytes are slightly larger than mature red blood cells, and they retain aggregates of ribosomal RNA. The role of the RNA is to synthesize hemoglobin, which is needed by mature red blood cells for oxygen transport.

The maturation time of reticulocytes in the circulating blood depends on the body's demand for he-

TABLE 19.5 The Correlation Between Hematocrit and the Maturation Time of Reticulocytes

Hematocrit (%)	Maturation Time of Reticulocytes (days)
45	1.0
35	1.5
25	2.0
15	2.5

moglobin. When hemoglobin is low, the maturation time is longer, allowing more hemoglobin production by the ribosomal RNA in the reticulocytes. Not surprisingly, maturation time is correlated inversely with hematocrit. (See Table 19.5.)

The amount of ribosomal RNA is greatest when reticulocytes are first formed. It declines as they age. Generally, the younger the reticulocyte, the more diffuse and marked is the network of RNA. Ribosomal RNA is completely absent from mature red blood cells. As Figure 19.7 shows, the ribosomal RNA is seen as dense blue granules or filaments when reticulocytes are stained with brilliant cresyl blue, new methylene blue, or Nile blue sulfate. These are called supravital stains because they stain only living cells, not dried blood smears. The incubation time will vary according to the type of supravital stain used.

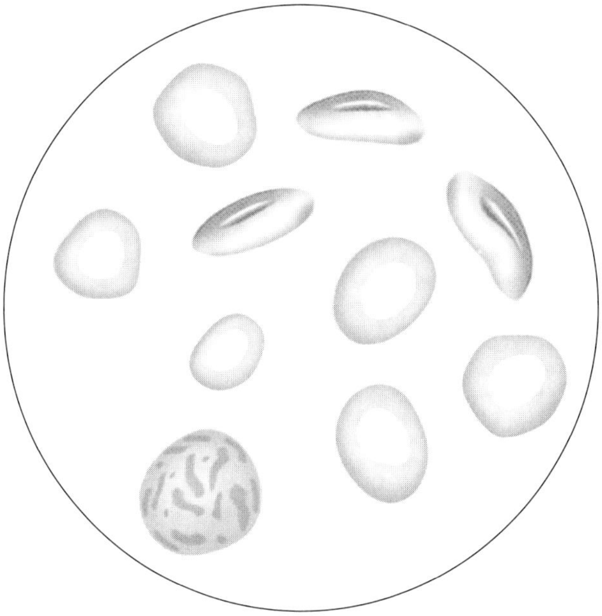

✦✦ Reticulocyte Count Procedures

Reticulocytes are counted on stained blood smears under the oil-immersion objective.

Preparing the Smear. Using a brilliant cresyl blue stain and test tube, place three drops in the small test tube. Add six to eight drops of capillary blood or EDTA-anticoagulated venous blood to the tube. If capillary blood is used, increase the amount of stain to prevent clotting. The blood need not be fresh. Blood that has been stored at 4 degrees Celsius for up to twenty-four hours produces a satisfactory reticulocyte preparation.

Figure 19.7. A stained reticulocyte.

✦ ✦ ✦   Note   ✦ ✦ ✦

Particles of stain adhering to the surface of mature red blood cells may be a serious source of error in reticulocyte counts. You must observe strictly the recommended incubation time for the blood-stain mixture. The longer you allow the mixture to stand beyond this recommended time limit, the greater the possibility of stain adhering to mature blood cells and causing erroneous counts.

Incubate the mixture for ten to twenty minutes at 37 degrees Celsius, and then prepare a blood smear in the usual manner and allow it to air dry. The smear should be thin, and it should not be counterstained with a polychromatic stain, such as Wright's stain or quick stain.

Using a Unopette Kit. The principle underlying the Unopette method for performing a reticulocyte count is similar to the principle underlying the method just described. The test kit contains a 7 mL dropper bottle of supravital stain (new methylene blue N) and a 25 μL capacity Unopette capillary pipette. The supravital stain is stable until the expiration date if the dropper bottle is recapped after each use and stored below 30 degrees Celsius. The blood-stain mixture is incubated for exactly ten minutes. Thin blood smears are prepared in the same manner as was followed in the brilliant cresyl blue stain method.

Counting Reticulocytes. Examine the slide under the oil-immersion objective in the body region of the smear. Both mature erythrocytes and reticulocytes have a light greenish blue background in a correctly prepared smear. You can distinguish the reticulocytes from the erythrocytes by their deep blue granules and filaments of ribosomal RNA. Count a total of 1,000 red blood cells including both reticulocytes and mature erythrocytes. You may use one slide for the entire count, or you may use two slides by counting 500 red blood cells on each slide.

Sources of Error in the Procedure. There are several potential sources of error in performing a reticulocyte count. Avoid these pitfalls when you perform the procedure:

- *Overincubation of the blood-stain mixture:* too much staining makes viewing difficult and may result in mature red blood cells being counted as reticulocytes.
- *Unfiltered stains:* without frequent filtering, stains form precipitations on the smears that may be confused with reticula and bias the count upward.
- *Undercounting reticulocytes:* overlooking reticulocytes with small amounts of cellular reticular material in the count biases the count downward.

♦ ♦ ♦   Note   ♦ ♦ ♦

The following cell features may be confused with reticular material:

- *Howell-Jolly bodies,* which are composed of nuclear fragments.
- *Heinz bodies,* which are composed of denatured hemoglobin.
- *Stippling, or spotting,* which occurs in basophilic red blood cells in some types of anemia.

- *Too few cells counted:* counting too few cells can lead to a count that is unrepresentative of the sample.
- *Nonsystematic counting of the cells in the counting area:* unless a systematic pattern of counting the cells is followed, some cells may be counted twice and others may be overlooked, producing a miscount.
- *Artifacts counted as reticula:* numerous cell artifacts may be confused with reticula and may bias the count upward.

♦♦ *Calculations*

The number of reticulocytes may be reported in two ways: as the percent of reticulocytes of all red blood cells counted or as the absolute number of reticulocytes counted.

The Percent of Reticulocytes. The percent of reticulocytes of all red blood cells counted is calculated as:

$$\text{Percent of reticulocytes} = \frac{\text{No. of reticulocytes counted} \times 100}{\text{No. of erythrocytes counted}}$$

Whenever 1,000 erythrocytes are counted, the following shorthand formula may be used:

$$\text{Percent of reticulocytes} = \frac{\text{No. of reticulocytes counted}}{10}$$

Assume, for example, that 40 reticulocytes were observed out of 1,000 erythrocytes counted on a smear. The calculation is:

$$\text{Percent of reticulocytes} = \frac{40 \times 100}{1,000}$$

$$= 4 \text{ percent reticulocytes}$$

The Absolute Number of Reticulocytes. The absolute number of reticulocytes counted is equal to the percentage of reticulocytes times the RBC count:

$$\text{Absolute no. of reticulocytes}$$
$$= \text{percent of reticulocytes} \times \text{RBC count}$$

Assume, for example, that the RBC count is 4,000,000 per cubic millimeter and that reticulocytes make up 2 percent of the red blood cells. The calculation is:

$$\text{Absolute no. of reticulocytes} = 2\%$$
$$\times \ 4{,}000{,}000 \text{ reticulocytes/mm}^3$$
$$= 80{,}000 \text{ reticulocytes/mm}^3$$

Which Calculation Should You Use? The absolute number of reticulocytes can be used directly to assess bone marrow response to anemia. It has more clinical significance than the percent of reticulocytes, which must be correlated with other hematological parameters to be useful clinically. Many POLs report the reticulocytes only as a percentage. Some report both the percentage and the absolute number. The latter is the recommended format.

◆◆ *The Normal Values for Reticulocyte Counts*

To interpret individual patient-test results for the reticulocyte count, you need to be familiar with normal values for both percent and absolute number of reticulocytes.

The Percent of Reticulocytes. Normal values for the percent of reticulocytes vary by age and sex. See Table 19.6.

The higher value for females is due to replacement of blood lost during menstruation. The newborn value drops to the adult value by two to five days after birth.

The Absolute Number of Reticulocytes. The average for the absolute count is 60,000 reticulocytes per cubic millimeter. This is the basal value. The maximum response under appropriate circumstances is considered to be seven times the basal rate.

◆◆ *Clinical Applications*

Reticulocytopenia, which is a lowering of the number of circulating reticulocytes, usually is found in patients with pernicious anemia, aplastic anemia, or bone marrow failure. A satisfactory response to therapy in these conditions is a rise in the reticulocyte count, which is used as an index of red blood-cell production. In patients with pernicious anemia, for example, an increase in reticulocytes usually is seen by the fourth day following specific therapy, and the maximal response generally is reached by the eighth to tenth day. This is followed by a gradual decline in reticulocytes coupled with a steady increase in the erythrocyte count and hemoglobin level until normal values are reached.

If anemia is known to exist and the bone marrow is not responding as indicated by an increase in reticulocytes, the cause must be investigated. Possibilities include vitamin B_{12} deficiency, folate deficiency, and invasion of the bone marrow by malignant cells.

In patients with low hematocrits, the percent of reticulocytes may appear to be elevated even if an unchanging number of reticulocytes is produced each day and the absolute number of reticulocytes is normal. This apparent reticulocytosis is due to the relatively small number of red blood cells, not to an increase in the number of reticulocytes. The lower the hematocrit, the greater the degree of apparent reticulocytosis. If the hematocrit is half of the normal value, for example, erythrocyte production can be assumed to be increased only if the percent of reticulocytes is consistently greater than twice normal, say, in the range of 5 to 6 percent. By comparison, in nonanemic patients, erythrocyte production is considered to be increased if the reticulocyte count is consistently greater than 2.5 to 3.0 percent.

Occasionally, the percentage of reticulocytes may be increased by factors other than an increased rate of erythropoiesis. For example, there may be premature release of reticulocytes from the bone marrow. This occurs acutely in response to massive hemorrhage.

TABLE 19.6 Normal Values for the Percent of Reticulocytes

Age/Sex	Percent Reticulocytes
Adult males	0.5 to 1.5
Adult females	0.5 to 2.5
Newborns	2.0 to 6.0

PROCEDURE

19.1

The Wintrobe Erythrocyte Sedimentation Rate

Goal

- After successfully completing this procedure, you will be able to set up a Wintrobe erythrocyte sedimentation rate and read the result at the end of one hour.

Completion Time

- 1 hour, 10 minutes

Equipment and Supplies

- impermeable jacket, gown, or apron
- disposable latex gloves
- hand disinfectant
- paper towels and tissues
- biohazard container
- EDTA-anticoagulated venous blood
- disposable Pasteur pipette
- Wintrobe sedimentation tube
- Wintrobe sedimentation rack
- One-hour timer with alarm
- notepad and pencil

Instructions

Read through the list of materials that you will need and the steps of the procedure. Be sure that you understand each step before you begin. Then complete each step correctly and in the proper order. If your completion time is too long, repeat the procedure until you increase your speed.

1. Put on a jacket, gown, or apron; wash your hands with disinfectant, dry them, and put on gloves.

2. Follow the Universal Precautions.

3. Collect and prepare the appropriate equipment.

4. Verify identification of the specimen and label the container.

5. Mix the blood sample well.

6. Fill the Pasteur pipette.

7. Fill the Wintrobe sedimentation tube to the zero mark. Proceed from the bottom of the tube upward to prevent bubble formation.

8. Place the Wintrobe sedimentation tube in the sedimentation rack in a level position away from vibrations, sunlight, and temperature extremes. Check the leveling bubble in the rack to ensure that the tube is perfectly vertical.

9. Set the timer for exactly one hour.

10. In exactly one hour, read the sed rate markings on the tube that measure the distance from the top of the plasma column to the top of the red blood cells.

11. Report the result in millimeters per hour on your notepad.

12. Discard disposable equipment.

13. Disinfect other equipment and return it to storage.

14. Clean the work area following the Universal Precautions.

S = Satisfactory	U = Unsatisfactory	S	U

15. Remove the jacket, gown, or apron, and gloves; wash your hands with disinfectant, and dry them.

OVERALL PROCEDURAL EVALUATION

Student's Name _____

Signature of Instructor _____ **Date** _____

Comments

PROCEDURE

19.2

◆

The Sediplast Disposable Westergren Erythrocyte Sedimentation Rate

Goal

- After successfully completing this procedure, you will be able to set up an erythrocyte sedimentation rate using the Sediplast Westergren system and read the result at the end of one hour.

Completion Time

- 1 hour, 10 minutes

Equipment and Supplies

- impermeable jacket, gown, or apron
- disposable latex gloves
- hand disinfectant
- surface disinfectant
- paper towels and tissues
- biohazard container
- EDTA-anticoagulated venous blood
- disposable Pasteur pipette
- Sediplast kit (disposable Westergren sedimentation tube, diluent, Sedivial, and rack)
- one-hour timer with alarm
- notepad and pencil

Instructions

Read through the list of equipment and supplies that you will need and the steps of the procedure. Be sure that you understand each step before you begin. Then complete each step correctly and in the proper order. If your completion time is too long, repeat the procedure until you increase your speed.

1. Put on a jacket, gown, or apron; wash your hands with disinfectant, dry them, and put on gloves.

2. Follow the Universal Precautions.

3. Collect and prepare the appropriate equipment.

4. Verify identification of the blood specimen and label the container.

5. Mix the blood sample gently and well.

6. Remove the cap on the Sedivial, which is prefilled with 3.8 percent sodium citrate.

7. Using a Pasteur pipette, fill the Sedivial to the indicated fill line with 0.8 mL of blood.

8. Mix the blood and sodium citrate solution together by replacing the pierceable stopper in the Sedivial and gently invert several times.

9. Place the sample in the rack in a level position away from vibrations, sunlight, and temperature extremes.

10. With a slight twisting motion, gently insert the Westergren sedimentation tube into the Sedivial of blood. Be sure that the tube is inserted all the way to the bottom of the Sedivial to ensure an accurate reading (blood will rise to the top of the sedimentation tube and excess will overflow into the reservoir compartment at the top of the tube).

11. Set the timer for one hour.

12. In exactly one hour, read the length of the plasma column on the sedimentation tube.

13. Report the result in millimeters per hour on your notepad and turn in to your instructor.

14. Discard disposable equipment.

15. Disinfect other equipment and return it to storage.

16. Clean the work area following the Universal Precautions.

17. Remove the jacket, gown, or apron, and gloves; wash your hands with disinfectant, and dry them.

OVERALL PROCEDURAL EVALUATION

Student's Name _____

Signature of Instructor _____ Date _____

Comments

PROCEDURE

19.3 Unopette Reticulocyte Determination by Manual Methods

Goal

- After successfully completing this procedure, you will be able to prepare a reticulocyte stain, count the reticulocytes present, and report the results.

Completion Time

- 40 minutes

Equipment and Supplies

- impermeable jacket, gown, or apron
- disposable latex gloves
- hand disinfectant
- surface disinfectant
- paper towels and tissues
- biohazard container
- glass-marking pen
- glass slide
- drop of fresh capillary blood or EDTA-anticoagulated venous blood
- methylene blue N stain
- Unopette capillary pipette with shield
- microscope with oil-immersion objective
- notepad and pencil

Instructions

Read through the list of equipment and supplies that you will need and the steps of the procedure. Be sure that you understand each step before you begin. Then complete each step correctly and in the proper order. If your completion time is too long, repeat the procedure until you increase your speed.

1. Put on a jacket, gown, or apron; wash your hands with disinfectant, dry them, and put on gloves.

2. Follow the Universal Precautions.

3. Collect and prepare the appropriate equipment.

4. Identify the specimen with a glass-marking pen.

5. Place a drop of fresh capillary blood or EDTA-anticoagulated venous blood on a clean glass slide. Beside it, place an equal amount of new methylene blue N stain.

6. Mix the blood and the stain with the tip of the capillary pipette shield. Wipe the tip to remove any remaining blood-stain mixture.

7. Remove the shield with a twist from the pipette assembly.

8. Collect the blood-stain mixture in the capillary pipette. Tip the slide slightly to facilitate this step.

9. Cover the capillary pipette with the shield, automatically forcing the blood-stain mixture into the overflow chamber. Let the mixture stand at room temperature for ten minutes. This time frame must be followed exactly.

10. Remove the shield from the capillary pipette.

11. Holding the tip of the capillary over the glass slide, fit the shield onto the open end of the overflow chamber. Advance the shield with a twisting motion to deliver the blood-stain mixture onto the slide.

12. Mix the blood-stain mixture on the slide again, using the tip of the glass capillary pipette.

13. Prepare a thin blood-stain smear.

14. Let the slide air dry.

15. Place the slide on the stage of the microscope and focus it under the oil-immersion objective, using the same focusing procedure as for other blood smears.

16. Count 1,000 erythrocytes and record the number of reticulocytes seen.

17. Calculate the percent of reticulocytes using the formula:

$$\text{Percent of reticulocytes} = \frac{\text{No. of reticulocytes} \times 100}{1,000}$$

18. Complete the necessary information on your notepad and give your results to your instructor.

19. Discard disposable supplies and equipment.

20. Disinfect other equipment and return it to storage.

21. Clean the work area following the Universal Precautions.

22. Remove the jacket, gown, or apron, and gloves; wash your hands with disinfectant, and dry them.

OVERALL PROCEDURAL EVALUATION

Student's Name _____

Signature of Instructor _____ **Date** _____

Comments

CHAPTER 19 REVIEW

Using Terminology

Match the term in the right column with the appropriate definition or description in the left column.

_____ 1. condition with spherical red blood cells

_____ 2. large cell

_____ 3. low in hemoglobin

_____ 4. low number of reticulocytes

_____ 5. mean cell hemoglobin

_____ 6. mean cell hemoglobin concentration

_____ 7. mean cell volume

_____ 8. normal in hemoglobin

_____ 9. sedimentation rate

_____ 10. stains living cells

a. ESR

b. hypochromic

c. macrocyte

d. MCH

e. MCHC

f. MCV

g. reticulocytopenia

h. normochromic

i. supravital

j. spherocytosis

Define the following terms in the spaces provided.

11. Erythrocyte indices: _____

_____

_____

12. Erythrocyte sedimentation rate (ESR or sed rate): _____

_____

_____

13. Mean cell volume (MCV): _____

    _____

14. Mean cell hemoglobin (MCH): _____

    _____

15. Mean cell hemoglobin concentration (MCHC): _____

    _____

    _____

Acquiring Knowledge

Answer the following questions in the spaces provided.

16. What three blood parameters are used to calculate the erythrocyte indices?

    _____

17. When did the erythrocyte indices become a routine part of the complete blood count? Why not until then?

    _____

    _____

    _____

18. How should you check the validity of the erythrocyte indices?

    _____

    _____

19. What is the formula for calculating MCV?

    _____

20. What two blood parameters determine MCH?

    _____

21. What ratio expresses MCHC?

    _____

22. What are the normal adult ranges for the erythrocyte indices?

    _____

    _____

23. What does a deviation of more than one unit from the normal range of an erythrocyte index usually mean?

    _____

24. What conditions lead to an increase over normal in the value of MCV? to a decrease?

_____

_____

_____

_____

25. When is the value of MCH likely to be greater than normal?

_____

26. Why is a very high MCHC value suspect?

_____

_____

_____

_____

27. When can the shorthand formula be used to calculate the platelet count?

_____

28. List several potential sources of error in performing manual platelet counts using the direct method.

_____

_____

_____

_____

_____

29. How can you check the validity of a platelet count?

_____

_____

_____

30. Describe the three stages of erythrocyte sedimentation. Which stage is the most significant for the ESR?

_____

_____

_____

_____

_____

_____

31. Compare the pros and cons of the Wintrobe and Westergren methods of estimating the ESR.

_____

_____

_____

_____

_____

_____

_____

32. What sources of error should be avoided in performing an ESR test?

_____

_____

_____

_____

_____

33. What red blood-cell factors influence the sed rate?

_____

_____

34. What plasma factors influence erythrocyte sedimentation? How do they respond to acute infections?

_____

_____

_____

_____

35. Name several potential sources of error in performing reticulocyte counts.

_____

_____

_____

_____

36. Explain why the reticulocyte count is a valuable indicator of erythropoiesis.

_____

_____

_____

37. Describe the clinical applications of the reticulocyte count.

_____

_____

_____

_____

_____

_____

38. Why is it recommended that the absolute number of reticulocytes be reported routinely?

_____

_____

_____

Applying Knowledge—On the Job

Answer the following questions in the spaces provided.

39. A patient has just reported to the laboratory for a reticulocyte count. Both the absolute number and the percentage of reticulocytes have been requested. What will the physician learn directly from these reports?

_____

_____

_____

_____

_____

40. You will need to stain the reticulocytes before counting them. How will you do this?

_____

_____

_____

_____

_____

_____

41. You have just received a request for a Westergren sed rate. What equipment and reagents will you need? How long will it take? What units will it be reported in?

_____

_____

_____

_____

_____

42. You have read two Wintrobe sed rates at exactly one hour. One has a reading of 50 mm/hr, the other of 5 mm/hr. Which is abnormal and which is normal?

_____

_____

43. A patient in the clinic where you work has the following blood parameters: RBC of 4.1 million/mm^3; Hgb of 6.4 g/dL; and Hct of 25 percent. Calculate the erythrocyte indices for this patient and make a tentative diagnosis.

_____

_____

_____

_____

44. The physician has requested a platelet count for a patient. You counted 162 platelets using the direct method (dilution = 1:100). What platelet count will you report to the physician?

_____

45. You just performed a reticulocyte count for a patient who has an RBC count of 3,500,000. You observed 43 reticulocytes out of 1,000 erythrocytes on the smear. What is the percent of reticulocytes? What is the absolute number of reticulocytes?

_____

_____

20

Blood Coagulation

COGNITIVE OBJECTIVES

After studying this chapter, you should be able to

- use each of the vocabulary terms appropriately.
- explain the role of hemostasis as an aspect of homeostasis.
- name the three mechanisms by which hemostasis comes about.
- identify the intravascular, vascular, and extravascular phenomena of hemostasis.
- describe the two pathways through which coagulation is initiated.
- explain how blood clots form.
- identify several diseases of coagulation and explain their causes.
- discuss the management of coagulation diseases.
- identify the three types of coagulation tests performed in POLs and specify when each type is appropriate.
- discuss the differences among bleeding time, prothrombin time, and activated partial thromboplastin time.

PERFORMANCE OBJECTIVES

After studying this chapter, you should be able to

- perform a bleeding time test, using the template method or Duke's bleeding time.
- perform a prothrombin time determination.
- perform an activated partial thromboplastin time determination.

TERMINOLOGY

activated partial thromboplastin time (APTT): a coagulation procedure that tests for coagulation factors II, V, VIII, IX, X, XI, and XII, all of which are involved in the intrinsic pathway of coagulation. It is used to evaluate the effect of administration of anticoagulant drugs.

bleeding time: the time it takes a small, standardized incision to stop bleeding.

cerebrovascular accident: stroke. A cerebrovascular accident is characterized by sudden loss of consciousness followed by possible paralysis. Cerebrovascular accidents may be caused by an embolus or thrombus that occludes a cerebral artery, among other causes.

clotting disorder: a coagulation disease in which clots form in the blood spontaneously.

coagulation: the process of clotting, which depends on the presence of several coagulation factors, including prothrombin, thrombin, thromboplastin, fibrinogen, and calcium.

coagulation factor: one of twelve compounds required for the coagulation process. Coagulation factors must be present in appropriate amounts for clotting to occur effectively.

coumarin: a group of drugs, including warfarin, used to prevent and treat clotting disorders. Coumarin drugs act in the liver, where they interfere with the synthesis of vitamin K-dependent coagulation factors (II, VII, IX, and X).

embolism: the sudden obstruction of a blood vessel by an embolus.

embolus: an undissolved mass, in a blood or lymphatic vessel. It is usually a blood clot but may consist of fat globules, bacteria, or other debris. About 75 percent of emboli arise in the deep veins of the legs.

fibrin: the whitish, filamentous protein formed by the action of thrombin on fibrinogen. Other formed elements in the blood become entangled in the interlacing filaments of fibrin, thus forming a blood clot.

fibrinogen: coagulation factor I; a compound in plasma that is converted to fibrin by thrombin in the presence of calcium.

Fibrometer®: an instrument commonly used to test clot formation for prothrombin time tests. It automatically detects and times fibrin clot formation.

hemophilia: one of a group of diseases in which excessive bleeding occurs because of inherited deficiencies in blood coagulation factors; characterized by uncontrolled hemorrhaging, possibly even from the slightest injury.

hemophilia A: classic hemophilia; the most common type of hemophilia, caused by a recessive sex-linked gene that leads to the inability to synthesize coagulation factor VIII, antihemophilic factor (AHF).

hemophilia B: Christmas disease; the second most common type of hemophilia, caused by a recessive sex-linked gene that leads to the inability to synthesize coagulation factor IX, plasma thromboplastin component (PTC).

hemophilia C: a relatively uncommon type of hemophilia, which is caused by a dominant autosomal gene, leading to inability to synthesize factor XI, plasma thromboplastin antecedent (PTA).

hemorrhagic disease: any of several diseases in which excessive bleeding occurs because blood fails to clot.

hemorrhagic disease of the newborn: a bleeding disease due to lack of vitamin K-producing intestinal flora in less than 1% of newborns, occurring between the second and seventh day after birth. Hemorrhagic disease of the newborn is treated by administration of vitamin K. Vitamin K is necessary to the formation of several clotting factors including prothrombin.

hemostasis: the arrest of bleeding.

heparin sodium: a widely used anticoagulant drug for the management of clotting disorders. It works by inhibiting the conversion of prothrombin to thrombin.

myocardial infarction: an infarct, or area of necrosis (tissue death), in the myocardium. Myocardial infarction is usually due to occlusion of a coronary artery. Myocardial infarction is associated with pain, shock, cardiac failure, and frequently death.

myocardium: the middle, muscular layer of the walls of the heart.

platelet plug (white thrombus): a clump of platelets that adhere to an injured vessel to help stop bleeding; often sufficient to stop the flow of blood in capillary wounds.

prothrombin: coagulation factor II; a compound in circulating blood that is converted to thrombin by the action of thromboplastin.

prothrombin time (PT): a coagulation procedure that tests for coagulation factors I, II, VII, and X, all of which are involved in the extrinsic pathway of coagulation. Prothrombin time is used to evaluate the effect of administration of anticoagulant drugs.

serotonin: a potent vasoconstrictor, which is released by platelets adhering to a wounded blood vessel.

template method (Ivy bleeding time): a method of testing bleeding time. The template method standardizes the size and depth of the incision with a template device called a Simplate.

thrombin: an enzyme formed from the conversion of prothrombin by thromboplastin and other coagulation factors. Thrombin joins soluble fibrinogen molecules into long, hairlike molecules of insoluble fibrin.

thrombocytopenia: a hemorrhagic disease due to a deficiency of platelets, which results in many small hemorrhages.

thrombophlebitis: the inflammation of a vein due to a blood clot. Thrombophlebitis is a common problem in elderly, immobile patients.

thromboplastin: coagulation factor III; the immediate initiator of the blood-clotting mechanism. Thromboplastin interacts with other coagulation factors to convert prothrombin to thrombin.

thrombosis: the formation of a blood clot, or thrombus, within the vascular system. Thrombosis is treated with anticoagulants.

thrombus: a blood clot within the vascular system.

vascular phenomenon: one of three major components of hemostasis. The term *vascular phenomenon* refers to the vascular response to bleeding, which is vasoconstriction.

vasoconstriction: the constricting, or narrowing, of a blood vessel.

warfarin: one of the coumarin group of anticoagulants used to prevent and treat clotting disorders. Warfarin also is used as rodent poison.

● ● ● ● ● ● ● ● ● ● ● ● ● ● ● ● ● ●

This chapter describes the processes of **hemostasis,** or the arrest of bleeding, and blood **coagulation,** or clot formation. It also describes diseases that affect coagulation and laboratory tests of coagulation.

HEMOSTASIS AND BLOOD COAGULATION

Hemostasis is part of the process of homeostasis, the dynamic balance, or equilibrium, of the internal body environment that is maintained by feedback and regulation. The balance that must be maintained in hemostasis is between fluid blood, which must circulate, and coagulated blood, which prevents blood loss. Death can occur when either bleeding or clotting is uncontrolled.

Blood coagulation is one of three mechanisms by which hemostasis comes about. The other two mechanisms are **vasoconstriction,** which is a narrowing of the injured blood vessel, and the formation of a platelet plug, which is a clump of platelets that adhere to the site of injury.

◆◆ *Components of Hemostasis*

The process of hemostasis, which Figure 20.1 shows, can be divided into three types of phenomena: vascular, extravascular, and intravascular.

The Vascular Phenomenon. The **vascular phenomenon** is the reaction of the injured blood vessel itself. The injured vessel undergoes vasoconstriction, an immediate response that decreases blood loss until clotting can occur. It is probably enhanced and prolonged by **serotonin,** a potent vasoconstrictor, which is released by platelets adhering to the wounded blood vessel.

The Extravascular Phenomena. The extravascular phenomena are those that occur outside the in-

Vascular: blood vessel contracts

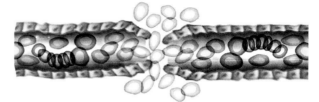

Extravascular: platelet plug formation triggered by mixture of tissue juices and exposed platelets

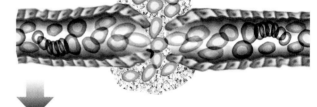

Blood clot activation in plasma

↓

prothrombin activator

↓

in presence of calcium

↓

prothrombin

↓

thrombin

↓

fibrinogen

↓

other clotting factors

↓

fibrin

↓

blood clot formation

↓

Intravascular: liquid blood turns to solid clot that plugs wound

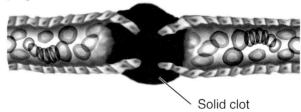

Solid clot

Figure 20.1. The process of hemostasis.

jured blood vessel. They consist of physical and biochemical reactions of the surrounding tissues, including release of **thromboplastin,** a compound that triggers coagulation. The tissue reactions activate other vascular and intravascular phenomena of hemostasis.

The Intravascular Phenomena. The intravascular phenomena are the processes that occur within the blood vessel. First, platelets adhere to the damaged site and accumulate to form a **platelet plug,** also called a **white thrombus.** The platelet plug may be sufficient to stop the bleeding if the site of bleeding is very small. If not, coagulation occurs next, through an extremely complex pathway of biochemical changes that transform liquid hemorrhaging blood into a solid clot around the platelet plug. Coagulation normally seals the injured vessel and stops the bleeding.

The process of coagulation requires twelve different compounds, called **coagulation factors,** which must be present in appropriate amounts for clotting to occur effectively (see Table 20.1).

◆◆ *Coagulation*

The initiation of coagulation occurs by one of two pathways—the extrinsic or the intrinsic. The extrinsic pathway is followed when blood comes into contact with traumatized tissues. The intrinsic pathway is followed when there is trauma to the blood itself, due, for example, to slow circulation, bacterial endotoxins, or vascular diseases. Each pathway has several steps, and both pathways end with formation of coagulation factor III, or thromboplastin, which is the immediate initiator of the blood-clotting mechanism.

The rest of the coagulation pathway is the same for both pathways. A clot is formed as follows:

- Thromboplastin interacts with other coagulation factors, such as factors IV and V, to convert **prothrombin** to **thrombin.**
- Thrombin joins soluble **fibrinogen** molecules into long, hairlike molecules of insoluble **fibrin.**
- Fibrin filaments form a meshlike network of strands, trapping cells and small amounts of serum, thus forming the clot.

TABLE 20.1 Coagulation Factors

Factor	Synonym
Factor I	Fibrinogen
Factor II	Prothrombin
Factor III	Thromboplastin
Factor IV	Calcium
Factor V	Labile factor (accelerator globulin)
Factor VI	—*
Factor VII	Serum prothrombin conversion accelerator (SPCA)
Factor VIII	Antihemophilic factor (AHF)
Factor IX	Plasma thromboplastin component (PTC)
Factor X	Stuart factor or Prower factor
Factor XI	Plasma thromboplastin antecedent (PTA)
Factor XII	Hageman factor (contact factor)
Factor XIII	Fibrin stabilizing factor
Platelet factor	Cephalin

*Factor VI is no longer considered a separate entity, but a form of Factor V.

DISEASES AFFECTING COAGULATION

Diseases that affect coagulation fall into two opposing categories—hemorrhagic diseases and clotting disorders. In **hemorrhagic diseases,** there is failure of the blood to clot. In **clotting disorders,** on the other hand, blood clots form spontaneously. Either extreme may be life threatening. Some blood-coagulation diseases are inherited, while others are acquired later in life. In general, the inherited disorders are more easily studied and better understood.

♦♦♦ Diseases and ♦♦♦ Hemostasis

Given the complexity of the process, it is not surprising that hemostasis is affected by diseases of several different organs and tissues; for example:

- *Bone marrow diseases* may reduce bone marrow production of platelets so that fewer are available for platelet plug formation.
- *Connective tissue diseases* may encourage hemorrhaging due to weakness and ease of trauma to blood vessels and other tissues.
- *Circulatory diseases* may impair circulation and encourage clot formation.
- *Liver diseases* may adversely affect coagulation because the liver synthesizes blood-coagulation factors, including prothrombin and fibrinogen.
- *High blood pressure* may lead to hemorrhaging.
- *Infections* may lead to tissue damage and bleeding.

♦♦ *Hemorrhagic Diseases*

The category of hemorrhagic diseases includes the hemophilias and several other disorders in which excessive bleeding occurs.

The Hemophilias. The **hemophilias** are a group of diseases in which excessive bleeding occurs because of inherited deficiencies in blood-coagulation factors. They are characterized by uncontrolled hemorrhaging, possibly even from the slightest injury.

Most cases of hemophilia are sex linked; that is, they are caused by a defective gene on the X chromosome, which is one of two sex chromosomes, X and Y. Females have two X chromosomes and males have one X chromosome and one Y chromosome.

Males with a defective gene on their one X chromosome have the disease hemophilia. Because the hemophiliac gene is recessive, only females with defective hemophiliac genes on both of their X chromosomes are affected by the disease. Females with one normal and one defective X chromosome, on the other hand, do not have the disease. Instead, they are carriers of hemophilia, because they can pass the defective gene on to their children. Because males need only one hemophilia gene to be affected by the disease, while females need two, the sex-linked forms of the disease affect males far more frequently than they do females. This is why female hemophiliacs are extremely rare. One in 10,000 males is born with hemophilia.

There are several types of hemophilia, each associated with the absence of a different clotting factor. Eighty percent of cases are **hemophilia A,** or classic hemophilia, in which a recessive sex-linked gene leads to inability to synthesize factor VIII, antihemophilic factor (AHF). Another 15 percent of cases are **hemophilia B,** or Christmas disease, in which a recessive sex-linked gene leads to inability to synthesize factor IX, plasma thromboplastin component (PTC). The remaining 5 percent of cases are due to deficiency of other coagulation factors. **Hemophilia C,** for example, is due to an autosomal (nonsex chromosome) dominant gene that leads to inability to synthesize factor XI, plasma thromboplastin antecedent (PTA).

The adverse effects of hemorrhaging associated with hemophilia are numerous. Bleeding into the soft tissues, the gastrointestinal tract, kidneys, and joints can have grave consequences. Bleeding into a joint, for example, can cause swelling, stiffening, and permanent crippling of the joint. The leading cause of death in hemophiliacs is intracranial bleeding.

Hemophiliacs need constant protection from injuries and blood loss. Whenever they receive injections, for example, small-gauge needles should be used, and pressure should be applied to the injection site afterward. The injection site should be monitored until all danger of hemorrhaging is past. Even small cuts are potentially life threatening and require medical attention. Hemophilia is much better controlled today than it was in the past, due to the availability of clotting factors derived from donated whole blood. Severe bleeding may require transfusion of normal fresh plasma or of the missing clotting factor.

Other Hemorrhagic Diseases. Vitamin K is important because it stimulates liver cells to synthesize prothrombin and several other clotting factors. It is stored in the liver. Vitamin K deficiency leads to the lack of prothrombin, which in turn results in prolonged blood-clotting time and increased hemorrhaging. Lack of vitamin K, which is essential to formation of factors II, VII, IX, and X, also causes **hemorrhagic disease of the newborn,** which occurs in less than 1% of newborns between the second and seventh day after birth. Administration of vitamin K corrects this condition until vitamin-K producing bacterial flora become established in the newborn.

Hypofibrinogenemia is a hemorrhagic disease caused by a deficiency of clotting factor I (fibrinogen). It may be inherited or acquired after severe liver damage. Generally, it is a mild disorder. **Thrombocytopenia** is a hemorrhagic disease due to a deficiency of platelets, which are also called thrombocytes for their role in clot formation. Without platelets to form platelet plugs, many small hemorrhages result.

♦ ♦ ♦ Drugs and ♦ ♦ ♦ Blood Clotting

The process of blood coagulation is adversely affected by a variety of drugs, such as aspirin, other analgesics, and antihistamines. Aspirin, for example, prevents platelets from adhering to one another. Patients with hemophilia should be especially careful when using drugs such as these.

♦♦ *Clotting Disorders*

In clotting disorders, clots form in the blood spontaneously. A clot that obstructs blood flow creates a serious condition and can result in death.

Thrombus Formation. Thrombosis refers to the formation of a blood clot, or **thrombus,** in the vascular system. A thrombus may arise spontaneously in the blood for a variety of reasons, including slowed blood flow and roughened or injured inner linings of blood vessels. Increased platelet activity or an elevated concentration of procoagulants also may be involved in the spontaneous formation of blood clots. If a clot arises within a major blood vessel or in the brain, death may occur because blood flow—and hence oxygen and nutrients—are blocked from vital areas.

The body has some natural defenses against thrombosis. They include phagocytic cells, which may engulf a clot, and inhibitors of the coagulation factors, such as antithrombin, a substance that opposes the action of thrombin.

Embolisms. Embolism refers to the sudden obstruction of a blood vessel by an **embolus,** which is usually a blood clot but may be fat globules, bacteria, or other undissolved matter. About three-fourths of emboli arise in the deep veins of the legs, where they may cause **thrombophlebitis,** or inflammation of the vein due to the clot. This is a common problem in elderly, immobile patients. Emboli that obstruct blood flow in the extremities may result ultimately in necrosis and gangrene.

Often, emboli tear loose and move through the circulatory system, lodging in vital organs, such as the lungs, heart, or brain. In the heart, they may cause **myocardial infarction,** which is an infarct, or area of necrosis, in the **myocardium** (middle wall of the heart), due to cessation of blood supply. Myocardial infarction is usually caused by occlusion of a coronary artery. It is associated with pain, shock, cardiac failure, and frequently death. In the brain, an embolus may cause a **cerebrovascular accident,** or stroke, which is accompanied by sudden loss of consciousness followed by paralysis.

Anticoagulant Drugs. Anticoagulants are drugs that prevent coagulation. They are used in the management of patients with a history of clotting disorders, such as thrombosis, thrombophlebitis, pulmonary embolism, acute myocardial infarction, and stroke.

Heparin sodium occurs naturally in the body and is obtained from domestic animals for use as a therapeutic drug. It interferes with coagulation by forming an antithrombin compound and preventing platelets from releasing thromboplastin, thus inhibiting conversion of prothrombin to thrombin.

The **coumarin** group of drugs, including **warfarin,** are ingested orally, absorbed from the gastrointestinal tract, and then carried to the liver. Here, they interfere with the synthesis of vitamin K-dependent coagulation factors (II, VII, IX, and X).

The effectiveness of anticoagulants may be increased by drugs such as aspirin and decreased by others, such as barbiturates. Alcohol intake and physiological processes also may affect their efficacy.

♦ ♦ ♦ Antidote for ♦ ♦ ♦ Warfarin Poisoning

Warfarin is used as not only an anticoagulant but also a rodent poison. In this form, it has been ingested accidentally by children. Overdosage of warfarin anticoagulant also sometimes occurs. The antidote in both cases, and for coumarin overdose in general, is administration of vitamin K.

Underdosage of anticoagulant drugs may lead to a life-threatening blood clot, while overdosage can cause a fatal hemorrhage. For these reasons, patients taking anticoagulant drugs require routine monitoring with laboratory tests.

LABORATORY TESTS OF COAGULATION

Several different types of laboratory tests monitor coagulation, including general tests of bleeding time, specific tests of coagulation factors, and screening tests for presurgical patients.

◆◆ General Tests of Bleeding Time

The single best test of the body's ability to maintain hemostasis is **bleeding time,** the time it takes a small incision to stop bleeding. This type of test is inclusive of any factor causing failure of hemostasis, but it cannot distinguish among possible causes.

◆ ◆ ◆ Aspirin Advisory ◆ ◆ ◆

Because aspirin ingestion may increase bleeding time, you should advise patients not to ingest aspirin or related analgesics for several days before a test of bleeding time.

For a general test of bleeding time, capillaries are punctured with a small, clean incision to produce a source of bleeding. After the incision begins to bleed, the time is noted, and welling blood around the cut is removed every fifteen to thirty seconds with filter paper, taking care not to disturb the platelet plug. As clotting proceeds, the circles of blood on the filter paper become smaller, until no fluid blood is left on the paper, marking the end of bleeding (see Figure 20.2). The interval between the beginning and end of bleeding is reported as the bleeding time.

◆ ◆ ◆ Note ◆ ◆ ◆

In order for bleeding time to be normal, the platelet count must be over 80,000, with platelets showing normal adherence and aggregation.

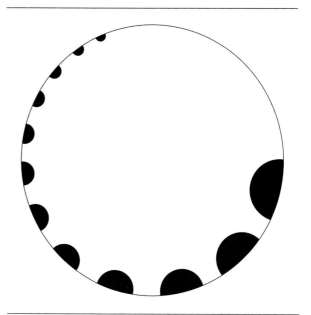

Figure 20.2. As clotting proceeds, the circles of blood on a filter paper become smaller.

General bleeding times tend to be imprecise because of variations in lab worker technique, external conditions, and the site of incision. For example, decreased bleeding time may result from failure to cleanse the incision site or from low temperature in the limb selected for the incision. On the other hand, increased bleeding time may result from pressure applied to the incision area or to a red flush in the limb selected. Because of variations such as these, it is not unusual for duplicate bleeding times performed on the same individual to vary by two or three minutes. For this reason, more standardized methods have been developed, including the template method and Duke's bleeding time.

The Template Method. The **template method,** also known as the **Ivy bleeding time,** standardizes the size and depth of the incision by using a template device called a Simplate, which is shown in Figure 20.3. The incision is made in the forearm above the wrist in an area cleaned with 70 percent alcohol. The area should be free of skin disease and obvious veins. In order to stabilize capillary pressure, a blood-pressure cuff is placed above the elbow, inflated to 40 mm, and maintained in place throughout the procedure. With the first appearance of blood from the incision, a stop watch is started. Then, every thirty seconds, blood from the cut is blotted onto a round of filter paper in a circular, rotating pattern. The time is noted when the blood flow stops. Bleeding time is the interval required for the bleeding to stop.

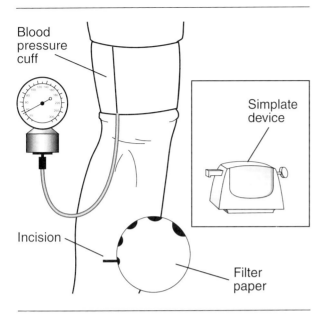

Figure 20.3. Ivy bleeding times are performed on adults by making an incision with a Simplate device, which standardizes the depth and length of the incision. Pressure in the cuff remains at 40 mm throughout the procedure. Normal range is 2.3 to 9.5 minutes.

Duke's Bleeding Time. The Duke's bleeding time test is less standardized and less precise than the template method, but it may be used with children. Bleeding times usually are not done on children because hairline scars and keloid formations may occur at incision sites. The incision site for this test is the earlobe. The lobe of the ear is warmed by gentle rubbing with a cotton ball, cleansed with 70 percent alcohol, and punctured with a device that gives a standardized wound. The same technique of blotting with filter paper is used that was described for the template method. Again, bleeding time is the interval required for bleeding to stop.

✦✦ *Specific Tests of Coagulation Factors*

Laboratory tests of specific elements of the coagulation process that are simple enough to be performed in POLs include the prothrombin time (PT) and the activated partial thromboplastin time (APTT). Results from these two tests, when correlated with the results of other tests, such as platelet counts, help determine the cause of coagulation problems. Both tests also are used routinely to monitor the coagulation status of patients on heparin and coumarin therapy.

Prothrombin Time. A prothrombin time (PT) tests coagulation factors I, II, VII, and X, all of which are involved in the extrinsic pathway of coagulation. A citrated plasma sample is added to a solution of calcium and tissue extract from an animal brain that contains thromboplastin. Prothrombin time is measured as the time required for clot formation. Normal PT is 11 to 13 seconds.

Activated Partial Thromboplastin Time. Activated partial thromboplastin time (APTT) tests coagulation factors II, V, VIII, IX, X, XI, and XII, all of which are involved in the intrinsic pathway of coagulation. A solution of calcium, a platelet substitute, and an activator are added to a plasma sample. The time needed for fibrin clot formation is measured as the activated partial thromboplastin time.

Methods. There are special instruments and specimen collection techniques for performing prothrombin times and activated partial thromboplastin times. Clot formation in the PT and APTT procedures can be tested manually by tilting the tube until clot formation is noted or by using a wire loop to detect the newly formed clot. It is preferable, however, to test clot formation with instruments like the commonly used **Fibrometer**®, shown in Figure 20.4. Compared with manual methods, this inexpensive instrument offers the advantages of higher accuracy, greater speed, less labor, and no manual pipetting. The instrument consists of three parts:

- *precision coagulation timer:* automatically detects and times formation of the fibrin clot
- *thermal block:* prewarms reagents and specimens to body temperature (37 degrees Celsius)
- *automatic pipette:* dispenses the 0.1 mL or 0.2 mL volume normally used in coagulation testing

With a fibrometer, clot formation is detected with an automatic wire loop. When the clot is formed, it completes an electrical circuit, stopping the timing mechanism. Also available are cups and pipette tips designed specifically for use with the instrument. These are disposable, made to the correct dimensions, and allow heat transfer from the heat block.

> ✦✦✦ **Note** ✦✦✦
>
> There is another instrument available for testing clot formation, the Abbott Vision instrument, which is described in Chapter 23. It uses a photo-optical method of detecting and timing clot formation.

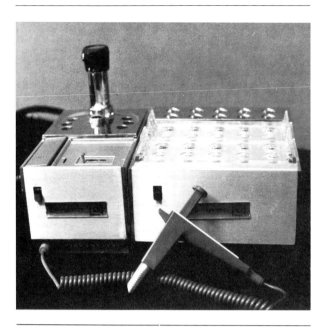

Figure 20.4. The Fibrometer® performs prothrombin times (PT) and activated partial thromboplastin times (APTT) more accurately and efficiently than manual methods. Photo by Mark Palko.

Use venous blood, collected with the anticoagulant trisodium citrate (blue-capped tube), for prothrombin and activated partial thromboplastin times. Use a clean glass or plastic tube for collection. If you use a vacutainer tube, fill it completely with blood to assure that the anticoagulant-to-blood ratio is 1:9. The blood must flow without interruption into the collection tube to prevent microclotting.

♦ ♦ ♦ Glass or Plastic? ♦ ♦ ♦

Prothrombin times and activated partial thromboplastin times are affected by the type of container—glass or plastic. Therefore, it is important to use consistently one or the other type of tube for collecting specimens for these coagulation procedures.

Centrifuge the specimen immediately after collection at a speed of 1,600 g for ten minutes. If centrifugation must be delayed, place the specimen on ice to maintain the integrity of the coagulation factors.

♦ ♦ ♦ PPP ♦ ♦ ♦

PPP refers to "platelet-poor plasma," a phrase occasionally seen in POL test instructions. It is plasma that has been centrifuged at high speed (1,600 to 2,000 g) for five to ten minutes. Plasma prepared in this way is required for most coagulation studies.

After centrifuging, pipette the plasma into a labeled plastic tube, cap it, and, if possible, test immediately. During pipetting, avoid the area near the buffy coat between the plasma and packed red blood cells. A concentration of platelets is there. If testing must be delayed, refrigerate the specimen for up to two hours or freeze it rapidly at −20 degrees Celsius or lower.

♦♦ *Screening Tests*

Prospective surgery patients often are screened to identify those with a hemorrhaging tendency. The battery of tests ordered commonly includes a scan of platelets on a blood film, a bleeding time, a prothrombin time, and an activated partial thromboplastin time. For patients whose history and platelet scan suggest abnormalities, an electronic or manual platelet count also may be ordered.

♦♦ *Quality Control and Safety*

As with all laboratory procedures, careful attention to sample collection and handling and other details of procedure is necessary to maintain quality control. Standardization, such as the use of the template method for bleeding time, also helps maintain quality control. Duplicates of controls and patient samples should be tested for prothrombin times and activated partial thromboplastin times. CLIA 1988 requires that two levels of daily control test results be maintained for permanent quality-control records.

Whenever you perform coagulation studies, keep in mind that both patient specimens and control specimens are potentially biohazardous. Always follow the Universal Precautions. For example, dispose of all used glass and plastic ware according to the rules concerning biohazardous waste.

PROCEDURE

20.1 Prothrombin Time Determination

Goal

- After successfully completing this procedure, you will be able to perform a prothrombin time using an automatic wire loop coagulation instrument. The following set of instructions should be used when a Fibrometer® instrument is used. The procedure may vary slightly with a different automated wire loop coagulation instrument.

Completion Time

- 30 minutes

Equipment and Supplies

- disposable latex gloves
- impermeable apron
- hand disinfectant
- surface disinfectant
- paper towels and tissues
- biohazard container
- 4 patient plasma samples
- thromboplastin reagent and control
- 6 test tubes
- disposable Pasteur pipette
- automatic wire loop coagulation instrument
- 10 pipette tips, sizes 0.1 mL and 0.2 mL
- 10 instrument cups
- heat block at 37 degrees Celsius
- pen and laboratory form

Instructions

Read through the list of equipment and supplies that you will need and the steps of the procedure. Be sure that you understand each step before you start. Then complete each step correctly and in the proper order. If your completion time is too long, repeat the procedure until you increase your speed.

1. Wash your hands with disinfectant, dry them, and put on gloves and apron.

2. Follow the Universal Precautions.

3. Collect and prepare the appropriate equipment.

4. Switch on the heat block. Allow fifteen minutes for temperature to stabilize at 37 degrees Celsius.

5. Reconstitute the thromboplastin reagent according to manufacturer's instructions, placing the reconstituted thromboplastin in a clean test tube labeled "reagent."

6. Reconstitute the control according to manufacturer's instructions, placing the reconstituted control in a clean test tube labeled "control."

7. Place both the reagent and control tubes in the heat block at 37 degrees Celsius for at least five minutes.

8. Place the patient plasma in a clean test tube labeled "patient." Put the patient tube in the heat block for at least five minutes.

9. Plug the automatic pipette into the automatic wire loop coagulation instrument, leaving the pipette switch in the "off" position.

10. Put the pipette on the 0.2 mL position and pipette 0.2 mL of reagent into each of four instrument cups (two cups for the patient sample and its duplicate and two cups for the control and its duplicate). Be sure to change pipette tips when you change from the patient plasma to the control or vice versa.

11. Raise the arm on the automatic wire loop and set the timer to zero.

12. Place one 0.2 mL cup of reagent in the well under the probe.

13. Switch the automatic pipette to the 0.1 mL position, being sure the automatic pipette switch is still in the "off" position. Change pipette tip to 0.1 mL size.

14. Draw up 0.1 mL of the control or patient plasma into the automatic pipette.

15. Change the automatic pipette switch to "on."

16. Hold the tip of the automatic pipette over the cup of reagent under the raised probe.

17. Dispense the 0.1 mL of control or patient plasma in the pipette into the reagent cup. This will activate the arm of the probe to drop into the reagent cup after a 0.5 to 1.8 seconds' delay, which allows time to remove the tip from under the probe (failure to remove the tip may damage the probe).

18. When the reaction between the thromboplastin and plasma forms a clot and the instrument shuts off automatically, raise the probe and carefully clean the electrodes with a clean tissue.

19. Remove the reagent cup and dispose of the clot in the biohazardous waste container.

20. Record the time in seconds, including parts of seconds, and reset the timer.

21. Repeat steps 12–20 with the other three samples. If duplicate samples differ by more than 0.5 seconds from each other, repeat the test. Normal prothrombin time for most controls is eleven to thirteen seconds.

22. Complete the necessary information on the laboratory requisition form and route it to the proper place.

23. Discard disposable equipment.

24. Disinfect other equipment and return it to storage.

S = Satisfactory   U = Unsatisfactory

	S	U
25. Clean the work area following the Universal Precautions.		
26. Remove your gloves and apron; wash your hands with disinfectant, and dry them.		

OVERALL PROCEDURAL EVALUATION

Student's Name _____

Signature of Instructor _____ Date _____

Comments

CHAPTER 20 REVIEW

Using Terminology

Define the following terms in the spaces provided.

1. Coagulation: _____
   _____

2. Bleeding time: _____
   _____

3. Cerebrovascular accident: _____
   _____

4. Clotting disorder: _____
   _____

5. Coagulation factor: _____

_____

6. Coumarin: _____

_____

7. Embolism: _____

_____

8. Fibrin: _____

_____

9. Fibrinogen: _____

_____

10. Hemophilia: _____

_____

11. Hemorrhagic disease: _____

_____

12. Hemostasis: _____

_____

13. Platelet plug (white thrombus): _____

_____

14. Prothrombin: _____

_____

15. Serotonin: _____

_____

16. Template method (Ivy bleeding time): _____

_____

17. Thromboplastin: _____

_____

18. Thrombus: _____

_____

19. Vasoconstriction: _____

_____

20. Warfarin: _____

_____

Acquiring Knowledge

Mark each of the following statements as true or false, and rewrite the false statements to make them true.

21. The mechanisms by which hemostasis comes about are coagulation, vasoconstriction, and erythropoiesis.

_____

_____

_____

22. The process of hemostasis can be divided into three types of phenomena: intravascular, vascular, and extrinsic.

_____

_____

_____

23. The vascular phenomenon that occurs when a blood vessel is injured is called vasoconstriction.

_____

_____

24. Thromboplastin interacts with other coagulation factors to convert prothrombin to fibrinogen.

_____

_____

25. Thrombin joins insoluble fibrinogen molecules into long, hairlike molecules of soluble fibrin.

_____

_____

26. Diseases that affect coagulation fall into two opposing categories: hemorrhagic diseases and bleeding diseases.

_____

_____

_____

27. Most cases of hemophilia are acquired.

_____

_____

28. Female hemophiliacs are extremely rare because the female sex hormone, estrogen, protects females from this disease.

_____

_____

29. Vitamin D, an antihemorrhagic factor normally present in blood, aids in blood coagulation and is necessary for the formation of thromboplastin.

_____

_____

_____

30. Thrombocytopenia is a hemorrhagic disease due to a deficiency of platelets.

_____

_____

Answer the following questions in the spaces provided.

31. What is thrombosis and how is it treated?

_____

_____

32. How are myocardial infarction and cerebrovascular accident similar?

_____

_____

_____

33. How do the drugs heparin and warfarin work to prevent clot formation?

_____

_____

_____

_____

34. Name two general tests of bleeding time and two specific tests of coagulation factors.

_____

_____

_____

35. How does a wire loop coagulation instrument detect the formation of blood clots?

_____

_____

_____

36. How is quality control maintained in blood-coagulation testing?

_____

_____

_____

_____

_____

Applying Knowledge—On the Job

Answer the following questions in the spaces provided.

37. A patient has come into the lab where you work for a bleeding time test, which was just ordered by the physician. The patient mentions that his arthritis has been acting up, so he has been taking aspirin for a few days. How does this information relate to the patient's test? What should you do?

_____

_____

38. An elderly patient has been told to come to the lab routinely for blood tests to monitor his medication. The patient has a history of thrombosis and recently suffered a mild stroke. What type of medication is the patient most likely taking? What test or tests will the physician probably routinely order on this patient's blood?

_____

_____

_____

39. Your coworker in the lab has just taken a sample of plasma from the refrigerator to run a prothrombin time. He is in a hurry because his shift ends in ten minutes, so he proceeds to run the test immediately on one sample. What errors has your coworker made? How will they affect the test results?

_____

_____

_____

_____

40. A patient in the clinic where you work is scheduled for major surgery tomorrow, so the physician has ordered screening tests to see if she has a hemorrhaging tendency. What tests are likely to be checked off on the requisition form for this patient? What further test might be requisitioned if the platelet scan appears abnormal?

_____

_____

_____

UNIT

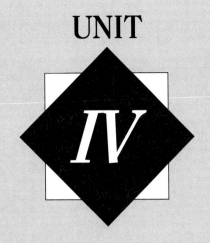

IV

Blood Chemistry

21 *Photometry*

COGNITIVE OBJECTIVES

After studying this chapter, you should be able to

- use each of the vocabulary terms appropriately.
- state Beer's law and explain how it is related to the use of photometry.
- describe how colorimeters and spectrophotometers work and how they differ from each other.
- explain the underlying principles of reflectance photometry.
- identify when reflectance photometry is used in POLs.
- describe the relationships of absorbance, transmittance, and reflectance of light with the concentration of a substance.
- list the parts and identify their functions for photometers commonly used in POLs.
- discuss how quality control is maintained with photometry in POLs.

PERFORMANCE OBJECTIVE

After studying this chapter, you should be able to

- establish a standard curve using a colorimeter or spectrophotometer.

TERMINOLOGY

Beer's law: the law stating that the extent to which a light beam is absorbed as it passes through a solution depends only on the number of absorbing molecules in the light path.

colorimeter: the type of photometer that filters light with colored glass. It measures the transmis-

sion of light through a solution to determine its concentration.

direct relationship: the relationship when two variables change in the same direction; for example, when the concentration of a solution increases, absorbance of light by it increases.

dry reagent (solid-phase) chemistry: a lab test, such as a urine reagent-strip test (dip stick), in which a dry reagent on a strip is used for a chemical reaction.

galvanometer: a device for measuring electric current. In a photometer, a galvanometer measures the amount of electricity produced by the photocell.

inverse relationship: the relationship when two variables change in opposite directions; for example, when the concentration of a solution increases, transmission of light through it decreases.

linear relationship: the relationship when two variables exhibit a constant relationship so that for each unit by which one variable changes, the other variable changes by a constant amount; for example, for each unit by which the concentration of a solution increases, its absorbance of light also increases by one unit.

monochromatic light: light of one color (just one or a small range of wavelengths).

photocell (photoelectric cell): a device for converting light to electric current. In a photometer, a photocell converts the light transmitted through the sample solution to a small electric current.

photometer: an instrument for measuring the intensity of light.

photometry: the measurement of the intensity of light, or brightness, with a device called a photometer. Photometry is used in POLs to assess the concentration of substances, such as hemoglobin and glucose in blood.

reflectance photometer: the type of photometer that measures the amount of light reflected back from a solid, such as a reagent pad. A reflectance photometer is used in dry reagent chemistry tests.

spectrophotometer: the type of photometer that filters light with a diffraction grating device or prism. A spectrophotometer measures the transmission of light through a solution to determine its concentration.

• • • • • • • • • • • • • • • • • • •

Photometry is the measurement of intensity, or brightness, of light, with a device called a **photometer.** Photometers are used in POLs to assess the concentration of substances, such as the concentration of hemoglobin and glucose in blood.

Two types of photometers are used in POLs. One type measures the intensity of light passing through a solution. It includes **colorimeters** and **spectrophotometers** (see Figure 21.1). The other type measures the intensity of light that is reflected back from a solid, such as a reagent pad. This is the **reflectance photometer.**

In either type of photometry, the wavelength of

light is an important variable because different substances absorb different wavelengths of light. When the wavelength most strongly absorbed by a substance is known, then the amount of transmitted or reflected light at that wavelength can be used to identify the amount of substance present.

> ♦ ♦ ♦ **Wavelength and Color** ♦ ♦ ♦
>
> The human eye can detect light waves that range from about 400 nanometers, which appear violet, to about 700 nanometers, which appear red. The rest of the visible spectrum falls between these two extremes. Wavelengths lower than 400 nanometers fall into the ultraviolet range and wavelengths higher than 700 nanometers fall into the infrared range, neither of which can be detected by the human eye.

COLORIMETERS AND SPECTROPHOTOMETERS

To understand how colorimeters and spectrophotometers work, you need to know their underlying principles. The operation of colorimeters and spectrophotometers is based on **Beer's law,** which states that the extent to which a light beam is absorbed as it passes through a solution depends only on the number of absorbing molecules in the light path. As a result, the more concentrated a solution, the more absorbing molecules and the more light that is absorbed. The less concentrated the solution, the fewer absorbing molecules and the less light that is absorbed.

This relationship between concentration and absorbance, which Figure 21.2 illustrates, is an example of a **direct relationship**—the two variables, absorbance and concentration, vary in the same direction. When one increases, the other increases. The relationship between absorbance and concentration also is a **linear relationship,** as indicated by the straight line in the figure. This means that for each unit by which concentration increases, absorbance increases by a constant amount.

Concentrated solutions, because they absorb more light, let less light pass through; that is, they transmit less light than do dilute solutions. Figure 21.3 shows the relationship between concentration and transmittance. This is an example of an **inverse relationship;** that is, the two variables, transmittance and concentration, vary in opposite directions.

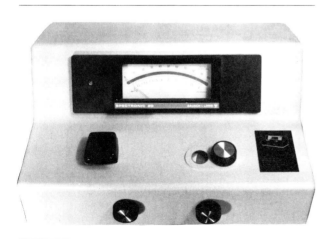

Figure 21.1. An all-purpose spectrophotometer. Photo by Mark Palko.

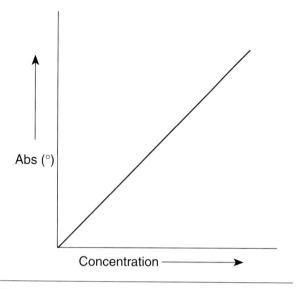

Figure 21.2. The relationship between the concentration and absorbance (°Abs) of light by a solution.

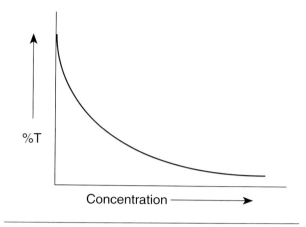

Figure 21.3. The relationship between concentration and transmittance (%T) of light through a solution.

TABLE 21.1. %T—Absorbance Conversion Table

%T	A	%T	A
1	2.000	26	0.585
2	1.699	27	0.569
3	1.523	28	0.553
4	1.398	29	0.538
5	1.301	30	0.523
6	1.222	31	0.509
7	1.155	32	0.495
8	1.097	33	0.482
9	1.046	34	0.469
10	1.000	35	0.456
11	0.959	36	0.444
12	0.921	37	0.432
13	0.886	38	0.420
14	0.854	39	0.409
15	0.824	40	0.398
16	0.796	41	0.387
17	0.770	42	0.377
18	0.745	43	0.367
19	0.721	44	0.357
20	0.699	45	0.347
21	0.678	46	0.337
22	0.658	47	0.328
23	0.638	48	0.319
24	0.620	49	0.310
25	0.602	50	0.301

✦✦ *How They Work*

Colorimeters and spectrophotometers have the following essential parts, which Figure 21.4 illustrates schematically for colorimeters and Figure 21.5 illustrates schematically for spectrophotometers:

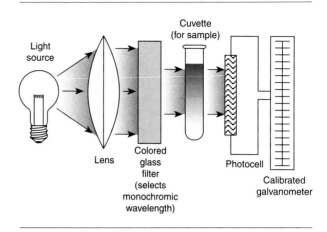

Figure 21.4. A schematic of colorimeters, showing the five essential parts and a sample cuvette.

TABLE 21.1. %T—Absorbance Conversion Table (continued)

%T	A	%T	A
51	0.292	76	0.119
52	0.284	77	0.114
53	0.276	78	0.108
54	0.268	79	0.102
55	0.260	80	0.097
56	0.252	81	0.092
57	0.244	82	0.086
58	0.237	83	0.081
59	0.229	84	0.076
60	0.222	85	0.071
61	0.215	86	0.066
62	0.208	87	0.061
63	0.201	88	0.056
64	0.194	89	0.051
65	0.187	90	0.046
66	0.181	91	0.041
67	0.174	92	0.036
68	0.168	93	0.032
69	0.161	94	0.027
70	0.155	95	0.022
71	0.149	96	0.018
72	0.143	97	0.013
73	0.137	98	0.009
74	0.131	99	0.004
75	0.125	100	0.000

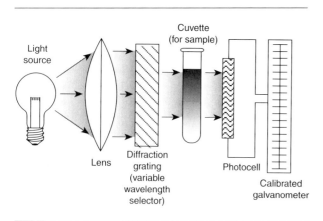

Figure 21.5. A schematic of spectrophotometers, showing the five essential parts and a sample cuvette.

- light source

- lens

- colored glass filter (colorimeter) or diffraction grating device or prism (spectrophotometer)

- photoelectric cell, or photocell

- galvanometer or similar device

Light from an electric bulb or other source is focused by the lens and filtered by the colored glass, diffraction-grating device, or prism, before passing through a cuvette of sample solution. Filtering produces **monochromatic light,** which is light of one color (just one or a small range of wavelengths). The color of light selected is the one most strongly absorbed by the substance in solution.

Any unabsorbed light that is transmitted through the solution is picked up by the **photocell,** or **photoelectric cell,** which converts the light to a small electric current. The strength of the current is directly proportional to the intensity of the light. The **galvanometer,** in turn, measures the amount of electricity produced, thus giving an electrical reading of the amount of light transmitted by the solution.

The amount of light transmitted through the solution of unknown concentration is compared with the light transmitted through solutions of known concentration of the same substance, with which the photometer has been calibrated. Most photometers make these comparisons automatically and then print out the final result as concentration value, saving lab workers this step in the procedure.

·· *The Difference Between Colorimeters and Spectrophotometers*

The only significant difference between colorimeters and spectrophotometers is how the wavelengths of light are selected. Colorimeters have colored glass filters that transmit light in a limited number of broad bands of wavelengths. Spectrophotometers, on the other hand, use a diffraction-grating device, or prism, that can transmit a large number of very narrow bands of light, each of a single wavelength. Spectrophotometry can best determine the specific wavelengths of light most strongly absorbed by particular substances.

REFLECTANCE PHOTOMETERS

The reflectance photometer is a modification of the colorimeter and spectrophotometer that was developed for use with **dry reagent (solid-phase) chemistry,** in which the solid substances used do not transmit light.

·· *Historical Note*

The first dry reagent chemistry tests developed were urine reagent-strip tests (dip sticks). Dry reagent blood-chemistry tests, including blood-glucose tests, also were developed. Until the development of reflectance photometry, dry reagent chemistry results were obtained by visual matching of the color of the reacted reagent strip to a chart of color blocks, and the human eye functioned as the photometer. The results were subjective and, because of individual variation in visual acuity, were not always reproducible. Also, because the number of color blocks was limited, the results were only semiquantitative. Reflectance photometry to read reagent strip-test results provided objective, quantitative results.

·· *Underlying Principles*

In reflectance photometry, the light measured is the light that reflects off the surface of the reaction pad, not the light that is transmitted through a solution. The amount of light reflected is inversely proportional to the amount of color change generated by the reaction, which in turn is proportional to the amount of analyte present in the sample tested. In other words, the greater the concentration of the analyte in the specimen, the greater the reaction and the greater the amount of light absorbed on the reagent pad. The more light that is absorbed, the less light that is reflected away from the pad.

◆◆ *How They Work*

As Figure 21.6 shows, filtered light is focused on a reagent pad. Any unabsorbed light is reflected off the reagent pad and strikes a photocell, which generates electrical current. The strength of the current is directly proportional to the intensity of the light and inversely proportional to the concentration of the analyte. Reflectance photometers calculate the amount of analyte present from the electrical current generated by the photocell.

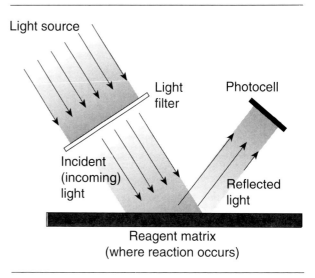

Figure 21.6. Reflectance photometry is utilized in all dry-reagent (solid-phase) chemistry instruments.

QUALITY CONTROL

The use of photometers in POLs completely removes personal judgment from the measuring process. The instrument, not the operator, determines the intensity of light being measured. All photometers can give good quality, reproducible results if the instrument is:

- properly constructed to eliminate any extraneous light from striking the photocell.
- used with good controls for purposes of comparison.

The accuracy of photometric instruments can be checked by testing control samples. If control samples with known values are run on a daily basis and the instrument reading for the control is the same as the expected value for the control, then the instrument is working properly. All manufacturers of blood-chemistry instruments, for example, recommend running a control sample at least once daily. Many recommend testing three levels of controls, including abnormally high values, normal values, and abnormally low values.

PROCEDURE

21.1 — Establishing a Standard Curve Using a Colorimeter or Spectrophotometer

Goal

- After successfully completing this procedure, you will be able to produce a standard curve using a photometric instrument by making the proper dilutions, reading the percent of transmittance on a photometer, converting the transmittance on the photometer to absorbance values, and plotting the absorbance values of each solution on a graph.

Completion Time

- 45 minutes

Equipment and Supplies

- automatic pipette filled with distilled water or 10 mL TD volumetric pipette and a suction bulb
- 1 mL of hematoxylin stain or methylene blue
- 7 clean, dry 50 mL test tubes
- 1 test tube rack
- 1 Pasteur pipette
- paper towels and lint-free tissues
- colorimeter or spectrophotometer with appropriate cuvettes
- ruler and pen
- graph paper (follows procedure)
- conversion table − %T to absorbance

Instructions

Read through the list of equipment and supplies that you will need and the steps of the procedure. Be sure that you understand each step before you begin. Then complete each step correctly and in the proper order. If your completion time is too long, repeat the procedure until you increase your speed.

	S	U

1. Label the seven test tubes as follows and place them in the test tube rack in this order: *B* (for reagent blank), *C* (for concentrated solution), and the numbers *5, 10, 15, 20,* and *25.*

2. Using the automatic pipette or the volumetric pipette, add 10 mL of distilled water to each of the seven test tubes. If you use an automatic pipette, do not hold the test tube under the nozzle while pulling up the plunger. If you use a TD volumetric pipette, draw the distilled water into the pipette with a suction bulb and allow the pipette to drain into each tube. Do not force the water out of the tip of the pipette.

3. Add 1 mL of hematoxylin stain or methylene blue to the distilled water in the test tube labeled *C.* Mix the stain and water by holding the test tube with your thumb and index finger and striking the bottom of the test tube with a downward stroke of your index finger on the other hand. The solution should swirl and form a small whirlpool.

4. Holding the Pasteur pipette horizontally, add drops of dye mixture from the test tube labeled *C* to each of the test tubes labeled with a number. Do not add dye mixture to the test tube labeled *B.* The number of drops that you add to each tube should correspond with the number on the test tube: five drops in the tube labeled *5,* ten drops in the tube labeled *10,* and so on. Mix each tube as instructed in step 3.

5. Set the wavelength of the photometer at 460 nm.

6. Transfer approximately 5 mL of distilled water from the tube labeled *B* into a cuvette. Clean the outside of the cuvette with a clean, lint-free tissue.

7. Place the cuvette in the instrument according to the manufacturer's instructions.

8. Adjust the instrument so that the percent of transmittance (%T) reads 100 with the *B* solution in the instrument. Note that on the ° A or OD scale, the value is 0.000, so this is sometimes referred to as zeroing the instrument.

9. Transfer approximately 5 mL of solution from the tube labeled *5* into another cuvette. This is a sample solution.

10. Replace the *B* solution cuvette with the sample solution cuvette, read the percent of transmittance, and record the result.

11. Repeat steps 9 and 10 using each sample solution (*10*, *15*, *20*, and *25*). Allow the cuvette to drain clean between samples by holding the cuvette upside down and touching the tip to a clean paper towel. Do not handle the bottom half of the cuvette. Oil from your fingers may distort the light path. Wipe this part of the cuvette with a clean, lint-free tissue if it is not completely clean.

12. Using the conversion table (see Table 21.1) convert each transmittance value (percent) to an absorbance value (degree).

13. Plot each of the absorbance values on the graph paper (Figure 21.7).

14. Discard disposable equipment and used reagents.

15. Clean other equipment and return it to storage.

16. Clean the work area.

17. Wash and dry your hands.

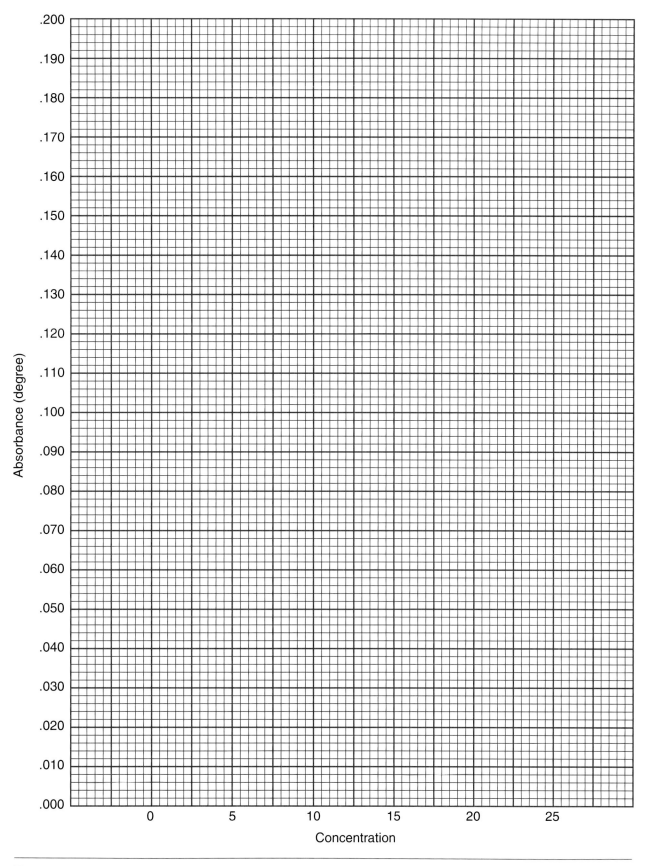

Figure 21.7. Graph paper for plotting absorbance values.

OVERALL PROCEDURAL EVALUATION

Student's Name _____

Signature of Instructor _____ **Date** _____

Comments

CHAPTER 21 REVIEW

Using Terminology

Define the following terms in the spaces provided.

1. Beer's law: _____

_____

2. Direct relationship: _____

_____

3. Dry reagent (solid-phase) chemistry: _____

_____

4. Galvanometer: _____

_____

5. Inverse relationship: _____

_____

6. Monochromatic light: _____

_____

7. Photocell (photoelectric cell): _____

_____

8. Photometer: _____

_____

9. Reflectance photometer: _____

_____

10. Spectrophotometer: _____

_____

Acquiring Knowledge

Answer the following questions in the spaces provided.

11. How are photometers used in POLs?

_____

_____

12. Explain how Beer's law is related to the use of photometry in POLs.

_____

_____

_____

_____

13. Describe how colorimeters and spectrophotometers work.

_____

_____

_____

14. Explain how colorimeters and spectrophotometers differ from each other.

_____

_____

_____

_____

15. Explain the underlying principles of reflectance photometry.

_____

_____

_____

_____

16. When is reflectance photometry used in POLs?

_____

_____

17. Describe the relationship between the absorbance of light and the concentration of a solution.

_____

_____

18. How are transmittance of light and concentration of a solution related?

_____

_____

19. How is the reflectance of light related to the concentration of an analyte on a reagent pad?

_____

_____

_____

20. What is the role of photocells in photometers?

_____

_____

21. What device in spectrophotometers selects the correct wavelength of light?

_____

_____

22. What is the role of galvanometers in photometers?

_____

_____

_____

23. In dry reagent chemistry, what is directly proportional to the color change on the reagent pad? What is inversely proportional to the color change?

_____

_____

_____

24. Discuss how quality control is maintained with photometry in POLs.

_____

_____

_____

_____

_____

_____

25. How is the wavelength of light related to the use of photometry in POLs?

_____

_____

_____

_____

26. What determines the strength of the current produced by the photocell in colorimeters or spectrophotometers?

_____

_____

_____

_____

27. Before the development of photometry, how were color changes detected in analytic chemistry? Why is use of a photometer superior to use of the older method?

_____

_____

_____

_____

_____

28. If the color of a reaction is to be detected by visual inspection, within what range of wavelengths must it fall? Why?

_____

_____

_____

_____

29. How does the amount of light passing through a solution change as the concentration of the solution increases?

_____

_____

30. How does the amount of light reflected back from a reagent pad change as the concentration of analyte increases?

_____

_____

Applying Knowledge—On the Job

Answer the following questions in the spaces provided.

31. In the lab where you work, you have been asked to read urine test strips. What instrument should you use? Why can't you use the same instrument that you use to read hemoglobin tests?

_____

_____

_____

_____

_____

32. Your laboratory supervisor has assigned you the task of establishing a standard curve for one of the chemistry tests performed with the spectrophotometer. You are to use a reagent blank and six different concentrations of the control. What is the reagent blank for? Why must you use so many different concentrations of the control?

_____

_____

_____

_____

33. You have been asked by your lab supervisor to run three control tests on the spectrophotometer in the POL where you work. What three levels of control should you run? How should you use the control test results?

_____

_____

_____

_____

CHAPTER 22

Blood Glucose: Measuring and Monitoring

COGNITIVE OBJECTIVES

After studying this chapter, you should be able to

- use each of the vocabulary terms appropriately.
- describe how glucose is metabolized and stored.
- identify the normal range of blood glucose for nonfasting and fasting samples.
- list causes of abnormally low and high blood-glucose levels.
- explain the cause of diabetes mellitus.
- distinguish between insulin-dependent diabetes mellitus (IDDM) and noninsulin-dependent diabetes mellitus (NIDDM).
- list several clinical and biochemical characteristics of IDDM.
- compare and contrast blood-glucose tests performed in POLs.
- describe how to care for a glucose meter and blood-glucose reagent strips.
- explain the role of patient monitoring of blood glucose in the management of IDDM.

PERFORMANCE OBJECTIVE

After studying this chapter, you should be able to

- perform a quality-control test and a whole blood-glucose test using a glucose meter.

TERMINOLOGY

acidosis: the acidity of body fluids.

diabetes mellitus: a syndrome caused by inadequate production or utilization of insulin, leading to impaired carbohydrate, protein, and fat metabolism. Diabetes mellitus occurs in two different forms—noninsulin-dependent diabetes mellitus (NIDDM) and insulin-dependent diabetes mellitus (IDDM).

Exton and Rose glucose-tolerance test: the glucose-tolerance test in which fasting blood and urine specimens are tested to obtain a baseline, followed by tests of two more samples, each thirty minutes after a 50 gram glucose load.

fasting blood-sugar (FBS) test: the blood-glucose test performed on a specimen collected after the patient has fasted for eight to twelve hours. The FBS test is usually scheduled for early morning, before the first meal of the day.

fructose: a simple, six-carbon sugar in fruit and honey.

galactose: a simple, six-carbon sugar derived from lactose, or milk sugar.

gestational diabetes: a transient form of diabetes that develops in response to the metabolic and hormonal changes of pregnancy in previously asymptomatic women.

glucagon: the hormone produced by the alpha cells in the islets of Langerhans of the pancreas; called the fasting hormone because it increases when blood-glucose levels are low and stimulates the liver to break down stored glycogen.

glucose: a simple, six-carbon sugar found in many foods. Glucose metabolism provides most of the energy needed for normal growth and functioning.

glucose meter: an instrument to measure blood glucose. Examples include the Glucometer 3 (Miles, Inc., Diagnostic Division) and the

Accu-Chek III (Boehringer Mannheim Corporation).

glycogen: a carbohydrate formed from excess glucose that is stored in liver and muscle cells. Glycogen serves as a source of stored energy for the body.

glycogenolysis: the process of breaking down stored glycogen into glucose. Glycogenolysis occurs in the liver when stimulated by the hormone glucagon.

glycosuria: the presence of glucose in the urine.

glycosylated hemoglobin (G-hemoglobin, G-Hgb): hemoglobin with an attached glucose residue.

glycosylated hemoglobin test: a recently developed blood-glucose test based on the amount of glycosylated hemoglobin in the blood. The glycosylated hemoglobin test detects hyperglycemia that may be missed in IDDM patients who have wide swings in their blood-glucose levels.

hyperglycemia: an abnormally high blood-glucose level, most commonly caused by diabetes mellitus.

hypertriglyceridemia: an excessive amount of triglycerides in the blood.

hypoglycemia: an abnormally low blood-glucose level. Hypoglycemia may be caused by hyperfunction of the islets of Langerhans or injection of excessive amounts of insulin.

insulin: the hormone secreted by the beta cells of the islets of Langerhans of the pancreas. Insulin helps transport glucose molecules across cell membranes so that glucose metabolism can occur.

insulin-dependent diabetes mellitus (IDDM): a severe form of diabetes mellitus, which usually requires administration of insulin for control. IDDM is characterized by rapid onset, typically before age twenty-five.

lactose: the sugar found in milk. Lactose breaks down into glucose and galactose.

lipolysis: fat decomposition.

monosaccharide: a simple, six-carbon sugar that is found in many foods. Monosaccharides include glucose, fructose, and galactose.

noninsulin-dependent diabetes mellitus (NIDDM): a mild form of diabetes mellitus, which usually can be controlled by diet alone. NIDDM typically has gradual onset after age forty. It is often associated with obesity.

polydipsia: excessive thirst.

polyphagia: excessive food intake.

polyuria: passage of large volumes of urine.

pruritus: severe itching.

random blood-sugar test: the test of blood glucose on a sample of blood, which is collected from a nonfasting patient during a routine visit to the doctor's office.

standard oral glucose-tolerance test (GTT or OGTT): the glucose test in which fasting blood and urine specimens are collected before the test starts to serve as a baseline and then specimens are collected over several hours after consumption of a glucose load.

two-hour postprandial blood-sugar (two-hour PPBS) test: the blood-glucose test administered two hours after the patient has consumed a meal containing 100 grams of carbohydrate or has drunk a 100 gram glucose-load solution.

● ● ● ● ● ● ● ● ● ● ● ● ● ● ● ●

Measuring the blood level of **glucose**, a simple sugar, is probably the most commonly performed blood-chemistry test in POLs. This chapter explains how and why blood glucose is measured.

♦ ♦

GLUCOSE

To understand why glucose is tested, it is important for you to know what glucose is and how it is normally metabolized and stored in the body.

♦♦ *What Glucose Is*

Glucose is one of several **monosaccharides,** or simple, six-carbon sugars that are found in many foods. Other monosaccharides in food include **fructose,** which is found in fruit and honey, and **galactose,** a derivative of milk sugar, or **lactose.** These simple sugars are converted to glucose before they are utilized by cells.

♦♦ *How Glucose Is Metabolized and Stored*

Glucose is metabolized in the cells, where it is broken down into carbon dioxide and water. See Chapter 24 for a detailed discussion of glucose metabolism. When glucose is metabolized, it releases stored energy, which the cells of the body use for virtually all their normal growth and functioning.

♦ ♦ ♦ Where the Energy ♦ ♦ ♦ Stored in Glucose Comes From

In plants, glucose is formed from water and carbon dioxide with energy from the sun and the help of the plant enzyme chlorophyll. This reaction is known as photosynthesis. The light energy stored in the glucose molecule is released when glucose is metabolized.

When the glucose from food is not needed for energy, it is stored in the form of **glycogen,** a carbohydrate. Most of the glycogen in the body is stored in liver and muscle cells. When these cells become saturated with glycogen, excess glucose is converted to fat and stored as adipose tissue. Fat can be converted back to glucose with the aid of enzymes.

If there is a decrease in the level of blood sugar, the pancreatic hormone, **glucagon,** called the fasting hormone, increases. Glucagon is produced by alpha cells in the islets of Langerhans. It stimulates the liver to increase the breakdown of stored glycogen to glucose in a process called **glycogenolysis.** Although glucagon is important in maintaining blood glucose at normal levels, it cannot do the job alone. The other major pancreatic hormone, **insulin,** also is required.

♦ ♦ ♦ Note ♦ ♦ ♦

In addition to stimulating glycogenolysis, glucagon may enhance the synthesis of glucose from amino acids, found in proteins, and from fatty acids found in lipids. Glucagon also is administered to relieve comas due to excessively low blood sugar.

The Role of Insulin. Insulin controls the rate at which glucose is metabolized because it is needed to transport glucose molecules through cell membranes into the cells where glucose metabolism occurs. Unless glucose can get from the circulating blood into the cells, it cannot be metabolized. Insulin is produced by the islets of Langerhans in the pancreas, specifically by the beta cells, which make up about 75 percent of the pancreatic structure.

♦ ♦

BLOOD GLUCOSE AND DISEASE

The normal glucose level in a random blood sample is 70 to 110 mg/dL. If the patient has fasted before the test, the normal level is 70 to 90 mg/dL.

♦ ♦ ♦ Characteristics ♦ ♦ ♦ of IDDM

Clinical characteristics of IDDM include the following:

- rapid weight loss
- **polyuria**
- **glycosuria**
- **polydipsia**
- **polyphagia**
- drowsiness and lethargy
- dehydration
- vomiting
- deep breathing
- a sweet, fruity odor on the breath
- warm but dry skin
- predisposition to infection
- **pruritus**

Biochemical characteristics of IDDM include the following:

- continued secretion of free glucose by the liver, despite hyperglycemia
- inhibited entry of free glucose into muscle and adipose tissue, preventing the storage of glucose as glycogen and fat
- increased **lipolysis**
- entry of uncontrolled amounts of free fatty acids into the blood
- conversion of free fatty acids into ketone bodies, causing a sweet odor on the breath
- severe **acidosis,** due to nonmetabolized ketone bodies
- severe **hypertriglyceridemia,** due to conversion of some of the free fatty acids to triglycerides, resulting in plasma with the appearance of thick cream
- spillover of glucose into the urine from the blood, which occurs when the plasma glucose level rises above the renal threshold of about 180 mg/dL

Blood glucose always is lowest in a fasting state. Blood glucose levels outside the normal range may indicate pathology.

An abnormally low blood-glucose level is referred to as **hypoglycemia.** It may be caused by hyperfunction of the islets of Langerhans or injection of excessive amounts of insulin. An abnormally high blood-glucose level is referred to as **hyperglycemia.** It may be caused by hyperthyroidism or adrenocortical dysfunction but most commonly is due to diabetes mellitus.

Diabetes mellitus is a syndrome caused by inadequate production or utilization of insulin, leading to impaired carbohydrate, protein, and fat metabolism. It occurs in two different forms:

- noninsulin-dependent diabetes mellitus (NIDDM), which usually can be controlled by diet alone

- insulin-dependent diabetes mellitus (IDDM), which requires administration of insulin to manage the disease

NIDDM is the milder form of the disease and the more common of the two, comprising 90 to 95 percent of all cases of diabetes mellitus. It usually has a gradual onset and generally affects adults over age 40. Patients with this form of the disease often are obese.

The more severe form of diabetes, IDDM, comprises only 5 to 10 percent of all cases of diabetes mellitus. It is characterized by rapid onset and typically strikes before age twenty-five.

BLOOD-GLUCOSE TESTS

Blood-glucose levels are tested to diagnose diabetes and other abnormalities of carbohydrate metabolism. They also are used to monitor the effects of insulin dosage in IDDM patients. Blood-glucose testing can be done in a variety of ways (see Table 22.1).

◆◆◆ Note ◆◆◆

The words *blood-glucose test* and *blood-sugar test* are used interchangeably in the POL.

◆◆ *The Random Blood-Sugar Test*

In a **random blood-sugar test,** a sample of blood is collected from a nonfasting patient during a routine visit to the doctor's office. The patient does not require any special preparation, and the length of time since the last meal is not important. The objective is

---

TABLE 22.1 Laboratory Tests That Measure Glucose Metabolism

Test	Description
Random blood-sugar test	A sample is taken at any time, while the patient is at the doctor's office.
Fasting blood-sugar test	A sample is taken with the patient in a fasting state eight to twelve hours after the last food and tobacco have been consumed.
Two-hour postprandial blood-sugar test	A sample is taken two hours after a meal.
Standard oral glucose-tolerance test	Fasting blood- and urine-glucose specimens are taken. Then the patient ingests 100 grams of glucose. Blood and urine specimens are taken at thirty minutes and each hour, as decided by the doctor. The test may be shorter but lasts no longer than six hours.
Exton and Rose glucose-tolerance test	This is a modification of the oral glucose-tolerance test. Fasting blood- and urine-glucose tests are performed. Glucose ingestion is divided into two parts. Thirty-minute and one-hour blood- and urine-glucose samples are tested.
Glycosylated hemoglobin test	Tests the glucose residue on hemoglobin to provide a measure of long-term blood-glucose levels.

to find out the patient's blood-glucose level under normal, ordinary conditions. Diabetes is indicated if the glucose level is greater than 200 mg/dL.

◆◆ The Fasting Blood-Sugar Test

A **fasting blood-sugar (FBS) test** is performed on a specimen that is collected when the patient is in a fasting state. The patient should not smoke, eat, or drink anything other than water for eight to twelve hours before the test. It is usually easiest for the patient if the test is scheduled for early morning, before the first meal of the day.

A normal FBS test virtually eliminates false positives that are caused by elevated blood glucose in random samples collected after carbohydrates have been consumed. Such cases of apparent diabetes can be diagnosed if the level of blood glucose is elevated even after the patient has fasted. Diabetes is indicated if on two or more occasions:

- venous plasma fasting specimens have glucose levels of 140 mg/dL or greater
- venous whole-blood fasting specimens have glucose levels of 120 mg/dL or greater

◆◆ Glucose-Tolerance Tests

When fasting blood-glucose levels are not definitive for a diagnosis of diabetes or when there is unexplained glycosuria, a glucose-tolerance test (GTT) may be ordered. Glucose-tolerance tests assess the ability to utilize carbohydrates by measuring the body's response to a challenge load of glucose. The results are interpreted by the physician. Figure 22.1 shows responses to the glucose load in a glucose-tolerance test for patients with a variety of conditions.

A glucose-tolerance test often is performed when there is some reason to suspect diabetes. Examples include obese patients with family histories of diabetes and patients with unexplained vascular, neurologic, or infectious illnesses. Glucose-tolerance tests also may be administered during pregnancy to screen for **gestational diabetes,** a transient form of diabetes that develops in response to the metabolic and hormonal changes of pregnancy in previously asymptomatic women. Gestational diabetes can adversely affect both mother and fetus. Women are considered to be at special risk of developing gestational diabetes if they have one or more of the following:

- a family history of diabetes
- glycosuria

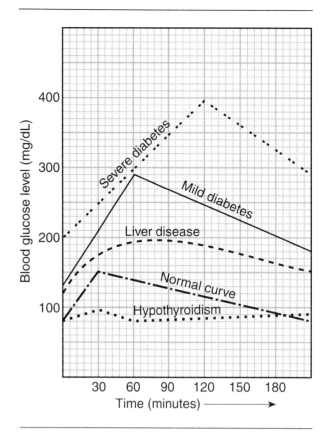

Figure 22.1. Typical glucose-tolerance curves, showing the responses of different types of patients.

- a previous fetal loss
- a previous birth of an unusually large infant

Three types of glucose-tolerance tests are performed in POLs:

- the two-hour postprandial blood-sugar test
- the standard oral glucose-tolerance test
- the Exton and Rose glucose-tolerance test

All three glucose-tolerance tests require that the patient be in a fasting state for the test. They also require that the patient consume at least 150 grams of carbohydrate per day for three days prior to the test. In addition, the patient must have had no alcohol intake.

The Two-Hour Postprandial Blood-Sugar Test. In the **two-hour postprandial blood-sugar (two-hour PPBS) test,** the patient is required to consume a meal that contains 100 grams of carbohydrate or to drink a 100-gram glucose-load solution. Two hours later, a blood specimen is collected from the patient. Some physicians also request a urine specimen to test for glycosuria. A plasma glucose concentration above 200 mg/dL suggests diabetes and warrants further evaluation. Whole blood samples show somewhat lower levels of glucose.

Standard Oral Glucose-Tolerance Test.

In the standard oral glucose-tolerance test (GTT or OGTT), fasting blood and urine specimens are collected before the test starts to serve as a baseline, and then repeated specimens are collected over several hours after consumption of a glucose load. The glucose-load solution usually contains 100 grams of glucose, but the amount may be tailored to body size. If so, either 1.75 grams of glucose per kilogram of body weight or 50 grams per square meter of body surface are administered.

◆ ◆ ◆ Note ◆ ◆ ◆

The collection of urine specimens in the standard oral glucose-tolerance test is useful for evaluating how much glucose spills over into the urine at a given level of blood glucose. If glycosuria is observed in the absence of high levels of blood glucose, the patient should be evaluated for abnormal renal tubular function.

Typically in the standard oral glucose-tolerance test, blood and urine specimens are collected hourly for up to six hours after the glucose is consumed. Most physicians also request a set of half-hourly specimens. Each specimen must be labeled with the exact time of collection. No further specimens are collected once the blood glucose drops back to the baseline level, usually within three or four hours.

During the test, the patient may drink water but must not consume any food or tobacco. It is common for patients to experience excessive perspiration and some weakness, even fainting, during the test. These are normal reactions to the drop in blood glucose that occurs as insulin is secreted by the pancreas in response to the glucose load.

The standard oral glucose-tolerance test is affected by many physiological variables, so careful preparation of patients is necessary for meaningful test results. Patients should be in a normal nutritional state and free of the following drugs: salicylates, diuretics, anticonvulsants, steroids, and oral contraceptives. Patients also should be free of excessive stress for good test results.

The standard oral glucose-tolerance test is subject to many different diagnostic interpretations, but some general criteria have been established. In normal patients, the blood-glucose level should return to the fasting level—70 to 90 mg/dL—within two hours. A blood-glucose level that remains elevated at two hours is considered abnormal. A modest two-hour glucose level that returns to baseline at three hours suggests impaired glucose metabolism but does not indicate diabetes. A diagnosis of diabetes mellitus is made when the two-hour specimen and at least one other specimen collected after ingestion of the glucose load meet or exceed 200 mg/dL for venous plasma or 180 mg/dL for venous whole blood.

A very sharp rise in the glucose level after ingestion of the glucose load followed by a decline to subnormal levels may indicate hyperthyroidism or alcoholic liver disease. Patients with gastrointestinal malabsorption may show false negative results because they cannot absorb the full glucose load.

It is important to take into account the age of patients when interpreting oral glucose-tolerance test results because the speed of glucose clearance declines with age. In normal patients, those without diabetes or a family history of the disease, two-hour blood-glucose levels are an average of 6 mg/dL higher for each decade over age thirty.

The Exton and Rose Glucose-Tolerance Test.

The **Exton and Rose glucose-tolerance test** is similar to the standard oral glucose-tolerance test, particularly in patient preparation, but the 100-gram glucose load is divided into two dosages, and the test lasts only one hour. As with the standard oral glucose-tolerance test, fasting blood and urine specimens are collected to establish a baseline. Then the patient is given 50 grams of glucose-load solution, and thirty minutes later blood and urine samples are collected. Immediately following the thirty-minute samples, the patient is given the second 50 gram dose of glucose. A second set of blood and urine specimens is collected thirty minutes later, about an hour after the start of the test.

Normal urine values for the Exton and Rose test are negative for glucose. Normal blood-glucose values are:

- fasting = 80 mg/dL
- thirty minutes = 150 mg/dL
- one hour = 160 mg/dL

◆◆ *The Glycosylated Hemoglobin Test*

The **glycosylated hemoglobin test** is a recently developed blood-glucose test now performed on some blood-chemistry analyzers in POLs. The test detects hyperglycemia that may be missed in IDDM patients who have wide swings in their blood-glucose levels.

The glycosylated hemoglobin test is based on a permanent change in the hemoglobin molecule that occurs when it is exposed to high levels of glucose. A glucose residue attaches to hemoglobin, forming **glycosylated hemoglobin (G-hemoglobin, G-Hgb)**, which persists for the remainder of the lifespan of the red cell—an average of 120 days.

> ◆ ◆ ◆ **Note** ◆ ◆ ◆
>
> Glycosylation does not impair the oxygen-carrying function of the hemoglobin molecule.

In individuals with repeated periods of hyperglycemia, 18 to 20 percent of the hemoglobin is glycosylated, compared with only 3 to 6 percent in normal individuals. In IDDM patients, a high level of glycosylated hemoglobin indicates inadequate diabetic control in the preceding three to five weeks. Once blood-glucose levels are brought under control, the G-hemoglobin level returns to normal in about three weeks.

USING A GLUCOSE METER

Blood glucose frequently is measured in POLs with a **glucose meter,** such as the Glucometer 3 by Miles Inc., Diagnostic Division and Accu-Chek III by Boehringer Mannheim Corporation. The test takes only a few minutes, so glucose meters may be used as initial screening devices, even if a complete panel of blood chemistries, including a glucose test, is ordered. When used correctly, glucose meters give good, quantitative measures of blood glucose. Both the Glucometer 3 and Accu-Chek III, for example, provide accurate results across a broad range of blood-glucose levels (20 to 500 mg/dL), and both can use their memory capabilities to store ten test results, which can be recalled and averaged.

◆◆ *Methods*

Glucose meter tests use dry reagent chemistry, involving an enzymatic reaction specific for glucose. Whole blood from either a finger stick or venipuncture is placed on the pad of a reagent strip. The pad is wiped off at the end of the reaction time and inserted into the meter. The degree of color change on the pad indicates the amount of glucose present. The darker the reaction, the more glucose is in the sample.

> ◆ ◆ ◆ **Note** ◆ ◆ ◆
>
> The blood-glucose test-strip reaction may be influenced by very high blood levels of cholesterol, triglycerides, ascorbic acid, and uric acid.

Glucose meters use reflectance photometry to read the intensity of color change on the reagent pad. The meters also calculate the result, which appears in the display window. Alternatively, the reaction can be read visually by comparing the test strip to a chart of color blocks on the side of the test-strip bottle. The visual reading is less precise than the photometer reading because of the limited number of color blocks for comparison. Nonetheless, the two readings should be in the same range.

◆◆ *Glucose Meter Controls*

CLIA 1988 requires that two glucose control levels be performed each day before a patient's blood glucose is checked on the glucose meter. The controls should include a normal value control and an abnormal value control.

◆◆ *Care of the Instrument and Reagent Strips*

Glucose meters are precision instruments that must be handled with care to give accurate results. Dropping may damage the internal electronics and cause a malfunction. Glucose meters also must be protected from humidity greater than 85 percent and temperatures outside a range of 59 to 95 degrees Fahrenheit for prolonged periods.

Periodic instrument cleaning is required to ensure accurate and reliable operation. The outside should be cleaned with a tissue moistened with clean water, carefully keeping water away from the display window and button. The slot where the reagent strip is placed for reading should be cleaned according to the manufacturer's instructions.

The reagent strips for glucose meters are sensitive

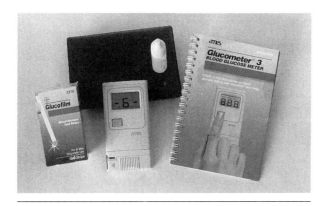

Figure 22.2. A Glucometer 3® blood-glucose meter with a Glucofilm® reagent on the left and a normal control and User's Manual on the right. Photo by Mark Palko.

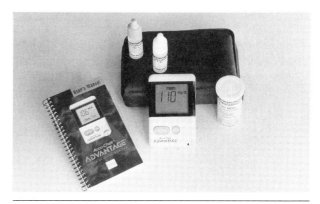

Figure 22.3. An ACCU-CHECK® ADVANTAGE blood-glucose meter with a User's Manual, test strips, Level 1 and Level 2 controls, and a meter check chip. Photo by Mark Palko.

to heat, light, and moisture, so they must be properly stored to prevent deterioration. When a test strip is removed from the bottle, the cap should be replaced immediately and kept tight to prevent moisture from entering the bottle. A desiccant in the bottle also helps absorb any excess moisture. Deteriorated test strips appear dark or discolored and should be discarded. Any questionable test strips should be tested with a glucose control solution.

PATIENT MONITORING OF BLOOD GLUCOSE

Blood-glucose meters are used not only in POLs but also in home monitoring by diabetics. Figures 22.2 and 22.3 show home glucose meters. Home blood-glucose monitoring is especially important for IDDM patients, for whom regularly scheduled blood testing helps effectively regulate insulin dosage and diet. A fasting blood-glucose level performed in the morning before breakfast is probably the best overall indicator of the degree of control in diabetes management. Good management helps IDDM patients avoid the extremes of hypoglycemia and hyperglycemia.

The task of instructing patients in diabetes management, including blood-glucose testing, frequently is the responsibility of medical assistants. Medical

assistants therefore must thoroughly understand the proper techniques of collecting and testing samples as well as the importance of quality-control checks. In addition to the mechanics of blood-glucose testing, diabetic patients must be instructed in the physical and emotional conditions that can affect glucose levels. Then, patients will know when extra testing is needed to ensure that their diabetes is still under control.

IDDM patients should keep a permanent log of test results for blood glucose and for urine glucose, if tested. The following information should be recorded in the log for each test:

- the date and time
- the test results
- whether or not a control was run
- whether or not the control was in the accepted range
- the number of hours since last eating
- the time of the last insulin injection or oral hypoglycemic medication
- whether or not the patient was under any physical or emotional stress
- the amount of exercise performed recently by the patient

22.1

Using a Glucose Meter to Test Blood Glucose

Goal

- After successfully completing this procedure, you will be able to perform a quality-control test and a whole blood-glucose test with an Ames Glucometer 3 and read the test results both visually and with the reflectance photometer in the glucose meter. If you use another glucose meter, follow the steps in the user guide.

Completion Time

- 10 minutes

Equipment and Supplies

- disposable latex gloves
- impermeable apron, lab jacket, or gown
- hand disinfectant
- surface disinfectant
- alcohol
- paper towels and tissues
- biohazard container
- blood-glucose meter and user's guide
- glucose control liquid
- glucose test strips
- glucometer check paddle
- lancet device and lancet for finger puncture
- pen and notebook

Instructions

Read through the list of equipment and supplies that you will need and the steps of the procedure. Be sure that you understand each step before you begin. Then complete each step correctly and in the proper order. If your completion time is too long, repeat the procedure until you increase your speed.

S = Satisfactory	U = Unsatisfactory	S	U

1. Put on a protective jacket, gown, or apron; wash your hands with disinfectant, dry them, and put on gloves.

2. Follow the Universal Precautions.

3. Collect and prepare the appropriate equipment.

4. Inspect the meter, read the user's guide, and familiarize yourself with the functions of the meter. *Note:* The Glucometer has only one button, which controls all functions.

Checking the Meter-Paddle Test

5. Turn on the meter by pressing the "on" button. Two displays will appear, one after the other.

6. Open the test slide and remove the check paddle from its container.

7. Press the button again and watch the display until twenty seconds have elapsed.

8. Insert the check paddle with the check (✔) side up.

9. Close the test slide and wait for the display on the screen.

10. Compare the reading to the range found on the label inside the plastic container for the paddle. If the reading is within the range, record it in your notebook. If the reading is outside the range, check the paddle for fingerprints and mars; then rerun the paddle test procedure, steps 7–10. If the paddle test result still is outside the range, or if the "ERR" (for error) signal appears, call the 800 number given in the user's guide for technical assistance.

11. Remove the paddle from the test slide and replace it in its container. Close the test slide, taking care not to scratch or mar the paddle.

12. Open the test slide and watch the display window until the letter *d* appears.

13. Press the button to delete the paddle-test result from memory. This prevents mix-ups between paddle-test results and patient-test results.

Running a Quality-Control Test

14. Press the button and watch the "888" symbol change to a program number (between 1 and 8). Press the button until the program number on the display matches the number printed on the bottle of test strips.

15. Open the test slide. The number 60 will appear and remain in the display.

16. Holding the test strip by its handle, apply a drop of control solution to the test pad, completely covering it.

17. Immediately press the button to start the countdown.

18. At twenty-five seconds, pick up a tissue and lay the test strip on it, ready to wipe at the signal given at twenty seconds.

19. At twenty-two and twenty-one seconds, when the machine beeps, fold the tissue over the handle, ready to wipe the control solution away.

20. At twenty seconds, quickly wipe the control solution from the test pad with the folded tissue over the test strip, using a motion like cleaning a table knife blade with a cloth. Do not pat or blot the solution on the test pad.

21. Immediately insert the test strip all the way into the test slot. Be sure that the test area faces upward, facing the display screen.

22. Immediately close the test slide before the countdown reaches 1.

23. When the test result is displayed, remove the test pad from the instrument.

	S	U

24. Compare the test strip pad to the color blocks on the control bottle for an approximate reading. Record the control-test results in your notebook. Control test results must fall within the accepted range given for the control.

25. Delete the test result from memory following steps 12 and 13. Store only patient test results in the memory of the instrument.

Running a Blood-Glucose Test

26. Wash your hands in soapy water, rinse them, and dry them thoroughly. Reglove.

27. Fold a tissue in half and load the lancet device with a new lancet.

28. Remove one test strip from the reagent bottle, lay it on a clean surface next to the tissue, and immediately close the reagent bottle tightly.

29. Press the meter's button and match the program number on the meter to the number on the bottle of test strips by pressing the button. See step 14.

30. Open the test slide. The number 60 will appear and remain in the display.

31. Choose another student for a partner and stick his or her finger with the lancet device or remove a glove and stick your own finger. Gently squeeze the finger to form a drop of blood.

32. Hold the strip by the handle and apply the blood to the test pad until the test area is covered completely.

33. Immediately press the button to begin the countdown.

34. At twenty-five seconds, pick up the folded tissue and lay the strip, pad side up, in the middle. Fold the tissue over the handle.

35. Listen for the beeps at twenty-two and twenty-one seconds to alert you to prepare to wipe the test pad.

	S	U

36. At twenty seconds, quickly wipe the blood from the test pad with firm pressure, using one smooth stroke. See step 20.

37. Immediately insert the test strip all the way into the test slot, with the test pad toward the display screen.

38. Close the test slide quickly before the countdown reaches one second.

39. Wait until the test result is shown in the display window and record the result in your notebook.

40. Press the button to store the test result in memory and turn off the meter.

41. Open the test slide, remove the test strip, and close the slide.

42. Compare the test strip to the color blocks on the bottle of test strips and record the results.

43. Discard disposable equipment.

44. Disinfect other equipment and return it to storage.

45. Clean the work area following the Universal Precautions.

46. Remove your jacket, gown, or apron, and gloves; wash your hands with disinfectant, and dry them.

OVERALL PROCEDURAL EVALUATION

Student's Name _____

Signature of Instructor _____ **Date** _____

Comments

CHAPTER 22 REVIEW

Using Terminology

Match the terms in the right column with the appropriate definition or description in the left column.

_____ 1. after-meal

_____ 2. breaking down glycogen

_____ 3. excessive thirst

_____ 4. carbohydrate

_____ 5. glycosylated

_____ 6. hormone from alpha cells

_____ 7. hormone from beta cells

_____ 8. increased food intake

_____ 9. low blood-glucose level

_____ 10. simple sugar

a. G-hemoglobin
b. glucagon
c. glucose
d. glycogen
e. glycogenolysis
f. hypoglycemia
g. insulin
h. polydypsia
i. polyphagia
j. postprandial

Define the following terms in the spaces provided.

11. Acidosis: _____

_____

12. Diabetes mellitus: _____

_____

13. Fructose: _____

_____

14. Gestational diabetes: _____

_____

15. Galactose: _____

_____

16. Hyperglycemia: _____

_____

17. Hypertriglyceridemia: _____

_____

18. Monosaccharide: _____

_____

19. Standard oral glucose-tolerance test (GTT or OGTT): _____

_____

_____

20. Lipolysis: _____

_____

Acquiring Knowledge

Mark the following statements true or false and rewrite the false statements to make them true.

21. Glucagon is a hormone produced by the beta cells of the islets of Langerhans of the pancreas.

_____

_____

22. A glucose-tolerance test assesses the ability to utilize carbohydrates by measuring the patient's response to a challenge load of glucose.

_____

_____

23. A fasting blood-glycogen test is based on the amount of glycosylated hemoglobin in the blood.

_____

_____

24. Glucose is metabolized in the cells, where it is broken down into carbon dioxide and oxygen.

_____

_____

25. When the glucose from food is not needed for energy, it is stored in the form of starch in liver and muscle cells.

_____

_____

_____

Answer the following questions in the spaces provided.

26. How is glucose metabolized in normal individuals?

_____

_____

27. Where and in what form is glucose stored in the body?

_____

28. What are the normal ranges of blood glucose for nonfasting and fasting samples?

_____

_____

29. What may cause hypoglycemia?

_____

_____

30. What may lead to high blood glucose? What is the most common cause?

_____

_____

31. What causes diabetes mellitus?

_____

_____

32. Compare and contrast insulin-dependent (IDDM) and noninsulin-dependent (NIDDM) forms of diabetes mellitus.

_____

_____

_____

_____

33. List the clinical characteristics of IDDM.

_____

_____

_____

_____

34. What biochemical characteristics of IDDM produce the clinical features of the disease?

_____

_____

_____

_____

_____

_____

_____

_____

_____

35. Compare and contrast random and fasting blood-glucose tests.

_____

_____

_____

36. Describe the similarities and differences among the three glucose-tolerance tests commonly performed in POLs.

_____

_____

_____

_____

_____

_____

37. When is a diagnosis of diabetes mellitus made in a standard oral glucose-tolerance test?

_____

38. What type of chemistry is used by glucose meters? How are the results read?

_____

_____

39. What test probably is the best overall indicator of control in the management of IDDM?

_____

_____

40. Explain the role of patient monitoring of blood glucose in the management of IDDM.

_____

_____

_____

Applying Knowledge—On the Job

Answer the following questions in the spaces provided.

41. The lab where you work does blood-glucose tests to monitor pregnant women at risk of developing gestational diabetes. What items of medical history identify those women at special risk?

_____

_____

_____

_____

42. One of your jobs in the physician's office where you work is to give patients instructions in how to prepare for lab tests. What instructions would you give to Ms. Talbot, who is going to have a fasting blood-sugar test performed tomorrow morning? What instructions would you give to Mr. Chen, who is going to have a glucose-tolerance test in three days?

_____

_____

_____

_____

_____

43. Today, in the POL where you work, a patient's glucose concentration remained above 200 mg/dL at the end of the second hour of his glucose-tolerance test. How would you interpret this result?

_____

_____

_____

44. The reagent strips that you use with the glucose meter in the POL where you work have turned a dark color. What should you do?

_____

_____

45. A new patient with IDDM needs instructions in home monitoring of blood-glucose levels. The doctor has asked you to explain to the patient how to keep a permanent log of blood-glucose testing. What information should you tell the new patient to record in the log?

_____

_____

_____

_____

23 *Blood-Chemistry Analyzers*

COGNITIVE OBJECTIVES

After studying this chapter, you should be able to

- use each of the vocabulary terms appropriately.
- state the advantages of using automated blood-chemistry analyzers in POLs.
- name the types of automated blood-chemistry analyzers and explain their major differences.
- describe the main features and operation of Vision, Ektachem DT, and Reflotron Plus automated blood-chemistry analyzers.

PERFORMANCE OBJECTIVE

After studying this chapter, you should be able to

- devise a general program for calibration and quality control of an automated blood-chemistry analyzer.

TERMINOLOGY

automated blood-chemistry analyzer: an instrument that performs blood-chemistry test procedures automatically.

continuous flow analysis system: a blood-chemistry analyzer in which samples and reagents flow through the instrument, one after the other. One test or a variety of tests may be performed on the same sample in a single operation of the instrument.

discrete (noncontinuous) analysis system: a blood-chemistry analyzer in which samples and reagents for each test are placed in separate containers, in which the tests are performed.

There are two different types—wet chemistry and dry chemistry.

discrete centrifugal analyzer: a blood-chemistry analyzer that uses centrifugation of reagents in liquid form for wet chemistry procedures. An example is the Vision system (Abbott Laboratories).

discrete solid-phase analyzer: a blood-chemistry analyzer that uses dry reagents layered on slides for solid-phase chemistry procedures. Examples are the Ektachem DT System (Eastman Kodak) and the Reflotron Plus System (Boehringer Mannheim Corporation).

hydrophilic: literally, water-loving; refers to materials that dissolve in water.

ion-selective electrode (ISE): a conductor that is sensitive to the activity of a particular ion in solution.

lyophilized: freeze-dried.

potentiometric test: an analytic chemistry test in which the concentration of an analyte is measured by electrical potential.

profile: a group of tests performed to help diagnose pathology of a specific organ or system.

• • • • • • • • • • • • • • • • • •

This chapter describes **automated blood-chemistry analyzers,** instruments that perform a variety of blood-chemistry test procedures automatically. Specific topics include the advantages of automated methods over manual methods, how automated analyzers work, the types of tests they perform, and how quality control is maintained.

THE ADVANTAGES OF AUTOMATION

Automated blood-chemistry analyzers in POLs improve diagnosis and treatment by providing physicians with a great deal of information. Automated analyzers can perform single tests or **profiles**, groups of tests, to help diagnose pathology of a specific organ or system. Automated analyzers increase POL efficiency by reducing turnaround time in test performance. Patients often prefer in-office testing because of its immediate results, and this is why many physicians add blood-chemistry testing to their labs. This has been a major influence in the development of chemical analysis instruments for POLs and has led to the production of reliable, simple-to-operate, and relatively inexpensive instruments that are small enough to fit on a lab bench. To help prevent obsolescence, many instrument manufacturers accept trade-ins of older models as part of the purchase price of upgraded models.

THE TYPES OF BLOOD-CHEMISTRY ANALYZERS

Automated blood-chemistry analyzers are based on one of two types of technology: continuous flow analysis or discrete (noncontinuous) analysis.

◆◆ Continuous Flow Systems

In **continuous flow analysis systems,** samples and reagents flow through the instrument, one after the other. One test or a variety of tests may be performed on the same sample in a single operation of the instrument. Samples of whole blood, plasma, or serum are placed in small sample cups, the number depending on the number of tests to be run. The cups are placed in a circular tray, which rotates automatically so that the samples are introduced, reacted upon, and read by the instrument at precise time intervals. The specific chemical methods used by the instrument are the same as those used in manual methods.

Instruments that use continuous flow analysis can perform eight to twenty different tests on a single sample. They generally are not used in POLs, but

---

> ### ◆◆◆ Which Blood- ◆◆◆ Chemistry Analyzer to Select
>
> Consider the following questions when selecting a blood-chemistry analyzer for a POL:
>
> - Does the instrument perform tests that are needed frequently for diagnosis?
> - How accurate are the test results?
> - How long does each test take?
> - Will additional staff be required?
> - How difficult is the instrument to maintain?
> - How difficult is the instrument to calibrate?
> - How difficult is the quality-control program?
> - What special training is needed to operate the instrument?
> - How much space is needed for the instrument?
> - How long are the reagents stable?
> - Do the reagents require refrigeration or freezer storage?
> - How much does the instrument cost initially?
> - How much do the reagents cost to run each test?
> - How much will Medicaid and Medicare reimburse for each test?
> - Will this addition to the lab be in keeping with the level of complexity at which the lab is certified? Check the most recent CLIA regulations.

---

they are common in hospital labs, where larger numbers of samples are tested.

◆◆ Discrete Analysis Systems

In discrete (**noncontinuous**) **analysis systems,** samples and reagents for each test are placed in separate containers, in which the tests are performed. The chemical method used by discrete analysis systems may be either wet chemistry, which involves centrifugal analysis of liquid reagents, or dry chemistry, which involves solid-phase analysis of dry reagents.

The Vision System. The Vision system by Abbott Laboratories (see Figure 23.1) is a **discrete centrifugal analyzer** that uses reagents in liquid form for wet chemistry procedures. The Vision system is very suitable for small laboratories like POLs. It can perform ten different tests per operation, with an average of eight minutes per analysis.

Reagents for the Vision system are prepackaged in separate compartments of test-pack cassettes, which

---

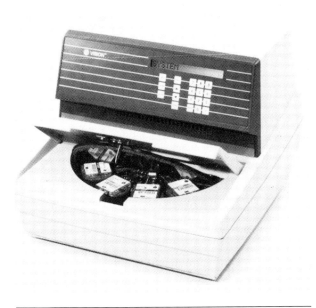

Figure 23.1. An Abbott Vision Chemistry Analyzer. Photo courtesy of Abbott Laboratories.

are stable for ninety days if refrigerated. The compartments are connected by tubelike passages, and centrifugation forces materials from one compartment to another in established sequences. The correct reaction time is allowed for each step before the next reagent is added, including allowance for incubation times when needed. The compartment in which the final reactions take place is a cuvette, and the final reaction product is read by the instrument's spectrophotometer at the proper wavelength.

Samples used by the instrument may be whole blood, plasma, or serum, collected by either finger stick or venipuncture. When whole blood is used, the cells are removed from the plasma by a cell-separation chamber in the test pack. Some tests, such as hemoglobin, require the red cells to remain as part of the sample during reactions. Two drops of sample are added to the sample well on the test pack, using a transfer pipette supplied by the manufacturer. Overfilling should be avoided.

A bar code on the front of the test pack, which is read by the instrument when the test pack is introduced, programs the instrument in all the parameters needed for operation. It tells the instrument

- which test to perform
- the sequence of rotations
- the centrifuge speed
- the incubation time

- the wavelength for the spectrophotometer to read the final reaction

At present, the Vision system can perform thirty-two different procedures, including profiles for:

- cardiac evaluation
- lipid group
- cardiac injury
- hepatic group
- hypertension group
- renal group
- metabolic group
- pancreatic group

This broad menu allows for either discrete or organ-specific testing. Specific procedures are listed at the end of this chapter.

Part of the protocol for maintenance of the Vision system is a once-a-month self-check for:

- incubator temperature
- centrifuge speed
- direction of rotation
- spectrophotometer wavelength and reading time

The instrument prints out the areas that do not pass the check. Some problems can be corrected using the troubleshooting section of the operator's manual. Others may require service by the manufacturer. An 800 number is available for technical assistance. If the instrument requires repair, a replacement will be loaned out by the manufacturer.

The manufacturer of the Vision analyzer also provides quality-control samples for checking the reliability of the instrument. Controls should be run daily for each type of test that is performed on patient samples. CLIA 1988 requires that controls include both normal and abnormal samples. Calibration with calibrators supplied by the manufacturer is required whenever the quality-control samples are out of the accepted value range for a particular test.

The manufacturer supplies quarterly proficiency-testing samples as part of its Quality Commitment Program (QCP). POLs analyze the samples and return the results to Abbott Laboratories for accuracy verification. Whenever POL results are more than two standard deviations away from accepted values, a technical representative from Abbott Labs visits the POL to review procedures and to check the instrument.

The Ektachem DT System. The Ektachem DT system by Eastman Kodak (see Figure 23.2) is a **discrete**

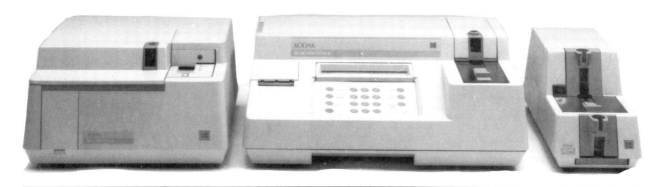

Figure 23.2. The Kodak Ektachem DT System. In the center of the photo is the Kodak Ektachem DT60 Analyzer. To the left is the Kodak Ektachem DTSC module, and to the right is the Kodak Ektachem DTE module. Photo courtesy of Eastman Kodak Co.

solid-phase analyzer. It is a bench-top model well suited for POLs. The dry reagents are layered on two-inch by two-inch slides, which are wrapped separately and come in boxes of twenty-five. The reagents are stable for one year if the slides are refrigerated or frozen.

The Ektachem DT system uses either serum, plasma, or, for hemoglobin determinations, whole blood. Anticoagulated whole blood must be spun down to separate the cells from the plasma. A clotted sample also must be processed to separate the serum. A sample size of 10 μL is spotted on the slide with an automatic pipette supplied by the manufacturer. The pipette has a battery-powered motor that aspirates and dispenses the sample (see Figure 23.3).

The complete Ektachem DT system has three modules: the DT60 Analyzer Module, the DTSC Module, and the DTE Module. The specific procedures that they can perform are listed at the end of the chapter. The DT60 Analyzer module is the heart of the Ektachem DT system, providing the commands for all three modules, which can operate independently of each other. Some POLs purchase the DT60 module first and add the other two modules later.

The DT60 module has a keyboard, a two-line LCD alphanumeric display, and a printer. It can perform fifteen different colorimetric tests and report up to sixty-five results per hour. To use this module, unwrap a slide and place it on the slide track of the loading station (see Figure 23.4). Introduce the slide into the instrument by pushing the slide advance lever to its stop on the slide loader. The instrument then reads the bar code on the slide and prints out the name of the test and the lot number for operator verification. You also are requested to enter the patient's ID, although this step is optional.

Next, the sample is aspirated with the automatic pipette as follows:

- The plastic tip is pressed into the pipette adapter.
- The tip is dipped into the sample.
- The button on the top of the pipette is pressed, and the pipette aspirates 10 μL of sample. A beep signals when aspiration is completed.
- The pipette tip is withdrawn from the sample immediately.

About two seconds later, the pipette draws in a 2 μL volume of air, which ensures that no sample is wicked out of the pipette when the operator wipes the outside of the pipette tip to remove excess sample.

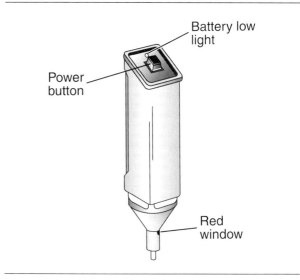

Figure 23.3. A battery-powered pipette. Courtesy of Eastman Kodak Co.

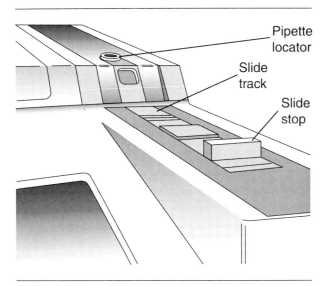

Pipette locator

Slide track

Slide stop

Figure 23.4. The slide loader of the DT60 Analyzer Module. Courtesy of Eastman Kodak Company.

The filled pipette is placed in the pipette locator, also called the spotting station. The spotting station seats the pipette for proper location of the tip over the center of the test slide. An optical sample-drop detector observes the reflection of infrared radiation from the slide surface, and the instrument beeps to verify correct spotting of the sample on the slide. The power button on the pipette dispenses the sample. Drop detection initiates the test process after a twenty second delay to ensure uniform spreading of the spot.

The slide automatically moves back and drops into an incubator at 37 degrees Celsius. Once a slide enters the incubator, the operator is no longer needed, unless another slide is to be loaded. The incubator holds up to six slides, and the incubation time for all tests is five minutes. Slides for different tests may be run in any order. The bar code on the slide tells the instrument which test to perform.

When the bottom slide in the incubator has incubated for five minutes, it is automatically pushed back into the reading station, where it is read by reflectance photometry at the proper wavelength. The bar code on the slide instructs the analyzer module to activate the light-emitting diode (LED) required for the colorimeter to operate. When the next slide has incubated for five minutes, it moves into the reading station. The process continues until all of the slides have been read. Slides that have been read are pushed automatically into a waste bin at the back of the instrument. Results of the completed tests appear on the printer tape.

The DTSC module operates on the same principles as the DT60, except that it can incubate and process only one slide at a time. The DTSC module can perform thirteen different special chemistry tests at a rate of twenty per hour.

The DTE module performs **potentiometric tests,** in which the concentration of an analyte is measured by electrical potential. **Ion-selective electrodes (ISEs),** which are sensitive to the activity of a particular ion in solution, are used to test for blood electrolytes, including sodium, potassium, chloride, and carbon dioxide. Test results are available at a rate of fifteen per hour.

One side of the dual manual pipette supplied by the manufacturer for this module is used to aspirate 10 µL of sample. The other side of the pipette is used to aspirate reference fluid. There are two active areas on each slide, one for the sample, the other for the reference fluid. Tests are run at 25 degrees Celsius.

The Ektachem DT system must be calibrated when it is first installed and then at least once every three months—minimally every six months, per CLIA regulations. More frequent calibration is required by CLIA 1988 if any of the following occurs:

- Control values drift out of range.
- The lot number of slides for a specific test changes.
- The lot number of the electrolyte reference fluid changes.

The DT60 microcomputer automates the calibration calculations, stores parameters, and warns of any unacceptable results.

Three calibrator samples are required to establish the calibration curve for the reflectrometric tests in the DT60 and DTSC modules, and two are needed for the potentiometric test in the DTE module. The DT60 calibrators are supplied in **lyophilized,** or freeze-dried, form and have a shelf life of at least one year. They are reconstituted with 3 mL of diluent, using a special 3-mL pipette supplied by the manufacturer. Reconstituted calibrators are stable for twenty-four hours if refrigerated.

In addition to calibration, quality control depends on routine checking of instrument settings through tests of control samples. Two levels of controls for specific tests must be run every day—or every eight hours, per CLIA regulations—that the tests are run on patient samples.

Reflotron Plus System. The Reflotron Plus (Boehringer Mannheim Corporation) (see Figure 23.5) is another discrete solid-phase analyzer well suited for POLs. The Reflotron Plus makes quantitative determinations of sixteen different clinical parameters

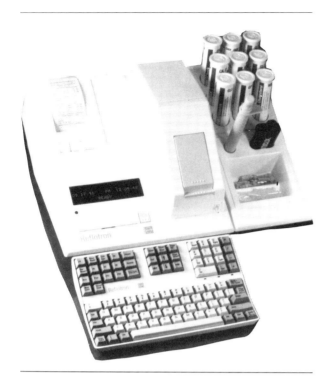

Figure 23.5. The Reflotron® Plus™ is an automated chemistry unit. Photo courtesy of Boehringer Mannheim Corp.

from whole blood, serum, plasma, or urine. Specific procedures are listed at the end of the chapter. Test results are available within a few minutes.

The Reflotron Plus system includes reagent carriers for each of the individual parameters tested. The reagent carriers have a shelf life of eight months to one year at room temperature. The Reflotron Plus system also has a reflectance photometer, controlled by a microprocessor, for reading test results. The manufacturer provides a pipette or glass capillary tube for dispensing the 30 µL of sample that is required for each test.

All but one of the reagent carriers in the Reflotron Plus system incorporate a plasma-separating layer of

---

♦ ♦ ♦ **Note** ♦ ♦ ♦

In the Reflotron Plus reagent carrier for hemoglobin determination, there is no glass-fiber plasma-separating layer. Instead, there is a layer of material impregnated with saponin, a lysing material containing cyanide. The saponin ruptures the red blood cells, releasing hemoglobin and forming cyanmethemoglobin.

---

glass-fiber fleece. Erythrocytes and other cellular constituents of whole-blood specimens are retained in the fleece, while analyte and plasma are drawn off by capillary forces. This allows whole blood to be used as the sample. Beneath the separation layer are layers of reagents for preliminary reactions, which vary by parameter tested. Preliminary reactions may consist of the elimination of interfering substances or the preincubation of the sample with activators or auxiliary reagents.

Reflotron Plus reagent carriers also contain a plasma-transporting layer. Like the plasma-separating layer, it is composed of glass-fiber fleece. However, because of differences in fiber composition and orientation, the capillary forces in the plasma-transporting layer are much stronger than those in the plasma-separating layer, acting like a sponge to draw the plasma through the separating layer. The transporting layer also acts as a reservoir for the plasma. Once collected in the transporting layer, the plasma is ready for testing.

Testing begins by pressing the reaction zone of the reagent carrier into the plasma reservoir. The reagents required for each specific test are arranged in the correct sequence in the carrier. Some may be stored in carrier paper or tissues or in **hydrophilic**, water-loving, films that dissolve completely when pressed into the plasma reservoir.

♦ ♦ ♦ **Note** ♦ ♦ ♦

Most of the encoded information needed for test performance is constant for a particular parameter, with the exception of the characteristic data for calculating results from the reflectance measurements. These are determined each time a new lot of reagent carriers is used.

The reflectance photometer reads the test results. Proper wavelengths and reading times are encoded in the magnetic tape on the reverse side of the reagent carrier. The magnetic tape also encodes other information needed for test performance, including:

- type of test
- duration of plasma separation
- preincubation, aeration, and reaction phases
- formula for calculating results from the reflectance measurement
- limits of the measurement range

- factors for converting the values obtained for the enzyme activities from 37 degrees Celsius to 30 and 25 degrees Celsius
- factors for converting international units into conventional units and vice versa

Correct reading of the magnetic code is checked by an internal test code. Test results are printed on the printer tape, along with information provided by the operator, such as patient ID.

◆ ◆ ◆ Note ◆ ◆ ◆

CLIA 1988 requires that two levels of control samples for each parameter be performed and recorded each day that a patient sample is tested for that parameter. Control samples should include a normal value and an abnormal value.

A calibration procedure, which is performed by the manufacturer on each lot of reagent carriers, brings the results of the Reflotron system into close agreement with current manual methods. The instrument checks calibration each time a test is performed, using information stored on the magnetic tape of the reagent carrier.

◆ ◆ ◆ Specific Procedures Performed by Automated Blood-Chemistry Analyzers

The following lists show the specific procedures performed by the Vision, Ektachem DT, and Reflotron Plus automated blood-chemistry analyzers.

Vision System (Abbott Laboratories)

- alkaline phosphatase
- cholesterol
- glucose
- triglycerides
- blood urea nitrogen (BUN)
- uric acid
- creatinine
- serum glutamic-oxaloacetic transaminase (SGOT, AST)
- serum glutamic-pyruvic transaminase (SGPT, ALT)
- total protein

- albumin
- calcium
- amylase
- HDL cholesterol
- whole-blood HDL cholesterol
- glutamyltranspeptidase (GGTP)
- creatine kinase (CK)
- lactic acid dehydrogenase (LDH)
- thyroxine (T4)
- phenytoin
- theophylline
- C-reactive protein (CRP)
- hemoglobin
- total bilirubin
- prothrombin time
- potassium
- LYTE potassium
- glycate hemoglobin Hg A, C

Ektachem DT System (Eastman Kodak)
Ektachem DT60 II Analyzer Module:

- ammonia
- amylase
- total bilirubin
- blood urea nitrogen (BUN)
- cholesterol
- creatinine
- glucose
- HDL cholesterol
- hemoglobin
- lactate
- magnesium
- phosphorus
- total protein
- triglycerides
- uric acid

Ektachem DTSC II Module:

- albumin
- alkaline phosphatase (ALKP)
- serum glutamic-pyruvic transaminase (SGPT, ALT)
- serum glutamic-oxaloacetic transaminase (SGOT, AST)
- calcium
- cholinesterase

- creatine kinase isoenzyme (CKMB)
- creatinine
- gamma glutamyltranspeptidase (GGT)
- lactic acid dehydrogenase (LDH)
- lipase
- theophylline

Ektachem DTE II Module:

- carbon dioxide
- chloride
- potassium
- sodium

Reflotron Plus System (Boehringer Mannheim Corporation)

- hemoglobin
- glucose

- cholesterol
- triglycerides
- HDL cholesterol
- LDL (calculated)
- uric acid
- bilirubin
- serum glutamic-pyruvic transaminase (SGPT, ALT)
- serum glutamic-oxaloacetic transaminase (SGOT, AST)
- gamma glutamyltranspeptidase (GGT)
- amylase (AMYL)
- blood urea nitrogen (BUN)
- creatinine (CR)
- potassium
- creatine kinase (CK)

CHAPTER 23 REVIEW

Using Terminology

Match the term in the right column with the appropriate definition or description in the left column.

_____ 1. Abbott Vision system

_____ 2. freeze-dried

_____ 3. group of tests

_____ 4. ion-selective electrode

_____ 5. measuring electrical potential

_____ 6. noncontinuous

_____ 7. Reflotron Plus system

_____ 8. water-loving

a. centrifugal analyzer

b. discrete

c. hydrophilic

d. ISE

e. lyophilized

f. potentiometric

g. profile

h. solid-phase analyzer

Acquiring Knowledge

Mark each statement true or false and rewrite the false statements to make them true.

9. Automated blood-chemistry analyzers are based on one of two types of technology: discrete analysis or centrifugal analysis.

_____

_____

10. In discrete analysis systems, samples and reagents flow through the instrument, one after the other.

_____

_____

11. Chemical methods used by discrete analysis systems may be either wet or dry chemistry.

_____

_____

12. The Kodak Ektachem DT analyzer is a discrete wet chemistry analyzer.

_____

_____

13. The DT60 Analyzer module controls the other two modules of the Kodak system.

_____

_____

14. The DTSC module of the Kodak Ektachem DT analyzer has the special function of blood-electrolyte testing.

_____

_____

_____

Answer the following questions in the spaces provided.

15. What are the major advantages of using automated blood-chemistry analyzers in POLs?

_____

_____

_____

16. What are some of the questions that must be addressed in selecting an automated blood-chemistry analyzer for a POL?

_____

_____

_____

_____

_____

_____

_____

_____

_____

_____

17. What is the basic difference between continuous flow and discrete blood-chemistry analyzers?

18. Briefly describe how continuous flow blood-chemistry analyzers test samples.

19. What two chemical analysis methods are used by discrete blood-chemistry analyzers?

20. How are reagents packaged for the Abbott Vision, Kodak Ektachem DT, and Reflotron Plus analyzers?

21. What is the role of centrifugation in discrete centrifugal analyzers?

22. Describe how the DT60 Analyzer module of the Kodak Ektachem DT analyzer is operated.

23. What special tests are performed by the DTE module of the Kodak Ektachem DT analyzer? What method is used?

_____

_____

_____

_____

_____

24. What is the purpose of the glass-fiber fleece layers in the Reflotron Plus analyzer?

_____

_____

_____

25. Briefly describe how to run a test on the Reflotron Plus analyzer.

_____

_____

_____

_____

26. How are tests read on solid-phase blood-chemistry analyzers, such as the Ektachem DT and Reflotron Plus?

_____

_____

27. In addition to the manufacturer's recommended calibration schedule, what conditions should lead to recalibration of blood-chemistry analyzers?

_____

_____

_____

28. What does the once-a-month self-check of the Abbott Vision analyzer check for?

_____

_____

_____

29. Do the methods used by automated blood-chemistry analyzers for chemical analysis differ from manual methods?

_____

_____

30. What test profiles can be performed by the Abbott Vision blood-chemistry analyzer?

_____

_____

_____

_____

Applying Knowledge—On the Job

Answer the following questions in the spaces provided.

31. Your coworker in the lab is testing samples with the Kodak Ektachem DT analyzer. The box of slides is empty, so she opens a new box with a different lot number from the old box and stores the new box in a cupboard. She removes the wrapper from the slide that she has kept out of the new box and proceeds to spot the sample on the slide and complete the procedure. Your coworker has made two mistakes. What should she have done instead?

_____

_____

_____

_____

32. In the POL where you work, you sometimes perform blood tests with the Abbott Vision analyzer. You have just put the instrument through its monthly self-check, and the printout indicates that there is a problem with the spectrophotometer. What should you do?

_____

_____

_____

_____

33. Your lab supervisor has asked you to develop a protocol for quality control of the new Abbott Vision analyzer that the lab just purchased. What should the protocol include?

_____

_____

_____

_____

_____

_____

_____

_____

24 The Physiology of Blood Chemistry and the Relationship to Pathology

COGNITIVE OBJECTIVES

After studying this chapter, you should be able to

- use each of the vocabulary terms appropriately.
- list the hormones that regulate glucose metabolism and identify how they affect blood-glucose levels.
- identify the major causes of hypoglycemia and hyperglycemia.
- distinguish between postprandial hypoglycemia and fasting hypoglycemia.
- describe the three types of biologically important lipids.
- explain the classification of lipoproteins on the basis of density.
- discuss the clinical significance of lipid and lipoprotein levels and proportions.
- describe the composition and role of proteins in the body.
- explain how serum proteins are measured.
- identify nonprotein nitrogen compounds in the blood that are assessed in POLs.

PERFORMANCE OBJECTIVES

After studying this chapter, you should be able to

- interpret abnormal blood-glucose levels.
- evaluate lipid and lipoprotein proportions.

TERMINOLOGY

acromegaly: a growth abnormality caused by overproduction of growth hormone by the pituitary gland.

adipose tissue: the connective tissue in which fat is stored in cells.

albumin: the most abundant plasma protein. Albumin is responsible for maintaining osmotic pressure at the capillary membrane.

amino acid: one of twenty different compounds in humans that are the building blocks of proteins. Each amino acid contains an amine group and an acidic carboxyl group.

atherosclerosis: the condition in which cholesterol deposits in the blood vessels.

blood urea nitrogen (BUN): the concentration of nitrogen in the blood, which is used as an indirect measure of urea in the blood.

cholesterol: the sterol of primary biological significance. High levels of cholesterol in the blood are linked with increased risk of cardiovascular disease.

conjugated lipid: a compound made up of fat and another compound, such as phosphoric acid (phospholipids) or a carbohydrate (glycolipids).

creatine: a nonprotein nitrogen compound found in muscle tissue. Creatine is synthesized primarily in the liver from three amino acids. It combines readily with phosphate to store energy for muscle contractions.

creatinine: the end product of the metabolism of creatine.

Cushing's syndrome: the condition caused by hypersecretion of the adrenal cortex.

disaccharide: a twelve-carbon sugar. Disaccharides include sucrose, lactose, and maltose.

globulin: the second most abundant type of plasma protein. Globulin has a diversity of functions, including transporting other substances and acting as a substrate.

gluconeogenesis: the formation of glycogen from noncarbohydrate sources.

HDL cholesterol: the cholesterol content of the HDL fraction of plasma lipoproteins.

high density lipoprotein (HDL): a lipoprotein that has high density because it is low in fat content.

hyperthyroidism: hyperactivity of the thyroid gland, leading to increased production of thyroxine.

insulinoma: a tumor of the beta cells of the pancreas.

LDL cholesterol: the cholesterol content of the LDL fraction of plasma lipoproteins.

lipid: fat; one of a group of organic compounds made up mainly of carbon, hydrogen, and oxygen. Lipids are used to store energy and as structural materials in the cells.

lipoprotein: a macromolecule of triglycerides, phospholipids, and cholesterol complexed with specialized proteins.

low density lipoprotein (LDL): a lipoprotein that is low in density because it contains large amounts of fat, primarily in the form of cholesterol.

oral hypoglycemic drug: a drug that decreases the amount of glucose in the blood by stimulating beta cells to secrete more insulin, inhibiting glucose production, or facilitating the transport of glucose to muscle cells.

plaque: a thickened region in an artery wall that prevents blood from flowing freely. Plaques may lead to heart attack or stroke.

polysaccharide: a carbohydrate composed of many molecules of simple sugars. Polysaccharides include starch in plants and glycogen in animals.

protein: one of a large group of complex, nitrogen-containing organic compounds, consisting of amino acids joined together by peptide bonds.

ribosome: a cellular structure on the surface of rough endoplasmic reticula that synthesizes protein.

saturated fat: a triglyceride in which the fatty acids are saturated with hydrogen atoms. Saturated fats form straight chain molecules that tend to pack together tightly, appearing like the dense white fat in bacon.

thyroxine: the thyroid hormone that raises the level of blood glucose.

triglyceride: a compound made up of fatty acids and glycerol.

unsaturated fat: a triglyceride in which the fatty acids are not saturated with hydrogen atoms. Unsaturated fats tend to be liquids at room temperature.

urea: a small molecule, formed from ammonia in the liver, which can move freely into both extracellular and intracellular fluid. Urea is concentrated in the urine for excretion.

uremia: a high level of urea in the blood.

uric acid: the end product of the metabolism of purine, an important constituent of nucleic acids.

● ● ● ● ● ● ● ● ● ● ● ● ● ● ● ●

The blood transports numerous substances related to metabolic processes. This chapter describes the substances most frequently measured in POLs as part of a general assessment of body metabolism. These substances include carbohydrates, lipids, and proteins. Some of the substances analyzed provide information about specific organs or systems, while others reveal the summed effects of numerous metabolic events involving more than one organ or system.

CARBOHYDRATES

Carbohydrates are a large group of sugars, starches, celluloses, and gums that contain only carbon, hydrogen, and oxygen and that are in approximately the proportions $1:2:1$, respectively. Carbohydrates are the main source of energy for all body functions, and they are needed to process other nutrients. They are formed by all green plants.

◆◆ *Glucose*

The body gets most of its energy from the oxidative metabolism of the carbohydrate glucose, a simple, six-carbon sugar, or monosaccharide, described in Chapter 22. Glucose is found in the diet most often as part of more complex sugars, including the **disaccharides,** or twelve-carbon sugars, which include sucrose, table sugar, which usually comes from sugar cane; lactose, milk sugar; and maltose, found in malt and sprouting seeds and formed from starch. Glucose also is found in the diet as the major constituent of

polysaccharides, which are carbohydrates composed of many molecules of simple sugars. Polysaccharides include starch in plants and glycogen in animals.

♦ ♦ ♦ Fatty Acids as ♦ ♦ ♦ an Energy Source

In addition to glucose, many cells can derive some energy by burning fatty acids, which are acids found in some fats. Fatty acids are a less efficient energy source than glucose, however, and their metabolism generates acid metabolites that are harmful when accumulated.

The body uses enzymes to release glucose from these more complex carbohydrates. Glucose that is not used directly for energy by the cells is stored in the liver and muscles as glycogen or in adipose tissue as **triglycerides.** The latter are compounds made up of fatty acids and glycerol, an alcohol. Glucose also can be converted by the liver into **amino acids,** which are the components of **proteins,** the main building materials of the body. The liver can convert the unused glucose through intermediary compounds into amino acids. Indeed, the liver is pivotal in regulating the distribution of glucose as needed for energy, storage, and structural purposes.

♦♦ Hormones That Regulate Blood-Glucose Levels

Because glucose is so important as an energy source, maintaining adequate blood levels of glucose is a high priority for homeostasis, involving many different hormones. The four hormones most significant for glucose regulation are the pancreatic hormones insulin and glucagon, the adrenal hormone epinephrine, and the thyroid hormone **thyroxine.** Insulin acts to lower blood-glucose levels, while the other three hormones all work to raise them.

Insulin, which is produced by beta cells in the pancreas, lowers blood-glucose levels by:

- enhancing the entry of glucose into the cells
- enhancing the storage of glucose as glycogen or fatty acids
- enhancing the synthesis of proteins and fatty acids
- suppressing the breakdown of proteins into amino acids and fat into free fatty acids

Glucagon, which is produced by alpha cells in the pancreas, raises blood-glucose levels by:

- enhancing the release of glucose from glycogen
- enhancing the synthesis of glucose from amino acids and fatty acids

Epinephrine originates in the medulla of the adrenal gland. It raises blood-glucose levels by enhancing the release of glucose from glycogen and fatty acids from adipose tissue. Thyroxine from the thyroid gland raises blood glucose by enhancing the release of glucose from glycogen. It also enhances the absorption of sugars from the intestine.

♦♦ Abnormal Blood-Glucose Levels

Blood-glucose levels are measured to assess the adequacy of the hormonal regulation of glucose metabolism and storage. Blood-glucose levels that are either too high or too low signal faulty homeostasis and the need to search for causes.

Hyperglycemia. As defined in Chapter 22, hyperglycemia refers to a higher than normal blood-glucose level. Recall that normal, nonfasting blood-glucose levels are between 70 and 110 mg/dL. The most common cause of hyperglycemia is diabetes mellitus, which occurs in two forms: insulin-dependent (IDDM) and noninsulin-dependent (NIDDM). In IDDM, the insulin receptors on the cells are normal, but the beta cell mass in the pancreas is markedly reduced. As a result, patients with IDDM have no measurable circulating insulin. They do not respond to **oral hypoglycemic drugs,** which work in a variety of ways to decrease the amount of glucose in the blood. Instead, patients with IDDM must take daily insulin injections.

♦ ♦ ♦ Hypoglycemic Drugs ♦ ♦ ♦

Contrary to popular belief, oral hypoglycemic drugs are not an oral form of insulin, although their purpose is the same—to decrease the amount of glucose in the blood. They work through several mechanisms, including:

- stimulating the beta cells of the pancreas to secrete more insulin
- inhibiting glucose production
- facilitating the transport of glucose to muscle cells

In NIDDM, on the other hand, beta cell mass is reduced only modestly, and insulin is present in the blood at low, normal, or even high levels. The insulin receptors on the cells are reduced or ineffective. Patients with NIDDM usually respond to oral hypoglycemic drugs, and some can control their disease with diet and exercise alone.

In addition to diabetes mellitus, several other conditions can cause hyperglycemia. They include:

- **hyperthyroidism,** or hyperactivity of the thyroid gland, which increases the production of thyroxine

- **Cushing's syndrome,** which is caused by hypersecretion of the adrenal cortex

- elevated levels of the hormones estrogen, epinephrine, or norepinephrine

- **acromegaly,** a growth abnormality caused by overproduction of growth hormone by the pituitary gland

- obesity, defined as weight gain of 20 percent greater than ideal weight for height and body build

- treatment with adrenal steroids, thiazide diuretics, or oral contraceptives

- severe liver or kidney damage, which impairs normal carbohydrate metabolism

- alcoholism, which causes liver damage and dysfunction

Hypoglycemia. As defined in Chapter 22, hypoglycemia refers to abnormally low levels of glucose in the blood. It is diagnosed only when blood glucose is below 50 mg/dL at the same time that the patient is experiencing symptoms of hypoglycemia. Which specific symptoms are experienced depend on how quickly blood-glucose levels fall. When blood glucose falls rapidly, it leads to increased epinephrine secretion, which produces sweating, trembling, weakness, anxiety, and, if prolonged, delirium and loss of consciousness. When blood glucose falls gradually, the symptoms include headache, irritability, and lethargy. In true hypoglycemia, a return to normal blood-glucose levels eliminates the symptoms.

The most common cause of hypoglycemia is insulin overdose in patients with unstable IDDM. Correcting the condition involves ingestion of a source of sugar, such as sugar cubes, candy, or orange juice, preferably as soon as symptoms appear. Other conditions that cause high levels of circulating insulin also can produce hypoglycemia. These include large tumors behind the peritoneum and tumors of the beta cells of the pancreas, called **insulinomas.**

There are two types of hypoglycemia: postprandial and fasting hypoglycemia. Postprandial hypoglycemia, also called reactive hypoglycemia, occurs several hours after food is ingested. Symptoms generally last no more than thirty minutes, and they resolve without further carbohydrate intake. Postprandial hypoglycemia appears to be due to a delayed or exaggerated response to the insulin that is secreted when sugar is ingested. It may occur early in the development of NIDDM, due to a mismatch between pancreatic insulin production and cellular insulin receptors, but most cases have no known physiological cause. The latter cases of postprandial hypoglycemia are considered to be functional disease, that is, disease in which no anatomical changes can be observed to account for the symptoms.

Fasting hypoglycemia is detected by measuring blood-glucose levels after a twelve or twenty-four hour fast. In contrast to postprandial hypoglycemia, fasting hypoglycemia usually is associated with recognizable anatomical changes in an organ or tissue. The major cause is liver disease. Alcoholics, for example, frequently develop fasting hypoglycemia if their carbohydrate intake is low. Their glycogen stores are depleted and alcohol metabolites interfere with **gluconeogenesis**—the formation of glycogen from noncarbohydrate sources. Pancreatic tumors also may cause fasting hypoglycemia.

＊＊

LIPIDS

Lipids, or fats, are a group of organic compounds made up mainly of carbon, hydrogen, and oxygen. The concentration of energy in lipids is twice that of carbohydrates, so they provide a good source of stored energy for the body. They also are used as structural materials in the cells.

＊＊ *Types of Lipids*

Three types of lipids are biologically important: neutral fats, conjugated lipids, and sterols. Neutral fats are triglycerides, fatty acids plus glycerol. **Conjugated lipids** are compounds made up of fat and another compound, such as phosphoric acid (phospholipids) or a carbohydrate (glycolipids). Sterols are steroid alcohols. **Cholesterol** is the sterol of primary biological significance.

Triglycerides. Each molecule of triglyceride contains a three-carbon glycerol molecule bonded to three fatty acids. Fatty acids are the major form of fat used by the body to store energy. They are found in **adipose tissue,** which is connective tissue in which fat is stored in cells. Fatty acids enter and leave adipose tissue as needed to provide raw material for gluconeogenesis and direct combustion as an energy source.

Most fatty acids are synthesized by the liver from carbohydrates and proteins. Those that cannot be synthesized are called essential fatty acids, because they must be consumed in the diet. They are found in vegetables in the form of linoleic and linolenic acids. One tablespoon per day of corn or olive oil fulfills the daily requirement for essential fatty acids, which are needed for proper functioning of all tissues. Essential fatty acids also are the precursors of prostaglandins, hormonelike fatty acids that perform a number of important functions, including:

- stimulating contractility of uterine and other smooth muscles
- lowering blood pressure
- regulating acid secretion of the stomach
- regulating body temperature
- regulating platelet aggregation
- controlling inflammation and vascular permeability

Symptoms of essential fatty acid deficiency include growth retardation, scaliness of the skin, infertility, and, possibly, kidney abnormalities and increased susceptibility to infections.

There are two basic types of triglycerides: saturated fats and unsaturated or polyunsaturated fats. **Saturated fats** are triglycerides in which the fatty acids are saturated with hydrogen atoms (that is, they are bonded to as many hydrogen atoms as possible). As a result, they form straight chain molecules that tend to pack together tightly, appearing like the dense white fat in bacon. **Unsaturated fats** are triglycerides in which the fatty acids are not saturated with hydrogen atoms. They have kinks—not straight chain structures—so they cannot pack together as tightly. As a result, unsaturated fats tend to be liquids at room temperature. Nutritional research suggests that it is more healthful to consume unsaturated fats, like canola, safflower, and olive oils, than saturated fats, such as butter and lard.

Phospholipids. Phospholipids, which include primarily lecithin, sphingomyelin, and cephalin, comprise the largest fraction of plasma lipids. Circulating phospholipids generally are in the ratio 70 percent lecithin, 20 percent sphingomyelin, and 10 percent cephalin and others. Up to age thirty, the plasma concentration of phospholipids is between 150 and 300 mg/dL. While all cells in the body are capable of synthesizing phospholipids, most circulating phospholipids probably are produced in the liver and intestinal mucosa.

Phospholipids play many important roles in body function. Phospholipids help stabilize other lipids being transported through the blood and are the major constituents of cell membranes. Circulating phospholipids serve as a source of phosphate groups for intracellular metabolism and play an essential role in blood coagulation. Both lecithins and sphingomyelins act as mild detergents. Unlike fatty acids, however, phospholipids seldom are used for energy storage.

Cholesterol. Cholesterol contains a hydroxyl radical ($-OH$) like all other alcohols. Cholesterol is an important component of cell-membrane structure and of the materials that make skin waterproof. The adrenal cortex, ovaries, and testes use cholesterol for the manufacture of steroid hormones, and the liver uses cholesterol to form bile acids, or salts.

It is likely that very little dietary cholesterol enters directly into metabolic reactions. Instead, cholesterol undergoes continuous synthesis, degradation, and recycling in the body. Virtually every type of body tissue can manufacture cholesterol from simple carbon compounds, but those that are particularly active in cholesterol production include the liver (primarily), adrenal cortex, ovaries, testes, and the intestinal epithelium.

The rate at which the liver produces cholesterol appears to be related inversely to the amount of circulating chylomicron cholesterol—microscopic cholesterol particles circulating in the blood after fat digestion. When the chylomicron cholesterol level is low, the liver increases its cholesterol production. This occurs with bile duct obstruction, which leads to a reduction in the amount of bile salts reaching the gut to emulsify fats for digestion. As a result, there is less circulating chylomicron cholesterol. The liver responds by doubling or tripling its production of cholesterol.

While the body can synthesize cholesterol with great ease, it has much more difficulty degrading it. Estrogen tends to promote the transport and excretion of cholesterol, while testosterone seems to have the opposite effect or no effect. This hormonal difference in cholesterol excretion may help explain why males have higher rates of **atherosclerosis,** or cholesterol deposits in the blood vessels, than do females, whose estrogen levels are much higher.

❖❖ Lipoproteins

Lipids are soluble in organic solvents like benzene, chloroform, and ether, but insoluble in water. They therefore require transport mechanisms for circulation in the blood. The main lipid components of serum are in the form of **lipoproteins,** which are macromolecules of triglycerides, phospholipids, and cholesterol complexed with specialized proteins. A very small amount of free fatty acids also is present in the blood, complexed with albumin, a simple protein. Lipids are detected and measured in the blood in lipoprotein forms.

Lipoproteins are classified on the basis of density. Because lipids are lower in density—have lower specific gravity—than are proteins, lipoproteins with many lipid molecules also tend to have low density. Conversely, lipoproteins with only a few lipid molecules have higher density. The three types of biologically significant lipids—triglycerides, phospholipids, and cholesterol—also vary in density, with triglycerides being the least dense. Lipoproteins with very high concentrations of triglycerides have specific gravities below plasma, so they rise to the top of a volume of plasma when centrifuged (see Table 24.1).

Lipoproteins with the lowest density are called very low density lipoproteins, or VLDL. They consist mainly of fat with very little protein, and virtually all the fat is in the form of triglycerides. **Low density lipoproteins,** or LDL, contain large amounts of fat, primarily in the form of cholesterol. The high cholesterol content is a potential cause of cardiovascular disease. **High density lipoproteins,** or HDL, have the lowest fat content of all the lipoproteins, being composed equally of protein and fat.

❖❖ Clinical Applications

Many physicians think that an adequate lipid assessment should include the following measurements:

- total cholesterol
- **HDL cholesterol,** the cholesterol content of the HDL fraction
- serum triglyceride level
- chylomicron concentration

The level of **LDL cholesterol,** the cholesterol content of the LDL fraction, can be determined by measuring the cholesterol remaining after the HDL fraction has been removed by precipitation.

The level of HDL cholesterol is higher, on average, in adult women than in adult men. It also tends to be inversely proportional to total triglyceride level (see Table 24.2).

The clinical significance of lipid measurements still is debated among researchers. While population-based studies reveal clear statistical associations between lipid levels and cardiovascular disease, establishing similar associations in individual patients is not always possible. Nonetheless, populations with high average total cholesterol have high rates of atherosclerosis. High levels of cholesterol in the blood lead to the formation of **plaques,** thickened regions in artery walls that prevent blood from flowing freely. Plaques in arteries of the heart may lead to heart attack and plaques in arteries of the brain may lead to stroke.

Again at the population level, HDL cholesterol concentrations above the normal range are associated with half the average risk for atherosclerosis, while HDL cholesterol concentrations below the normal

---

TABLE 24.1 The Composition of Lipoproteins

Lipoprotein	% Triglyceride	% Cholesterol	% Phospholipid	% Protein
Chylomicrons	85 to 95	3 to 5	5 to 10	1 to 2
Very low density (VLDL)	60 to 70	10 to 15	10 to 15	10
Low density (LDL)	5 to 10	45	20 to 30	15 to 25
High density (HDL)	Very little	20	30	50

TABLE 24.2 Normal Ranges for HDL Cholesterol

Age/Sex Group	HDL Cholesterol Concentration (mg/dL)
Adult females	30 to 80
Adult males	22 to 68

range are associated with twice or greater the average risk of atherosclerosis. That is why LDL cholesterol sometimes is called "bad cholesterol" and HDL is called "good cholesterol" and why patients with a low proportion of HDL cholesterol are encouraged to adopt healthful life-style habits that have been found to raise HDL cholesterol levels. This association between HDL cholesterol and atherosclerosis also explains why quantitative measurements of individual lipids generally are of less interest than are their proportions in plasma. The ratio of total cholesterol to HDL cholesterol or the ratio of HDL to LDL cholesterol is thought to have more clinical significance than is their absolute concentrations.

♦ ♦ ♦ Raising HDL Levels ♦ ♦ ♦

People who follow these healthful life-style habits are likely to increase their level of HDL cholesterol:

- regular exercise
- a diet low in saturated fats and high in foods like vegetables and fish oils
- maintenance of normal weight
- no smoking
- no heavy drinking

PROTEINS

Proteins are a large group of complex, nitrogen-containing organic compounds. The building blocks of proteins are amino acids, which are smaller molecules each containing an amine group $(-NH_2)$ and an acidic carboxyl group (COOH). Proteins consist of amino acids joined together by peptide bonds between the carbon of one amino acid and the nitrogen of the next. There are twenty different amino acids in humans, and they can be linked together in countless different combinations. As a result, there are numerous different kinds of protein molecules, as compared with just a few kinds of carbohydrate and lipid molecules. We all are different from each other because of our proteins, not because of our carbohydrates or fats.

♦ ♦ ♦ Diet Essentials ♦ ♦ ♦

All amino acids enter the body through dietary sources, but twelve of the twenty amino acids also can be synthesized in our cells. The remaining eight amino acids are called essential amino acids, because they cannot be synthesized by the human body and must be ingested in foods on a regular basis. Animal sources of protein contain all eight essential amino acids, but most plant sources are lacking in one or more.

Protein synthesis and degradation occur continuously in the body. Each day, approximately 20 to 30 grams of protein are irreversibly degraded. As a consequence, this same amount of protein must be ingested to maintain a metabolic steady state, called nitrogen balance. If nitrogen balance is positive, more amino acids are entering the body than are being excreted. If nitrogen balance is negative, on the other hand, excretion of amino acids or their nitrogen-containing metabolites exceeds ingestion. If negative nitrogen balance persists for very long, there will be an eventual loss of essential protein-mediated functions.

Protein synthesis occurs in all body cells on structures called **ribosomes,** located on the surface of rough (granular) endoplasmic reticula (ER). The process is controlled by the genes, which are found on the chromosomes within the cell nuclei. Individuals with faulty genes for a particular protein are unable to synthesize that protein correctly. For example, individuals with faulty genes for the blood protein hemoglobin are unable to synthesize normal hemoglobin. Depending on the exact nature of genetic defect, they may synthesize sickle-cell hemoglobin or some other abnormal form of the hemoglobin molecule.

◆◆ *The Role of Proteins in the Body*

Because protein molecules are so diverse, they are able to fill a great many different structural and functional roles in the body. Proteins that detect light in the eyes, for example, are very different in composition from proteins that detoxify poisons in the liver.

Structurally, proteins are the main building materials of the body, comprising three-fourths of the solid matter of the body. Proteins are the major components of muscles, blood, skin, hair, nails, and visceral organs.

Functionally, proteins play many important roles. They are needed to:

- form hormones, which act as chemical messengers to body organs
- form enzymes, which help biochemical reactions occur faster and control virtually all the life processes that go on in the cells
- form antibodies, which help protect the body against disease
- transport molecules, which carry substances through the body, such as the hemoglobin protein that transports oxygen in the blood

◆◆ *Blood Proteins*

The normal protein content of serum is 6 to 8 g/dL, of which approximately two-thirds is **albumin,** one third **globulin,** and a few percent fibrinogen. Albumin is responsible for maintaining osmotic pressure at the capillary membrane. Globulin has a diversity of functions, including transporting other substances and acting as a substrate. Fibrinogen is essential for blood-clot formation. For more on fibrinogen, see Chapter 20.

Liver cells, called hepatocytes, synthesize fibrinogen and albumin and between 60 and 80 percent of globulin. The remaining globulin consists of immunoglobulins, or antibodies, which are manufactured by the lymphoreticular system.

A general study of blood proteins usually measures total protein and the albumin and nonantibody globulin content of the serum. If either albumin or globulin is measured, the other can be calculated by subtraction from the total protein value. Results are given as the albumin to globulin ratio, A/G.

Most protein determinations actually measure nitrogen, which is found in all amino acids. Nitrogen content then is converted to protein concentration by multiplying by a conversion factor. This provides an accurate estimate of total protein unless hypoalbuminemia and hyperglobulinemia are present. Other lab tests can detect these conditions and provide the diagnostic information needed for patient assessment.

◆◆

NONPROTEIN NITROGEN COMPOUNDS

Nonprotein compounds in the blood that contain nitrogen include ammonia, urea, uric acid, and creatinine.

◆◆ *Ammonia*

Ammonia (NH_3) is a pungent, colorless, alkaline compound that results when proteins are degraded in intracellular protein turnover or in the colon by bacteria that aid in protein digestion. It is formed when amine groups ($-NH_2$) are removed from amino acids in a process called deamination. Ammonia travels to the liver, where it undergoes a series of reactions that convert it to urea.

◆◆ *Urea*

Urea is a small molecule that can move freely into both extracellular and intracellular fluid. It is concentrated in the urine for excretion. In stable nitrogen balance, about 25 grams of urea are excreted daily. In the blood, urea levels reflect the balance between urinary excretion of urea and hepatic production of urea from ammonia.

In labs in the United States, urea in the blood is measured indirectly as nitrogen, and the results are expressed as **blood urea nitrogen,** or **BUN.** The normal serum BUN value is 8 to 25 mg/dL. Nitrogen contributes about half of the total weight of urea, and the concentration of urea can be estimated by multiplying the BUN value by 2.14. The BUN may rise slightly following prolonged massive protein intake, but recent dietary intake does not affect random values.

A high level of urea in the blood is called **uremia.** The most common cause is impaired excretion due to renal failure. Postrenal uremia occurs when urea diffuses back into the bloodstream due to urethral obstruction by stones, tumors, or inflammation. Prerenal uremia refers to a high level of urea in the blood that is due to increased protein breakdown. This may be caused by shock, blood loss, dehydration, crush injuries, fever, or burns. A low level of urea in the blood may be caused by liver damage, but damage must be severe to affect BUN values.

◆◆ *Uric Acid*

Uric acid is the end product of the metabolism of purine, an important constituent of nucleic acids, which are the building blocks of DNA. Purine is found in the diet, especially in organ meats such as heart and kidney, legumes, anchovies, and yeast. The turnover of purine occurs continually in the body, producing much of the uric acid, even without purines in the diet. Most uric acid is synthesized in the liver and then carried by the blood to the kidneys, where filtration, absorption, and secretion affect its excretion. Normal daily excretion of uric acid varies from about 0.5 gram on a low purine diet to about 1.0 gram on a normal purine diet.

Uric acid dissolves poorly in water, and uric acid salts, or urates, may precipitate as calculi, or stones, in urine that has a high urate concentration. This may occur even if the serum urate concentration is normal. Patients with high serum urate concentrations often have urate deposits in the soft tissues, particularly the joints, producing a painful condition called gout. Conditions that may increase serum uric acid levels include cytolytic treatment of malignancy, especially leukemia and lymphoma; polycythemia; and sickle-cell anemia. Serum levels also are higher when excretion of uric acid is decreased, as it is with alcohol ingestion and renal failure due to any cause.

◆◆ *Creatinine*

Creatinine is the end product of the metabolism of **creatine,** a nonprotein nitrogen compound found in muscle tissue. Creatinine is picked up by the blood and transported to the kidneys for excretion. Blood concentration and total urinary excretion of creatinine fluctuate very little. Blood creatinine rises with kidney failure, but less steeply than the rise in blood urea.

◆ ◆ ◆ **Creatine** ◆ ◆ ◆

Creatine is synthesized in the liver from amino acids. Daily production of creatine remains fairly constant unless a crushing injury or degenerative disease causes massive muscle damage. Creatine combines readily with phosphate to form phosphocreatine, which stores high energy phosphates necessary for muscle contraction. The reaction is reversible, but small amounts of creatine are irreversibly converted to creatinine during the reaction.

▼ CHAPTER 24 REVIEW ▼

Using Terminology

Define the following terms in the spaces provided.

1. Albumin: _____

    _____

2. Amino acid: _____

    _____

3. Cholesterol: _____

    _____

4. Conjugated lipid: _____

_____

5. Creatine: _____

_____

6. Creatinine: _____

_____

7. Disaccharide: _____

_____

8. Globulin: _____

_____

9. High density lipoprotein (HDL): _____

_____

10. Low density lipoprotein (LDL): _____

_____

11. Oral hypoglycemic drug: _____

_____

12. Polysaccharide: _____

_____

13. Protein: _____

_____

14. Triglyceride: _____

_____

15. Urea: _____

_____

Match the term in the right column with the appropriate definition or description in the left column.

_____ 16. end product of purine metabolism

_____ 17. formation of glycogen

_____ 18. fraction of plasma lipoproteins

_____ 19. high level of urea in the blood

_____ 20. macromolecule of triglycerides, phospholipids, cholesterol, and specialized proteins

_____ 21. nitrogen concentration

_____ 22. stores fat

_____ 23. synthesizes protein

_____ 24. thickened regions in artery walls

_____ 25. triglycerides

a. adipose tissue
b. BUN
c. gluconeogenesis
d. HDL cholesterol
e. lipoproteins
f. plaques
g. ribosomes
h. fats
i. uremia
j. uric acid

Acquiring Knowledge

Answer the following questions in the spaces provided.

26. What hormones regulate glucose metabolism?

27. How do each of the hormones listed in question 26 affect blood-glucose levels?

28. What are the major causes of hypoglycemia?

29. What are some of the causes of hyperglycemia?

30. What are the differences between postprandial hypoglycemia and fasting hypoglycemia?

_____

_____

_____

_____

_____

_____

_____

_____

_____

31. What are the three types of biologically important lipids and how do they differ from one another?

_____

_____

_____

32. How are lipoproteins classified?

_____

_____

33. What is the clinical significance of lipid and lipoprotein proportions?

_____

_____

_____

_____

_____

_____

34. Describe the composition of proteins.

_____

_____

_____

35. What are some of the important roles played by proteins in the body?

_____

_____

_____

_____

_____

36. How are serum proteins measured?

_____

_____

_____

37. What nonprotein nitrogen compounds are found in the blood?

_____

_____

38. Where does the body get most of its glucose?

_____

39. Which sterol is most important biologically?

_____

40. In what form is most stored energy found in the body?

_____

41. Why is LDL cholesterol called "bad cholesterol" and HDL cholesterol "good cholesterol"?

_____

_____

_____

_____

42. What pathological condition results from high levels of circulating cholesterol over a long period of time?

_____

_____

_____

43. What is the difference between essential and nonessential amino acids?

_____

_____

_____

44. What are the two types of triglycerides? Which group is considered to be more healthful as a dietary component?

_____

_____

_____

45. What three food groups are the basis of most of the body's metabolism?

_____

_____

Applying Knowledge—On the Job

Answer the following questions in the spaces provided.

46. A patient with normal weight came to the laboratory for a repeat cholesterol test. Her previous blood-cholesterol level was elevated, and she had been following a special low fat, low cholesterol diet recommended by the physician. Why is the physician concerned about the patient's cholesterol level and fat intake?

_____

_____

_____

47. An overweight fifty-year-old female has reported for a postprandial blood-glucose test. Last week, she had a positive glucose-tolerance test. She has been taking oral hypoglycemic medication and following a diet and exercise program prescribed by the doctor. What disease does she most likely have?

_____

_____

48. A male patient with an attack of excruciating joint pain has come to the lab for a blood test. The physician suspects that the patient has gout. What blood test might be performed to help confirm the diagnosis? If the patient has gout, what will the test result likely be?

_____

_____

_____

49. A six-year-old girl is very low in weight for her age, even though she eats well because she is "always hungry." She also complains of fatigue and excessive thirst. What is the most likely cause of the girl's symptoms? What further testing might be done to confirm the diagnosis?

_____

_____

50. A patient with a history of chronic alcoholism suffers from hypoglycemia. What is the likely cause of his hypoglycemia?

_____

_____

_____

UNIT

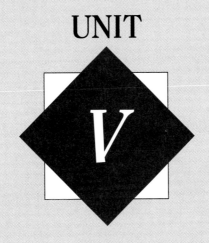

Immunology and Microbiology

25

Immunology Tests

COGNITIVE OBJECTIVES

After studying this chapter, you should be able to

- use each of the vocabulary terms appropriately.
- list and describe four types of nonspecific immune defenses in humans.
- explain the role of antigen-antibody reactions in specific immunity.
- distinguish between humoral immunity and cell-mediated immunity.
- describe three types of diseases of the immune system and give examples of each.
- explain how sensitivity and specificity relate to test accuracy.
- differentiate among the different types of immunology tests performed in POLs.
- describe how immune reactions are measured quantitatively.
- identify several ways in which quality control is maintained in immunology testing.
- describe the ABO and Rhesus blood groups and explain their clinical significance.

PERFORMANCE OBJECTIVES

After studying this chapter, you should be able to

- use a commercial agglutination kit to test for the presence of infectious mononucleosis antibodies.
- prepare and perform a human chorionic gonadotropin determination for detection of pregnancy by the ELISA method using urine.

- prepare and perform individual blood types of the ABO and Rhesus blood groups.

TERMINOLOGY

ABO blood group: one of two clinically important inherited blood groups; the ABO blood group has two antigens, A and B, and includes four blood types: A, B, AB, and O.

antibody: a protein molecule produced by the lymph system in response to a particular antigen.

antigen: short for antibody generating, a foreign substance that provokes a specific antibody reaction.

autoimmunity: the condition in which the immune system responds inappropriately to the wrong antigens—to self instead of nonself.

B-lymphocyte: B-cell; a lymphocyte that secretes short-lived antibodies involved in humoral immunity.

Candida: a genus of yeastlike fungus. Overgrowths can lead to female vaginal infections, and mouth and throat infections in infants and young children.

cell-mediated immunity: the type of specific immunity that is controlled by T-lymphocytes.

chlamydia: a bacterial disease, thought to be the most prevalent sexually transmitted disease in the United States.

Coomb's test: the antiglobulin test; used for monitoring the development of Rh incompatibility in Rh negative pregnant women.

C-reactive protein (CRP): an abnormal glycoprotein that appears in the acute stage of various inflammatory disorders.

endocytic and phagocytic response: the type of nonspecific immunity in which microorganisms and other foreign matter are engulfed and degraded by body cells.

flocculation: a precipitate in the form of downy tufts.

herpes: the common name for diseases caused by herpesvirus, a family of viruses, including those that cause cold sores and genital ulcers, *Herpes simplex I and II.*

human chorionic gonadotropin (hCG): the hormone produced by the villi of the placenta. Detecting it is the basis for early pregnancy tests.

humoral immunity: the type of specific immunity that involves the formation and activity of short-lived antibodies in body fluids.

hypersensitivity: allergy; exaggerated immune response to foreign antigens.

immunity: the body's resistance to foreign invaders, including microorganisms, cancer cells, toxins, and incompatible blood types from other individuals.

immunodeficiency: compromised immune response; the condition in which the immune system is compromised due to a congenital or acquired disorder; characterized by increased susceptibility to disease and poor recovery.

immunology: the branch of medical science that studies the physical and chemical aspects of immunity, or resistance to disease.

immunology test: a lab test that depends on immune reactions for results. Immunology tests include tests for pregnancy, many diseases, and blood types.

inflammatory response: a complex series of events, triggered by a wound or invasion by microorganisms, leading to redness, swelling, heat, and pain. Inflammatory response reduces the spread of infection and promotes healing.

Lyme disease: a bacterial disease transmitted by deer ticks.

nonspecific immunity: innate immunity; the general resistance to disease that characterizes a particular species. In humans, nonspecific immunity includes physical and anatomical barriers, physiological barriers, endocytic and phago-

cytic responses, and the inflammatory response.

physical and anatomical barriers: a type of nonspecific immunity; the body's first line of defense against foreign invaders. Physical and anatomical barriers include the skin, mucous membranes, body secretions, and benevolent bacteria.

physiological barrier: a type of nonspecific immunity; a chemical factor that kills pathogens gaining access to the body.

Rhesus (Rh) blood group: one of two clinically important inherited blood groups. Rh positive blood has the D antigen; Rh negative blood does not.

rheumatoid arthritis (RA): a chronic systemic autoimmune disease characterized by inflammation in the joints and crippling.

rubella: German measles; a mild systemic disease caused by the *Rubella* virus.

sensitivity: the ability of a lab test for a particular disease to identify correctly those who have the disease.

specific immunity: acquired immunity; immunity to a specific foreign antigen that is acquired after exposure to it.

specificity: the ability of a lab test for a particular disease to identify correctly those who do not have the disease.

syphilis: a devastating, sexually transmitted disease caused by the spirochete *Treponema pallidum.*

systemic lupus erythematosus (SLE): a systemic autoimmune disease that affects connective tissues and injures the skin, joints, kidneys, nervous system, and mucous membranes.

titer: the highest dilution, or lowest concentration, capable of producing an observable reaction.

T-lymphocytes: T-cells; the basis of cell-mediated immunity.

toxin: poison.

● ● ● ● ● ● ● ● ● ● ● ● ● ● ● ● ● ●

This chapter describes how the immune system protects individuals from disease and how immune reactions are used in POLs to diagnose disease and to type blood.

IMMUNOLOGY AND IMMUNITY

Immunology is the branch of medical science that studies the physical and chemical aspects of **immunity**—the body's resistance to foreign invaders. Foreign invaders include, most commonly, disease-causing microorganisms, like bacteria and viruses. They also include cancer cells, **toxins**, transfused blood, and transplanted tissue cells from other individuals.

Interest in immunity dates back to the earliest written accounts. A large volume of sacred scriptures outlined health laws and practices to avoid contamination, such as segregating individuals with certain diseases. Over the past three hundred years, the research of scientists like Leeuwenhoek, Jenner, Pasteur, and Koch has provided knowledge that led to modern laws of sanitation and aseptic medical practices.

♦ ♦ ♦ The Case of Smallpox ♦ ♦ ♦

Smallpox is a good example of how knowledge of immunity has advanced through time. The practice of immunizing against smallpox and thereby provoking the body into an immune response to the disease was begun many centuries ago. By the end of the 1700s, Edward Jenner began using the milder and safer cowpox vaccine to immunize against smallpox.

It was not until this century, with advances in microbiology and biochemistry, that the physiological mechanisms underlying vaccination were understood. By 1969, thanks to efforts in public health, the World Health Organization declared the world to be free of the smallpox virus, the first pathogen to have been eradicated by human efforts. Cultures of the smallpox virus now are kept in only a limited number of research laboratories. It is currently debated whether these last remaining smallpox organisms should be destroyed or kept for potential future research.

The typing of blood began in the first part of the twentieth century and laid the foundation for safe and effective blood transfusions. Today's understanding of the immune system has been increased greatly by research on organ transplants and HIV, the virus that causes AIDS, a disease of the immune system.

HOW THE IMMUNE SYSTEM WORKS

The human immune system is a complex system of cells and molecules that act in concert to distinguish foreign invaders from the body's own cells and to eliminate foreign invaders from the body. Immune system responses fall into two broad categories: nonspecific immunity and specific immunity.

♦♦ *Nonspecific Immunity*

Nonspecific immunity, sometimes called innate immunity, is the general resistance to disease that characterizes a particular species. In humans, it consists of four types of defense against foreign invaders: physical and anatomical barriers, physiological barriers, endocytic and phagocytic responses, and the inflammatory response.

Physical and Anatomical Barriers. **Physical and anatomical barriers** are the body's first line of defense against attack from foreign invaders, preventing most microorganisms from entering the body. They include:

- the skin
- mucous membranes
- body secretions like tears, saliva, and mucus
- benevolent bacteria

More specifically, the skin is somewhat acidic, thus preventing the growth of most microorganisms on its surface. Ciliated epithelial cells of the mucous membranes sweep microorganisms away from the respiratory and gastrointestinal tracts. Tears, saliva, and mucus all contain proteins that kill the microorganisms swept away. The gut and vagina have protective colonies of benevolent bacteria that prevent pathogenic strains from gaining a foothold in these areas.

Physiological Barriers. If microorganisms do gain entry to the body, they are met with a variety of **physiological barriers**—chemical factors that kill pathogens. For example, the very acidic environment of the stomach kills most microorganisms that reach it. Soluble chemical factors, which consist of a variety of proteins in the body, attack viruses and bacteria. Interferon, which is a protein formed when cells are exposed to viruses, helps protect noninfected cells against viral infection. Complement, a series of enzymatic proteins in serum, causes lysis of microorganisms and enhances the inflammatory response.

Endocytic and Phagocytic Responses. Microorganisms that evade the first two sets of barriers and penetrate blood or tissue are subject to **endocytic and phagocytic responses,** in which they are engulfed and degraded by body cells. Most body cells are able to ingest and degrade foreign molecules. Phagocytes can engulf and consume whole bacteria. Phagocytes include:

- *macrophages:* large cells of the reticuloendothelial system that are found in loose connective tissues and various organs of the body

- *monocytes* and *neutrophils:* two types of white blood cells

---

◆ ◆ ◆ Note ◆ ◆ ◆

Some microorganisms can evade phagocytosis by living within the blood cells. An example is the human immunodeficiency virus, HIV.

The Inflammatory Response. The **inflammatory response** is a complex series of events, triggered by a wound or invasion by microorganisms. It leads to redness, swelling, heat, and pain. This response isolates foreign matter and keeps it from spreading to other parts of the body. It also promotes healing.

◆◆ *Specific Immunity*

Specific immunity, or acquired immunity, refers to immunity from a specific foreign invader that is acquired after exposure to it. Specific immunity primarily involves lymphocytes.

The Basis of Specific Immunity. Specific immunity depends on the ability of the immune system not only to distinguish self from nonself but to "remember" encounters with foreign invaders. Because of this "memory," having once encountered a foreign molecule or microorganism, the immune system is capable of inducing a heightened state of immune reactivity when it encounters the foreign invader again.

The Antigen-Antibody Reaction. Foreign substances that provoke a specific immune reaction are called **antigens.** Most often, antigens are large protein molecules found on the surfaces of microorganisms, but they also include toxins and molecules on foreign blood cells and other tissues. The word *antigen* is short for "antibody generating." **Antibodies,** in turn, are protein molecules produced by the lymph system in response to a particular antigen.

◆ ◆ ◆ Note ◆ ◆ ◆

Antibodies are the globulin portion of serum proteins, which were described in Chapter 24. Antibodies also are called immunoglobulins. They are classified into the subgroups IgA, IgD, IgE, IgG, and IgM on the basis of molecular size and other characteristics.

Antibodies usually are specific for a particular antigen; that is, a given antigen stimulates the production of antibodies that react against just that antigen. Each type of antigen-antibody bonding is unique, like a lock and key, as Figure 25.1 shows. Even closely related microorganisms elicit somewhat different antibodies in a human host.

Once bonded, the antigen-antibody complex can be neutralized by precipitation or agglutination. Alternatively, antibodies may "tag" antigens for destruction by phagocytes or lysis by complement. (See page 457, Lysin Reactions.)

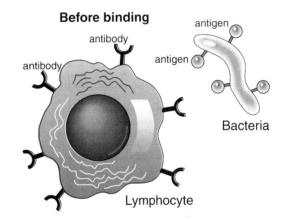

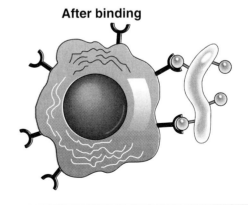

Figure 25.1. The antigen-antibody complex. This schematic representation shows the immune antibodies of the lymphocyte reaching out to the antigens on the covering of the bacterium.

Types of Specific Immunity. Specific immune responses are divided into two types—humoral immunity and cell-mediated immunity. **Humoral immunity** is the formation and activity of short-lived antibodies in the body's "humors," that is, in body fluids. Humoral antibodies are found in blood, lymphatic fluid, lymph nodes, the spleen, spinal fluid, and saliva. The lymphocytes involved in humoral immunity are **B-lymphocytes,** or B-cells. They originate in the bone marrow. They migrate to various lymphoid tissue where they proliferate and differentiate into antibody-secreting cells.

Cell-mediated immunity is controlled by **T-lymphocytes,** or T-cells, which also arise in the bone marrow. While still immature, T-cells migrate to the thymus where they mature and become immunocompetent, that is, capable of responding to foreign invaders. Immunocompetence is indicated by the appearance of antigen-specific receptors on the surfaces of mature T-cells. Immunocompetent T-cells leave the thymus and migrate to the lymph nodes and spleen, where antigens bind to their surface receptors.

This binding event sensitizes the T-cells to grow and multiply rapidly. They soon form an army of identical cells, called clones.

Some members of the T-cell clone become killer T-cells. These kill virus-infected, cancer, or foreign tissue cells by binding to them and releasing toxic chemicals (see Figure 25.2). Other members of the clone become helper T-cells, also called effector T-cells. These interact with B-cells and release chemicals, called lymphokines, that perform a number of immune functions, including:

- stimulating killer T-cells and B-cells to grow and divide
- attracting other types of white blood cells, such as neutrophils, into the area
- enhancing the ability of macrophages to ingest and destroy microorganisms

Finally, a few members of each T-cell clone become memory cells. These are long-lived cells that provide immunological memory of the antigen so

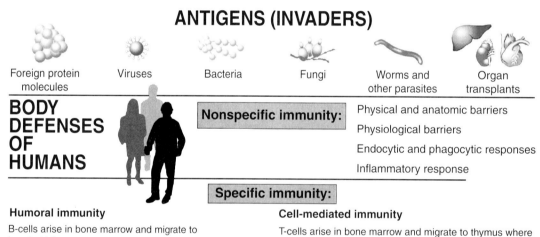

Figure 25.2. How the body defenses of humans attack antigens (invaders).

that the body can respond more quickly to its subsequent invasions. There are also memory B lymphocytes. This is how the immune system "remembers" encounters with foreign invaders.

DISEASES OF THE IMMUNE SYSTEM

Because the immune system is crucial to good health, when it becomes dysfunctional, serious illness usually results. Dysfunctions of the immune system include immunodeficiency, autoimmunity, and hypersensitivity.

✦✦ *Immunodeficiency*

Immunodeficiency, or compromised immune response, is characterized by:

- persistent or recurrent infections by organisms that do not ordinarily cause disease
- incomplete recovery from infections
- undue susceptibility to certain forms of cancer

Some immunodeficiency diseases result from congenital defects that interfere with normal development of the immune system. Others result from acquired conditions that damage the function of the immune system. An example of congenital immunodeficiency is hypogammaglobulinemia, an inherited deficiency of one or more types of immunoglobulin. Examples of acquired immunodeficiency include the weakening of body defenses by severe malnutrition, many types of cancer, and HIV. Immunodeficiency also can result from the administration of immunosuppressant drugs, which are prescribed to prevent rejection of transplanted organs.

✦✦ *Autoimmunity*

Autoimmunity refers to an inappropriate immune response to the wrong antigens—to self instead of nonself. The cause of autoimmune diseases is poorly understood, but several theories have been proposed, including:

- Mutations, viruses, drugs, or injuries alter body tissues so that they are no longer recognized as self.
- Normally inaccessible tissue antigens leak into areas where they come into contact with the immune system and stimulate the production of antibodies.

The inappropriate immune response in an autoimmune disease may be either localized or systemic. Systemic lupus erythematosus (SLE) is a systemic autoimmune disease. Hashimoto's thyroiditis, on the other hand, is localized. It affects just the thyroid gland. These and other human autoimmune diseases and the organs or systems that they affect are listed in Table 25.1.

✦✦ *Hypersensitivity*

Hypersensitivity is exaggerated immune response to foreign antigens. Hypersensitive reactions also are called allergic reactions. They may be systemic or localized.

There are two types of hypersensitivity: immediate hypersensitivity and delayed hypersensitivity. Immediate hypersensitivity, which involves B-cells, occurs within minutes after a sensitive individual is exposed to an antigen. Reactions range from mild to life threatening. Exposure to an antigen may cause temporary, localized hives, for example, or it may cause anaphylaxis, a potentially fatal, systemic hypersensitivity with symptoms of edema and choking. Delayed hypersensitivity, which involves T-cells, develops over a period of twelve to twenty-four hours. It is usually induced by infections of fungi, viruses, bacteria, and other microorganisms.

TABLE 25.1 Human Autoimmune Diseases

Disease	Organ or System Affected
Addison's disease	Adrenal cells
Autoimmune hemolytic anemia	Red blood-cell membrane
Grave's Disease	Thyroid gland
Hashimoto's thyroiditis	Thyroid gland
IDDM	Pancreatic beta cells
Multiple sclerosis (MS)	Central nervous system
Pernicious anemia	Gastric parietal cells
Rheumatoid arthritis	Connective tissue
Spontaneous infertility	Sperm
SLE	Connective tissue, any organ of the body

LABORATORY TESTS UTILIZING IMMUNE REACTIONS

Lab tests that depend on immune reactions for results are called **immunology tests.** Pregnancy, autoimmune diseases, diseases caused by microorganisms, and blood types are among the conditions that can be detected by immunology tests. Simple test kits are used in POLs to test for some of these conditions. Others usually are referred to reference laboratories.

♦ ♦ ♦ Historical Note ♦ ♦ ♦

The first tests involving immune reactions were called serological tests because serum was the body fluid tested when these tests were pioneered at the beginning of this century. Now, other body fluids, cells, tissues, and urine are tested for immune reactions, but the term *serology* is still used interchangeably with *immunology*.

♦♦ *Sensitivity and Specificity*

Immunology tests, like most other lab tests, vary in the accuracy of the results that they produce. Manufacturers often include information in their product inserts about the accuracy of their test products, frequently using the terms *sensitivity* and *specificity*. To judge the accuracy of the tests used in a POL, it is important to be familiar with the meaning of these two terms.

The **sensitivity** of a lab test for a particular disease refers to the ability of the test to identify correctly those who have the disease. If a test has a high degree of sensitivity, virtually all patients who have the disease will test positive. There will be few, if any, false negatives—people who have the disease but test negative—although the test may produce false positives—people who do not have the disease but test positive.

The **specificity** of a lab test for a particular disease refers to the ability of the test to identify correctly those who do not have the disease. If a test has a high degree of specificity, virtually all those who do not have the disease will test negative. There will be few, if any, false positives, although the test may produce false negatives.

The most accurate lab tests are both highly sensitive and highly specific, producing very few false positive or false negative results. Such tests identify vir-

tually everyone who has the disease and seldom if ever misidentify those who do not. Although most tests in POLs are not both highly sensitive and highly specific, they still give useful results when combined with other clinical findings. For example, a quick, inexpensive test with a high degree of sensitivity, but not specificity, may be used to screen individuals who are at risk of a disease. Being highly sensitive, the test is unlikely to produce false negatives, that is, to miss anyone who actually has the disease. False positives can be eliminated with a follow-up test that is more specific—and often more expensive and difficult.

♦ ♦ ♦ Biological ♦ ♦ ♦ False Positives

Biological false positives may be caused by the presence of other diseases, including acute infections, leprosy, and malaria. Biological false positives may persist for a short time or may last for many years. Long-lasting biological false positives may be presymptomatic indicators of collagen disease.

♦♦ *Immunology Tests*

Basically, all immunology tests consist of an antigen-antibody reaction and some form of measurable, often visible, indicator of the reaction. Based on the type of reaction and how it is detected, immunology tests can be placed in the following categories, which are described in detail below:

- *radioimmunoassay:* an antigen binds to a radioactive isotope and the level of radioactivity is measured
- *enzyme-linked immunosorbent assay (ELISA):* an antigen or antibody binds to an enzyme, producing a colored reaction
- *precipitin reaction:* antigen-antibody complexes precipitate out of solution, producing a visible residue
- *agglutinin reaction:* antigen-antibody complexes agglutinate, or clump together, in solution
- *lysin reaction:* antigen-antibody reaction causes lysis of cells

Radioimmunoassay. A radioimmunoassay tags an antigen with a radioactive isotope and then tests its presence or quantity in antigen-antibody reactions. This type of test is extremely sensitive, but it is available for use only in large laboratories.

Enzyme-Linked Immunosorbent Assay. In an enzyme-linked immunosorbent assay (ELISA), an antigen or antibody binds to an enzyme. The enzyme then generates a colored reaction product. The colored reaction may occur in a tube, coated on a dipstick or latex beads, or printed on a membrane. Unlike radioimmunoassays, ELISA tests are simple to use and are available in several different test kits for use in POLs. Tests for HIV and pregnancy, for example, are of the ELISA type.

Precipitin Reactions. Precipitin reactions depend on the formation of a precipitate when the antigen and antibody are in solution together. If a soluble antigen and antibody are placed in solution in optimal amounts, minute flakes or granules precipitate, which are visible to the naked eye. Precipitation may occur in the form of a ring at the bottom of the tube. The size of the ring indicates the quantity of antigen or antibody present, but it is not very precise. Some types of precipitin reactions produce **flocculation,** a precipitate in the form of downy tufts.

♦ ♦ ♦ Note ♦ ♦ ♦

Large amounts of antibody may prevent precipitin reactions from taking a visible form.

Agglutinin Reactions. Agglutinin reactions depend on the formation of clumps of antigen-antibody complexes in solution. Agglutinin reactions are common in tests of bacteria, yeast, and molds. They also occur in blood typing. Agglutinin reactions often are preferred to precipitin reactions because agglutination is easier to see than is precipitation. Agglutinin reactions also are far more sensitive. Precipitin reactions can be converted to agglutinin reactions by adsorbing antigens onto latex beads, red blood cells, or other particles.

Passive agglutinin reactions include an additional step. Two consecutive antigen-antibody reactions are used, the second to test if the first has occurred. Some drug tests use passive agglutinin reactions.

♦ ♦ ♦ Lab Lingo ♦ ♦ ♦

In the lab, immunology tests may be nicknamed "spot," "dot," or "floc" based on how the reaction is read. Make sure that you know which tests are referred to by any slang used in your POL.

Lysin Reactions. In lysin reactions, cells are lysed by an antigen-antibody reaction coupled with complement (serum enzymes). Red blood cells are lysed in transfusions of incompatible blood and in hemolytic disease of the newborn. Lysis also occurs when a bacterial membrane is destroyed by an attacking antibody.

♦ ♦ ♦ Note ♦ ♦ ♦

Different types of tests may be used for the same antigen-antibody reaction. For example, an antigen-antibody reaction that normally causes precipitation may be caused to agglutinate instead by adsorbing antigen into a medium such as latex beads or red blood cells. The same reaction may have an enzyme complex attached to it that changes color when the reaction occurs. The choice of test for a particular antigen-antibody reaction depends on factors like accuracy, simplicity, cost, and time.

♦♦ Quantitative Measurement of Immune Reactions

Most POL immunology tests are qualitative—the results are only positive or negative, indicating presence or absence of an antigen or antibody. To understand the course or severity of disease, sometimes it is important to know the quantity of an antigen or antibody. For example, a positive rheumatoid arthritis agglutination should be retested and reported quantitatively.

Quantitative reports of antigen-antibody reactions are expressed as titers. The **titer** is the highest dilution, or lowest concentration, still capable of producing an observable reaction. For an agglutinin reaction, for example, the titer is the highest dilution capable of producing agglutination.

In determining the titer, dilutions generally are graduated, with each dilution twice as great as the one before. Tubes for the desired number of dilutions are set up, labeled with their dilutions, and the same amount of diluent is added to each. Then, an equal amount of specimen is added to the first tube, producing a 1:2 dilution. After the first tube is mixed, a new pipette is used to move half the solution from the first tube to the second tube, then half the solution from the second tube is moved to the third tube, and so on, until the last tube is reached. Diluting in this manner ensures that each tube is twice as dilute, or half as concentrated, as the tube preceding it. The tubes then have the dilutions 1:2; 1:4, 1:8, 1:16, and so on. An alternative method sometimes used produces dilutions of 1:10, 1:20, 1:40, and so on.

After the dilutions of a positive testing specimen are prepared, each dilution is tested and read for a positive reaction, such as agglutination or color change, depending on the test. The highest dilution that still gives a positive reaction is the titer.

♦♦ *Quality Control*

As with all tests performed in POLs, controls should be run on immunology tests to check reagents and test procedures. Quality-control results of immunology controls should be written in the quality-control records for documentation purposes.

The Use of Controls. Control sera may be supplied with kits or purchased separately. To augment these, sera from positive patients sometimes are saved for use as controls. Both positive and negative controls should be run daily or with each batch of patient samples. Positive controls indicate if the test is working. Negative controls show if reactions are caused by some substance other than test sera. Both positive and negative controls also are used as standards for reading patient-test results.

Batch Size. Batches of tests must not be so large that there is too great a time lag between the reading of the first and last specimens. If there is a difference in the readings of controls run at the beginning and end of the batch, the batch size should be reduced.

The Manufacturer's Instructions. POL tests are researched thoroughly by large research laboratories, and manufacturer's instructions must be followed precisely to ensure accurate patient-test results. Variables such as temperature, humidity, and lighting must be as close as possible to those recommended by the manufacturer.

Most antigen-antibody tests must be performed at room temperature, so reagents and patient specimens must be allowed to come to room temperature before testing. If the climate is extremely dry, the humidity level may have to be increased.

Lighting is important for reading test results accurately. A black background is best for reading the agglutination of white latex beads, for example, while a white background is best for reading agglutination of dark colors. Reflected light usually is specified, but lighted translucent panels are used in reading blood-type agglutinations.

Other Considerations. Cross-contamination between patient specimens and controls must be avoided by using separate stirrers and pipettes for each specimen and control. Toothpicks or wooden applicator sticks may be used as disposable stirrers. Care must be taken to replace the correct caps on reagent bottles, because switching caps also can produce cross-contamination.

Reagents should be mixed well but not overmixed or shaken too vigorously, especially if the reagent is fragile. Latex beads and blood cells have protein coatings that may be damaged if mixing is too vigorous.

Patient specimens should not be lipemic or hemolyzed. If test results are questionable for particular specimens, they should be retested using the same method or a different method, or they should be sent to a referral laboratory for testing. If questions still remain, the manufacturer of the test kit or reagent should be contacted for assistance.

♦♦ *Conditions Tested With Antigen-Antibody Test Kits*

Producing the reagents needed for tests of antigen-antibody reactions is beyond the scope of POLs, so test kits from medical supply houses are used. Table 25.2 lists some of the immunology tests for which kits are available.

TABLE 25.2 Antigen-Antibody Test Kits Available for Use in POLs

Test	Disease or Condition
hCG	Pregnancy (hormone)
RPR (rapid plasma reagin)	Syphilis (bacteria)
Epstein–Barr (Heterophile antibodies)	Infectious mononucleosis (virus)
GAS (Group A strep)	Strep throat (bacteria)
GBS (Group B strep)	Neonate infection (bacteria)
Rheumatoid arthritis factor	Rheumatoid arthritis (autoimmunity)
Respiratory syncytial virus	Respiratory infection (virus)
Herpes simplex I and *II*	Cold sores and genital ulcers (virus)
Chlamydia	Sexually transmitted disease (bacteria)
Lyme disease	Disease transmitted by ticks (bacteria)
Allergens (miscellaneous)	Hypersensitivity (immunity)
Autoimmune antibodies	Systemic lupus erythematosus (autoimmunity)
Candida	Yeast infections (fungus)
C-reactive protein (CRP)	Acute inflammatory condition
Rubella	Rubella (German measles) (virus)
Febrile agglutinations	Typhoid, paratyphoid, brucellosis, Proteus infections, tularemia (bacteria)

♦ ♦ ♦ Storing Test Kits ♦ ♦ ♦

Many immunology test kits should be stored in the refrigerator between uses, but some may be stored at room temperature. Refrigerated kits generally have a longer period of use before the expiration date. Always check the expiration date and discard out-of-date test kits.

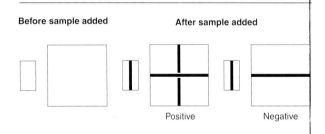

Figure 25.3. Test results from ready-purchased kits are easy to read. This pregnancy test result after sample is added shows up as the color development of a plus (+) or minus (−) sign. The control window at the left produces a colored straight line which shows that the test has been completed and has worked correctly. Some kits use a system of development of colored dots.

Pregnancy. Pregnancy can be ascertained as early as ten days after conception by testing for **human chorionic gonadotropin (hCG)**, a hormone produced by the chorionic villi of the placenta (see Figure 25.3). Most commercial test kits for this hormone use the ELISA method on either serum or urine specimens. Several pregnancy tests may be run at once, but separate pipettes must be used. Otherwise, hCG may be transferred from one test pad to another.

If urine is used, a first morning specimen is preferred because it contains higher levels of hCG, but any random specimen may be used. Urine should be collected in a clean, dry glass or plastic container. If serum is used, the specimen must not be hemolyzed. For both serum and urine, the specimen should be tested immediately, refrigerated for up to forty-eight hours, or frozen for later testing.

Chlamydia. The bacterial disease **chlamydia** is thought to be the most prevalent sexually transmitted disease in the United States. It also may be transmitted to infants from infected mothers through direct contact during or after birth. Chlamydia causes both urogenital disease and eye disease. Worldwide, it is the single leading cause of blindness. Because chlamydia is a bacterial disease, infections can be cured with broad-spectrum antibiotics and sulfonamides. However, chlamydia is hard to diagnose. The bacteria are very small and live only within the host's cells. An ELISA test now is available for chlamydia testing in POLs.

Strep Throat. Strep throat is caused by Group A strep (GAS), a hemolytic strain of *Streptococcus* bacteria that causes strep throat and, less commonly, rheumatic fever, an autoimmune disease. The latter may lead to endocarditis, or inflammation of the inner lining of the heart, and permanent damage to the heart valves. Other organs, including the kidneys and nerves, also may be affected. Without prompt treatment of the original strep infection with antibiotics, autoimmune disease may result.

The GAS test is an ELISA test that is easy to perform, but the steps must be followed precisely. Care should be taken not to mix up the reagents or use them out of order. First, the throat is swabbed with a sterile, nonabsorbent dacron-fiber or calcium-alginate swab. A cotton-tipped swab should not be used because cotton fibers may interfere with growth of strep organisms. The swab is inserted into a small container supplied with the kit, which treats the swab with reagents to extract the strep antigen. Then, the swab is discarded, the contents of the container are inserted into the ELISA test well, and the results are read.

> ♦ ♦ ♦ **Note** ♦ ♦ ♦
>
> Group B strep (GBS) is the nonhemolytic strain of *Streptococcus* that causes severe infections in newborns and infants. There is a separate test for this pathogen.

Infectious Mononucleosis. Also called "mono" and abbreviated IM, this serious disease most often affects teenagers and young adults. Because it is thought to be transmitted orally, infectious mononucleosis is sometimes also called the "kissing disease." It is caused by the Epstein–Barr virus, and it has flulike symptoms, including fever, fatigue, weakness, swollen lymph nodes, sore throat, and headache. Symptoms may be prolonged and lead to involvement of the liver, spleen, or other organs.

There are two types of lab tests for mononucleosis. The easiest is a screening test, which is used in POLs. It involves agglutination of the mononucleosis antibody on a slide. The other test is more difficult and likely to be performed in a larger laboratory. It uses lysis of blood cells through several dilutions of serum to give the titer of the heterophile antibody, which reacts with the Epstein–Barr virus. The screening test, if positive, often is followed by the titer test.

> ♦ ♦ ♦ **Note** ♦ ♦ ♦
>
> The infectious mononucleosis antibody may be present even in the absence of symptoms. This may occur for several months after the acute, febrile phase of the illness has passed or if the case is subclinical.

Syphilis. The devastating STD **syphilis** is caused by the spirochete, or spiral bacterium, *Treponema pallidum*. Without antibiotic treatment, syphilis persists for many years, leading to involvement of many organs and systems and, ultimately, death.

The immune system produces complex antibodies to the bacteria, and these provide the basis for the diagnostic tests. Two screening tests used in POLs are the RPR, rapid plasma reagin, and the VDRL, named for the Venereal Disease Research Laboratory. Both are flocculation tests that require a mechanical rotator.

False positives are frequent with syphilis screening tests, so positive results generally are verified with more accurate tests performed in larger laboratories. False positives may be caused by malaria, advanced pulmonary tuberculosis, pregnancy, or old age. False negatives also occur. They may be caused by a nonfunctioning immune system, alcohol consumption, or syphilis infection that is too recent to have triggered antibody production.

Rheumatoid Arthritis. A chronic systemic disease, **rheumatoid arthritis (RA)**, is characterized by inflammatory changes in joints and related structures that result in crippling deformities. The specific cause of rheumatoid arthritis is unknown, but generally it is thought that the pathological changes in the joints are related to an autoimmune antigen-antibody reaction.

The diagnostic test for rheumatoid arthritis detects the presence of rheumatoid factor, an immunoglobulin (IgM) found in the sera of many rheumatoid arthritis patients. The test uses agglutination on a latex-fixation slide to detect the presence of the immunoglobulin. False positives may be caused by acute viral infections and old age. When the rheumatoid arthritis test is positive, the serum is diluted and retested, and the result is reported as a titer.

Systemic Lupus Erythematosus. Systemic lupus erythematosus (SLE) is an inflammatory disorder primarily affecting women ages twenty to forty years. Depending on the severity of the disease, almost any organ of the body may be affected. SLE is considered to be an autoimmune disease that arises spontaneously, but viral infections and certain drugs also may be causal factors.

Laboratory tests for patients with SLE show a decrease in WBC and RBC counts and in the platelet count, along with an increased sed rate. Diagnosis is confirmed by positive test results for the presence of antinuclear antibodies (ANA).

Lyme Disease. Lyme disease is caused by the spirochete *Borrelia burgdorferi,* which is transmitted from host to host by small deer ticks. Symptoms, which are not definitive of Lyme disease, include fever, severe headache, fatigue, and muscle aches. Without antibiotic treatment, the disease may progress to arthritis and involvement of the heart and nervous system. Diagnosis is made with an ELISA test.

Herpes. Herpes is the common name for diseases caused by herpesvirus, a family of viruses including those that cause cold sores *(Herpes simplex I),* genital ulcers *(Herpes simplex II),* shingles *(Herpes zoster),* and chicken pox *(Varicella).* After the primary infection, herpesvirus may remain dormant for years and then establish a latent infection. The virus lives within the nerve cells, where it is protected from the immune system. It may become activated by any of a variety of factors, including stress, trauma, allergic reactions, and illness. Once activated, the virus multiplies and emerges as a sore on the skin. Cold sores commonly occur around the mouth. Genital ulcers occur on the penis in the male and on the perineum, vagina, and cervix in the female. Genital herpes is a sexually transmitted disease. An ELISA test is available for diagnosing active herpes. The procedure is similar to that for the GAS test described earlier.

Rubella. Rubella, or German measles, is a mild systemic disease caused by the *Rubella* virus. Symptoms include slight fever, drowsiness, swollen lymph nodes, sore throat, and a characteristic rash. The disease is similar to but generally milder than rubeola (measles). If a woman contracts rubella during the first trimester of pregnancy, the virus may damage the fetus, producing mental retardation, microcephaly, deafness, cardiac abnormalities, or generalized growth retardation. A latex agglutination card test is available to POLs to test for rubella.

Yeast Infections. *Candida,* a genus of yeastlike fungus, is part of the normal flora of the mouth, skin, intestinal tract, and vagina, but an overgrowth of *Candida* causes pathology. It may cause persistent vaginal yeast infections in females. In infants and young children it may cause yeast infections of the mouth and throat, a condition called thrush. A latex agglutination test is available for detection of the presence of *Candida.*

Inflammatory Conditions. The acute stage of various inflammatory disorders is characterized by an abnormal glycoprotein, called **C-reactive protein** (**CRP**). CRP is a general test for inflammation and is useful when correlated with other diagnostic information. A latex agglutination test is available for CRP testing in POLs.

Hemolytic Disease of the Newborn. Also known as *erythroblastosis fetalis*, hemolytic disease of the newborn (HDN) causes severe jaundice in newborns and may result in stunted growth, mental retardation, or death. The cause of HDN was unknown until the discovery of the **Rhesus (Rh) blood group.** It generally occurred only in second and succeeding pregnancies, not firstborn infants. It is now known that HDN is due to a blood-type incompatibility between mother and fetus. Rhesus antigen in the Rh positive fetus stimulates production of maternal antibodies in the Rh negative woman, who lacks the antigen. The maternal antibodies may cause severe hemolysis of fetal blood and high levels of bilirubin by the time of birth. Severely affected infants must be given a blood exchange to replace the hemolyzed blood with normal blood.

HDN has a chance of occurring whenever an Rh negative woman has a child with an Rh positive man because there may be an accidental exchange of blood between fetus and mother. Pregnant women routinely have Rhesus blood-type determinations to see if they are Rhesus negative and thus at risk for HDN. If the father tests negative for Rhesus antigen, there is no risk. If the father tests Rh positive, then the woman should be given HDN vaccine to prevent HDN in future pregnancies.

HDN vaccine contains antibodies from Rh negative individuals who have been sensitized to the Rh antigen. The vaccine is given to the Rh negative mother immediately after the birth of her first Rh positive child, before her immune system has had time to develop antibodies to the Rhesus antigen. As a result of the vaccine, the Rh negative mother's immune system does not produce the antibodies itself and develops no "memory" for the antigen. The vaccine antibodies are short lived so that, by the time of the next pregnancy, the woman no longer has circulating Rhesus antibodies.

Coomb's Test. Coomb's test, also known as the antiglobulin test, is used for monitoring the development of Rh incompatibility in at-risk pregnant women. It detects the presence of antierythrocyte antibodies on their red blood cells. If antibodies are present, red blood cells have been sensitized in vivo to the D antigen, and their fetuses are at risk of HDN.

The red blood cells of the patient are washed in a saline solution to remove the plasma, which has interfering substances. Then the red blood cells are mixed with antiglobulin serum that has been obtained from a medical supply house, centrifuged, and

checked for agglutination. Agglutination indicates that antibodies are present and sensitization has occurred. When the test result is negative, the sample is left for a few minutes at room temperature and then recentrifuged. If there is still no agglutination, a negative test result is reported. A control of red blood cells known to be sensitized is tested along with the patient's cells.

◆◆

CLINICALLY IMPORTANT INHERITED BLOOD TYPES

The Rhesus blood group is one of two clinically important inherited blood groups. The other is the **ABO blood group.** Although there are many other inherited blood groups, these two cause most of the problems with incompatibility.

When a transfusion of Rh positive blood is given to an Rh negative sensitized patient, the same hemolytic reaction may occur as the one just described for hemolytic disease of the newborn. In this case, the Rh negative individual most likely was sensitized by a previous transfusion of Rh positive blood. An Rh negative patient can receive only one exposure to Rh positive blood without a notable transfusion reaction. Therefore, only Rh negative blood can be given safely.

Exposure to incompatible ABO blood-group antigens occurs in ways in addition to transfusions of incompatible blood. By adulthood, most of us are sensitized to antigens of incompatible ABO blood types through exposure to bacteria that contain the same antigenic molecules.

In POLs, slide tests are sufficient for typing the ABO and Rhesus blood groups for diagnostic purposes. In blood banks, where blood is prepared for transfusions, a more complete analysis of blood compatibility is necessary. This includes tube typing and tube cross-matches, which analyze both antigens and antibodies. Blood transfusions are prepared only by qualified technicians with specialized training in blood banking.

◆◆ *Understanding Blood Types*

To understand why some blood types are compatible and others are not, you need to know more about the ABO and Rhesus blood groups. Keep in mind that Rh incompatibility must be considered separately from ABO incompatibility. A patient's own blood type is always preferred for a transfusion.

TABLE 25.3 Compatible ABO Blood Types

Recipient ABO Blood Type	Recipient Antigens	Recipient Antibodies	Compatible Donor Blood Types
AB	A, B	None	AB, A, B, O
A	A	B	A, O
B	B	A	B, O
O	None	A, B	O

Other blood types, if compatible, may be substituted during emergencies or shortages.

ABO. The ABO blood group has four different blood types—A, B, AB, and O. The letters signify the type of antigen that each type of blood has on the surface membranes of its red blood cells. Type A blood has A antigen, type B blood B antigen, and type AB blood has A and B antigens equally. Type O blood has neither type A antigen nor type B antigen.

People with blood types A, B, and O produce antibodies against the antigens they do not carry—type A against antigen B, type B against antigen A, and type O against antigens A and B. Therefore, patients with type A blood never should receive transfusions of type B or AB blood. Similarly, patients with type B blood cannot receive type A blood or type AB blood, and type O patients cannot receive type A, B, or AB blood. As Table 25.3 shows, Type O blood can be accepted by anyone. This is because it lacks both A antigens and B antigens. It is also why type O people are called universal donors. By contrast, people of type AB blood can accept blood of any type because they produce no antibodies. This is why they are called universal recipients.

Rhesus. The Rhesus blood group antigens are controlled by three closely linked pairs of genes. The antigens are grouped as follows:

- *C, D, and E:* called Rh positive factors because they produce an antibody response
- *c and e:* called Rh negative factors because they do not cause an antibody response

Antigen D is the most common and causes the strongest antibody reaction, so it is the most significant clinically. People with antigen D are called Rh positive; people without it are called Rh negative. About 15 percent of Euro-Americans are Rh negative. People with Rh negative blood cannot receive blood transfusions of Rh positive blood. People with Rh positive blood, on the other hand, can receive transfusions of either Rh positive or Rh negative blood (see Table 25.4).

TABLE 25.4 Compatible and Incompatible Rhesus Blood Types

Recipient Rhesus Blood Type	Recipient Antigen	Recipient Antibodies	Compatible Donor Rh Blood Types
Rh positive	D	None	Rh positive & Rh negative
Rh negative	None	Anti-D	Rh negative only

TABLE 25.5 Slide Reactions to Commercial Typing Antisera

Patient Blood Type	Anti-A-Sera	Anti-B-Sera	Rh Positive Sera
A positive	Agglutinated	—	Agglutinated
B positive	—	Agglutinated	Agglutinated
AB positive	Agglutinated	Agglutinated	Agglutinated
O positive	—	—	Agglutinated
A negative	Agglutinated	—	—
B negative	—	Agglutinated	—
AB negative	Agglutinated	Agglutinated	—
O negative	—	—	—

◆◆ *Testing for Blood Type*

POL tests for blood type are based on agglutinin reactions because blood-group antigen-antibody complexes normally agglutinate.

ABO and Rhesus Blood Types. ABO and Rhesus blood types usually are tested in POLs by the slide method. A drop of blood cells, either fresh or suspended in their plasma, is mixed with commercial antiserum and inspected for agglutination. Table 25.5 and Figure 25.4 show agglutination of different blood types.

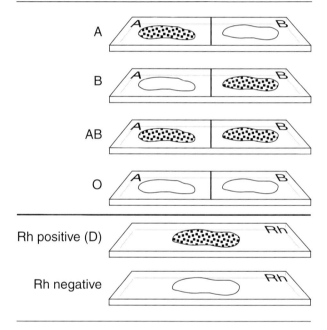

Figure 25.4. The agglutination of different ABO and Rhesus blood types with antisera.

PROCEDURE

25.1

Infectious Mononucleosis Agglutination Test

Goal
- After successfully completing this procedure, you will be able to use a commercial agglutination kit (Hycor Serascan Infectious Mononucleosis) to test for the presence of antibodies specific for infectious mononucleosis.

Completion Time
- 15 minutes

Equipment and Supplies
- disposable latex gloves
- impermeable jacket, gown, or apron
- hand disinfectant
- surface disinfectant
- paper towels and tissues
- biohazard container
- patient serum or citrated plasma sample
- commercial test kit for infectious mononucleosis
- positive and negative infectious mononucleosis controls
- paper and pencil

Instructions
Read through the list of equipment and supplies that you will need and the steps of the procedure. Be sure that you understand each step before you begin. Then complete each step correctly and in the proper order. If your completion time is too long, repeat the procedure until you increase your speed.

S = Satisfactory	U = Unsatisfactory	S	U
1. Put on a protective jacket, gown, or apron; wash your hands with disinfectant, dry them, and put on gloves.			

S = Satisfactory   U = Unsatisfactory   S   U

2. Follow the Universal Precautions.

3. Collect and prepare the appropriate equipment.

4. Verify the identification of the patient sample and label the container.

5. Unfold the test-kit instructions, ready for use. Lay the slides, pipettes, and applicator sticks from the test kit on the counter.

6. Allow the patient sample and the controls, reagents, and other test-kit materials to come to room temperature.

7. Fill the capillary pipette from the test kit two-thirds full with the patient sample.

8. Hold the capillary pipette in a perpendicular position about 1 inch above one section of the slide. Then deliver a free-falling drop of patient sample onto the slide.

9. Gently mix the positive control by inverting and squeezing the polyethylene container. Then hold it in a perpendicular position about 1 inch above another section of the slide and deliver a free-falling drop of the positive control onto the slide.

10. Repeat step 9 with the negative control.

11. Resuspend the infectious mononucleosis reagent by mixing the suspension gently until it is homogeneous, without apparent sediment.

12. Using the dropper assembly provided with the kit, add one drop of the reagent to each of the controls and to the patient sample.

13. Using separate stirrers for each sample, mix the patient and control sera with the reagent in a circular manner over the entire area of each section of the slide. Discard the stirrers into the biohazardous waste container.

14. Tilt the slide back and forth for one minute.

15. Place the slide on a flat surface and allow it to stand motionless for one minute. Do not move the slide.

16. After one minute, examine the samples for macroscopic agglutination with the naked eye under a reflected light.

17. Compare the patient sample with those of both controls. The positive control should show strong agglutination, and the negative control should show no agglutination. Refer to the manufacturer's insert for further information on assessing agglutination.

18. If no agglutination is present in the patient sample, report it as negative. If agglutination is present, report the agglutination of the patient sample from 1+ to 4+, where 1+ is the smallest, weakest clumping and 4+ is the largest clumping, with clear fluid in the background.

19. Disinfect the test slide and rinse it with distilled or deionized water; allow the test slide to dry for reuse with the kit. Do not use detergent on the slide, because the residue interferes with test results.

20. Replace the controls and reagent in the kit and store the kit in the refrigerator.

21. Discard disposable equipment in the biohazard container.

22. Disinfect other equipment and return it to storage.

23. Clean the work area, following the Universal Precautions.

24. Remove your jacket, gown, or apron, and gloves; wash your hands with disinfectant, and dry them.

OVERALL PROCEDURAL EVALUATION

Student's Name _____

Signature of Instructor _____ **Date** _____

Comments

PROCEDURE

25.2 ◆ **ELISA Pregnancy Test**

Goal

- After successfully completing this procedure, you will be able to prepare and perform a human chorionic gonadotropin (hCG) determination with urine for early detection of pregnancy by the ELISA method.

Completion Time

- 15 minutes

Equipment and Supplies

- disposable latex gloves
- impermeable jacket, gown, or apron
- hand disinfectant
- surface disinfectant
- paper towels and tissues
- biohazard container
- Abbott Testpack or another ELISA-type pregnancy test kit
- patient urine or serum sample
- paper and pencil

Instructions

Read through the list of equipment and supplies that you will need and the steps of the procedure. Be sure that you understand each step before you begin. Then complete each step correctly and in the proper order. If your completion time is too long, repeat the procedure until you increase your speed.

S = Satisfactory U = Unsatisfactory	S	U
1. Put on a protective jacket, gown, or apron; wash your hands with disinfectant, dry them, and put on gloves.		
2. Follow the Universal Precautions.		

3. Collect and prepare the appropriate equipment.

4. Verify the identification of the patient sample and label the container.

5. Remove the pregnancy test kit from the protective pouch and place it on a flat, dry surface.

6. Use the disposable transfer pipette supplied with the kit to dispense three drops of urine or serum into the sample well.

7. Wait until a red color appears in the "End of Assay" window (in approximately four minutes for urine).

8. Immediately read the test result window: a plus sign (+) indicates that the urine contains elevated levels of hCG; a minus sign (−) indicates absence of detectable hCG. Interpret any color on the vertical (patient) bar as positive for hCG.

9. If no color is visible in the "End of Assay" window or if the + /− indicator cannot be read in the test result window, retest the sample.

10. Complete the necessary information on the laboratory report.

11. Dispose of the patient sample and disposable equipment following waste disposal guidelines for biohazardous waste.

12. Disinfect other equipment and return it to storage.

13. Clean the work area, following the Universal Precautions.

14. Remove your jacket, gown, or apron, and gloves; wash your hands with disinfectant, and dry them.

OVERALL PROCEDURAL EVALUATION

Student's Name _____

Signature of Instructor _____ **Date** _____

Comments

PROCEDURE

25.3 ## ABO and Rhesus Blood-Type Determination

Goal

- After successfully completing this procedure, you will be able to prepare and perform individual blood types for ABO (Part A) and Rhesus (Part B) blood groups.

Completion Time

- 20 minutes (both parts)

Equipment and Supplies

- disposable latex gloves
- impermeable jacket, gown, or apron
- hand disinfectant
- surface disinfectant
- paper towels and tissues
- biohazard container
- glass microscope slides
- disposable wooden applicators or toothpicks
- commercial antisera for blood typing (anti-A, anti-B, and anti-Rh)
- view box with built-in light
- watch with second hand
- wax pencil
- Pasteur pipette
- blood sample
- paper and pencil

Instructions

Read through the list of equipment and supplies that you will need and the steps of the procedure. Be sure that you understand each step before you begin. Then complete each step correctly and in the proper order. If your completion time is too long, repeat the procedure until you increase your speed.

S = Satisfactory   U = Unsatisfactory

	S	U

1. Put on a protective jacket, gown, or apron; wash your hands with disinfectant, dry them, and put on gloves.

2. Follow the Universal Precautions.

3. Collect and prepare the appropriate equipment.

4. Verify the identification of the specimen and label the container.

❖❖ *Part 1: ABO Blood Type*

5. Divide a clean glass slide into two equal parts with a wax pencil and label the left side "A" and the right side "B," as in the illustration.

6. Holding the dropper about one-half inch from the slide, place a drop of A antiserum on the left (A) side of the slide. Do not contaminate the dropper by letting it touch the slide.

7. In the same way, place a drop of B antiserum on the right (B) side of the slide. Do not contaminate the dropper by letting it touch the slide.

8. Using a Pasteur pipette, place a drop of blood beside the antiserum on the left side of the slide; the drop should be about the same size as the drop of antiserum. Again, do not contaminate the pipette by letting it touch the slide or antiserum.

9. Repeat step 8 for the right side of the slide.

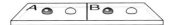

10. Using a circular motion and a disposable wooden applicator, thoroughly mix
    the blood and A antiserum together on the left side of the slide. Then dispose
    of the applicator in the biohazard container.

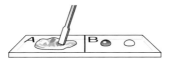

11. Repeat step 10 for the right side of the slide, using a new disposable wooden
    applicator.

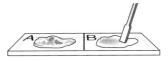

12. Turn on the view box and note the time.

13. Rock the slide gently back and forth for two minutes while observing the cells
    for agglutination. (*Note:* if a view box is unavailable, improvise with a strong
    light).

14. If agglutination occurs on the left side only, record the blood type on the
    laboratory report as type A. If agglutination occurs on the B side only, record
    the blood type as type B. If agglutination occurs on both sides, record the
    blood as type AB. If there is no agglutination on either side, record the blood
    as type O.

15. Discard the glass slide in the biohazard container.

❖❖ *Part 2: Rhesus Blood Type*

16. With a wax pencil, label a clean, dry glass slide with "Rh," as shown in the
    illustration.

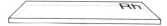

17. Holding the dropper about one-half inch from the slide, place a drop of Rh (D) antiserum on the slide. Do not contaminate the dropper by touching it to the slide.

18. Using a Pasteur pipette, place a drop of blood beside the Rh (D) antiserum. Make the drop of blood the same size as the drop of antiserum. Do not contaminate the pipette by letting it touch the slide or the antiserum.

19. Using a circular motion and a disposable wooden applicator stick, thoroughly mix the blood and the antiserum together on the slide. Then dispose of the wooden applicator in the biohazard container.

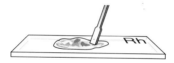

20. Check to see that the view box (or strong light) is on and note temperature. The surface temperature of the view box should be between 40 and 50 degrees Celsius. Place the slide on the warm view box, which should bring the slide to approximately 37 degrees Celsius.

21. For two minutes, rock the slide gently back and forth while observing the cells for agglutination.

22. If agglutination occurs, record the blood type as Rh positive on the laboratory report. If no agglutination occurs, record the blood type as Rh negative.

23. Dispose of the patient sample and disposable equipment following waste disposal guidelines for biohazardous waste.

S = Satisfactory	U = Unsatisfactory	S	U

24. **Refrigerate the antisera.**

25. **Disinfect other equipment and return it to storage.**

26. **Clean the work area following the Universal Precautions.**

27. **Remove your jacket, gown, or apron, and gloves; wash your hands with disinfectant, and dry them.**

OVERALL PROCEDURAL EVALUATION

Student's Name _____

Signature of Instructor _____ **Date** _____

Comments

Using Terminology

Match the term in the right column with the appropriate definition or description in the left column.

_____ 1. allergy	a. B-lymphocytes
_____ 2. antiglobulin test	b. Coomb's test
_____ 3. an autoimmune disease	c. CRP
_____ 4. cell-mediated immunity	d. flocculation
_____ 5. C-reactive protein	e. hCG
_____ 6. downy tufts	f. hypersensitivity
_____ 7. humoral immunity	g. immunodeficiency
_____ 8. increased susceptibility to disease	h. RA
_____ 9. rapid plasma reagin	i. RPR
_____ 10. pregnancy hormone	j. T-lymphocytes

Acquiring Knowledge

Mark the following statements as true or false and rewrite the false statements to make them true.

11. Specific immunity is the general resistance to disease that characterizes a particular species.

_____

_____

_____

12. Interferon is a protein that helps protect uninfected cells from viral infection.

_____

_____

13. Innate immunity refers to immunity acquired after exposure to a foreign invader.

_____

_____

14. Foreign substances that provoke a specific immune reaction are called antibodies.

_____

_____

15. B-cells are involved in humoral immunity.

_____

_____

16. A few members of each T-cell clone become memory cells.

_____

17. The sensitivity of a lab test for a particular disease refers to the ability of the test to identify correctly those who do not have the disease.

_____

_____

18. False positives are people who have the disease but do not test positive.

_____

_____

19. In a radioimmunoassay, an antigen binds to a radioactive isotope and the level of radioactivity is measured.

_____

_____

20. In determining titer, dilutions are graduated, with each dilution three times as great as the one before.

_____

_____

Answer the following questions in the spaces provided.

21. What are four types of nonspecific immune defenses in humans?

_____

_____

_____

22. What role do physical and anatomical barriers play in defending bodies from microorganisms? What are some examples?

_____

_____

_____

_____

_____

23. What are the physiological barriers of nonspecific immunity?

_____

_____

_____

24. Describe the inflammatory response.

_____

_____

_____

25. What is the role of antigen-antibody reactions in specific immunity?

_____

_____

_____

_____

_____

26. Distinguish between humoral immunity and cell-mediated immunity.

_____

_____

_____

_____

_____

_____

27. What is autoimmunity and what are some possible causes?

_____

_____

_____

_____

_____

_____

28. What conditions may bring about immunodeficiency?

_____

_____

_____

29. What characterizes patients with immunodeficiency?

_____

_____

_____

_____

30. What distinguishes immediate hypersensitivity and delayed hypersensitivity?

_____

_____

31. How do sensitivity and specificity relate to accuracy?

_____

_____

_____

_____

_____

_____

_____

_____

_____

32. For each of the following types of immunology tests, describe the reaction that occurs and give one example of a disease or condition that is diagnosed with that type of test: a. ELISA, b. precipitin reaction, c. agglutinin reaction, d. lysin reaction.

_____

_____

_____

_____

_____

_____

33. How are immune reactions measured quantitatively?

_____

_____

_____

_____

_____

34. Discuss quality control in immunology testing in POLs.

_____

_____

_____

_____

_____

35. Describe the ABO blood group, including all of the antigens and blood types.

_____

_____

_____

36. Which ABO blood types may donate to which types?

_____

_____

_____

_____

37. Describe the Rhesus blood group and blood types.

_____

_____

_____

_____

38. What Rhesus blood types can be received by an Rh positive patient? by an Rh negative patient?

_____

_____

_____

39. When and why does hemolytic disease of the newborn (HDN) occur?

_____

_____

_____

_____

_____

40. List four diseases or conditions that are tested by immunological methods.

_____

_____

_____

_____

41. Why is blood typed for Rh in POLs?

_____

_____

42. What causes the color reaction in an ELISA test?

_____

43. What is the most common sexually transmitted disease?

_____

Applying Knowledge—On the Job

Answer the following questions in the spaces provided.

44. You have just received a request for a rheumatoid arthritis test. What controls should you run with the patient test to be certain that the reagents are reacting as they should?

_____

_____

_____

45. A teenage patient came to the laboratory for a CBC, blood chemistries, and an immunology test. He has been very sick with flulike symptoms and is not recovering well. When you examine the stained blood differential slide you find many large, abnormal lymphocytes. What antigen-antibody test might the physician order to help diagnose this patient's condition?

_____

_____

46. A small child has been brought to the laboratory for a throat smear. The mother told you that the physician prescribed antibiotics to prevent a possible occurrence of rheumatic fever. What bacterial infection does the physician suspect? What immunology test might the physician order to diagnose it?

_____

_____

47. One of your patients has just submitted urine for a pregnancy test. What hormone will you test for?

_____

_____

48. One of the patients in the clinic received an allergy shot, and in just a few minutes she began to choke from severe edema of the larynx. What type of reaction did the patient have?

_____

49. You have just typed a pregnant woman's blood for both ABO and Rhesus blood groups. There were no agglutinations. What is her blood type?

_____

COGNITIVE OBJECTIVES

After studying this chapter, you should be able to

- use each of the vocabulary terms appropriately.
- explain the relevance of microbiology to POLs.
- describe how infectious diseases are diagnosed.
- list the reasons that viral diseases often are difficult to diagnose and treat.
- discuss differences that aid in the identification of bacteria species.
- describe the requirements of bacterial growth.
- discuss the role of sensitivity testing in selecting antibiotics for bacterial infections.
- identify several human diseases caused by fungal, protozoan, and helminth microorganisms.
- list aseptic techniques for working with microorganisms in POLs and explain why these techniques are important.

PERFORMANCE OBJECTIVES

After studying this chapter, you should be able to

- prepare a heat-fixed bacterial smear.
- prepare a Gram stain from an unstained bacterial smear.
- examine a prepared Gram-stained smear and classify the microorganisms by their morphology and Gram-stain reaction.

TERMINOLOGY

antibiotic: a drug administered to kill or inhibit the growth of bacteria.

aseptic technique: a lab technique that ensures the isolation of pathogenic microorganisms, including personal protective equipment and sterilization.

bacillus: a rod-shaped bacterium. Bacilli include the bacteria that cause tuberculosis and diphtheria.

bacitracin: an antibiotic used in cultures to give an early indication of the presence of Group A strep.

bacteria: single-celled microorganisms in the kingdom *Monera*. Bacteria cause many different infections in humans.

catalase test: the lab test in which hydrogen peroxide is added to urine cultures to distinguish strep from staph infections.

coagulase test: the lab test that demonstrates the presence of an enzyme produced by pathogenic staph organisms, thereby distinguishing them from nonpathogenic strains of staph.

coccus: a spherical or oval bacterium. Cocci include *Streptococcus* and *Staphylococcus*.

direct culture: a primary culture; a culture grown by inoculating patient specimens directly onto the culture medium.

fastidious bacterium: a bacterium that has very precise nutritional and environmental requirements for growth, including *Niesseria gonor-rhoeae.*

fungus: a plant of the phylum *Fungi,* which lacks chlorophyll. Fungi are microorganisms that include yeasts and molds, some of which cause disease.

gram negative: bacteria that stain pink or red with Gram stain, including *Escherichia coli* and *Neisseria gonorrhoeae.*

gram positive: bacteria that stain deep purple with Gram stain, such as staph and strep organisms.

Gram stain: the most commonly used stain for bacterial smears. Gram stain separates organisms into two clinically meaningful groups—gram-negative organisms and gram-positive organisms.

helminth: a true worm. Several species parasitize the human intestinal tract, including tapeworms and hookworms.

microbiology: the branch of science that studies microscopic organisms.

oxidase test: the lab test in which oxidase reagent is added to a colony of suspected *Niesseria gonorrhoeae* to confirm the presence of this organism.

protozoan: a single-celled animal. Several species of protozoa are pathogenic to humans, including *Giardia lamblia.*

pure culture: a culture that is grown from a single colony of bacteria, which was taken from a direct culture. A pure culture serves to further isolate the pathogen.

spiral bacteria: bacteria that include the bacteria that causes syphilis and Lyme disease.

urinary tract infection (UTI): an infection of the urinary tract caused by any of several different bacteria. A UTI is diagnosed when the urine bacteria concentration exceeds 100,000 organisms per milliliter.

virus: a simple organism that causes many diseases in humans, including colds and herpes. Viruses live and reproduce within the cells of a host.

● ● ● ● ● ● ● ● ● ● ● ● ● ● ● ● ●

Microbiology is the branch of science that studies microscopic organisms. This chapter shows how microbiology is relevant to POLs, describes disease-causing microorganisms, and outlines microbiology procedures.

◆ ◆

MICROBIOLOGY

The relevance of microbiology to POLs lies primarily in isolating and identifying disease-causing microorganisms. This is necessary for diagnosis and treatment of many infectious diseases.

◆◆ *How Infectious Diseases Are Diagnosed*

As is true with any disease, when a patient presents with an infectious disease, signs and symptoms often provide physicians with a tentative diagnosis. For example, measles, a viral disease, often is diagnosed by its characteristic rash.

A tentative diagnosis may be followed up with a lab test to confirm the diagnosis. A simple blood test may confirm the presence of a virus through detection of an antigen-antibody reaction. If a bacterial pathogen is suspected, as in a wound, a specimen from the infected area may be examined directly in a stained smear. Alternatively, culturing may be necessary to produce sufficient bacteria for identification.

◆◆ *Clinical Applications*

Few of today's POLs use all of the procedures for identifying microorganisms that are outlined in this chapter. Some POLs depend entirely on reference laboratories for microbiology testing. Nonetheless, the contents of this chapter are important for all POL workers for the following reasons:

- understanding the diagnosis and treatment of patients with infectious diseases
- practicing correct collection and handling of patient microbiology specimens
- following safety practices for microbiological hazards

To understand the diagnosis and treatment of patients with diseases caused by microorganisms, you should know the types of organisms involved and their characteristics and requirements. Knowledge of correct specimen-collection and specimen-handling procedures is important because virtually all POL workers collect and handle microbiology specimens, even when the testing is done in reference labs. The reports from reference labs can be only as good as the specimens they receive.

For their own safety and the safety of their patients, POL workers must follow appropriate aseptic practices when handling infectious disease organisms. In addition to the rise of AIDS and hepatitis, several other infectious diseases have made a resurgence over the past decade—tuberculosis, measles, and antibiotic-resistant strains of strep and staph, among others.

◆◆ Microbiology in Tomorrow's POLs

It is likely that many more microbiology tests will be performed in POLs in the future. Immunoassay techniques will become available to identify more and more microorganisms by their antigen-antibody reactions. Immunology tests are quick and easy compared with today's culturing of specimens.

Gene technology also promises to provide quick identification of microorganisms and some types of cancer, leading to quicker diagnosis and treatment. The tuberculosis pathogen, for example, might be detected in just twenty-four hours with gene technology, instead of today's culture of several weeks duration.

————————————————————— ◆ ◆

DISEASE-CAUSING MICROORGANISMS

Most disease-causing microorganisms, like other living things, are part of the Linnean system of clas-

---

◆ ◆ ◆ Classification ◆ ◆ ◆ of Living Things

In the Linnean system of classification, the largest subdivision of living things is the kingdom, followed by the phylum, class, order, family, genus, and species. The kingdom includes organisms that are only generally similar, whereas, at the other end of the hierarchy, the species includes only organisms of the same type. The scientific name of an organism consists of its genus and species names. *Candida albicans,* for example, is the genus and species of a yeast that causes vaginal infections.

---

sification, in which organisms are grouped according to their similarities. Organisms also may be classified clinically into pathogenic, disease-causing, and nonpathogenic, nondisease-causing, groups. Human pathogenic microbes include viruses, bacteria, fungi, and protozoa. In addition, large internal parasites, such as tapeworms, hookworms, and pinworms, produce microscopic eggs.

◆◆ Viruses

Although three hundred **viruses** have been identified to date, there still is debate over their classification. Many scientists do not place them in any of the kingdoms of living organisms because they do not consider them to be true organisms. Why? Viruses are simpler than bacteria, which are the simplest true organisms known today. Viruses also are the smallest living things, measuring about one twenty-billionth of a meter in diameter. In addition, viruses do not have cells or metabolic machinery. An individual virus particle, or virion, consists of nothing more than a thin protein coat wrapped around either RNA or DNA. All other living things have both RNA and DNA.

How do viruses grow and reproduce? They invade the cells of other organisms for shelter, nutrients, and the missing nucleic acids. Within a host cell, they take over the metabolic machinery, thrive, and multiply. When the host cell dies, they spread through the fluids surrounding the cell and infect new host cells. Some viruses can survive in the outside environment before infecting a new host.

The fact that viruses live within their hosts' cells makes viral illnesses difficult to treat. There are few effective virucides, drugs that kill viruses, because most chemicals that destroy viruses are toxic to the cells of the host. Antibiotics are useless against viruses, although they may be prescribed for opportunistic bacterial infections that sometimes occur when the body is weakened by viral infection. Viruses also get a head start on treatment because most viral infections do not produce symptoms until multiplication of the virus is under way. In addition, viruses that can survive extremes of humidity and temperature may be difficult to eliminate from the environment.

Some viruses produce a passing acute infection in the host. Rhinovirus, for example, which causes colds, generally produces an acute, self-limiting infection. Other viruses infect the host for life. Herpesvirus, for example, may produce cold sores throughout the life of the host, whenever the host's immunity is weakened. Similarly, the varicella virus that causes chicken pox may remain dormant in the host for years and resurface later in life as the disease shingles.

Because of their small size, viruses are not visible under light microscopes. Viruses are highly antigenic, however, so many can be identified immunologically. As you saw in Chapter 25, the viruses that may be detected in POLs with immunological tests include those that cause German measles, herpes, infectious mononucleosis, and AIDS. Other viral diseases seen in physicians' offices include colds (rhinovirus), mumps, influenza, hepatitis, chicken pox, shingles, encephalitis, and warts.

♦ ♦ ♦   More About Warts   ♦ ♦ ♦

Warts are caused by the papilloma virus and are spread from person to person by direct contact. Plantar's warts grow underneath the epidermis of the soles of the feet and often are very painful. Venereal warts are found on the genitals and are sexually transmitted.

♦♦ *Bacteria*

Bacteria are single-celled microorganisms that previously were classified as plants but now are placed in a kingdom of their own, the *Monera*. The smallest bacteria are only two-ten millionths of a meter (0.2 micrometers) in diameter. The size of bacteria puts them just within the range of light microscopes, so they may be observed directly in smears.

Bacteria reproduce by cell division at a very high rate—about once every twenty minutes for some species. It has been estimated that trillions of bacteria are in and on the average human body. Clearly, the total number of bacteria in the world must be astonishingly high. Fortunately, most bacteria are either beneficial or nonpathogenic to humans as long as they stay in their usual environments. However, most bacteria also are capable of causing disease if they breach the body's defenses. Any bacteria grown from a normally sterile site should be regarded as pathogenic until proven otherwise.

Bacterial species differ from one another in several ways. These ways include size, shape, appendages, motility, staining characteristics, chemical characteristics, and population growth patterns. Many of these differences are useful in determining which species are causing disease in patients. Identification is important for the administration of the appropriate an-

tibiotic treatment. Bacteria also vary greatly in the type of environment and nutrients that they require for growth. Lab workers must take these differences into account when culturing bacteria.

Morphology. As Figure 26.1 illustrates, bacteria have three principal shapes: spherical or oval (cocci), rod-shaped (bacilli), and spiral (spirilla and spirochetes).

The **cocci** (spherical or oval bacteria) may appear singly (micrococci) or in pairs (diplococci), chains (streptococci), or irregular grapelike clusters (staphylococci). They also may occur in square or cubical groupings (sarcinae). Cocci are incapable of independent motion. They include the bacteria that cause common strep and staph infections.

The **bacilli** (rod-shaped bacteria) may appear single or attached end to end in chains (streptobacilli). Bacilli also may occur in palisades, that is, attached side to side like boards in a fence. Most bacilli have appendages allowing independent motion. The appendages may be single or multiple, occurring either as whips or as tufts. They may be located at just one end of the organism, at both ends, or protruding from all surfaces. Bacilli include the bacteria that cause tuberculosis, typhoid fever, diphtheria, and leprosy.

The **spiral bacteria** may be comma-shaped (virbrios), rigid and spiral (spirilla), or very coiled and flexible (spirochetes). The flexible spiral bacteria

---

Forms of bacteria

Cocci (round)

Bacilli (rods)

Spiral (spirochetes and spirilla)

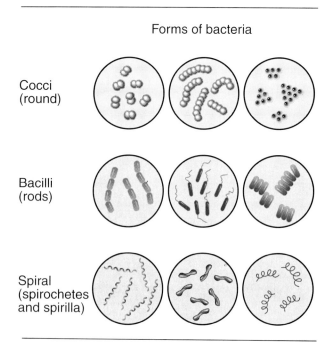

Figure 26.1. The three principal shapes of bacteria.

---

move by flexing, snapping, or bending. Spiral bacteria include the bacteria that cause syphilis, yaws, and Lyme disease.

Staining Characteristics. Another way of identifying bacteria is by their staining characteristics. Staining also is necessary to enhance the visibility of features of an individual bacterium. The most commonly used stain is the **Gram stain,** named for its originator. Using Gram stain is a four-step procedure (see Figure 26.2):

- staining with crystal violet, a deep purple dye
- intensifying the purple stain with iodine
- decolorizing with alcohol
- counterstaining with safranin, a pink dye

✦ ✦ ✦ Technique Tip ✦ ✦ ✦

Beware: gram-positive bacteria can be decolorized if the timing of the decolorization step of the procedure is too long.

On the basis of their staining affinities with Gram stain, bacteria can be divided into two groups—gram positive and gram negative. **Gram-positive** bacteria stain deep purple with crystal violet, because their thick cell walls retain the dye even when alcohol is added to the slide. **Gram-negative** bacteria are decolorized by the addition of alcohol because their cell walls are thinner. Instead, they stain pink or red with the safranin.

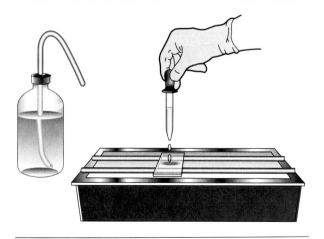

Figure 26.2. Creating a Gram stain.

✦ ✦ ✦ Some Gram-Positive ✦ ✦ ✦ and Gram-Negative Bacteria

Gram-Positive Bacteria (stain deep purple)

- *Diplococcus pneumoniae* (pneumonia)
- Staphylococcus group (boils, abscesses)
- Streptococcus group (sore throats, scarlet fever)
- *Clostridium tetani* (tetanus)
- *Clostridium perfringens* (gas gangrene)
- *Lactobacillus acidophilus* (nonpathogenic flora of the mouth, vagina, and intestines)

Gram-Negative Bacteria (stain pink or red)

- *Escherichia coli* (urinary tract infections)
- *Hemophilus influenzae* (bacterial meningitis in children)
- *Neisseria gonorrhoeae* (gonorrhea)
- *Proteus mirabilis* (urinary tract infections)
- *Pseudomonas aeruginosa* (infection in debilitated patients)
- *Salmonella typhosa* (typhoid fever)
- *Shigella dysenteriae* (dysentery)

The classification of bacteria into gram-positive and gram-negative groups is very useful clinically. Gram-positive and gram-negative bacteria not only react differently to chemical tests but also have different antibiotic sensitivities as well.

Many other bacterial stains are used for special purposes. A stain that is quick and easy to use is crystal violet. Crystal violet stain is added to smears for one minute and then rinsed off in a gentle stream of water. This is the first step in using Gram stain. This step can be done alone to identify the presence or absence of bacteria and show their shape.

✦ ✦ ✦ Capsule Formation ✦ ✦ ✦

Many bacteria form a layer of slimy, mucouslike material around each cell, called a capsule. The presence of a capsule is associated with the virulence of some pathogenic bacteria. Capsules can be seen in stained smears of bacteria.

Bacterial Metabolism. Bacteria produce enzymes that break down complex organic matter into simpler compounds. Some bacteria, called fermenters, break down sugars and other carbohydrates into alcohol and carbon dioxide. Other bacteria break down complex proteins into simpler nitrogenous compounds in a process called putrefaction. In the absence of air, these bacteria create foul odors in wound abscesses.

Enzymatic reactions such as these may be used to distinguish bacteria that have the same shape and staining characteristics. The nitrite test on the urine dipstick, for example, tests for the breakdown of nitrates into nitrites by bacteria present in the urine. Other such tests are conducted in culture tubes. A bacterial species may be identified by the type of sugar that it ferments, for example, or the color it produces when a particular chemical is added to the culture medium.

Toxin Production. Many bacteria produce toxins that are detrimental to the human host. Exotoxins are given off by the living bacterial cell to the surrounding tissues. Endotoxins are released as the bacteria die and disintegrate. Diseases caused by bacterial toxins include diphtheria, tetanus, and botulism (see Table 26.1).

Bacterial Growth. Like all living things, bacteria have the property of growth in a favorable environment. Aspects of the environment important for bacterial growth include nutrition, temperature, humidity, and pH. Knowledge of bacterial growth is essential in POLs, where colonies of bacteria may be grown from just one organism to supply enough bacteria to identify the species.

Some bacteria have very precise nutritional and environmental requirements for growth. These are

---

◆ ◆ ◆ **Note** ◆ ◆ ◆

The following environmental requirements are necessary for bacterial growth:

Nutrition

Physical environment

- Temperature
- Humidity
- Atmosphere (free oxygen, oxygen compounds, or carbon dioxide)

Chemical environment

- pH
- Proteins
- Carbohydrates (simple and complex sugars)
- Mineral salts
- Vitamins
- Water

---

called **fastidious bacteria.** An example is *Neisseria gonorrhoeae*, which causes gonorrhea. It requires an atmosphere of 3 to 10 percent carbon dioxide and special nutrients, including hemolyzed blood. In addition, inhibitors must be added to the culture medium to prevent rampant growth of nonpathogenic bacteria that also grow in the genitourinary tract.

When bacteria are grown under ideal conditions, the pattern of population growth of the colony may help in its identification. Many bacteria, such as *Escherichia coli*, multiply every twenty minutes, pro-

---

TABLE 26.1 Some Exotoxin-Producing Bacteria and Related Diseases

Bacterial Species	Disease
Bacillus cereus	Food poisoning
Clostridium botulinum	Botulism (food poisoning)
Clostridium tetani	Tetanus
Corynebacterium diphtheriae	Diphtheria
Escherichia coli	Urinary tract infections
Staphylococcus aureus	Pyogenic (pus-forming) infection
Streptococcus pyogenes	Pyogenic infection, scarlet fever
Salmonella typhosa	Typhoid fever

ducing an exponential rate of growth. Growth will continue at this rate until nutrition is exhausted or the environment is altered unfavorably.

Figure 26.3 shows an idealized population growth curve for a colony of bacteria. Following are the phases of population growth:

I. *Lag phase:* population growth is not yet apparent

II. *Exponential phase:* the population is experiencing very rapid growth, doubling each time it reproduces

III. *Stationary period:* the population growth ceases as a balance is reached between cell division and cell death

IV. *Death acceleration:* the death rate accelerates as nutrients are depleted and/or waste materials collect

V. *Death phase:* The colony is reduced to just a few organisms

Most bacteria derive their food from organic sources; however, some live on nonliving organic matter and are referred to as saprophytes. Saprophytic bacteria are nonpathogenic and are considered to be benevolent because necessary processes of decay depend on them. Bacteria that survive on living organic matter are called parasites. They often cause disease in their hosts.

Most bacteria require free oxygen to live. Bacteria of this type are called aerobes. Some aerobes prefer free oxygen but can survive on oxygen obtained from chemical compounds. Other bacteria are called anaerobes. They are able to grow in the absence of oxygen (O_2). Obligate anaerobes can grow only in the absence of oxygen. Facultative anaerobes, on the other hand, prefer an atmosphere without oxygen but can grow in oxygen as well. These distinctions are important for culturing bacteria because an oxygen-free environment must be provided for anaerobes.

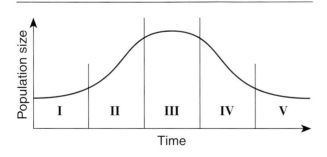

Figure 26.3. Idealized population growth curve for a colony of bacteria.

The fastidious bacterial species *Neisseria gonorrhoeae* that causes gonorrhea is also anaerobic. It requires carbon dioxide for optimal growth. Atmospheric carbon dioxide for the organism can be produced in several ways:

- a carbon dioxide-producing tablet inserted into an airtight plastic bag containing the culture

- a lighted candle placed in the upper part of an airtight jar containing the culture

- a vacuum pump that removes the oxygen, which is replaced with carbon dioxide (only in larger POLs)

If the bag or jar is opened to inspect the culture, a new tablet or lighted candle must be used to reestablish the carbon dioxide atmosphere.

Most pathogenic bacteria prefer a temperature near human body temperature (37 degrees Celsius), but many saprophytic bacteria have optimum growth over a wider range of temperatures. Some species of bacteria can survive in temperatures that range from subfreezing to 70 degrees Celsius. The typhoid bacterium, *Salmonella typhosa*, for example, can remain frozen for months and, after thawing, it still can cause disease.

The spores of some bacteria can survive more extremes of temperature, necessitating the use of autoclaves and dry ovens for sterilization. Although scientists know the temperature above which many bacteria cannot live, a more useful concept is thermal death time, the length of time required to kill a particular type of bacteria at a certain temperature. For example, sterilization with moist heat at 250 degrees Fahrenheit for thirty minutes is the thermal death time for many bacteria grown in laboratories. Incineration also is effective against bacteria (see Figure 26.4).

Moisture is essential for the growth of all bacteria, although different species vary in their ability to tolerate dryness. Moisture is needed in order for nutrients to enter the cells and wastes to leave them, because these processes depend on diffusion. Diffusion is the passing of molecules in aqueous solution through a membrane from a region of high concentration to a region of lower concentration.

The majority of human pathogenic bacteria living on the skin and in the body cavities prefer a pH near neutral—7.2 to 7.5. Although an occasional pathogenic bacterial species can withstand extremely acidic or alkaline conditions, generally strong acids and bases are quickly lethal to microorganisms.

Antibiotics. Antibiotics are drugs that are administered to either kill bacteria (bactericides) or inhibit their growth by preventing reproduction (bacterio-

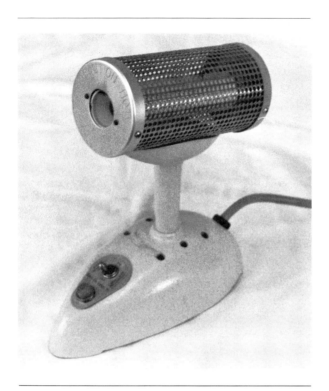

Figure 26.4. This bacterial loop incinerator can quickly and safely sterilize inoculation loops, needles, and culture tube mouths. OSHA requires that bacterial loops be sterilized in this type of incinerator to avoid splattering of material from the loop. Photo by Mark Palko.

static antibiotics). Sensitivity tests determine which particular antibiotic to use against a given bacterial pathogen.

In sensitivity tests, the antibiotics being considered for treatment are placed in a culture medium. If the culture does not grow, the drug is considered to be effective. If the culture grows in abundance, the drug is considered to be ineffective. This mode of testing is based on the assumption that bacteria will respond to antibiotics *in vivo* (in the body) in the same way they have been demonstrated to respond *in vitro* (in an artificial environment). Antibiotic sensitivity testing is not recommended for POLs unless quantitative dilutions of the drug and pathogen are used. The amounts of both pathogen and drug affect the outcome.

Antibiotic sensitivity testing is important in preventing the development of antibiotic-resistant strains of bacteria, which is a major treatment problem. Because bacteria reproduce so quickly and exchange DNA molecules, they can evolve multiple drug-resistant strains. This is most likely to occur when patients are treated with ineffective antibiotics

or when they prematurely discontinue treatment with antibiotics that are effective.

Culturing Bacteria. When bacteria are not easily seen on a direct smear, a culture may be attempted. Some types of bacteria cannot be cultured in laboratories, so even this procedure may not produce a positive identification. Because of limitations in staff, space, and equipment, it is generally recommended that small POLs limit their bacterial cultures to three types of specimens:

- throat swabs for Beta Group A strep (causative agent for strep throat)

- urine, cervical, and urethral exudates for the gonorrhea bacterium

- midstream, clean-catch urine specimens for a variety of organisms

The organisms likely to grow in these three cultures can be managed safely in POLs.

Specimens not recommended for culture in small POLs include stool, sputum, skin lesions, wounds, body fluids, and ear and eye exudates. Instead, these specimens should be collected and sent to a referral laboratory. If the referral laboratory is close by, pa-

---

✦ ✦ ✦ Types of Bacterial ✦ ✦ ✦ Culture Media

Examples of different types of bacterial culture media include the following:

- *Basic media:* used for routine purposes

- *Selective media:* contain deterrents that discourage growth of microbes other than those being studied

- *Enriched media:* have additives to encourage the growth of fastidious organisms

- *Differential media:* contain additives that permit visual differentiation of bacteria; for example, MacConkey media contain lactose and a color-key indicator to distinguish lactose-fermenting bacteria (red) from others (pale pink or colorless)

- *Transport media:* protect pathogens during transport; may contain charcoal to absorb bactericidal waste substances

- *Carbohydrate-metabolism media:* have a specific carbohydrate and indicator added

- *Proteolysis media:* a variety of media that test for the splitting of various proteins into their components; often have colored indicators that depend on a secondary chemical reaction

tients may be referred there for specimen collection as well as culturing. Not only does culturing these specimens require more staff, space, and equipment than generally are found in smaller POLs, but the organisms involved are more difficult to identify. These tests may also exceed the level of complexity at which the lab is registered. Current CLIA regulations have specific guidelines addressing these specifically.

To culture a specimen, a nutritional medium must be selected. It may be a liquid, such as beef broth, or a solid, such as gelatin or agar, a seaweed component that gives a gelatin-like consistency. The medium also may be semisolid or semiliquid, depending on the amount of gelatin, agar, or both. Agar provides a good base for isolating bacterial colonies. In fact, one of the best media for bacteria is blood agar, which is a solution of 5 percent sheep cells and agar. Specialized media may be made by adding ingredients that inhibit or promote the growth of individual bacterial species or have other special functions.

Media should be stored in the refrigerator to prolong their usefulness. Before use, they should be allowed to warm to room temperature. There should be no growth on media or other signs of contamination or deterioration.

Contamination of cultures by nonpathogenic strains is a common problem in POLs. It is important to remember to always store agar plates with the agar side on top to prevent condensation contamination.

A colony is a group of bacteria grown from a single parent cell. Sometimes colonies are divided and grown on several types of media to study their growth patterns. When grown under different conditions they may differ in appearance and have distinctive odors.

Bacterial colonies can be described in terms of their shapes in cross section, their patterns of growth, and the types of margins that they have. In cross section, the shape of a bacterial colony may be flat, convex, pulvinate (very convex), or umbilicate (dimpled). The growth pattern of a colony may be crenated (notched), circular, filamentous, spindle-shaped, or irregular. The margin of the colony may be swarming (covers entire plate), lobed, undulating (wavy), filamentous, curled, or eroded.

Automation. Automated panels now are available for use in larger POLs for testing bacteria for both chemical reactions and antibiotic sensitivities. Each panel, measuring about 4 by 6 inches, contains many numbered microcuvettes, which may be inoculated simultaneously using a diluent dispenser module. There are separate panels for gram-positive and gram-negative bacteria.

To use the panels, the specimen first is grown on isolation media where the suspected pathogen is isolated and identified as gram positive or gram negative. Then a colony is transferred to a broth medium. If it is a rapidly growing bacteria, it is inoculated into the appropriate panel—gram-positive bacteria into a gram-positive panel, and gram-negative bacteria into a gram-negative panel. If it is a slowly growing bacteria or has not incubated long enough, it is incubated for two to four hours before inoculation into the appropriate panel. The suspension of bacteria is standardized according to turbidity standards so the amount of bacteria inoculated is standardized.

The microcuvettes contain dehydrated nutrients and chemicals to support thirty-two different growth patterns and/or chemical reactions of bacteria. On the gram-negative panel, for example, the chemical reactions include the fermenting of various sugars. The panel is incubated for eighteen to twenty-four hours and then each microcuvette is "read," either manually or by instrument, according to a key that interprets the color or reaction as positive or negative. (Figure 26.5 shows a viewing instrument.) The particular combination of positive cuvettes that results identifies the microbe being investigated. The combination key can be found in a manual.

An antimicrobic susceptibility panel of microcuvettes also is inoculated at the same time and incubated. Again, panels are available for both gram-positive and gram-negative bacteria. In addition to dehydrated nutrients, the microcuvettes in this panel

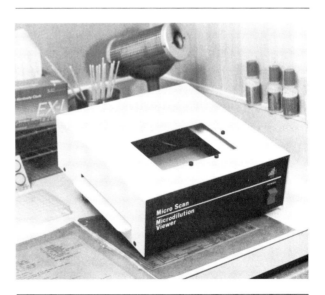

Figure 26.5. This microdilution viewer permits viewing of the bacterial growth or chemical reaction in each microdilution culture tube. Photo by Mark Palko.

contain various dilutions of thirty-seven different drugs used to treat bacterial infections.

❖❖ Fungi

Fungi is a group of microorganisms that includes yeasts and molds. (Figure 26.6 shows some examples.) Only a few species cause disease in humans. Fungi that cause disease often are divided into dermatophytes, which infect only the skin, and systemic fungi, which can cause disease within deeper tissues and organs of the body. Diseases caused by parasitic fungi include histoplasmosis, coccidioidomycosis, and dermatomycosis. Yeast is part of the normal flora of the intestines and skin, but overgrowths commonly cause infections. Thrush is a common infection caused by overgrowth of yeast.

Histoplasmosis. Histoplasmosis is a systemic respiratory disease acquired by inhaling dust contaminated with *Histoplasma*, a genus of parasitic fungi. *Histoplasma* is especially common in the rural Midwest. The disease ranges from a mild, self-limiting infection to a fatal disease. Antibiotic treatment is prescribed.

Coccidioidomycosis. Also known as San Joaquin Valley fever, coccidioidomycosis is caused by a fungus that grows in hot, dry areas, especially in the southwestern United States. It ranges from an acute, self-limiting disease involving the respiratory organs to a progressive, chronic disease that may involve almost any part of the body. Antibiotic treatment is needed for the progressive form of the disease.

Dermatomycosis. Dermatomycosis, also called tinea or ringworm, is any fungus infection of the skin.

It may occur on various parts of the body. There are several common names for skin infections caused by fungi, depending on the part of the body infected. Athlete's foot refers to a fungal skin infection of the foot; jock itch refers to a fungal infection of the groin and perineum. The fungi thrive on moisture, so the affected areas should be kept clean and dry. Treatment generally is with topical fungicides.

Thrush and Other Yeast Infections. Yeast infections frequently are seen in POLs. Generally yeast infections are caused by *Candida albicans*, a gram-positive pathogenic strain. Thrush is a yeast infection of the mouth that often occurs in infants. Vaginal yeast infections also are common, especially in pregnancy, with antibiotic use, and in patients with diabetes mellitus. In addition to a well-balanced diet and good hygiene, treatment of these infections includes fungicidal drugs and antibiotics.

Tests for Fungal Infections. To test for fungal infections of the nails, skin, and vagina, a specimen is collected from the infected area. Vaginal specimens are described here, but the same general procedure applies to specimens from other parts of the body.

The physician collects the vaginal specimen by holding two swabs together and swabbing the cervix, fornix, and vaginal walls. The specimen is placed in a small amount (about 0.5 mL) of saline solution in a tube. The swabs are mixed and squeezed against the wall of the tube to make certain that the solution contains all of the collected specimen. Then, a drop of the saline solution is transferred with one of the swabs to a microscope slide. One drop of 10 percent potassium hydroxide (KOH) solution is added to the drop on the slide. The liquid on the slide is covered immediately with a coverslip, and the underside of the slide is heated over a light bulb or flame. Boiling is avoided.

After the slide cools, it is examined under both low-power and dry high-power objectives for fungal

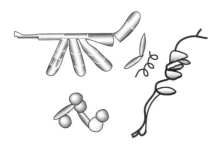

Figure 26.6. Fungi specimens may show a variety of forms, such as threads, buds, and hyphae.

❖ ❖ ❖ Preparing and Storing ❖ ❖ ❖ KOH Solution

Prepare 10 percent potassium hydroxide solution by dissolving 5 grams of KOH in 40 mL of deionized or distilled water. Add enough water to make 50 mL of solution. Store the solution at room temperature in a glass or plastic bottle. Keep a small amount for convenience in a small bottle with a dropper cap. Take care to properly label all containers.

cells, hyphae (mold filaments), and yeast cells. Under the microscope, fungi may appear as a tangled mat. Fungal cells generally are larger than are bacterial cells, and they have definite, thick walls. Fungal cells vary in both size and shape (round, ovoid, or elongated). Hyphae look like filamentous, branching chains. Although yeast has a characteristic appearance (rounded single cells with buds), it may be mistaken for red blood cells in urine specimens. Closer inspection reveals different cells sizes and budding.

✦✦ *Protozoa*

Protozoa are single-celled organisms in the animal kingdom. There are several species pathogenic to humans, including *Entamoeba hystolytica, Giardia lamblia,* and *Trichomonas vaginalis.*

Entamoeba hystolytica. This protozoan parasite causes amoebic dysentery, which is characterized by diarrhea, intestinal bleeding, and fatigue. It is spread by contaminated water and food and by flies. Amoebic dysentery is common in third world countries, and occasional cases are seen in the United States.

Similar nonpathogenic organisms may be confused with this pathogen. Diagnosis is made from stool specimens in reference laboratories.

Giardia lamblia. This protozoan may cause malabsorption syndrome and weight loss as well as diarrhea and gastrointestinal discomfort. Stool specimens processed by POLs may be analyzed in a reference laboratory for the presence of cyst and trophozoite stages of the giardia's life cycle.

Trichomonas vaginalis. This protozoan is transmitted sexually. It infects the vagina of females and the prostate gland of males. While it may be asymptomatic in males, in females it causes profuse vaginal discharge, with intense burning, chafing, and itching.

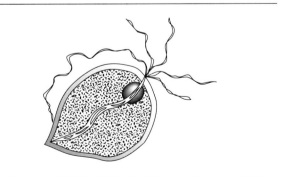

Figure 26.7. *Trichomonas vaginalis.*

Once diagnosed, both sexual partners are treated for infection. Although asymptomatic, a male may reinfect his female partner if he is not treated.

Trichomonas pathogens are easy to observe in saline solution under a coverslip. The specimen should be examined immediately because the parasites quickly lose their mobility and then resemble white blood cells. Occasionally, *Trichomonas* are seen alive in urinary sedimentation examinations. It is a relatively large microorganism, with four anterior antenna and an undulating membrane (see Figure 26.7).

✦✦ *Helminths*

Helminths are true worms as opposed to the larval forms of insects. A number of helminth species parasitize the human intestinal tract, including tapeworms, hookworms, pinworms, whipworms, and roundworms. The majority of worm infestations occur in tropical areas, but they may be found worldwide.

Diagnosis of helminth infestations involves identifying either the microscopic eggs or the adult worms, most commonly in fecal specimens. Without specialized training, it is difficult to distinguish the eggs from other fecal matter. Except for detection of pinworms, which is an easy test, fecal specimens should be analyzed in reference laboratories. State, regional, and local health departments often provide diagnostic services for helminth infestations as well. Mailing tubes usually are supplied by the diagnostic laboratory, but they also can be purchased from supply houses.

Tapeworms. Tapeworm infestations are caused by several different species of worms in the subclass *Cestoda*. Tapeworms vary in length from a few millimeters to several meters. Adult tapeworms live in the small intestine, anchored to the intestinal wall by a scolex—the so-called head, which has hooks and suckers for attachment. Tapeworms absorb food from the intestinal tract of the host through their skin. Their eggs are excreted in the host's feces and may be ingested by intermediate vertebrate hosts such as cows, pigs, or fish. The eggs develop into larvae in the muscle tissues of the intermediate hosts. Human infection occurs when inadequately cooked meat from an infected animal is eaten.

Hookworms. Hookworm infestations are caused by species belonging to the class *Nematoda*. Larval forms enter the body through bare feet and then migrate through the blood stream to the lungs. Eventually, the larvae are coughed up and then swallowed, thereby entering the intestinal tract. In the intestines, they attach to the intestinal wall and suck blood for nourishment. Hookworm infestations can cause lethargy, abdominal pain, and microcytic hypochromic anemia.

Pinworms. Pinworm infestations are caused by the species *Enterobius vermicularis,* also in the class *Nematoda.* They live in the colon unattached to the host. The eggs are deposited in the perianal region, where they may cause itching and come into contact with the hands and fingernails of the host. From there, they may be carried to the mouth, where they are swallowed and reinfect the host's intestinal tract. Other family members may be infected through contaminated clothing and bedding. Infections are more common in children than in adults. Good hygiene is the best prevention for pinworm infestations.

Pinworms are often transmitted on playgrounds where ova have been deposited. The play of the children causes ova to become airborne in the dust. The ova are then inhaled into the gastrointestinal tract via the nose and mouth. Care must be taken not to label pinworms as strictly a hygiene problem. In spring, play areas such as sandboxes and playgrounds are possible sites of contamination—for even the cleanest children.

Diagnosis of pinworm infestations is based on the microscopic detection of the eggs or worms trapped on a sticky swab, which may be purchased for this purpose or improvised from cellophane tape and a tongue depressor.

To collect a pinworm specimen, construct a collection system:

- tear off several inches of cellophane tape.
- place the tape over the end of a disposable wooden tongue depressor, sticky side out.
- press the sticky side of the tape to the perianal area.
- tape is then placed sticky side down on a microscope slide. The tongue depressor is discarded.
- press on the tape to remove air bubbles. Carefully wash your hands.
- the collections should be made by the patient (or the patient's parent if the patient is a child) over three consecutive mornings before rising (see Figure 26.8).

Examine the slide under low power. Because the slide may contain living larvae, it should be handled carefully and placed in a biohazard container when the procedure is done.

Whipworms. Whipworm infestations are caused by the species *Trichuris trichuria,* another Nematode.

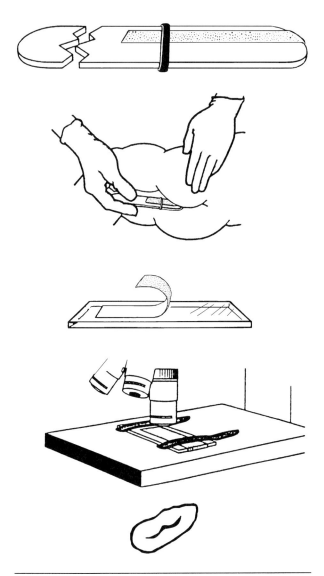

Figure 26.8. Collecting a pinworm specimen. 1. Attach a piece of cellophane tape to a wooden spatula. 2. Early in the morning, before the child is awake, the parent should touch the tape to the child's perianal area. 3. Remove the cellophane tape from the wooden spatula. Attach the cellophane tape sticky side down to a microscope slide. 4. Press the tape to the slide so it can be viewed under the microscope. 5. Eggs and, occasionally, an adult worm may be seen.

Whipworm occurs primarily in the southeastern United States. Like pinworm infestations, whipworm infestations are best prevented through good hygiene.

The worms develop as larvae in the small intestine and move to the colon when they reach adulthood. A heavy infestation may cause bloody or mucoid diarrhea, abdominal pain, and weight loss. Diagnosis is made by detecting whipworm eggs in the feces of the infected patient.

Roundworms. Roundworm infestations are caused by the species *Ascaris lumbricoides,* a large Nematode. Eggs are passed in the feces of infected hosts, incubate in the soil, and are ingested by new hosts. The adult form lives in the small intestine and may cause abdominal pain and vomiting.

MICROBIAL TECHNIQUES

This section describes procedures and materials needed to identify microorganisms in POLs. Because safety is of primary importance when dealing with potentially infectious microorganisms, this subject is addressed first.

◆◆ *Safety*

Safety must always be a top priority in microbiology work. Even when the strains of microorganisms being handled are not considered highly pathogenic, there is risk of serious infection. This may occur if:

- the specimen contains other, unsuspected pathogens
- the suspected pathogen has mutated into a more virulent strain
- individuals coming into contact with the pathogen are unusually susceptible due to compromised immunity

The best safeguards against accidental microbial infection in POLs are knowledge of the dangers involved and careful attention to aseptic techniques.

Aseptic Technique. The practice of **aseptic techniques** ensures that pathogens remain isolated. Isolation prevents accidental exposure of lab workers and patients as well as contamination of specimens by unwanted organisms from the outside. When dealing with potentially infective microorganisms, lab workers always should wear appropriate personal protective equipment, including:

- disposable latex gloves
- plexiglass face shields to protect the face from spatters
- laboratory jackets, aprons, or gowns to absorb spatters

The immediate work area should be covered with paper towels that are disposed of immediately after the task is completed. When performing microbiology collections and procedures, all spills should be wiped up immediately with disinfectant. Counters, work surfaces, and refrigerators should be disinfected daily with surface disinfectant. All contaminated equipment and instruments should be sterilized as they are used. Specimens and cultures should be sterilized by autoclave or incineration. The wire loop that is used to manipulate specimens and cultures should be sterilized with an electric incinerator. Alternatively, disposable plastic loops may be used. These save time and labor. Sterile containers always should be used, as should sterile media and swabs, which are available from supply houses.

◆◆ *Tools Needed for Microbiology Procedures*

Several specialized instruments and supplies are needed for microbiology procedures in POLs. Some were shown in Figure 3.1.

Loops and Needles. Loops are used to manipulate very small amounts of specimen. They come in different sizes, most commonly 10 μL (0.01 mL) and 1.0 μL (0.001 mL). There are reusable wire loops and disposable plastic loops. Wire loops may be made of platinum iridium, a very expensive metal, or nickel chromium, which is cheaper. Loops always must be sterile.

By touching a colony with a loop, a lab worker can lift small amounts of microorganisms from one solid medium onto another and can streak the microbes in thin ribbons on the second medium to start a new culture. The loop can be used to move colonies to and from broth for incubation and study. It also can be used to transfer drops of water or saline solution to slides to mix with bacteria for smears.

Alternatively, needles are used for inoculating media with microorganisms for culturing. The same precautions should be taken in using inoculating needles as other needles used in POLs. Needles should also be sterilized after every use.

Swabs and Media. The swabs and media used in microbiology work in POLs usually are purchased sterile and prepackaged from commercial supply houses. Both must remain sterile and free of all contaminants until use. Only then can lab workers be certain that the growth of bacteria on culture media is of pathogens and not contaminants. In addition, media should be kept in a dark refrigerator until just before use, when they should be allowed to come to room temperature.

Testing Microbiology Specimens

After a microbiology specimen is collected, the swab should be enclosed in a sterile tube. A small amount of sterile distilled water or saline solution may be added to the tube to prevent drying. The swab should be squeezed against the sides of the tube to extract all of the specimen into the liquid.

Smears. In order to study microbes under the microscope, a smear must be made. This may be a direct smear, made from a swab of the affected area to provide a quick view of the specimen, or the specimen may be cultured first and then a smear made from the cultured organisms.

◆ ◆ ◆ Technique Tip ◆ ◆ ◆

If there is just one swab to make both a direct smear and a culture, use a sterile slide for the direct smear. If two swabs are used, use one for the smear and the other to inoculate the culture medium.

A direct smear is made by rolling a specimen swab across the surface of a sterilized glass slide. A clean slide can be sterilized by heating it in a flame until it is hot and then allowing it to cool. The smear should be air dried and then heat fixed by quickly passing the slide, specimen side up, through a flame two or three times. The slide should be quite warm but not too hot to be touched. Heat fixing coagulates the protein in the bacteria, fixing them to the slide so that they will not wash away when the smear is stained.

After the slide has cooled, the smear is stained with Gram stain. Then, the slide is placed under the high-power (oil-immersion) objective of the microscope. The morphology, stain affinity, density, and other notable characteristics of the specimen are reported.

A smear from a culture is made by first preparing the slide to accept the pathogen. A small drop of distilled water is added with a sterile loop to the top of the slide. Then, the loop is resterilized, touched to an isolated culture, and a very small amount is withdrawn and mixed with the water on the slide to make an emulsion. The emulsion is spread thinly on the slide so that it is about as wide as a dime or nickel. Then it is fixed, stained, and viewed in the same way as a direct smear.

Cultures. A **direct culture**, or primary culture, is grown by inoculating patient specimens directly onto the culture medium. The specimen swab is rolled on the medium to get as much as possible of the specimen from the swab. A **pure culture** is one that is grown from a single colony of bacteria, which was taken from the direct culture. Pure cultures generally are preferred to direct cultures because they further isolate the pathogen.

Whenever inoculating a medium, lab workers should avoid breathing directly toward the medium and should perform the inoculation in an area free of dust. The cover of the petri dish containing the medium should be lifted only partway to inoculate and observe the culture. It should be kept closed at all other times.

◆ ◆ ◆ Technique Tip ◆ ◆ ◆

When removing covers from sterile containers such as the caps of tubes, hold them in your other hand. Do not lay them down. If you must lay a cover down, make sure to face the inner surface upward, away from the counter. Dispose of waste immediately without touching the counter.

Throat Cultures for Group A Streptococcus

While viruses cause some sore throats, Group A strep is considered to be the major cause of sore throats due to bacterial infection. If possible, the diagnosis of strep throat is made during the patient's office visit with an antigen-antibody test. However, if only a few strep organisms are present, a false negative may result. In this case, a confirmatory test is made by culturing for the Group A strep organism. Diagnosis is based on hemolysis of blood in the culture medium by streptolysin, an enzyme produced by the strep organism that lyses red blood cells.

Collecting and Handling Specimens. A sufficient sample of microorganisms must be collected to grow a representative throat culture. This is done by taking a throat swab with a sterile Dacron or calcium alginate swab. A cotton swab should not be used because it may inhibit the growth of the strep organism.

With the tongue held down with a tongue depressor, the specimen should be taken directly from the back of the throat and tonsils. The swab should be rubbed on these areas, not just patted. This can be accomplished quickly and relatively easily by using a horizontal, or lazy 8, motion or a large O with the swab. Two swabs should be done at the same time so that if one swab is used for the enzyme test and is negative, the second swab is available for a culture to be planted. This is especially important with children and patients with a sensitive gag reflex.

The teeth and inside of the mouth must be avoided when the swab is inserted and withdrawn. If the swab touches them, the culture may be representative of the flora of the mouth, not the throat.

If the specimen is to be forwarded to a reference laboratory, the swab should be placed immediately in a sterile collection tube containing holding media. The tube should be labeled with the patient's name and chart number, and the specimen should be processed according to the instructions provided by the reference laboratory.

Culturing Specimens. Throat cultures are grown on 5 percent sheep-blood agar. This medium provides good growth potential and is best for showing the hemolytic activity of Group A strep. The culture medium may have inhibitors added to suppress the growth of normal throat flora for better growth of the strep organism (see Figure 26.9).

To inoculate the throat swab onto the blood-agar plate, follow these steps:

- Label the bottom of the agar plate with the patient's name and chart number. (The container will be stored upside down.)

- Using the throat swab, inoculate a small area of the plate by rolling the swab over it. Then discard the swab in disinfectant or a biohazard container.

- Use a sterile loop to streak one-fifth of the outside area of the plate, overlapping some of the area where the swab was rolled.

- Stab the loop into the agar.

- Without sterilizing or withdrawing the loop, proceed to the next area.

- Continue around the plate in a clockwise direction until you cover most of the outside surface, stabbing into the medium between quadrants. Make the final quadrant into a "fishtail" streak.

- Immediately sterilize the loop if it is wire or discard it into disinfectant or a biohazard container if it is plastic. Do not lay the contaminated loop down on the counter.

Some laboratories place a disk of the antibiotic **bacitracin** in the center of the first quadrant of the agar plate to give an early indication of the presence of Group A strep. A zone of growth inhibition

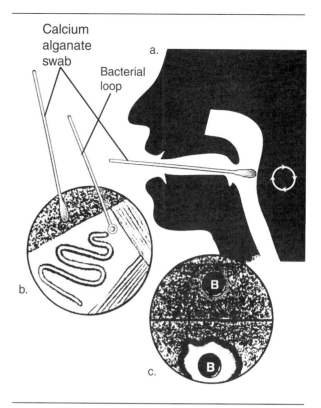

Figure 26.9. Collecting and processing a throat culture. a. Swab (do not just touch) the throat area. Swab any white patches on the tonsils. b. Inoculate the throat culture by first swabbing an area and then using a loop to streak the organisms into a more isolated pattern. c. Bacitracin, an antibiotic, will inhibit the growth of Group A strep and can be used to give a presumptive identification.

around the disk is indicative of Group A strep because bacitracin inhibits the growth of this organism.

For a pure culture, a single colony of the pathogen is taken from the first culture with a sterile loop. The colony then is streaked onto a new blood-agar plate. A bacitracin disk is placed in the center of the streaked area. If need be, pure cultures for more than one patient can be grown on the same agar plate.

Interpreting the Results. Cultures are read for evidence of Group A strep after they incubate for eighteen to twenty-four hours. Diagnosis is based on beta hemolysis of the blood agar by the streptolysin enzyme. Blood agar normally is semiopaque, and beta hemolysis makes it translucent. After beta hemolysis, there are large, colorless, translucent zones surrounding the colonies, both on the surface of the agar and within the stabs. The colonies themselves appear translucent to slightly opaque and are about the size of pinpoints.

Other bacteria, including staphylococcus, produce beta hemolysis, but their colony morphology is different from that of strep. Normal throat bacteria produce a different type of hemolysis, called alpha hemolysis, which leads to distinctive greenish zones around the colonies. Colonies with no change in opacity or color in the agar surrounding them are those of nonhemolytic organisms.

Quality Control. Quality control for strep throat cultures requires careful attention to procedures and manufacturer's instructions. It also involves proficiency testing, maintenance of quality-culturing materials, and documenting quality-control results in the quality-control records.

New shipments of media should be checked on arrival for visible signs of contamination and deterioration, such as cracking, drying, hemolysis, leaking, and bubbling. Media lot numbers should be kept as part of the quality-control record. Sleeves of agar plates should be stored agar-side up and kept in the plastic sleeves until needed. Opening too soon can allow drying or contamination. Each new vial of bacitracin disks should be checked for effectiveness by testing a disk on a known beta Group A strep culture.

◆◆ Genitourinary Cultures for Gonorrhea

Gonorrhea is a prevalent, sexually transmitted disease caused by the bacterium *Neisseria gonorrhoeae*. Symptoms include inflammation and pus. Early diagnosis is important for successful treatment because, without treatment, gonorrhea can lead to sterility and other complications.

◆◆◆ Note ◆◆◆

This section applies only to genitourinary tract specimens, not those collected from the eye, rectum, or throat. Specimens from the latter areas should be sent to a reference laboratory.

By law, a positive test for gonorrhea in POLs must be reported to the state health department. A positive POL test for gonorrhea also should be confirmed by a reference laboratory if:

- it appears to be an antibiotic-resistant strain
- the clinical picture is at odds with the test result
- legal issues are involved (for example, the patient is a child)

Culturing *Neisseria gonorrhoeae*. Gonorrhea often can be diagnosed from a direct smear of penile exudate, but when a direct smear fails to reveal the organism, a culture may be made. For a specimen culture of suspected gonorrhea, Thayer-Martin or New York City agar medium should be used. Both are enrichment media that enhance the growth of *Neisseria gonorrhoeae* while inhibiting competitive organisms from the genitourinary area. The media may be purchased separately or as part of self-contained kits that also contain carbon dioxide-generating capsules. Recall that this pathogen requires a carbon dioxide atmosphere.

The specimen swab should be plated as soon as possible after the sample is collected because the pathogen can survive just thirty minutes away from the moisture and warmth of the human body or a substitute medium. This also is why *Neisseria gonorrhoeae* specimens and cultures never should be refrigerated.

In inoculating the plate, all areas of the swab are rolled over the medium which has been brought to room temperature. Then, the swab is discarded into a biohazard container. A sterile loop is used to streak the specimen back and forth across the medium. The inoculated plate should be placed immediately in the incubator at 37° C in an atmosphere of 3 to 10 percent carbon dioxide.

After the culture has incubated for twenty-four to forty-eight hours, it is examined for the presence of *Neisseria gonorrhoeae*. If the culture is negative, it should be incubated for another twenty-four hours (or a total of seventy-two hours) and examined again before being discarded.

Identifying *Neisseria gonorrhoeae*. Colonies of *Neisseria gonorrhoeae* are small, smooth, translucent, and grayish. However, colony morphology is insufficient for positive identification of the pathogen. Several other microorganisms, including both bacteria and yeast, may grow on the inhibitory media and present a similar appearance. Positive identification of *Neisseria gonorrhoeae* is based on two additional factors. The organisms must:

- test gram negative and look like coffee beans facing each other
- test positive on the oxidase test

In the **oxidase test,** oxidase reagent is added to a

colony of suspected *Neisseria gonorrhoeae*. One or two drops of reagent may be added directly to the colony on the culture. Alternatively, one or two drops of reagent may be used to moisten filter paper and a loop may be used to smear microbes on the moistened paper. Instructions from the manufacturer of the oxidase reagent should be followed. If a black or dark blue color occurs within thirty seconds of adding the reagent, the result is positive and the organism is *Neisseria gonorrhoeae*.

♦ ♦ ♦ Caution! ♦ ♦ ♦

Certain wire loops may give positive results on the oxidase test because iron in the wire reacts with the reagent.

Quality Control. Quality control in *Neisseria gonorrhoeae* testing requires adherence to proper techniques, occasional proficiency testing of unknown samples, and maintenance of the quality of the culture media and oxidase reagent. Remember to document the quality-control results in the quality-control journal.

Each new batch of culture media must be tested by inoculation with both *Escherichia coli* and *Neisseria gonorrhoeae*. The media should grow *Neisseria gonorrhoeae* and inhibit *Escherichia coli* after twenty-four hours of incubation. Alternatively, pretested media can be obtained from reference laboratories, which also supply documentation of the quality-control testing. This documentation must be kept in the quality-control records of POLs.

The oxidase reagent must be checked each day it is used. This is done by testing a known sample of *Neisseria gonorrhoeae*.

♦♦ *Urine Cultures*

Urine cultures usually are made to diagnose **urinary tract infection** (UTI). The urinary tract is predisposed to infection because urine has nutrients capable of supporting bacterial growth. If urine is not completely voided from the bladder at each urination (as occurs in some medical conditions), bacteria may grow in the bladder. The ureter is only about 1.5 inches long in adult females, so their bladders are relatively accessible to bacteria. That is why UTIs are more common in women than in men.

Urine cultures differ from strep throat and gonor-rhea cultures in that the number of bacteria present are more important in diagnosis than are the type of bacteria present. A bacterial concentration of over 100,000 organisms per milliliter indicates UTI, while a concentration below 10,000 per milliliter indicates no infection. A concentration between 10,000 and 100,000 organisms per milliliter is inconclusive and must be confirmed by another culture or by clinical evidence.

Microorganisms That Cause Urinary Tract Infections. Most UTIs result from migration of the patient's own intestinal tract flora to the urinary tract. Intestinal tract flora are predominantly gram negative. *Escherichia coli*, a gram-negative organism, accounts for 80 percent of UTI. Most of the remaining 20 percent of UTIs are due to the gram-negative species *Klebsiella pneumoniae*, *Enterobacter aerogenes*, and species of *Proteus* and *Pseudomonas*. Gram-positive organisms, like strep and staph, account for very few UTIs.

**♦ ♦ ♦ Reducing the ♦ ♦ ♦
Risk of UTI**

Female patients should be encouraged to follow hygienic practices that reduce the risk of UTIs. After using the toilet, they always should wipe from front to back. This helps prevent contamination of the ureter by bacteria from the intestinal tract.

Collecting and Handling Specimens. Patients must be instructed in how to obtain a midstream, clean-catch urine specimen. The urine specimen should not be centrifuged before culturing. Other urinalysis tests of the same specimen should be postponed until after the culture is made in order to prevent contamination of the culture.

Gram Staining. A Gram stain can provide a valuable guide to the type of antibiotic that should be prescribed for a UTI. Antibiotics are classified according to the type of bacteria against which they are most effective. Some antibiotics are most effective against gram-negative organisms, while others are most effective against gram-positive organisms.

Several methods are available for culturing urine for a Gram-stain test. In the traditional method, a known amount of uncentrifuged urine is measured with either a 0.01 mL or 0.001 mL loop and placed on two different media:

- general purpose sheep-blood agar
- gram-positive inhibiting media (either MacConkey or EMB medium)

The media are streaked in a crisscross pattern and incubated for twenty-four hours. Then, the colonies are counted and the concentration of bacteria is calculated with the following formula:

$$\text{Bacteria/mL} = \frac{\text{No. of colonies}}{\text{Quantity of urine}}$$

Alternatively:

$$\text{Bacteria/mL} = \text{No. of colonies} \times \text{Conversion factor}$$

where the conversion factor is 100 for the 0.01 mL loop and 1,000 for the 0.001 mL loop.

Two types of commercial culture kits are available for urine testing—the dipstick paddle and the coated tube. The dipstick paddle has a selective medium for gram-negative organisms on one side and a nonselective medium on the other side that grows both gram-negative and gram-positive organisms. The media are inoculated by pouring urine over the paddle or by dipping the paddle in urine. After inoculation, the paddle is replaced in its sterile bottle and incubated at 37 degrees Celsius for eighteen to twenty-four hours.

The coated-tube culture has a special enriched medium and color indicators on its inner surface. Urine is poured into the tube and then poured out. The cap is placed on the tube, and the urine residue is incubated in the same way as in other urine cultures.

For both commercial culture kits, the manufacturer's inserts include color charts and instructions for counting colonies and calculating bacteria concentration. When identification and colony counts are made from the comparison chart, the growth should be reported as "presumptive." This is particularly important when Gram stains and isolation of the bacteria are not performed as additional tests. (Precise identification requires more complex testing to differentiate between strains of bacteria.) The term *presumptive* is a precaution in keeping with CLIA and the registration status of moderate-level POLs. It indicates to the medical staff the extent of testing. If needed, bacteria grown with the kits may be used for additional testing, transferred to other cultures, or sent to reference laboratories for further study.

Chemical Tests. Chemical tests are available to identify the organisms found in urine cultures. The **catalase test** uses hydrogen peroxide to distinguish strep from staph, both gram-positive organisms. Staph produces bubbles when exposed to 30 percent hydrogen peroxide. Strep does not.

The **coagulase test** demonstrates the presence of an enzyme produced by pathogenic staph organisms. Nonpathogenic strains, such as those found on the skin, lack the enzyme and test negative. In the test, staph organisms are mixed with a drop of rabbit plasma. Clotting indicates a positive result—the presence of the enzyme.

◆ ◆ ◆ **Note** ◆ ◆ ◆

Forward unusual organisms growing in a urine culture to a reference laboratory for further identification.

Quality Control. Quality control in urine cultures is maintained by the same general methods used in other types of cultures. Media quality is maintained by visual inspection, proper storage, and usage before the expiration date. Reagent quality is maintained by testing. Vials of catalase and coagulase should be checked upon receipt. Catalase can be checked with a known staph species or a drop of blood. Coagulase is checked with *Staphylococcus aureus*. Remember to document your quality-control results in the quality-control journal.

◆ ◆ ◆ **Contaminated** ◆ ◆ ◆
Cultures

Individual UTIs usually are caused by one type of bacteria. If a culture shows a mix of three or more different organisms, then you should suspect contamination.

◆ ◆ ◆ **Caution!** ◆ ◆ ◆
Treat all urine cultures as biohazardous at all times and discard them in a biohazard container.

PROCEDURE

26.1 ◆ ## Heat-Fixing a Bacterial Smear

Goal

- After successfully completing this procedure, you will be able to prepare a heat-fixed bacterial smear with microorganisms supplied by the instructor or from a swab of normal microflora in your mouth.

Completion Time

- 15 minutes

Equipment and Supplies

- disposable latex gloves, impermeable apron or laboratory jacket
- hand disinfectant
- surface disinfectant
- paper towels and tissues
- biohazard container
- source of microorganisms
- alcohol lamp or Bunsen burner
- glass slides
- sterile cotton swab or sterilized loop
- distilled water or saline solution
- forceps

Instructions

Read through the list of equipment and supplies that you will need and the steps of the procedure. Be sure that you understand each step before you begin. Then complete each step correctly and in the proper order. If your completion time is too long, repeat the procedure until you increase your speed.

	S	U

1. Put on a protective jacket, gown, or apron; wash your hands with disinfectant, dry them, and put on gloves.

2. Follow the Universal Precautions.

3. Collect and prepare the appropriate equipment.

4. Prepare the work area by covering the counter with paper towels, slightly dampened with disinfectant.

5. Using a sterile loop or swab, place one loop or a small drop of water or saline solution on a clean glass slide.

6. With a sterile swab, rub your teeth and gums gently, turning the swab to cover all sides with mouth microflora. Alternatively, use a sterile loop or swab to obtain a small sample of microorganisms from the instructor. If you use a nondisposable loop, sterilize it before and after in an incinerator until it is red hot.

7. Place the mouth swab, or the microorganism specimen, in the drop of liquid on the slide; turn the swab gently to mix the microorganisms into the liquid.

8. Stir the liquid and mouth microflora, or microorganism specimen, until they form a thin emulsion about the size of a dime or nickel.

9. Set aside the slide and allow it to air dry to avoid scattering microorganisms; do not wave or blow on the slide.

10. After the slide has air dried, heat fix it by passing it two or three times over the Bunsen burner or alcohol lamp. Hold the slide with forceps to prevent burning your hands in the flame, but do not let the slide get too hot to touch.

11. Lay the slide aside to cool before using Gram stain. See Procedure 26.2. Go immediately to Procedure 26.2 or to step 12.

12. Discard disposable supplies and equipment in the biohazard container.

	S	U
13. Disinfect other equipment and return it to storage.		
14. Clean the work area following the Universal Precautions.		
15. Remove your gloves, jacket, gown, or apron; wash your hands with disinfectant, and dry them.		

OVERALL PROCEDURAL EVALUATION

Student's Name _____

Signature of Instructor _____ Date _____

Comments

PROCEDURE

26.2 Gram-Staining a Bacterial Smear

Goal

- After successfully completing this procedure, you will be able to prepare a Gram-stained smear from an unstained bacterial smear.

Completion Time

- 15 minutes

Equipment and Supplies

- disposable latex gloves, impermeable apron or laboratory jacket
- hand disinfectant
- surface disinfectant
- paper towels and tissues
- biohazard container
- unstained, heat-fixed smear of microorganisms from Procedure 26.1
- staining rack
- squeeze bottle or beaker of tap water
- Gram-stain kit containing reagents (crystal violet, iodine, ethyl alcohol or acetone and safranin)
- eyedropper or Pasteur pipette
- forceps

Instructions

Read through the list of equipment and supplies that you will need and the steps of the procedure. Be sure that you understand each step before you begin. Then complete each step correctly and in the proper order. If your completion time is too long, repeat the procedure until you increase your speed.

S = Satisfactory	U = Unsatisfactory	S	U

1. Put on a protective jacket, gown, or apron; wash your hands with disinfectant, dry them, and put on gloves.

2. Follow the Universal Precautions.

3. Collect and prepare the appropriate equipment.

4. Read the manufacturer's instructions. If they differ from the steps described below, follow the manufacturer's instructions instead.

5. Place the unstained, fixed smear on the staining rack, with the smear side up.

6. Flood the slide with crystal violet solution and let it stand one minute.

7. At the end of one minute, rinse the stain off with tap water from a plastic squeeze bottle or beaker; drain off the excess water.

8. Flood the smear with iodine solution and let it stand for one minute.

9. At the end of one minute, wash the smear with tap water. Drain off the excess water.

10. Pick up the slide and decolorize (with ethyl alcohol, acetone, or both) for about five seconds until the dye no longer runs off the smear except in the thickest portion.

11. Wash the slide briefly with tap water.

12. Apply safranin for ten seconds to counterstain.

13. Wash it gently and briefly with tap water. Clean the back of the slide and blot the front dry with a paper towel. Either go immediately to Procedure 26.3 or to step 14.

S = Satisfactory	U = Unsatisfactory	S	U

14. Discard disposable supplies and equipment in the biohazard container.

15. Disinfect other equipment and return it to storage.

16. Clean the work area, following the Universal Precautions.

17. Remove your jacket, gown, or apron, and gloves; wash your hands with disinfectant, and dry them.

OVERALL PROCEDURAL EVALUATION

Student's Name _____

Signature of Instructor _____ Date _____

Comments

PROCEDURE

26.3 ◆ Microscopic Examination of a Gram-Stained Smear

◆ Goal

- After successfully completing this procedure, you will be able to examine a prepared Gram-stained smear and report the morphology and Gram-stain reaction of the microorganisms.

◆ Completion Time

- 15 minutes

◆ Equipment and Supplies

- disposable latex gloves, impermeable apron or laboratory coat
- hand disinfectant
- surface disinfectant
- paper towels and tissues
- biohazard container
- microscope
- immersion oil
- lens paper
- Gram-stained bacterial slide

◆ Instructions

Read through the list of equipment and supplies that you will need and the steps of the procedure. Be sure that you understand each step before you begin. Then complete each step correctly and in the proper order. If your completion time is too long, repeat the procedure until you increase your speed.

S = Satisfactory U = Unsatisfactory	S	U
1. Put on a protective jacket, gown, or apron; wash your hands with disinfectant, dry them, and put on gloves.		
2. Follow the Universal Precautions.		

3. Collect and prepare the appropriate equipment.

4. Secure the slide, stained side up, on the microscope stage.

5. Focus the slide under the 10X objective.

6. Focus the slide under the 45X objective.

7. Move the 45X objective out of the way and place a drop of immersion oil on the slide.

8. Move the 100X objective into place and focus with the fine-focus adjustment knob until the bacteria come into view. Adjust the light as necessary.

9. If you cannot adjust the focus, check to see that the slide is right side up, then return to the 10X objective and repeat steps 5 through 8.

10. Scan the slide to find thin areas. Thick areas do not show cell morphology well.

11. Identify the type of bacteria by shape such as coccus, bacillus, and spirochete, and describe any other morphology, such as chains, clusters, and palisades. Record the results.

12. Classify the bacteria by stain reaction (purple are gram positive and pink or red are gram negative). Record the results.

13. Wipe the immersion oil off the slide with a soft tissue if it is to be saved.

14. Discard disposable supplies and equipment in the biohazard container.

15. Clean and store the microscope in its proper storage area.

16. Clean the work area, following the Universal Precautions.

17. Remove your jacket, gown, or apron, and gloves; wash your hands with disinfectant, and dry them.

OVERALL PROCEDURAL EVALUATION

Student's Name _____

Signature of Instructor _____ Date _____

Comments

CHAPTER 26 REVIEW

Using Terminology

Define the following terms in the spaces provided.

1. Virus: _____
   _____

2. Coccus: _____
   _____

3. Spiral bacteria: _____
   _____

4. Gram positive: _____
   _____

5. Gram negative: _____
   _____

6. Fastidious bacteria: _____

_____

7. Catalase test: _____

_____

8. Coagulase test: _____

_____

9. Helminth: _____

_____

10. Fungus: _____

_____

11. Protozoan: _____

_____

12. Aseptic technique: _____

_____

13. Direct culture: _____

_____

14. Pure culture: _____

_____

15. Oxidase test: _____

_____

16. Bacitracin: _____

_____

17. Urinary tract infection (UTI): _____

_____

18. Microbiology: _____

_____

19. Antibiotic: _____

_____

20. Bacteria: _____

_____

Acquiring Knowledge

Answer the following questions in the spaces provided.

21. Identify several types of microorganisms that cause disease in humans and name some of the diseases that they cause.

22. Explain the relevance of microbiology to POLs.

23. Describe how infectious diseases are diagnosed.

24. Why are viral diseases sometimes difficult to diagnose?

25. Why are viral diseases often difficult to treat?

26. Discuss the use of Gram stain in identifying bacteria.

27. What role does morphology play in distinguishing among species of bacteria?

_____

_____

_____

28. Besides staining and morphology, what differences among bacterial species aid in their identification?

_____

_____

_____

29. What factors must be appropriate for optimal growth of a given bacterial species?

_____

_____

_____

30. What are the differences between saprophytic and parasitic bacteria?

_____

_____

_____

_____

31. How do obligate anaerobes differ from facultative anaerobes?

_____

_____

_____

32. What temperature do most pathogenic bacteria prefer? Why?

_____

_____

_____

33. Discuss the role of sensitivity testing in selecting antibiotics for bacterial infections.

_____

_____

_____

_____

_____

_____

34. Identify several human diseases caused by fungi.

_____

_____

_____

35. What treatment usually is prescribed for fungal infections?

_____

_____

36. What diseases in humans are caused by protozoan microorganisms?

_____

_____

37. What are some helminth infestations in humans?

_____

38. Explain the role of sanitation and hygiene in the transmission of helminth diseases.

_____

_____

_____

_____

_____

_____

39. List the aseptic techniques for working with microorganisms in POLs.

_____

_____

_____

_____

_____

_____

40. Why are aseptic techniques important when working with microbial pathogens?

_____

_____

_____

_____

Applying Knowledge—On the Job

Answer the following questions in the spaces provided.

41. The father of a preschooler brought in a piece of scotch tape on a tongue depressor to be analyzed. It had been applied to the child's rectum in the morning. What pathogen should the specimen be examined for? How will you process the specimen?

42. A suspected gonorrhea specimen has been collected in the clinic where you work. How should you process it?

43. You have been asked to examine a blood-agar culture for the growth of Group A strep. What should you look for?

44. Your laboratory just received a new supply of media for bacterial cultures. Where and how should you store them until they are used?

45. The physician has requested that a Gram stain be made of the discharge from an infected sore to determine if the infecting organism is staphylococcus. How should you make and stain the smear? What do you expect to see if it is a staph infection?

Universal Precautions and Other Safety Information ◆

UNIVERSAL PRECAUTIONS

1. Treat all biological material as biohazardous and capable of transmitting HIV, HBV, and other diseases. Isolate and contain biological material from collection, through testing, to disposal.
2. Utilize the best personal protective equipment and engineering controls available. Wear gloves and laboratory coats. Wear a face shield if spatters are likely. Keep specimens enclosed when possible in covered containers. Use a biological safety cabinet for procedures that produce aerosols or droplets.
3. Sanitize equipment and work surfaces before and after procedures, after spills, and at the end of the day. Apply the principles of sanitation to all general laboratory work. Avoid careless techniques that scatter pathogenic contaminants through the laboratory.
4. Decontaminate blood and body fluid spills immediately. Use 10 percent household bleach or another approved disinfectant.
5. Do no mouth pipetting. Avoid sharp instruments. Do not handle used needles with your hands.
6. Wash your hands often—between each activity and whenever you touch biohazardous material. Contaminated hands provide a bridge for pathogens to escape from one area to another.
7. Keep your hands, pencils, etc. away from your face and hair. Touching one's face is often a habit—a dangerous one. The eyes, nose, and mouth are lined with mucous membranes, which may be penetrated by pathogens.
8. Do not eat, drink, groom, or mix nonlaboratory activities within the laboratory even when relaxing or saving time. Do not store food, drink, or other nonlaboratory items in the laboratory area used for collecting, testing, or reagent storage. Leave pencils, laboratory jackets, and work gear in the laboratory. These provide bridges for pathogens to escape from the work area.
9. Keep informed about current developments concerning serious communicable diseases, including HIV (AIDS), HBV (Hepatitis B), and tuberculosis. Know the infection probability, the means of prevention, and the effectiveness of treatment. Consider the benefits of a Hepatitis B vaccination.
10. Keep safety in mind. Incorporate into your laboratory routine a safety review schedule that provides automatic reminders.

CHEMICAL SAFETY

1. Respect chemicals. Treat them as toxic unless they are known to be harmless.
2. Store chemicals in appropriate containers and cabinets. Flammable chemicals should be stored in fireproof cabinets. Reactive and caustic chemicals should be stored separately, in shatterproof containers.
3. Wear appropriate personal protective equipment. This includes suitable shoes to protect your feet, long sleeves, and gloves, where needed.
4. Avoid fumes and physical contact with chemicals. Never smell or taste a chemical. Wash your hands after handling chemicals.
5. Discard unidentified, contaminated, questionable, or out-of-date chemicals.
6. Use good inventory and storage techniques. Keep on hand only what is needed in an up-to-date inventory.

PHYSICAL SAFETY

1. Avoid electrical and physical accidents by anticipating and removing hazards before accidents happen.
2. Maintain an emergency plan. Display a drawing of the fire-escape routes in the building.
3. Do not block exits with furniture or storage. In case of fire, these items present a hazard.
4. Maintain a safety manual and review it periodically.

APPENDIX B
Laboratories Subject to the Clinical Laboratory Improvement Amendment (CLIA 1988) ◆

1. Accredited hospital-based facilities
2. Nonaccredited hospital-based facilities
3. Federal hospitals, such as military, Veterans Administration, and Public Health Service hospitals
4. Independent laboratories
5. Physicians' office laboratories
6. Skilled-nursing facilities
7. End-stage renal disease facilities
8. Intermediate-care facilities, including those for individuals with mental retardation
9. Ambulatory surgical centers
10. Rural health clinics
11. College of American Pathologists (CAP) accredited, NY State approved, and low-volume exempt laboratories
12. Insurance laboratories
13. City, county, and state laboratories
14. Federal clinics
15. Drug-screening laboratories
16. Mobile laboratories
17. Any other facilities, including Planned Parenthood clinics, pharmacies, and health fairs that perform qualitative or screening-test procedures or examinations

APPENDIX C
CLIA's Levels of Certification ◆

As of April 1997 CLIA has three levels of certification for POLs: waiver, moderate complexity, and high complexity. Laboratories certified for waiver testing can perform only tests classified as waiver-level tests. Laboratories that certify as moderate complexity may do moderate-level tests plus waivered tests. Laboratories certified as high complexity may do high-complexity plus all waivered and moderate-level tests. Figure C.1 shows a laboratory request form for one POL.

WAIVERED—14 TESTS ◆◆

1. Dipstick or tablet reagent urinalysis (nonautomated) for:
   - bilirubin
   - hemoglobin
   - leukocytes
   - protein
   - specific gravity
   - glucose
   - ketone
   - nitrite
   - pH
   - urobilinogen
2. Fecal occult blood
3. Ovulation—visual color comparison tests for human lutenizing hormone
4. Urine pregnancy—visual color comparison tests
5. Erythrocyte sedimentation rate (nonautomated)
6. Hemoglobin-copper sulfate (nonautomated)
7. Blood glucose, by glucose monitoring devices cleared by the FDA specifically for home use
8. Spun microhematrocrit
9. Hemoglobin (automated) by single analyte instruments with self-contained or component features to perform specimen-reagent interaction, providing direct measurement and readout
10. Cholesterol testing—by cholesterol monitoring devices cleared by the FDA
11. Boehringer Manneheim Chemstrip Micral test—monitors low urine concentrations of albumin, which aids in early detection of renal diseases in at-risk patients
12. *Helicobacter pylori* tests—bacterial or antibody identification for causative gastric ulcers; various methods
13. Strep A tests—for rapid identification of Group A streptococcal (GAS) antigen; aids in diagnosing *Group A Streptococcus*, the causative agent of strep throat, tonsillitis, and scarlet fever; various methods
14. All qualitative color comparison pH testing of body fluids (except blood)—pH detection (acid-base balance) in body fluids such as semen, amniotic fluid, and gastric aspirates; various methods

CLARKSVILLE MEDICAL GROUP, P.A.
MISCELLANEOUS LAB

DX _____

Drawn Time: _____ Drawn By: _____

Reference Lab (NHL)

____ OB (COBIC)	_____ RUBELLA
____ DNAGC	_____ COOMBS
____ DNA CHLAMDIA	_____ VDRL
____ HEALTH SURVEY	_____ HIV
____ OTHER	_____ T7

A	B	C	E	F	G	H	I	J	K	SID:

HEMATOLOGY	OTHER	CHEMISTRY

HEMATOLOGY

____ CBC   _____ PLT
____ RBC   _____ OTHER
____ WBC   _____
____ HGB   _____
____ HCT
____ MAN DIFF
BASO _____
EOSIN _____
MUELO _____
META _____
BAND _____
SEG _____
LYMPH _____
MONO _____

RBC: MORPH:
ANISO _____
POIKI _____
HYPO _____
_____
_____
____ ESR _____

____ PT _____
CONTROL _____
____ STREP _____

____ GRAM STAIN _____
_____
____ GUAIAC _____
_____
____ POST VAS _____
_____
MONO _____
_____
FERN TEST _____
_____
____ PREG (URINE) _____
____ PREG (SERUM) _____

OTHER

____ UA   _____ ROUTINE VOID
             _____ CLEAN CATCH
             _____ SPEC FROM HOME
____ DIPSTICK ONLY
COLOR _____
CLARITY _____
GLU _____
BILI _____
KETO _____
SG _____
PH _____
PRO _____
URO _____
NIT _____
BLO _____
LEU _____

____ MICRO ONLY
WBC _____
RBC _____
CASTS _____
BACTERIA _____
YEAST _____
TRICH _____
CRYSTALS _____
EPICELLS _____
MUCOUS _____

____ CULTURE _____
SOURCE _____
____ WET PREP _____
WBC _____
RBC _____
BACT _____
TRICH _____
YEAST _____
EPITH _____

____ KOH _____
_____
_____

CHEMISTRY

____ NA	_____ PHOS
____ K+	_____ T.PROT
____ ALB	_____ TRIG
____ ALT/SGPT	_____ UREA/BUN
____ AST/OT	_____ URIC A.
____ T. BIL	_____ ALP
____ CA	_____ CHEM 12
____ CHOL	_____ LIVER
____ CREAT	_____ LIPIDS
____ LDH	_____ TSH
____ GLU	_____
____ HDL	
____ LDL	
____ MAG	

OTHER _____
_____

	URINE	
____ GTT	GLU	KETO
____ O'SULLIVAN		
FBS		
½ HR		
1 HR		
2 HR		
3 HR		
4 HR		
5 HR		

_____ TECH
_____ DATE

Figure C.1. A POL laboratory test request form. Used with permission of Clarksville Medical Group PA.

TESTS OF MODERATE COMPLEXITY—7,500 TESTS IN THE FOLLOWING CATEGORIES

- Automated chemistry
- Automated blood gases
- Automated hematology
- Manual differential counts (identify normal cells only)
- Microscopic urinalysis
- Slide and care agglutination tests
- Direct antigen tests
- Urine culture and colony count kits
- Throat culture screens

TESTS OF HIGH COMPLEXITY—2,500 TESTS IN THE FOLLOWING CATEGORIES

- All cytology, cytogenics, histopathology, histocompatibility
- Nonautomated chemistry
- Flame photometry
- Radioimmunoassay
- Bone marrow examination
- Manual hematology procedures
- Differential count (identify abnormal cells)
- Isolation and identification of bacteriology cultures

APPENDIX D
Preparing the Physician's Office Laboratory for Inspection

Preparation for CLIA 1988 inspection should begin six to eighteen months ahead of the inspection date. OSHA inspections are unannounced.

STEP 1

The laboratory director should request that you make a complete laboratory inventory. This inventory should include a complete evaluation of all test procedures, including the instruments that support them. The laboratory director will seek to identify the deficiencies that must be corrected and eliminate out-of-date, costly, and seldom-used tests. All tests must be within the certification level of the POL.

STEP 2

Use OSHA and CLIA guidelines in the following areas to ensure there is:

- an adequate quality assurance program for all tests
- an adequate safety program in place

- a written documentation for all tests

The safety program must include a written plan that reduces the risk of:

- occupational exposure to bloodborne pathogens (Universal Precautions)
- occupational exposure to hazardous chemicals

The following safety documentation will be needed:

- job classification and biohazardous tasks list for each laboratory employee
- OSHA personnel categorization file that shows the level of exposure to bloodborne pathogens for each job level
- Hepatitis B immunization certificate or signed waiver of vaccination for each employee
- proof of biological safety training
- sanitation, waste-disposal, and housekeeping plans
- a file documenting any employee's accidental occupational exposure to biohazards or toxic chemicals and records of medical follow-up

STEP 3

Register the physician's office laboratory with HCFA (Health Care and Finance Administration). *Use HCFA form 109* and do the following:

- Name a qualified laboratory director (in some instances, this may be the physician/employer).
- List job titles of personnel who perform tests and their certification and level of education.
- List each test performed along with the instrument and reagents or kits used.
- List specialty areas of testing (hematology, chemistry, microbiology, etc.).
- List the number of patient tests performed annually in each speciality area.

STEP 4

Organize an efficient documentation system. (*Remember:* If it isn't written down, it wasn't done.) All steps of the laboratory testing loop must have the following written documentation: physician's requisition, specimen collection, test procedure, quality control, instrument and reagent maintenance, and final reporting of the test result. Documentation may begin with a written and signed order of the physician in the patient's record. Laboratory manuals must document test collection, test procedures, instrument and reagent maintenance, quality control, and problem correction. The loop ends with the reporting of the patient-test results to the physician and charting on the patient's record.

STEP 5

Develop an effective quality-control program. Include every test performed in the laboratory.

- Record each test-control result in the log on the same day that the test control is performed.
- Perform a statistical analysis *monthly*. This statistical analysis should include the mean, standard deviation, coefficient of variation, and a Levey-Jennings graph. These calculations are sometimes performed automatically by electronic instruments or they may be provided by instrument manufacturers or the control providers.
- Maintain a remedial action log to document problems and their resolution. Record events such as unacceptable results, rejected specimens, statistical trends and shifts, and routine operating problems (for example, specimen loss or mix-up).

STEP 6

Apply for certification after the documentation procedures are in place and the tests are running smoothly.

STEP 7

If you cannot complete the preceding steps yourself, obtain the guidance of a laboratory consultant.

APPENDIX E
Normal Values of Laboratory Tests

The normal values given for each test in the following tables may vary according to the test procedure being utilized by the laboratory. Values obtained from plasma or serum will vary from those of whole blood. Different populations and localities may have variations in normal values. Also note that the same test value may be expressed in different metric units or SI units. Normal values for laboratory tests are also referred to as reference values or ranges.

URINE

The average urine volume of adults = 600 − 1600 mL/24 hr.

Routine Urinalysis	Normal Values	Clinical Significance
Albumin	Negative	Kidney function
Bilirubin	Negative	Liver function
Blood, occult	Negative	Kidney function
Glucose	Negative	Carbohydrate metabolism
Hemoglobin	Negative	Kidney function
Ketones	Negative	Fat metabolism disorder
pH	4.6–8.0	Acid/base balance
Protein	Negative	Kidney function
Urobilinogen	0.1-1.0 E.U.*/dL	Liver function

*Ehrlich units

Test	Normal Values	Clinical Significance
CBC		
Hemoglobin	Varies with age: Ten years = 12–14.5 g/dL Adult female = 12.5–15 g/dL Adult male = 14–17 g/dL	Increases with polycythemia, high altitude, chronic pulmonary disease Decreases with anemia, hemorrhage
Hematocrit	Varies with age: Newborn = 50–62% One year old = 31–39% Adult female = 36–46% Adult male = 42–52%	Increases with dehydration and polycythemia Decreases with anemia and hemorrhage
White blood cell count	Varies with age: Adults = 4,500–12,000/mm^3	Increases with acute infection, polycythemia and other diseases Extremely high counts in leukemia Decreases in some viral infections and other conditions
Red blood cell count	Varies with age: Adult female = 4.0–5.5 million/mm^3 Adult male = 4.5–6.0 million/mm^3	Increases with polycythemia and dehydration . Decreases with anemia, hemorrhage, and leukemia
Erythrocyte sedimentation rates		
Sediplast (Westergren autozero system)	F < age 50 = 0–20 mm/1 hour F > age 50 = 0–30 mm/1 hour M < age 50 = 0–15 mm/1 hour M > age 50 = 0–20 mm/1 hour	Increased in infections, inflammatory diseases, and tissue destruction Decreased in polycythemia and sickle-cell anemia
Wintrobe sedimentation rate	F 0–15 mm/1 hour M 0–7 mm/1 hour	Increased in infections, inflammatory diseases, and tissue destruction Decreased in polycythemia and sickle-cell anemia

Test	Normal Values	Clinical Significance
Platelets	140,000 – 400,000/mm^3	Increases with hemorrhage Decreases with leukemias
Blood chemistries		
Albumin	3.2–5.5 gm/dL	Decreases in kidney disease and severe burns
Alkaline phosphatase	30–115 mU*/mL	Assists in diagnosis of liver and bone diseases
ALT (SGPT)	0–45 mU*/mL	Used to detect liver disease
Amylase	25–125 U*/L	Elevated in acute pancreatitis, mumps, intestinal obstructions
AST (SGOT)	0–41 mU*/mL	Used to detect tissue damage Increases with myocardial infarction, other conditions Decreases in some diseases
Total bilirubin (serum)	0.3–1.1 mg/dL	Increases in conditions causing red blood-cell destruction or biliary obstruction
BUN (blood urea nitrogen)	8–25 mg/dL	Used in diagnosis of kidney disease, liver failure, other diseases
Calcium	8.5–10.5 mg/dL	Used to assess parathyroid functioning and calcium metabolism and to evaluate malignancies
Total cholesterol	Average = 120–200 mg/dL* (varies with age and sex of individual)	Cardiovascular disease

*A cholesterol level of less than 200 mg/dL is recommended by the American Heart Association for both males and females of all ages.

		Increases in diabetes mellitus and hypothyroidism
		Decreases in hyperthyroidism, acute infections, and pernicious anemia
HDL cholesterol	30–85 mg/dL*	

*Varies with the age and sex of the individual.

LDL cholesterol	50–210 mg/dL*	

*Varies with the age and sex of the individual.

Creatinine	0.4–1.5 mg/dL	Used as a screening test of renal functioning
Fasting blood sugar	70–110 mg/100mL	Used as a screening test for carbohydrate metabolism
GTT (glucose-tolerance test)	FBS 70–110 mg/dL 30 min 120–170 mg/dL 1 hr 120–170 mg/dL 2 hr 100–140 mg/dL 3 hr less than 125 mg/dL	Used to detect disorders of glucose metabolism
LDH (Lactate dehydrogenase)	100–225 mU*/mL	Assists in the diagnosis of myocardial infarction and differential diagnosis of muscular dystrophy and pernicious anemia

Test	Normal Values	Clinical Significance
Triglycerides	40–170 mg/dL	Used to evaluate suspected atherosclerosis
Uric acid	2.2–9.0 mg/dL	Used to evaluate renal failure, gout, leukemia
Electrolytes		
Carbon dioxide (CO_2)	22–26 mEq/L	Diagnosis of acid/base imbalance
Chloride	96–110 mEq/L	Helps in diagnosing disorders of acid/base balance
Potassium	3.5–5.5 mEq/L	Used to diagnose disorders of water balance and acid/base imbalance
Sodium	135–145 mEq/L	Diagnosis of acid/base imbalance occurring in many conditions

*U = Unit (International enzyme unit)

APPENDIX F
Blood Chemistry Tests Arranged by Panels/Profiles ◆

✦✦ General Metabolism

- AST/SGOT
- Bilirubin
- BUN
- Creatinine
- Cholesterol
- Triglycerides
- Glucose
- LDH
- Potassium
- Uric acid

✦✦ Cardiac and Circulatory

- ALT/SGPT
- AST/SGOT
- Cholesterol
- Triglycerides
- CPK
- LDH
- Potassium

✦✦ Diabetic Screening

- Glucose
- Possibly renal panel

✦✦ Hepatic (Liver Functions)

- ALT/SGPT
- AST/SGOT
- Bilirubin
- LDH

✦✦ Renal

- BUN
- Creatinine
- Cholesterol
- Potassium
- Uric acid

✦✦ Lipid

- Cholesterol
- Triglycerides

APPENDIX G
Vocabulary of the Clinical Laboratory ◆

Clinical laboratories, like other medical specialties, have their own standard vocabulary to be mastered for efficient work. Accuracy and efficiency that promote quality assurance are emphasized. Variation is not permitted if it hinders work or might result in misunderstanding. However, standard abbreviations are used routinely for both tests and reagents. The rules of standard medical terminology, with root words, prefixes, and suffixes, apply to many terms. These may describe laboratory equipment, tests, and the diseases being treated. Reagents are named by the rules of chemistry.

Laboratory vocabulary can be divided into the general areas of metric measurement, laboratory equipment, reagents, tests, and clinical diseases. The general types of vocabulary within each division follow:

- Metric measurement (SI) uses the prefixes and units of the metric system. The prefixes designate the multiple or fraction of the metric unit. These prefixes, units, or abbreviations must always use the correct letter and capitalization.

- Laboratory equipment is often named by prefixes and word roots based on the rules of medical terminology. (An example is the photometer, which consists of the two root words: *photo*, meaning

light, and *meter*, meaning measure). However, automated instruments and test kits are often known by the tradenames assigned by the manufacturer.

- Laboratory reagents are denoted by their chemical names, symbols (which are chemical abbreviations), or initials. Trade names may also be used. Inorganic compounds are generally identified by their chemical symbols or name. Complex organic compounds are often designated by the initials or names of their chief components. The concentration level of a reagent, if needed, is included along with the name.

- Tests are generally signified by the analyte or parameter being measured. However, the name may be derived from the procedure itself.

- Names of the clinical diseases associated with particular tests often follow the rules of standard medical terminology. (These rules may be found in medical terminology textbooks. Abbreviated lists of word roots, prefixes, and suffixes are found in various medical textbooks and medical dictionaries.)

Common Abbreviations in the Physicians' Office Laboratory follow:

AIDS: acquired immunodeficiency syndrome
BUN: blood urea nitrogen
B-cell: a type of lymphocyte
Ca: chemical symbol for calcium
CBC: complete blood-cell count
CDC: Centers for Disease Control
Cl: chemical symbol for chloride
CLIA '88: Clinical Laboratory Improvement Amendment of 1988.
CMA: certified medical assistant
CO$_2$: carbon dioxide
EDTA: a blood anticoagulant (ethylenediaminetetraacetic acid)
epith: epithelial
ESR: erythrocyte sedimentation rate
GTT: glucose-tolerance test
HBV: Hepatitis B virus
Hct: hematocrit
HDL: high density lipoproteins

Hb, Hgb: hemoglobin
HIV: human immunodeficiency virus
H$_2$O: water
HPF: high-power field of the microscope
IDDM: insulin-dependent diabetes mellitus
K: chemical symbol for potassium
LDL: low density lipoproteins
LPF: low-power field of the microscope
mEq: milliequivalent (a chemical measurement)
MLT: medical laboratory technician
MT (ASCP): medical technologist certified by the American Society of Clinical Pathologists
Na: chemical symbol for sodium
NIDDM: noninsulin-dependent diabetes mellitus
OSHA: Occupational Safety and Health Administration

pH: a measure of acidity or alkalinity (hydrogen ion concentration)
PKU: phenylketonuria
POL: physician's office laboratory
PPBS: postprandial blood sugar
RA: rheumatoid arthritis
RBC: red blood cell, also called erythrocyte
RF: rheumatoid factors
RMA: registered medical assistant
RMT: registered medical technologist
sp gr: specific gravity
staph: staphylococcus
stat: immediately (emergency)
strep: streptococcus
T-cell: a type of lymphocyte, a white blood cell
UA: urinalysis
WBC: white blood cell, also called leukocyte

APPENDIX H
Bibliography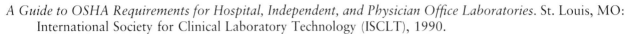

A Guide to OSHA Requirements for Hospital, Independent, and Physician Office Laboratories. St. Louis, MO: International Society for Clinical Laboratory Technology (ISCLT), 1990.

All About OSHA. U.S. Dept. of Labor. OSHA Publ. 2056, 1991.

Ames Modern Urine Chemistry, A Guide to the Diagnosis of Urinary Tract Diseases and Metabolic Disorders. Elkhart, IN: Miles Laboratories, Inc., 1979.

Bennington, J. L., Ed. *Saunders Dictionary & Encyclopedia of Laboratory Medicine and Technology.* Philadelphia: W. B. Saunders Co., 1984.

Berner, J. J. *Effects of Disease on Laboratory Tests.* Philadelphia: J. B. Lippincott Co., 1983.

Diggs, Sturm, and Bell. *The Morphology of Human Blood Cells,* 5th ed. Abbott Laboratories, PO Box 352, North Chicago, IL 60064-4000, 1985.

Flynn, J. C. *Procedures in Phlebotomy,* 1st ed. Philadelphia: W. B. Saunders Co., 1994.

Free, H. M., Ed. *Modern Urine Chemistry Manual.* Elkhart, IN: Miles Laboratories, Inc., 1979. Revised 1991.

Henry, J. B. H., Ed. *Todd, Sanford, and Davidsohn's Clinical Diagnosis and Management by Laboratory Methods,* 17th ed., Philadelphia: W. B. Saunders Co., 1984.

Hepler, Opal E. *Manual of Clinical Laboratory Methods,* 4th ed., 19th printing. Springfield, IL: Charles Thomas, 1975.

Hyun, B. H., J. K. Ashton, K. Dolan. *Practical Hematology Laboratory Guide with Filmstrips.* Philadelphia: W. B. Saunders Co, 1975.

Introduction to Phlebotomy. Denver, CO: Colorado Association for Continuing Medical Laboratory Education, 1983.

Kaplan, R., et al. *Clinical Chemistry—Interpretation and Techniques,* 4th ed. Baltimore: Williams & Wilkins, 1995.

Laboratory Medicine. Chicago, IL: American Society of Clinical Pathologists, monthly.

MAX (Miles: Assuring Excellence) in Physician-Office Testing. Quality Assurance Program. Elkhart, IN: Miles, Inc., Diagnostic Division, 1989.

National Committee for Laboratory Standards. *Physician's Office Laboratory Guidelines; Tentative Guidelines,* NCCLS 1–T. Villanova, PA: NCCLS, 1989.

Occupational Exposure to Bloodborne Pathogens. U.S. Dept of Labor. OSHA Publ. 3127, 1993.

Physician's Office Laboratory Technician (POLT) Handbook. International Society for Clinical Laboratory Technology. Suite 918, 818 Olive St., St. Louis, MO 63101, 1990.

Raphael, Stanley S. *Lynch's Medical Technology,* 4th ed. Philadelphia: W. B. Saunders Co., 1983.

Seventh Annual Medical Office Laboratory Conference Syllabus. San Diego, CA: Jan., 1994.

Spivak, J. L., Ed. *Fundamentals of Clinical Hematology,* 2nd ed. Philadelphia: Harper & Row, 1984.

Technical Manual of the AABB (American Association of Blood Banks), 11th ed. 8101 Glenbrook Road, Bethesda, MD 20814, 1993.

Tietz, N. W., Ed. *Clinical Guide to Laboratory Tests.* Philadelphia: W. B. Saunders Co., 1983.

Urinalysis Today. Boehringer Mannheim Corporation. Fax 1-800-428-4674. PO Box 50100, Indianapolis, IN, 1991.

Widmann, F. K. *Clinical Interpretation of Laboratory Tests,* 9th ed. Philadelphia: F. A. Davis & Co., 1983.

Chapter Review Answers
Chapter 1

1. Aerosolization: the conversion of a liquid, such as blood or blood products, or a solid, such as powdered chemical, into a fine mist that travels through the air.

2. Biohazard: anything contaminated by biological specimens from humans and having a potential for transmitting disease.

3. Biological specimen: a specimen that originates from a living organism. Examples are blood, blood products, body fluids such as cerebrospinal fluid or urine, biopsy samples, bacterial smears, and bacterial cultures.

4. Chain of transmission: the line of transmission of a disease from one host with the disease to a new host.

5. Engineering control: a device that keeps biohazards away from laboratory workers.

6. Exposure incident: a situation in which a lab worker is exposed to a potentially hazardous substance, such as blood or a toxic chemical.

7. Material Safety Data Sheet: a sheet included with all shipments of hazardous laboratory chemicals. It should be checked for necessary precautions.

8. HBV (hepatitis B virus): the virus that causes hepatitis B, a type of severe hepatitis transmitted by sexual contact, by needle sharing, or through contaminated blood, blood products, or other body fluids.

9. HIV (human immunodeficiency virus): the virus that causes AIDS (acquired immunodeficiency syndrome).

10. ICP (infection-control program): a program that provides the maximum protection for health care workers against occupational sources of disease.

11. OSHA (Occupational Safety and Health Administration): a federal agency under the supervision of the U.S. Department of Labor, OSHA works to assure the safety and health of workers.

12. PPE (personal protective equipment): clothing and other equipment that shield workers from outside contaminants. PPE includes gloves, uniforms, fluid-proof aprons, masks, and eye-shields.

13. Universal Precautions: a set of recommendations formulated by the Centers for Disease Control and Prevention to protect workers against HIV. The precautions impose isolation of all specimens of blood, blood products, and other body fluids capable of transmitting HIV.

14. Work-practice control: a method that incorporates safety into laboratory procedures.

15. The Universal Precautions assume that *all* blood and body fluids capable of carrying HIV are potentially infectious and, therefore, must be isolated. They heighten worker awareness about the need for protection against all such specimens. Protection is provided by engineering controls, disinfection, work-practice controls, and personal protective equipment.

16. A wide variety of diseases can be contracted in the laboratory through blood contamination, fecal material, direct patient contact, and microorganisms present in smears and cultures. Some of the diseases are hepatitis B, AIDS, tuberculosis, typhoid, strep and staph infections, pneumonia, and influenza.

17. Laboratory workers should realize that a high level of stress is a contributing factor in many accidents. Workers should try to identify and then reduce the source of stress. If the stress level is affecting laboratory work, it may be dealt with in several ways, depending on the problem. The work may be made more efficient with good scheduling. Too many demands should be dealt with by pointing out the impossibility of complying. The problem may be discussed with other personnel.

18. Always do pipetting with a suction device or mechanical pipette, never by mouth. Dispose of used needles and lancets as quickly as possible. When handling is necessary, use tools, never your hands. Manipulate biohazards that spatter inside a biohazard cabinet or behind a spatter screen. A facial shield also may be worn.

19. Biohazards should be quickly apparent to those who work around them.

20. No certain way exists to determine if a particular biospecimen poses a health threat. Many apparently healthy persons carry deadly viruses, such as the hepatitis B virus and HIV. Therefore, in order to exclude all possible biohazards, all biospecimens must be treated as potential carriers of deadly microbes such as HBV and HIV.

21. All of these body fluids are capable of transmitting HIV, if contaminated. Therefore, all should be handled according to the Universal Precautions.

22. A vaccine against HBV (hepatitis B virus), which immunizes most laboratory workers, is made available to laboratory workers by their employers. However, no such vaccine exists against HIV and a number of other serious diseases.

23. A written exposure incident report is required by OSHA. Follow-ups of exposure incidents and a report to OSHA of a positive HBV or HIV test are required if they are traced to an injury or exposure incident.

24. Following are some ways to prevent exposure to toxic chemicals when it is necessary to use them in the laboratory:

   • Assume that all chemicals are toxic unless you know otherwise. Use OSHA's list of toxic chemicals to check toxicity.
   • Avoid unnecessary exposure. Never breathe the fumes or smell or taste a chemical to identify it. Avoid undue exposure to all chemicals.
   • Keep an orderly lab, clearly labeling all reagents and storing them correctly in leakproof containers.
   • Store chemicals as recommended by the manufacturer—flammable chemicals in a metal cabinet and caustic chemicals in leakproof, unbreakable containers.
   • Wear protective personal equipment, such as gloves, long-sleeved jackets, and enclosed shoes.
   • Read labels for toxicity and storage usage precautions.
   • Purchase, store, and use only the minimum amount of chemicals necessary for efficient laboratory work.
   • Keep an up-to-date inventory. Do not store out-of-date chemicals. Discard them.

25. New employees should be given an explanation of:

   • the epidemiology and symptoms of HBV and HIV infections.
   • the modes of transmission of HBV and HIV.
   • the POL's infection control program, including engineering controls, work practices, and PPEs.
   • how the HBV vaccine works.
   • the procedure to follow in case of an exposure incident, how to report the incident, and the available medical follow-up.
   • the signs, symbols, and color(s) used to denote biohazards.

26. Physical hazards include slippery floors, dangling electrical cords, fire hazards, and security breaches. Vigilant attention to correct details and good housekeeping are the best ways to prevent most accidents. Complacency should be guarded against with a program of reminders and scheduled safety reviews.

27. Freshly prepared bleach dilutions from 1:10 to 1:100 are used for disinfection. A 1:100 dilution is used to disinfect smooth, nonporous, already cleaned areas. A stronger solution of up to 1:10 is used for tough cleanup jobs such as biohazard spills or hard-to-clean porous surfaces.

28. Attitude is probably the most important component of laboratory safety. Alertness prevents accidents. A continuous safety program that includes safety education, monitoring, and periodic reviews is the best safeguard. Complacency, on the other hand, is a major

cause of laboratory accidents and occupational disease exposure.

29. Laboratory workers should wash their hands often. They should wash their hands before donning gloves and after removing them, between patients, and between different procedures. They should also wash their hands before leaving the laboratory. Hand washing prevents the transfer of pathogens from one area to another.

30. Laboratory workers must never contaminate this sensitive area by putting objects near their face or hair while in the laboratory. The mouth, eyes, nose, and other body entrances should be protected against exposure to disease-causing microbes. This protection is violated by chewing on pencils and fingers or applying makeup.

31. Laboratory workers should follow the rules in the safety manual for disposing of each group of waste materials. Biohazards should be bagged in protective bags marked with the biohazard symbol and disposed of as prescribed by OSHA. Chemicals should be flushed down the sink or disposed of as prescribed by local codes.

32. In the case of fire, all routes should be apparent and open in case they are needed. There is not time to remove supplies or furniture in the case of fire.

33. Needle sticks are best avoided by not touching the contaminated needle. Handle the needle only as required and then only with a tool, such as forceps, that keeps the needle away from your hands and body.

34. Wear gloves to prevent exposure to chemicals or biohazards that may otherwise enter the body through abrasions or wounds in the skin. Wear gloves for any task where they offer protection, but especially when handling blood and other biohazards.

35. First, Jane should report the accident in writing to her supervisor.

- The employer will see that the exposure incident is documented and will find out the HBV and HIV status of the source patient, if known.
- A confidential medical evaluation and follow-up will be given to Jane.
- Her blood will be drawn as soon as possible and tested for HBV and HIV.
- The source patient, if known, will be contacted and requested to give consent for a blood specimen to be tested for HIV and HBV.
- The employer will offer Jane follow-up testing for HIV 6 weeks, 12 weeks, and 6 months after the exposure.
- Follow-up of Jane's exposure incident will include counseling, medical evaluation of any acute febrile illness

within 12 weeks post-exposure, and standard post-exposure medical treatment.

36. Because you already practice Universal Precautions, the routine should not be varied unless you feel the need for extra precautions as a psychological support. You should wear new, disposable gloves to draw the blood. You should exercise usual care to prevent a needle stick. Keep the blood sample covered and take care not to spill or spatter the specimen. This patient has the same infection potential as other patients whose positive HIV status has not been revealed to you.

37.
- Sharps containers are properly placed in the lab.
- Workers wear gloves when they handle all potentially hazardous materials.
- Workers use protective shields when working with procedures that may cause aerosolization to occur.
- Workers wash their hands frequently.
- Food and drink are prohibited in the laboratory area.
- Workers wear protective lab coats or aprons if they are working with materials that are frequently spattered.
- All hazardous materials are identified with proper labels.
- At least one sink in the lab has an eyewash station.

38. Tasks a, d, and i.

39.
- Fire exits were clearly marked and there was an alternate fire exit.
- The fire extinguisher was in proper working order.
- The lab had a fire blanket, which could be used if someone's clothes were accidentally ignited.

Chapter 2

1. e   2. d   3. b
4. c   5. a   6. g
7. f
8. a. ocular, or eyepiece
   b. nosepiece
   c. objective
   d. condenser
   e. focus control
   f. light
   g. base
9. Care must be exercised in the focusing of the oil-immersion lens because the working distance is very short. Only the fine focus adjustment knob should be used. It should never be forced, because forcing can damage the objective.
10. Most microscopic specimens require staining to render their details easily visible under the microscope. An unstained microscopic specimen is generally colorless, with little contrast, and details are difficult or impossible to differentiate.

11. The compound microscope, the one commonly used in a POL, has two lens acting together as one to magnify the image.

12. Multiply the magnification of the objective lens by the magnification of the ocular lens to get the total magnification. Since the ocular is usually ten, 10 × power of objective = total magnification.

13. The binocular microscope has two oculars (eyepieces).

14. The lens systems are mounted at opposite ends of the barrel of the microscope.

15. The total magnification of the microscopic specimen you are viewing is obtained by multiplying the power of the objective being used by the power of the ocular (usually a power of 10). Total magnification changes when you change the objective.

16. You should request that the supplier obtain light bulbs and other replacements made for your model of microscope from the original manufacturer of the microscope. Otherwise, the replacement parts may not fit or work properly.

17. The red cell is enlarged 450 times. The objective enlarges it to a size 45 times larger, and then the eyepiece remagnifies this 45X image to a size 10 times larger. Ten (the eyepiece magnification) times 45 (the objective magnification) gives a magnification size of 450X (X = times) the original size of the specimen.

18. The specimen must be transparent. It must be thin enough to allow light from the lamp below to pass through it and into the objective and eyepiece of the microscope.

19. Staining enhances the qualities of color and contrast. If the slide had no different colors or contrasts, you could not differentiate the details of crystals, cell structures, or similar characteristics under the microscope.

20. You can distinguish the structures of only one layer of cells with ease. More layers cause overlapping and crowding, which obscures the details of the individual cells.

21. You should alternate between looking through the oculars and looking sideways at the objectives when focusing and when changing the objectives. This avoids damaging the objective by crushing it on the slide.

22. The term *aperture*, from the Latin word meaning "to open," describes an opening, referring in this case to the microscope stage.

23. The term *working distance* describes the space between the objective and specimen. The lowest power objective has the greatest working distance, the 45X has a medium working distance, and the

highest power objective, the oil-immersion objective, has the least.

24. You should always use the coarse focus adjustment knob with the lowest power objective to begin the focusing process. It covers a greater distance faster and is more efficient in finding the image.

25. To bring the focus into its clearest possible image, use the fine focus adjustment knob. The fine focus adjustment knob will turn the objective only a short distance for each revolution, giving you better control.

26. You should always use the fine focus adjustment knob to focus the oil-immersion lens because the working distance is very short with this lens. The fine focus adjustment knob moves the objective only a short distance, which is safer with a short working distance.

27. The specimen side of the slide must always face upward for viewing. The specimen cannot be focused on the bottom side of the glass slide. Attempting to do so will crush the objectives.

28. The oil-immersion (100X) objective has a very short working distance and therefore requires focusing with the fine focus adjustment knob.

29. Lens paper must always be used to clean microscope lenses because cheaper tissues may scratch and damage the lenses. Many manufacturers' warranties are voided if lens paper is not used.

30. The microscope lenses must be wiped clean with lens paper after each period of use before storing. When needed, blow away dust with an infant's ear syringe or use a camel hair brush. Any stubborn debris that cannot be brushed away is removed by gently rubbing with a lens paper moistened in alcohol or lens cleaner.

31. A microscope should be stored away from the light in a place where it will not be bumped or jarred.

32. A rheostat is a device that controls the amount of current entering the light of the microscope.

33. +

34. +

35. The working distance is the distance between the objective and the specimen.

36. +

37. +

38. +

39. +

40. Resolution refers to the ability of a set of lenses to distinguish fine detail.

41. +

42. Located in the condenser, the iris diagram controls the amount of light entering through the aperture in the stage.

43. +

44. The higher the magnification, the shorter the working distance.

45. The coarse focus adjustment knob causes the objective to move farther for each complete turn of the knob.

46. +

47. +

48. As is true with any other piece of expensive equipment, records should be kept of routine maintenance and other service procedures on the microscope.

49. +

50. +

51. +

52. Susan probably smudged the ocular with her eyelashes, leaving an oily film on it. Melissa should clean the ocular with lens paper moistened with lens cleaner.

53. She should call the company that sold the microscope and ask for a representative to service the microscope. She might also ask the local hospital laboratory personnel for the name of their microscope service representative if they are pleased with the service.

54. Brenda should mention to her coworker that she should coverslip liquid specimens of urine to prevent damage to the objectives and biohazardous contamination of the POL. If the coworker does not cooperate, Brenda should report it to the lab supervisor.

55. You should mention that the microscope may be bumped where it is and that its position next to the centrifuge will cause it to vibrate excessively when the centrifuge is in operation. Suggest that the sturdy table away from vibrations and traffic is a more suitable place.

56. Tell Jamie that the light is deficient. Trace the path of light up through the microscope, making adjustments and eliminating possible obstructions. You can increase the light intensity by adjusting the rheostat, raising the condenser, opening the iris diaphragm, and adjusting the nosepiece.

57. There are two possibilities: the slide is stained too darkly or the slide is too thick. When the cells appear very crowded and indistinct, it is likely that the smear is too thick. A smear should have only one layer of cells.

58. Tim should have noted and written down the position of the cells on the x and y axes of the mechanical stage. Then, he could have returned quickly to the exact location of the blood cells.

59. The eyepieces will become scratched and fuzzy, destroying the clarity of the magnified image. Oil and other debris may loosen the cement around the objectives, throwing the image out of alignment. The microscope soon will be useless if this type of care continues.

Chapter 3

1. d 2. k 3. c
4. a 5. b 6. i
7. e 8. j 9. f
10. g 11. h

12. Beaker: a deep glass container with a wide mouth, often with a lip for pouring.

13. Flask: a container with a broad base and a narrow neck for holding liquids or mixing reagents.

14. Meniscus: the downward curve at the surface of a liquid in a container, due to the attraction of molecules of liquid to the side of the container. The bottom of the curve always is used for reading the amount of liquid in the container.

15. Pipette: an instrument for measuring small, accurate quantities of laboratory samples or reagents.

16. The autoclave sterilizes instruments with steam under pressure.

17. A drying oven is used to dry glassware.

18. To heat fix a bacterial smear, quickly pass the bottom of a slide over the tip of a Bunsen burner flame, coagulating the smear, sealing it on the slide, and preventing it from washing off during staining.

19. A wire loop is used to transfer bacteria from one location to another—for example, from a patient smear to agar gel in a petri dish.

20. Celsius also is called Centigrade because it has 100 equal divisions, or degrees, between the freezing and boiling points of water.

21. It should read 4 degrees Celsius in the refrigerator or −20 degrees Celsius in the freezer.

22. Normal human body temperature, 37 degrees Celsius. Human bacteria are genetically programmed by natural selection to thrive at the normal temperature of their human hosts.

23. Graduated containers are used for measuring liquids when very precise measurements are not required. Volumetric containers are used for measuring liquids for tests of controls and standards when very precise measurements are required. They are manufactured to contain only a certain, very exact amount.

24. Volumetric flasks and pipettes are preferred because they measure the most accurately.

25. If you pipette by mouth you risk ingesting the pipetted material, which may be biohazardous or toxic.

26. A conical centrifuge tube.

27. A sterile petri dish or a sterile screw-capped bottle.

28. A cylinder is useful in measuring variable amounts of liquid when extreme accuracy is not necessary.

29. Put the glassware into a disinfectant solution to soak until it can be washed. Use the appropriate automatic washer or wash it by hand using laboratory detergent. Rinse it thoroughly in tap water and then rinse it in distilled water to remove any chlorine or other chemicals. Sterilize it in a dry heat oven or an autoclave.

30. Low temperature preserves reagents. Body temperature maximizes enzyme activity and bacterial growth. High temperature sterilizes and dries equipment.

31. Cuvettes.

32. The hemacytometer is filled by touching the tip of a blood pipette to the *v*-shaped depression and allowing fluid to flow by capillary action into the space under the coverslip.

33. It is obvious that the POL staff is overworked. More workers could be hired or some lab practices could be changed to reduce the work load. Disposable equipment, though more expensive, would reduce the work load. So would sending some tests out to a reference lab. With the time saved, the inventory could be kept up to date, waste from outdated reagents could be reduced, and the time could be allotted to disinfecting the POL.

34. In this case, close watch of inventory is crucial to avoid shortages. The person in charge of inventory and ordering should take special care to anticipate usage rates and allow an extra margin for unexpectedly heavy usage. Extra stocks of nonperishable supplies should be kept if possible. Reagents that expire, especially expensive ones, should be checked frequently so that new supplies can be ordered and shelved before old ones are used up.

35. The supervisor is responsible for the quality and efficiency of the POL and is correct in pointing out Victoria's deviation from procedure—all POL procedures should be followed exactly for quality control reasons. In the case of pipettes, Victoria was in error—using the wrong pipette could affect the test results.

36. First, Jan should acquaint herself with the laboratory manuals, especially the procedures manual. She should read over the procedures that she is responsible for several times to become familiar with them. She should take every opportunity to work through the procedures on the actual equipment used. Jan should keep a notebook to record the information that she receives throughout the work day. After work, she should sort it out and make a list of questions to ask the next day.

37. The supervisor is correct. Such practices waste supplies and equipment, require more work in the long run, increase the cost of POL operation, and create hazards for lab workers. A trained laboratory worker is expected to take care of equipment, conserve supplies, and not contaminate the surroundings.

Chapter 4

1. b   2. c   3. i
4. h   5. j   6. g
7. e   8. f   9. d
10. a   11. e   12. d
13. c   14. i   15. g
16. b   17. f   18. h
19. a

20. Concentrate: a substance, either liquid or solid, that is strong because it has had fluid removed from it.

21. Diluent: an agent that reduces the strength of a substance to which it is added.

22. Dilution: a solution that has been weakened by addition of a diluent.

23. Solute: the substance dissolved in a liquid to form a solution.

24. Solvent: the liquid in which substances are dissolved to form a solution.

25. Total volume: the amount of a solution, including both solute and solvent.

26. Kilograms are the appropriate metric unit to measure body weight. One kilogram is approximately 2.2 pounds. The wavelengths of light are measured in nanometers; the POL disinfectant is measured in liters or milliliters. A blood specimen is measured in either milliliters or microliters.

27. Arranged from large to small:
kilo- = 1,000;
deci- = 1/10;
centi- = 1/100;
milli- = 1/1,000;
micro- = 1/1,000,000,
and femto- =
1/1,000,000,000,000,000 of the basic unit being measured. The micro- and femto- prefixes are easier to express in scientific notation. Micro- = 10^{-6} and femto- = 10^{-15}.

28. Set up an equation with equivalent fractions using the dilution fraction as one side and the percent as the other:

$\frac{1}{8} = \frac{x}{100\%};$ $8x = 100\%;$
     $x = 12.5\%$

$\frac{1}{4} = \frac{x}{100\%};$ $4x = 100\%;$
     $x = 25\%$

$\frac{1}{10} = \frac{x}{100\%};$ $10x = 100\%;$
     $x = 10\%$

29. 0.002 grams = 2 mg
0.000015 liter = 15 μL
$\frac{15}{1,000}$ liter = 15 mL

30. $\frac{\times \text{ solute required (numerator)}}{\text{desired volume (denominator)}} =$
     $\frac{\text{dilution}}{\text{ratio}} \left(\frac{\text{numerator}}{\text{denominator}}\right)$

31. $C_1 \times V_1 = C_2 \times V_2; C_2$

32. The level of accuracy of the answer should be the same as that of the original measurements. If the measurements can be made only to a tenth or hundredth of a unit, then that should be apparent from the answer.

33. Keep the same level of accuracy as in the original measurements; that is, keep the same number of digits to the right of the decimal point. Round up if the following digit is 5 or more. Round down if it is less than 5. Everyone must round the same way to assure accuracy and reproducibility of test results.

34. $\frac{1}{100}; \frac{1}{1,000}.$

35. The best way to learn and feel comfortable with the metric system is to use it. The more that you apply it, the more familiar and easy to understand it becomes. Use the metric ruler and the liquid volume containers in the student laboratory to become proficient with metric units of measurement.

36. The easiest way is to convert them to decimals first using the calculator. Divide the numerators by the denominators. Then add them as you would whole numbers, being sure that the decimals are in the correct place. Converted to decimals, these fractions are 0.5, 0.25, 0.1, 0.05, and 0.04. Their sum is 0.94.

37. The metric system is the most accurate because the English system never developed units for smaller amounts. Scientists use only the metric system, which can measure incredibly small amounts. Red blood-cell indices, for example, are reported in femtoliters and picograms.

38. The original basic units are the meter, which measures length; the liter, which measures volume; and the gram, which measures mass (weight). Prefixes are added to these as needed to measure larger or smaller amounts. SI now uses the kilogram as the basic unit of weight.

39. By adding more water or other solvent.

40. The unit "mm" stands for millimeters. The red cells of patient A settled 39 millimeters $\frac{39}{1,000}$ meters, or 0.039 meters in one hour, an abnormally high rate, indicating a pathological condition. The red cells of patient B settled 9 milliliters $\frac{9}{1,000}$ meters, or 0.009 meters in one

hour, a normal finding. The difference in their rates is 39 mm/hr − 9 mm/hr = 30 mm/hr.

41. This is a typical formula encountered in POLs. Substitute the values provided into the formula and perform the arithmetic functions with a calculator:

$$\text{Percent retic.} = \frac{\text{No. of retic. counted} \times 100}{\text{No. of RBC counted}}$$

$$\text{Percent retic.} = \frac{4}{500} \times 100 = 0.8\% \text{ retic.}$$

42. Before the calibration is needed, go to the appropriate manual and read over the instructions several times. On a separate notepad, write down any part of the procedure that you do not understand. Go to your supervisor, outline your plan for recalibration, and ask her to clarify any points that are hazy. Write down her answers. Then begin the recalibration.

43. Even though it is a very busy day, you must take time to find out why the figures vary from the usual range. Start your investigation by determining if the numbers entered into the formula appear abnormal. If so, look for errors in collecting and analyzing the specimen. If not, look for errors in your calculations. The patient's test result is then reported after verifying that there were no apparent errors.

44. Most patient tests require accurate and precise measurements for meaningful test results. Only metric and its revision, SI, have units capable of precisely measuring the very small amounts required.

45. You will use microliters (μL) to measure the specimen. This will enable you to perform the needed blood chemistry with a very small amount of blood.

Chapter 5

1. Mode: the value that occurs most often in a sample.

2. Coefficient of variation (CV): the relative standard deviation; the standard deviation expressed as a percent of the mean.

3. Median: the middle value in an ordered sample of values, with the same number of values below and above it.

4. Index: the small i under the summation sign. The index indicates the range over which the summation is to be performed.

5. Sigma (Σ, σ): the eighteenth letter of the Greek alphabet; used in statistics to represent the standard deviation (lowercase, σ) or summation (uppercase, Σ).

6. Mean: the arithmetic average of a sample of values.

7. Summation: represented by uppercase sigma, Σ: indicates addition of the numbers or variables that follow.

8. Range: the difference between the largest and smallest values in a sample.

9. Standard deviation (s or σ): a measurement of variation from the mean in a sample of values.

10. Statistics: the branch of mathematics dealing with the collection, analysis, and interpretation of numerical data.

11. Any difference from the mean of more than two standard deviations is too variant to be normal.

12. *Median* tells you where the middle of the set of samples falls.

13. The range of these samples is 10 (98.2 − 88.2).

14. You must calculate the mean and ±2 standard deviations.

15. 10^2 inverse = 10^{-2}, or $\frac{1}{10^2} = \frac{1}{100}$; 10^{-3} inverse = 10^3, or 1,000.

16. Exponents are used to write very small numbers in scientific notation. For example, the femtoliter is written as 10^{-15} of a liter. The same number written without exponents would be $\frac{1}{1,000,000,000,000,000}$. Using exponents in calculations helps prevent errors.

17. Sigma is the eighteenth letter in the Greek alphabet. It is used in statistics to indicate summation (Σ) and to represent the standard deviation (σ).

18. The mean is represented by $\bar{x}$, read "x bar." It is calculated with this formula:

$$\bar{x} = \frac{\sum_{i=1}^{n} x_i}{n}$$

The mean is the arithmetic average of a sample of values.

19. The range is not used because it is influenced too much by one or two extreme values.

20. The mean and standard deviation use whatever units the original data were measured in.

21. The formula is:

$$CV = \frac{s}{\bar{x}} \times 100$$

22. The purpose of calculating the coefficient of variation is to compare variation in two different samples of test results in order to assess the precision of two different methods for the same substances being tested, for example. The coefficient of variation standardizes the standard deviations for differences in sample means and units of measurement.

23. Another term is *relative standard deviation*.

24. The coefficient of variation is reported as a percent. It is otherwise a unitless measure.

25. Σ = sum of values; n = number of values in the sample; $\bar{x}$ = mean of the values; $\sqrt{}$ = square root.

26. a 27. g 28. f
29. c 30. d 31. e
32. b 33. h

34. First review the appropriate section of the quality-control manual—several times, if necessary. If you still do not understand the instructions, make notes of any points that are unclear. Attempt to work through sample problems. If you cannot, ask for help. Write down the explanation given.

35. You can explain this to Anne by referring to the example given in the chapter. A standard deviation of 2 mm represents far more variation when the mean is 4 mm than when the mean is 4 cm. To illustrate your explanation, draw lines with lengths of 2 mm, 4 mm, and 4 cm.

36. Although the coworker does not need to understand the working formula to use it, explain to him that the only difference in the formulas is in the numerators. The working formula squares each observation and then subtracts the square of the mean. This is equivalent to the numerator of the other formula, in which the mean is subtracted from each observation and then the difference is squared. Suggest to the coworker that he calculate a sample standard deviation using both forms of the equation to convince himself that they produce the same results.

37. To calculate the coefficient of variation for each sample, you should use the formula:

$$CV = \frac{s}{\bar{x}}$$

To calculate s, you should use the working formula for the standard deviation:

$$s = \sqrt{\frac{\sum_{i=1}^{n} x_i^2 - \dfrac{\left(\sum_{i=1}^{n} x_i\right)^2}{n}}{n - 1}}$$

To calculate $\bar{x}$, use the formula for the mean:

$$\bar{x} = \frac{\sum_{i=1}^{n} x_i}{n}$$

x_i = the individual values in each sample
n = the number of values (six in each sample)

Chapter 6

1. g   2. a   3. d
4. h   5. f   6. b
7. i   8. e   9. c

10. Accuracy: freedom from error.
11. Calibration: standardization of an instrument as required and recommended by the manufacturer.
12. Primary standard: a quality-control sample that is of the highest possible quality and accuracy.
13. Secondary standard: a quality-control sample that is developed in comparison with a primary standard.
14. Precision: the closeness of test results from the same sample.
15. Out of control: the description given to a quality-control procedure when test results are beyond the upper or lower limits of the accepted range or when they are on only one side of the mean, showing a shift or trend.
16. CLIA requires recording of test results of patients and quality controls daily and outside proficiency testing in POLs every three months (once a quarter). This entails receiving a sample from a CLIA-certified lab, analyzing it, and submitting the results to the proficiency-certifying agency.
17. About 68 percent of test results should fall within the range $\bar{x} \pm 1$ SD, about 95 percent within $\bar{x} \pm 2$ SD, and 99 percent within $\bar{x} \pm 3$ SD.
18. Terms with opposite meanings are: *precision* and *variability; accuracy* and *bias; mean* and *deviation.*
19. The formula for calculating the standard deviation of a sample of test results is:

$$s = \sqrt{\frac{\sum_{i=1}^{n}(x_i - \bar{x})^2}{n-1}}$$

20. Levey–Jennings quality-control charts (graphs) have the mean and upper and lower limits as horizontal lines across the page. The plotting of the daily quality-control tests quickly shows unusual patterns or wide deviations.
21. Random errors, shifts, and trends are quickly apparent on a Levey-Jennings chart. Random errors show on the chart as points far away from the mean, with no obvious pattern. Shifts suddenly move away from the mean and then parallel the mean. Trends move continuously farther from the mean.
22. The Clinical Laboratory Improvement Amendment (CLIA) of 1988 mandated that all clinical laboratories meet criteria for accurate testing of patient specimens by 1992. According to the CLIA, individual POLs must maintain adequate quality-control records and pass the proficiency testing requirements of an independent testing agency.
23. Bias refers to the skewing of test results away from the true value. Precision refers to the closeness of measurements to each other when the same sample is measured repeatedly. Precision must be present in accurate measurements, although precision is possible without accuracy in biased measurements.
24. Quality-control results should be recorded when they are obtained. The results may be lost or misinterpreted if posting is delayed. When results are recorded immediately, they can be compared with past results. For these reasons, CLIA mandates performing and reporting of quality-control test results the same day as patient-test results.
25. First, record the out-of-control result and then repeat the control test. If the next reading indicates the usual accuracy, you can consider the out-of-control result to be a random error, which may have numerous causes, such as a surge in the electrical current. However, if the next reading is also out of the acceptable range in the same direction, an instrument may be failing or reagents may be out of date. You must resolve the problem before you resume patient testing.
26. Inform Mrs. Smith that the POL has, by law, the same quality-control program as every other clinical lab nationwide. Explain that your POL, like every other clinical laboratory, meets stringent federal standards, which are monitored regularly.
27. Workers A and B are both consistent with acceptable QC test results. However, they are performing some part of the test procedure in a slightly different manner, such as timing, pipetting, or readying an instrument. Worker C is not showing consistent or accurate results. He or she is not duplicating the test procedure from one test to another. This variation could be due to poor eyesight, inattention, or sloppiness, among other causes.
28. Your coworker's suggestion is unethical, unprofessional, and illegal. Remind her that without quality-control monitoring, there is no way to assure accurate testing. Remind her that an inaccurate test report is worse than no test at all because it may be the basis for inappropriate patient diagnosis and treatment.
29. Dr. Tataglia intends to have you test occasional samples that are divided into two parts. She will send one part to a reference laboratory and you will test the other part in your lab. She will compare the two test results on the sample. If the results are very different, there may be a problem with the procedure in your POL.
30. Because the colorimeter is essential to the accuracy of tests performed with it, the problem must be corrected before patient testing can continue. Check the troubleshooting section of the instrument manual. It should be nearby with the record of upkeep and listings of support staff from the manufacturer. Check for defective plug-ins or other simple malfunctions. If simple troubleshooting does not solve the problem, call the support staff and describe the problem to them. Have the machine nearby so that you can carry out telephone instructions. You must reestablish the quality-control limits.
31. Dr. Arewa should buy the machine that comes as a package with technical support and service. He should think beyond the initial cost of the machine. Without appropriate quality control and upkeep, a machine is worthless for use in the POL.
32. She should admit her error, discard the control (no matter how expensive), and begin again the process of reconstituting a new concentrate, making certain to measure the diluting fluid accurately.

Chapter 7

1. Action value: also called panic value; a patient-test result requiring immediate medical attention.
2. Procedure: test instructions, a detailed written description of a testing process meant to standardize the manner in which the test is performed.
3. Manual: a laboratory handbook that contains instructions and recording forms for a particular aspect of laboratory work.
4. General policy manual: a laboratory manual that contains overall policies for every aspect of laboratory operation.
5. Record: a written account of a procedure or past event.
6. Requisition: a printed form used by a physician to request a laboratory test for a patient.
7. Standard operating procedure (SOP) manual: a lab manual containing instructions for each procedure performed in the POL.
8. Master laboratory log: the daily, chronological journal of all work done in a lab.
9. Computerized records are easy to store and retrieve, and manuals stored in computer files are easy to revise.
10. Even experienced lab workers should refer to the appropriate manual to ensure that they perform all lab tests according to exact specifications.

11. Quality-control results are recorded daily in both the master laboratory log and the quality-control manual.

12. A practicing physician is liable to lawsuits alleging malpractice. Daily recording of temperature controls in the POL is part of the proof that all possible precautions were taken to preserve quality control and integrity of testing.

13. Oral transmission should be avoided because it can compromise patient confidentiality. Also, oral transmission of information without written backup should be avoided because it lends itself to misunderstanding and loss of records.

14. The purpose of POLs is to furnish accurate and prompt patient-test results to physicians. However, the records must also support the legal requirements of the physician's office.

15. The POL's specimen-collection manual should contain the names of POL tests; the type of collection apparatus required for each test; and descriptions of any special collection techniques, handling requirements, and transportation and storage needs for each type of specimen.

16. Only the patient's physician has the right to order laboratory tests for a patient.

17. Requisition → specimen collection → collection information recorded in master laboratory log → specimen testing → test result recorded in master laboratory log → test result, if normal, is recorded in patient's chart with the normal range of a healthy individual. If the result is an action value, it is called immediately to the physician's attention then recorded in the chart.

18. Action values in the POL include high urine protein; high urine glucose and blood glucose; many white blood cells, red blood cells, or bacteria in fresh urine; grossly abnormal blood cells; pronounced anemia; and any indicator of malignancy.

19. Values for quality-control tests are recorded in the master laboratory log and the quality-control manual.

20. Proficiency testing records, as well as other quality-control records, must be kept on file for three years to satisfy CLIA regulations. State statute of limitation laws must also be considered.

21. A split specimen checks accuracy by sending part of a sample to another laboratory for analysis and retaining part for analysis in the home laboratory. The results of the two labs are compared for similarity.

22. The best way to prove that a POL is not negligent in a malpractice suit is to maintain good records of all patient-test and quality-control test procedures and results and of all calibrations.

23. The master laboratory log is a complete record of all work done in the POL, much of which is also recorded in other places. For example, quality-control test results are recorded both in the quality-control manual and the master laboratory log.

24. A statute-of-limitations law defines how many years must pass after a patient's treatment until a physician is free of professional liability and the possibility of malpractice suits. All lab records must be kept for at least this long.

25. A patient's laboratory-test results can be released legally only after written permission is given by the patient.

26. The general-policy manual should have this information.

27. Medical records, including laboratory records, must be protected against loss because they are valuable legal documents.

28. The physician has the ultimate authority and responsibility for the policies of a POL.

29. A typical requisition form when used also as a report form, contains the patient's name, the chart number, the type of test requested, the date and time the test was ordered, the name of the physician ordering the test, the date and time the specimen was collected, the name of the individual who collected the specimen, the date and time the specimen was tested, any unusual observations about the patient or specimen, the test result, and normal values for the test.

30. Patient-test results are recorded permanently in the progress notes of the patient's chart. They are part of the patient's permanent record.

31. Quality-control records safeguard the accuracy of laboratory-test results by ensuring that all test procedures produce results within accepted limits.

32. The master laboratory log provides a daily, chronological record of important POL events.

33. Action values, sometimes also called panic values, are patient-test results that indicate a need for immediate medical attention because they are so grossly abnormal.

34. The physician decides at which level of abnormality to treat patient-test results as action values. In fact, the physician must always interpret patient-test results because only the physician has the expertise and knowledge to assess their significance for a particular patient, based on the patient's symptoms and history.

35. The SOP (standard operating procedure) manual contains detailed, precise instructions to be followed in all patient testing procedures.

36. The mixup never should have occurred because all patient records are confidential. The master laboratory log, like all other medical records, should be kept in a private area of the POL instead of where patients can read it.

37. Dr. Paro's patients' confidentiality has been violated, and the doctor's professional reputation has been compromised. Dr. Paro should stress to her staff that they must not divulge confidential information either intentionally or through careless gossip.

38. Although Jera may be tempted to placate Mr. Boroughs by drawing his blood, she should not do it until Mr. Boroughs has fasted. Jera should report the situation to her supervisor or the physician and let him or her deal with the patient if necessary. Jera should not have to put herself in a position where she feels threatened, nor should she feel forced to compromise her professionalism.

39. Anne should ask to see the clinic general-policy manual. It should address these employee concerns.

40. Debbie should check to see if the test results fall within the action-value range designated by the physician. If they do, she should follow the procedure that POL workers are to follow when a test result falls within the action-value range.

41. This problem could have been avoided if the lab worker who collected the blood had looked up the amount of blood needed for each test and collected the full amount the first time Mrs. Bond was there.

42. The POL staff should assemble all relevant records, including records of correspondence, the master laboratory log, and the patient's chart.

43. The evidence needed includes all relevant quality-control and urine-test reports of that time period. Medical authorities can judge if the quality-control documentation shows that the POL met acceptable medical standards.

Chapter 8

1. The urinary system
   a. kidneys   d. prostate
   b. ureters   e. urethra
   c. bladder

2. The kidney
   a. cortex   c. renal pelvis
   b. medulla   d. ureter

3. The nephron
   a. Bowman's capsule
   b. glomerulus
   c. afferent arteriole
   d. efferent arteriole
   e. loop of Henle
   f. proximal tubule

g. distal tubule
h. collecting tubule

4. The proximal convoluted tubule is the coiled part of the tubule leading away from the Bowman's capsule. The distal convoluted tubule is the coiled part merging with tubules from other nephrons and draining into a collecting tubule.

5. Nephropathy, nephrotic syndrome, nephrosis, nephritis, nephro cystitis, and pyelonephritis are diseases of the kidneys.

6. The suffix -uria means "in the urine"; glucosuria and proteinuria.

7. Micturition, voiding, and urination describe the passing of urine from the body.

8. Electrolytes regulated by the kidneys include sodium, potassium, chloride, and bicarbonate ions.

9. i   10. e   11. b
12. c   13. g   14. d
15. a   16. h   17. f

18. Three reasons for performing a urinalysis are screening, diagnosis, and monitoring.

19. Two diagnostic purposes for urinalysis are detecting metabolic abnormalities and detecting dysfunctions of the urinary system.

20. The first physician to make urinalysis a routine part of the medical exam was Richard Bright.

21. Complete urinalysis includes physical analysis, chemical analysis, and microscopic analysis.

22. Blood vessels, nerves, and the ureter enter the kidney through the hilum.

23. Urine from the nephrons drains into the renal pelvis, which drains into the ureter.

24. Blood enters the glomerulus through the afferent arteriole and leaves through the efferent arteriole.

25. The two parts of nephrons are the renal corpuscle and the renal tubule.

26. The primary functions of nephrons are removal of waste substances from the blood and regulation of water-electrolyte balance.

27. The roles of nephrons in the formation of urine include glomerular filtration, tubular reabsorption, and tubular secretion.

28. The rate of filtration by nephrons is directly proportional to the blood pressure—faster when blood pressure is high, slower when blood pressure is low.

29. Glomerulonephritis is a condition in which the glomerular capillaries are inflamed and permeable to proteins.

30. Proteinuria is protein in the urine.

31. Glucosuria denotes the presence of glucose in the urine.

32. Diabetes insipidus is a metabolic disorder caused by a deficiency of antidiuretic hormone (ADH). This leads to failure of water reabsorption by the nephron tubules. The result is a high volume of dilute urine.

33. The breakdown of proteins produces urea, which is excreted in the urine.

34. Normal urine output is considered to be between 50 and 60 mL (cc) per hour.

35. Electrolytes found in urine include sodium, potassium, chloride, and bicarbonates.

36. Women are more prone to bladder infections than men because the female urethra is shorter, providing a shorter pathway from outside for bacteria to travel.

37. Homeostasis is the body's ability to maintain equilibrium in a changing internal and external environment.

38. Numerous factors influence the volume of urine, including fluid intake, environmental temperature, relative humidity, respiratory rate, and emotional state.

39. Renal plasma threshold denotes the concentration that a substance may reach in the blood, above which it spills over into the urine. The term is often used in conjunction with diabetes mellitus and the spillover of glucose into the urine.

40. Renal failure is failure of the kidney to carry out functions that are necessary for life—excretion of toxic substances and water-electrolyte balance.

41. Arranged in order, the parts through which urine moves from formation to micturition are: proximal convoluted tubule, loop of Henle, distal convoluted tubule, collecting tubule, collecting duct, calyx, renal pelvis, ureter, urinary bladder, and urethra.

42. Diabetes insipidus has many of the same symptoms as diabetes mellitus but a different underlying cause. Treatments differ as a result. The patient's urine will appear watery because it is not concentrated.

43. Tell Mrs. Kinsey that cystitis means inflammation of the bladder, which accompanies bladder infections. Her prescription for an antibiotic should be suitable.

44. The patient's positive test for urine glucose creates a suspicion of diabetes mellitus, which should be confirmed with further testing. The glucose is present in the urine because the renal plasma threshold level was exceeded, causing the excess to spill over into the urine.

45. A high level of protein in urine may indicate a urinary tract disorder, such as glomerulonephritis. The level of protein shows the progress of the disease. The medical term for the condition in which there is protein in the urine is proteinuria.

Chapter 9

1. A urine specimen always collected at the clinic, never at home, is the midstream, clean-catch specimen used for urine cultures.

2. Catheterization is the process of collecting urine by inserting a tube through the urethra into the bladder. It is performed by a physician, usually when the urethra is blocked.

3. An eight-hour urine specimen is collected as soon as the patient arises in the morning.

4. The urine specimen from the middle part of a single urination is a midstream specimen.

5. The postprandial urine specimen is taken after meals. That is when glucose is most likely to spill over.

6. The random urine specimen is collected as needed at any time of day or night.

7. The perineum is the area of the body immediately surrounding the rectum and urethra.

8. Urinary casts are microscopic solid molds formed from protein in the renal tubules. They often are seen in renal disease.

9. Fluid intake is the amount of liquid, such as water and juices, drunk by a patient.

10. The twenty-four hour urine specimen is collected at home by the patient over a twenty-four hour period.

11. The glucose-tolerance test (GTT) assesses the ability of the patient to metabolize glucose.

12. A urine culture requires a sterile container.

13. Diabetes mellitus is characterized by glucose and ketones in the urine.

14. The pediatric collection system is used to collect specimens from infants and young children.

15. The twenty-four hour urine specimen must be either collected into a refrigerated container or chemically preserved from the beginning to prevent decomposition of urinary casts and red and white cells.

16. Urinalysis should be performed at room temperature. If the specimen has been refrigerated, it should stand until room temperature is reached and then mixed thoroughly.

17. In the glucose-tolerance test, a sample of both urine and blood is taken after the patient has fasted. Then, glucose is administered to the patient, and additional samples of urine and blood are

taken. Diabetes mellitus is characterized by spillover of glucose into the urine following glucose administration.

18. The eight-hour urine specimen (also known as the overnight, early morning, or first morning specimen) is best for microscopic examination and for tests of nitrite and protein because the urine has been concentrated for several hours without recent fluid intake. As a result, protein is at higher levels, making diagnosis of kidney malfunction easier. The urine also has had time to incubate bacteria, which are detected by microscopic exam and the nitrite test. A high level of bacteria or positive nitrite test indicates an infection that needs treatment.

19. The midstream, clean-catch specimen must be free of contamination because it is used to incubate bacteria. This is done to identify bacteria causing urinary infection. Extraneous (outside) bacteria easily can be confused with the disease-causing organisms if extraneous bacteria are allowed to contaminate the culture. The correct pathogen must be identified because a specific drug is prescribed for each type of bacteria.

20. Urinalysis is limited to a one-hour period after collection unless the specimen is refrigerated or chemically preserved. After this time, the urine may change due to bacterial and chemical decomposition.

21. A quantitative urine test measures the exact amount of a tested substance that is excreted over a given period of time. The amount of urine and its constituents must be measured with a twenty-four hour urine specimen.

22. A postprandial urine specimen is collected two hours following a meal. At that time, the blood glucose level is most likely to be elevated and may spill over into the urine if the renal plasma threshold is reached.

23. The preferred urine-collection container is a paper or plastic disposable cup with a capacity of 50 to 100 mL and an opening of at least 2 inches. It must be both scrupulously clean and completely dry. It should be sterile if the specimen is to be cultured.

24. Urine is collected from infants with a disposable collection apparatus consisting of a plastic bag with an adhesive backing around the opening. This is attached to the child so that the urine goes directly into the bag.

25. A urine container should be labeled with the patient's name, the patient's identification number, the name of physician, and the date and time of specimen collection.

26. Random specimens are so named because they are collected at random—at any time of day or night. They are convenient, easy, and useful for qualitative tests.

27. All urine specimens, including random ones, should be collected midstream because this reduces the potential for perineal contamination.

28. Menstruating females should insert a sterile tampon before collecting urine to avoid potential contamination with menstrual blood. They also should cleanse the inner labia and urethral opening.

29. A midstream, clean-catch specimen is the middle portion of a urination, collected after the patient has completed a thorough cleansing procedure.

30. The concentration of urine varies during a twenty-four hour period mainly because of variation in fluid intake and activity level.

31. When collecting a midstream, clean-catch sample, the patient should not touch the inside of either the lid or the container.

32. To protect laboratory workers against disease, the outside of the urine container is wiped with a disinfectant when first received from the patient. The specimen should also be capped.

33. Double-voided specimens, usually timed thirty minutes apart, are collected to compare the concentration of an analyte, such as glucose.

34. A two-hour postprandial urine specimen is taken two hours after a meal.

35. Bacteria digest glucose and ketones in urine after it stands a long time. Urea is converted to ammonia.

36. Bilirubin is reduced in light. Therefore, urine specimens should not be exposed to light.

37. A young child's urine specimen is collected with a pediatric collection apparatus consisting of a plastic bag with an adhesive backing. It is attached to the perineum, and the child voids directly into the bag.

38. The female patient should be instructed to follow the cleansing procedure for female patients. She first should insert a sterile tampon if she is menstruating.

39. You should call the patients and ask them to return to the doctor's office to give another specimen. Explain to them why. The collection process should be reviewed and provision be made for correct identification of all specimens immediately after they are collected. While situations such as this may occur even in well-managed laboratories, they should serve as a warning that better methods are needed.

40. The method and purpose of the test should be explained to the patient. The patient should be told to report to the lab two hours after a meal for a urine specimen to be collected.

41. First, you should find out if the specimen was collected as instructed and whether it is fresh or refrigerated. Also, you should obtain the proper identification and wipe the specimen container with disinfectant.

42. Elderly patients may need physical assistance to prevent falls. They also may require a more thorough explanation of how to collect the specimen.

43. Look in the specimen-collection manual for patient instructions if needed. Instruct the patient to collect all urine in the container provided for exactly twenty-four hours. Tell the patient to use a preservative or refrigeration to prevent the growth of bacteria. Tell the patient to bring the specimen in as soon as possible after collection.

44. Discard the remaining sample after the doctor has seen the patient and the results of the urinanalysis and has decided that no further testing is necessary.

Chapter 10

1. f   2. d   3. b

4. g   5. a   6. c

7. e

8. *Hematuria* describes the presence of erythrocytes (red blood cells) in urine.

9. Another term for "milky" urine is *opalescent*.

10. *Anuria* signifies the complete absence of urine excretion.

11. *Polyuria* refers to the excretion of excessive amounts of nearly colorless urine.

12. The term *oliguria* designates urine production of less than 400 mL per twenty-four hours. This scant amount is incompatible with life and must be corrected.

13. *Specific gravity* refers to the density of urine relative to the density of distilled water.

14. Dehydration results when the body loses more water than it takes in.

15. Urea is a nitrogenous end product of protein metabolism secreted from the body through the urine.

16. The urinometer measures the specific gravity of urine by the depth to which it sinks as it floats in urine. It is read on an upright scale.

17. *Turbid* describes urine that has suspended matter, which gives it a cloudy appearance. A change in pH may be the cause.

18. The curved surface at the top of the urine is the meniscus. You should always read the bottom of the meniscus in order to standardize measurements.

19. Routine urinalysis examines chemical, microscopic, and physical properties of urine.

20. The physical properties of urine include color, turbidity, odor, volume, and specific gravity.

21. Concentrated urine tends to have a darker color.

22. Orange color in urine may be due to bilirubin or certain drugs.

23. Black urine may be due to melanin or iron complexes.

24. A positive yellow foam test indicates bilirubin in the urine.

25. Urine with a sweet or fruity odor may indicate diabetes mellitus.

26. Patients with a urinary tract infection may void urine with the odor of ammonia.

27. Two congenital metabolic disorders that cause urine odors are phenylketonuria (PKU) and maple-syrup urine disease. PKU causes a mousy odor in urine and maple-syrup disease urine has a maple-syrup odor.

28. Some diuretics are caffeine, alcohol, thiazides, and oral hypoglycemic agents.

29. Minerals, salts, and organic compounds influence the specific gravity of urine.

30. A very low specific gravity that never rises indicates a marked impairment of renal function.

31. Diabetes mellitus, hepatic disease, diarrhea, and dehydration may produce a high specific gravity in urine.

32. Three methods of measuring specific gravity of urine are (1) with a urinometer, which uses the weight of urine; (2) with a refractometer, which uses the refraction of light; and (3) with a reagent strip, which measures the concentration of urine.

33. Normal urinary specific gravity ranges from 1.005 to 1.030. Readings of 1.010 to 1.025 are more common.

34. A reading of 1.000 specific gravity is obtained with distilled water.

35. As a capable laboratory worker, you must report any finding that will help the physician treat his or her patients. Diseases may alter the appearance or odor of urine, providing valuable clues for treatment. Therefore, you should report any unusual finding.

36. Bilirubin (a product of hemoglobin metabolism) and certain drugs will impart a bright orange or gold color to urine. Bilirubin will also cause a yellow foam. Hepatitis, including hepatitis B, may cause a high bilirubin.

37. This is turbid urine. Changes in pH, white blood cells, red blood cells, bacteria, or fat globules may create this appearance. Chemical and microscopic urinalysis will identify the cause.

38. Odor is usually not significant, but there are exceptions. Bacteria may produce an ammonia odor. Urinary infections require prompt treatment.

39. The quality-control measures that you will use depend on the procedures designated by your supervisor. If you use a urinometer, you should test it frequently in distilled water. The reading should be 1.000. Other solutions of known specific gravity also may be used. If you use a refractometer, you should calibrate it daily to 1.000 using distilled water. Test the reagent strips with a urine-control solution.

Chapter 11

1. b   2. a   3. c
4. g   5. d   6. f
7. h   8. i   9. e

10. Glucose: tests carbohydrate metabolism; detects diabetes mellitus, a disorder of carbohydrate metabolism.

11. Ketones: tests carbohydrate and fat metabolism; ketones are present in out-of-control diabetes mellitus and starvation.

12. Protein: tests kidney function; a high protein level indicates a kidney or urinary tract lesion.

13. Blood: the presence of blood indicates a lesion within the urinary tract.

14. Bilirubin: indicates excess destruction of red blood cells or a liver disorder.

15. Urobilinogen: increases in early hepatitis and certain types of jaundice.

16. Nitrite: a positive test indicates the presence of bacteria and consequently a urinary tract infection.

17. Leukocytes: a positive test indicates large numbers of leukocytes and a urinary tract infection.

18. Routine urinalysis is the most commonly performed laboratory procedure because it provides much valuable diagnostic information to physicians. It is noninvasive, poses no risk to patients, and is inexpensive.

19. Analytes included in routine urinalysis are pH, glucose, ketones, protein, blood bilirubin, urobilinogen, and sometimes nitrite and leukocytes.

20. A screening test is an inexpensive test (usually) that determines if a patient is within the normal reference range for the analyte tested. It is used to diagnose disease in a large population of patients not known to be at particular risk.

21. A confirmatory test is generally more expensive and time-consuming than a screening test, but it is also more specific and precise. It is used to verify a patient's test result that falls outside the normal test range on a screening test.

22. The concentration of hydrogen atoms in a solution is expressed as pH.

23. The acid−base balance of the body is also measured as pH.

24. The pH of acidic urine is less than 7.0.

25. The pH of alkaline urine is more than 7.0.

26. The type of sugar most often found in urine is glucose.

27. The chief cause of glucosuria is diabetes mellitus.

28. Patients with diabetes mellitus have a deficiency of insulin, the substance that enables glucose to cross cell membranes. As a result, glucose remains in the blood, where it reaches the renal threshold and spills over into the urine.

29. Reagent strips test only for glucose.

30. The form of energy utilized by body cells is glucose.

31. Ketoacidosis develops when the body uses fats as the primary energy source.

32. An abnormal increase of protein in urine is indicative of renal disease.

33. Jaundice is yellowing of the eyes and skin. It is caused by a high level of bilirubin in the blood.

34. The nitrite test detects bacteria in a first morning specimen.

35. Bence Jones protein is not detected in the reagent-strip test. It is present in the urine of patients with multiple myeloma and other conditions.

36. Screening is performed with reagent strips. If results are positive, confirmatory tests are done.

37. Mr. Gomez's acidic urine could be due to a number of different factors, including a high-protein diet, uncontrolled diabetes mellitus, and respiratory diseases involving carbon dioxide retention.

38. Antibiotics used to treat urinary tract infections are most effective when the urine is alkaline.

39. The reagent-strip test is specific for glucose. The CLINITEST® reagent tablet is not specific for glucose and will give a positive reaction to any type of simple sugar in the urine, including galactose and lactose. The physician may be seeking evidence in the urine for galactosemia or lactose intolerance. Galactosemia, an intolerance to the sugar galactose, is a lethal metabolic disorder. It must be identified and treated by excluding galactose and lactose from the diet.

40. (a) Marked proteinuria. Possible causes include nephrotic syndrome and glomerulonephritis.
    (b) Moderate proteinuria. Possible causes include bladder stones and pre-eclampsia of pregnancy.
    (c) Minimal proteinuria. Possible causes include pyelonephritis and polycystic kidney disease.

41. A urinary bacterial infection may cause these symptoms. A very alkaline urine with the odor of ammonia may occur as bacteria decompose uric acid into urea. Bacteria convert nitrates into nitrites. A positive leukocyte esterase test occurs when the number of white blood cells that fight bacteria increases.

42. The reagent strip tested primarily for the protein albumin. Mr. Chan may have signs and symptoms of multiple myeloma. The doctor may suspect that he has high levels of urinary protein despite the negative reagent-strip test. Bence Jones protein, elevated in patients with multiple myeloma, shows up only with a confirmatory test for protein.

43. Explain to Elaine that clinically significant levels of blood can be present in urine without being visible to the naked eye, either because the amount of blood is very small or because the red blood cells have lysed.

44. When not an outside menstrual contaminant, blood is an indication of infection of or injury to the renal system. It may occur as whole red blood cells or as free hemoglobin that has been released from red blood cells that have lysed. The latter is called occult blood. It is important to notify the physician of this finding.

45. A screening test with accurate negative results is often less expensive than is a confirmatory test. A screening test also requires less time and reagent. Most patients will test negative. However, the occasional patient who tests positive will need a confirmatory test which is more sensitive. Confirmatory tests also provide a valuable quality control for screening tests.

46. When bilirubin is present in urine, the patient may have infectious hepatitis. Always use extra care when handling such a urine specimen.

47. To assure the highest level of accuracy, take care to preserve the original quality of the specimen by prompt testing or refrigeration. Keep reagent strips closed when you are not using them, and away from strong chemicals or sunlight when you are using them. Time the readings exactly as recommended. Use daily quality controls to check the reagents. Use proficiency testing to provide a backup to the above methods.

48. Several tests are time dependent and must be accurately timed. If Jerry tests several urines at once, he may make an error in timing each test. The work load may justify an automatic test-strip reader.

Chapter 12

1. f	2. e	3. i
4. h	5. a	6. d
7. c	8. b	9. g

10. Lymphocyte: a nongranular white blood cell with a single nucleus.

11. Renal cast: formed from protein in the tubules of the kidney. A high number indicates disease.

12. Cylindruria: the condition characterized by large numbers of casts in the urine.

13. Crenated: shrunken; usually used to refer to shrunken red blood cells, which appear small and scalloped around the edges.

14. Phase microscopy: the type of microscopy in which differences in the refractive index are translated into differences in brightness; used to view unstained specimens.

15. Urine sediment: the solid material that settles to the bottom of urine when it stands or is centrifuged.

16. Microscopic examination of urine sediment is the part of urinalysis that is most difficult to perform accurately and consistently for several reasons, including patient variation in urine concentration, variation in centrifuging the urine specimen, variation in power of magnification under the microscope, and lack of reference standards for urine sediments.

17. Microscopic analysis of urine sediment can provide vital information for diagnosis because it contains all of the insoluble materials in urine, including red and white blood cells, casts, crystals, bacteria, fungi, and parasites. All are useful in diagnosing disease.

18. The analysis of urinary sediment is sometimes called "liquid biopsy" because, next to actual biopsies of kidney tissue, microscopic findings are the clearest indicators of intrinsic renal disease.

19. In decantation, the supernatant liquid is poured away from the sediment of a centrifuged specimen without disturbing the sediment.

20. Urine specimens are centrifuged before microscopic examination to concentrate the formed elements.

21. The microscopic examination is begun under low-power magnification (10X) using subdued lighting. As the magnification is increased, the lighting also is increased.

22. The slide should be examined first under low power with subdued lighting to locate the fields in which most of the casts and other formed elements are present.

23. Red blood cells, white blood cells, casts, and epithelial cells are identified with high-power (45X) magnification.

24. Red blood cells, white blood cells, and epithelial cells are reported as the number per HPF, or high-power field.

25. Other elements sometimes observed in urine sediment besides cells and casts include crystals, bacteria, parasites, mucous threads, and spermatozoa and fungi such as yeast.

26. A normal urine specimen has 0 to 1 cast per LPF (low-power field).

27. An abnormally high number of casts may be due to several factors, including decreased rate of tubular flow, increased acidity of urine, and decreased volume of urine with increased protein or salt concentration.

28. When an increase in urine red blood cells is found in conjunction with red blood-cell casts, the bleeding is renal in origin.

29. An increase in urine red blood cells without casts or proteinuria indicates an extrarenal source, such as the bladder.

30. Red blood cells in hypotonic urine will lyse.

31. Red blood cells in hypertonic urine will shrink, or crenate, to resemble shriveled balls.

32. Pyuria indicates a bacterial infection in the urinary tract.

33. More than 50 leukocytes (white blood cells) per HPF and/or clumps of white blood cells in the urine are indicative of an acute urinary tract infection.

34. The type of white blood cell most often observed in the urine is the neutrophil, so named because it stains with neutral dyes.

35. When the urine contains many white blood cells and also white blood-cell casts, their origin is renal.

36. Epithelial cells are clinically significant in urine sediment when they are being desquamated at a rapid rate.

37. The results of different types of urinalysis should agree. Therefore, if microscopic examination shows many red blood cells, chemical analysis should be positive for occult blood and, possibly, for protein.

38. Ampicillin and sulfa drugs may produce crystals in urine.

39. White blood cells are about twice as large as red blood cells. White blood cells also have a nucleus, while red blood cells do not.

40. The matrix of casts is glycoprotein produced by renal epithelial cells lining the ascending limb of the loop of Henle and the distal convoluted tubule.

41. Hyaline casts are colorless, homogeneous, and semitransparent. Granular casts are dark and are usually a degenerative form of hyaline casts. Granular casts may be fine or coarse grained. Granular casts are fairly rare except in disease, while hyaline casts are the commonest type and may show an increase for nonpathological reasons, such as emotional stress or strenuous exercise.

42. Abnormal conditions revealed by a microscopic examination of urine sediment might include:
    a. various kidney diseases, by the presence of casts of different types
    b. kidney and urinary tract infections, by the presence of white blood cells and bacteria

c. inflammation from a nonurinary tract disease, by the presence of hematuria and red blood cells

d. metabolic diseases such as homocystinuria, by urinary crystals

43. The average urine on microscopic examination would probably contain a few epithelial cells, 1 or 2 red blood cells per high-power field, and 1 or 2 white blood cells per high-power field. There also might be a few crystals, the type depending on the pH of the urine. An occasional mucous strand, artifacts such as clothing strands, and, in males, a few spermatozoa also might be found.

44. The findings of the two types of analysis should be in agreement, but they are not. If many white blood cells and bacteria are present in sediment, the reagent-strip test for leukocyte esterase and nitrite should be positive.

45. The report appears to be incorrect because the findings of the microscopic and chemical examinations do not agree. When many red blood cells are observed microscopically, the reagent-strip test should have produced a positive result for occult blood. The urine specimen should be tested again. If the microscopic examination still shows many red blood cells and the chemical analysis still results in a negative result for occult blood, the chemistry quality control should be checked. The possibility of yeast being mistaken for RBC should also be considered.

Chapter 13

1. b   2. c   3. a

4. Urine chemistry analyzers eliminate the variation in timing and reading reagent strips.

5. Other advantages associated with automated urinalysis include automatic calibration; time saved; highlighting abnormal values; and automatic printing of results, which eliminates transcription errors.

6. The Clinitek 100 urine chemistry analyzer completes all testing with reagent strips, including the leukocyte esterase test, within one minute. Up to one hundred specimen results can be stored in its memory bank. Results are printed by its thermal printer, or it can be interfaced with a computer printer.

7. The instrument is keyed to start, and a reagent strip that has been immersed in a urine specimen is laid on the strip table. The start key is pressed, and ten seconds later, the strip table is drawn automatically into the machine for reading.

8. Semiquantitative results (+ system) give a rough indication of how much of an analyte is present. Quantitative results

(mg/dL) give the precise concentration of the analyte.

9. Variation in the interpretation of reagent strips may result from individual differences in visual acuity and color vision.

10. Difference among workers in the interpretation of reagent strips can result in loss of precision and accuracy because it introduces variability in test results.

11. The Clinitek 100 automatically goes through a calibration cycle when it is turned on. A control sample also is tested daily using the regular testing procedure. The sample is identified as a control specimen, and the results are recorded in the quality-control record as well as compared with the expected values for that control specimen.

12. Precision and accuracy in laboratory work produce reliable test results.

13. The best way to assure reliability in laboratory testing is always to follow the procedures. This helps maintain precision and accuracy.

14. If not already in liquid form, urine controls must be reconstituted with the appropriate diluent, in accordance with manufacturer's directions.

15. Urine-control samples can be used only a limited number of times because each time a reagent strip is dipped into the control sample, some of the reagents are leached out of the pads into the control solution, thus contaminating the control.

16. The Clinitek 100 requires only routine cleaning of the strip table, which can be removed and washed with mild soap and rinsed with warm water. The strip table platform should be disinfected with a 5 percent bleach solution.

17. The Clinitek 100 marks abnormal test results with an asterisk (*).

18. In a proficiency-testing program, unknown samples similar to the daily known-value control samples are mailed to each participating laboratory. Results are compared for precision and accuracy.

19. POL proficiency-test results that are significantly different from those of other labs suggest a problem with the procedure, sample, reagent, or instrumentation.

20. Urine controls are used to check previously opened bottles of reagent strips and new bottles of reagent strips. They also can be used by new lab workers to check on the precision and accuracy of their work.

21. There are several ways to familiarize yourself with a new instrument, such as a urine chemistry analyzer, including (a) read the manufacturer's instructions, (b) watch a demonstration of the instrument, and (c) practice test procedures

using the instrument. If you run into problems, you should seek assistance from a coworker or your supervisor. If that fails, contact a manufacturer's representative.

22. Clarisse apparently does not realize that the new instrument analyzes only the chemical components and pH of urine, not physical characteristics such as color and clarity. The latter must be observed and entered in by the lab worker.

23. Jason should have reconstituted a new urine control to test the new box of reagent strips, and he should have recorded the results. Only then should he have gone on to analyze the urine specimen. Without first testing the new reagent strips with a fresh urine control, Jason has no way of knowing if the patient-test result is accurate. Quality control never should be sacrificed for the sake of expediency.

Chapter 14

1. Anticoagulant: an agent that prevents the clotting of blood.

2. Antecubital: in the inner arm at the bend of the elbow.

3. Capillary: a small blood vessel connecting arteries and veins.

4. Hematology: the study of blood cells, blood-forming tissues, and coagulation factors.

5. Hematoma: a subcutaneous mass of blood at a venipuncture site.

6. Autolet: a semiautomatic device with a disposable lancet for capillary puncture.

7. Blood chemistry: the quantitative analysis of the chemical composition of blood.

8. Plasma: liquid portion of unclotted blood.

9. Hemoglobin (Hgb): the oxygen-carrying molecule of red blood cells.

10. Infant capillary puncture site: the commonly used capillary puncture site for infants is either side of the heel. This site can provide sufficient blood while avoiding damage to the calcaneus (heel bone).

11. Capillary puncture: the puncture of a capillary for the purpose of drawing blood.

12. Hemoconcentration: the concentration of red blood cells due to decreased plasma volume.

13. Venipuncture: the puncture of a vein for therapeutic purposes or drawing blood. Note: Remember that intravenous transfusions and venous medications are given by means of venipuncture.

14. b   15. g   16. a
17. d   18. e   19. c
20. f   21. h

22. Capillaries are small blood vessels throughout the body that connect the smaller arteries to the smaller veins.

23. A capillary puncture is made 2 to 3 mm deep with a hand-held blood lancet or a semiautomatic device with a disposable lancet.

24. A sharps container is used for safe disposal of used needles, lancets, and syringes.

25. Tourniquets are used in the procedure of venipuncture to stop the flow of venous blood and to cause the veins to enlarge, making venipuncture easier.

26. Differently colored stoppers identify collection tubes needed for different types of samples—whole blood, plasma, and serum. The colors indicate which, if any, additives (anticoagulants and separator gel) are in the tubes.

27. Separator gel in a serum-collection tube makes the work of the laboratory faster and safer because it promotes the clotting of blood and allows the serum to be left in its original tube.

28. The centrifuge is used to separate cells from the liquid portion of blood.

29. The preferred site for venipuncture is the inside of the arm at the bend of the elbow.

30. Most referral laboratories provide instructions for processing and transporting patient specimens to the referral laboratory.

31. *Serum* and *plasma* both refer to the liquid portion of blood minus the cells. Plasma has fibrinogen; serum does not.

32. The label must be placed on the specimen container at the time of collection in order to avoid misidentification.

33. A blood-collection chair makes venipuncture easier for lab workers who are drawing the blood and more comfortable for patients. An armrest supports either arm at the correct angle and stores supplies so that they are readily available.

34. Place a venipuncture tourniquet on the upper arm. Leave it on no longer than two minutes before collecting the sample. Remove it before withdrawing the needle from the vein.

35. You should use a syringe for venipuncture with children and elderly patients. The syringe is easier to maneuver and requires less cooperation from the patient. In addition, you can control the amount of vacuum in the syringe, reducing the risk of collapsed veins in elderly patients.

36. Heparin is added to some blood samples to prevent coagulation.

37. When performing a capillary puncture, choose a finger that is not calloused because a calloused area is hard to penetrate with the lancet.

38. Squeezing a finger-stick site will dilute the sample with tissue fluid from outside the capillary and will affect test results. It may also cause hemolysis.

39. Information on a blood-specimen label should include the following: name of patient, patient identification number, the date, and the time (if critical to the test). In some laboratories, the time is recorded routinely.

40. You must release the tourniquet before withdrawing the needle from the vein to prevent a hematoma.

41. The Universal Precautions are important in blood collection because they are the best protection against acquiring diseases such as AIDS and hepatitis from occupational exposure to blood.

42. Hemolysis ruins a blood sample because the red pigment that is released when red blood cells break down interferes with optical tests. The breakdown of red cells also changes the composition of the plasma or serum, affecting the results of many different blood tests.

43. Fainting, nausea, convulsions, and excessive bleeding are adverse patient reactions to venipuncture that require immediate attention.

44. Explain to the patient that hematomas often occur when blood leaks from the vein into the outside tissue. Reassure her that it is not dangerous. Explain that hematomas may be the result of a difficult venipuncture, where the needle passes through the veins or where multiple punctures are made in the same vein. A tourniquet that is left on after the needle is removed will cause a hematoma. Hematomas may also occur when insufficient pressure is maintained after the venipuncture to allow the clotting to be completed. Elderly patients are especially likely to suffer hematomas because their veins are very fragile. Bleeding time also may be prolonged. In order to minimize incidents such as this, use capillary puncture if possible. If venipuncture is necessary, take extra care with the tourniquet and keep the pressure applied afterwards for 3 to 5 minutes or more, if needed, until the bleeding stops.

45. You should get assistance from the physician or from a more experienced lab worker because patients who have blood drawn frequently may need to have the puncture made at an unusual site.

46. You should try to prevent the patient from injuring himself. Do not leave him, but call for assistance. Alert the physician immediately. Do not put anything in his mouth except a soft tongue depressor, if needed, to prevent choking.

47. You should always use capillary puncture to draw blood from an infant. You should make the puncture in the heel

following the recommended procedure for obtaining good circulation and not injuring the heel bone. A parent should hold the child, or place the infant where he or she cannot fall.

Chapter 15

1. e   2. a   3. g

4. h   5. i   6. f

7. b   8. c   9. d

10. Buffy coat: the whitish-tan layer of white blood cells and platelets between the packed red blood cells and plasma in centrifuged whole-blood samples.

11. Stromatolytic agent: a compound that helps break down the spongy protoplasmic framework of red blood cells.

12. Microhematocrit: a method of determining the hematocrit. It uses just two or three drops of blood collected in a capillary tube.

13. Hemoglobin C: an abnormal hemoglobin that is relatively common in African-Americans.

14. Hemoglobin S: sickle-cell hemoglobin.

15. Hemolytic anemia: the anemia that is due to the breakdown of red blood cells.

16. Hemoglobin E: an abnormal hemoglobin that is prevalent in India, Southeast Asia, and Southeast Asian refugees of the United States.

17. Complete blood count (CBC): a battery of hematological tests often requisitioned in POLs.

18. Erythropoietin: The kidney hormone that triggers red blood-cell formation.

19. The functions of hemoglobin are to transport oxygen to the tissues from the lungs and, to a lesser extent, carbon dioxide to the lungs from the tissues.

20. The normal adult male has a hemoglobin concentration between 14 and 17 g/dL and a hematocrit ranging from 42 to 52 percent. The normal adult female has a hemoglobin concentration between 12.5 and 15 g/dL and a hematocrit ranging from 36 to 46 percent. The normal newborn has a hemoglobin concentration between 17 and 23 g/dL and a hematocrit ranging from 50 to 62 percent.

21. The cyanmethemoglobin method estimates hemoglobin using Drabkin's reagent, a photometer or spectrophotometer, and a sample of uncoagulated whole blood.

22. Whenever hemoglobin concentration or oxygen saturation declines, the kidney produces the hormone erythropoietin, which triggers red blood-cell formation in the bone marrow.

23. The volume of packed red blood cells in the hematocrit is expressed as a percent-

age of the total volume of whole blood in the sample.

24. The complete blood count is actually a battery of tests that includes hemoglobin concentration, hematocrit, white blood-cell count, differential white blood-cell count, red blood-cell count, and sometimes erythrocyte indices.

25. Iron-deficiency anemia causes a low hemoglobin concentration because iron is needed for hemoglobin formation. Red blood cells still are formed, however, so the hematocrit is normal.

26. Use the concentration of the hemoglobin standard (C_s) to calculate the hemoglobin concentration of a patient's blood:

$$C_u = \frac{A_u}{A_s} \times C_s$$

where A_u is the absorbance of the patient sample and A_s is the absorbance of the standard, both read from the spectrophotometer.

27. The hemoglobin molecule consists of four polypeptide chains called globins, each with an iron-containing heme group attached.

28. A normal hematocrit reading of 60 percent would characterize a newborn. A normal hematocrit reading of 50 percent would characterize an adult male.

29. The specific-gravity test for hemoglobin is performed by adding a drop of blood to a copper sulfate solution of known density and determining if the blood is more or less dense than the solution by observing its movement in the solution.

30. Two different copper sulfate solutions are required for the specific-gravity test because blood from female patients normally has a lower specific gravity than does blood from male patients.

31. The principle behind the cyanmethemoglobin test is the breakdown of red blood cells by the action of Drabkin's reagent, releasing hemoglobin into the plasma, where its concentration is measured photometrically.

32. Iron is an essential element in the hemoglobin molecule that must be furnished in the diet. A lack of dietary iron results in iron-deficiency anemia. Without iron, red blood cells are produced with insufficient hemoglobin.

33. Hemoglobinopathies are diseases due to inherited defects of the hemoglobin molecule.

34. Sickle-cell hemoglobin is the most common abnormal hemoglobin in the United States affecting primarily Afro-Americans. Sickle-cell anemia is relatively common in Africa, where malaria is prevalent.

35. Sickle-cell hemoglobin is so named because it distorts red blood cells to a sickle shape when oxygen tension is low.

36. Individuals who are homozygous for the sickle-cell hemoglobin gene produce only sickle-cell hemoglobin and are affected by sickle-cell anemia. Heterozygotes have normal hemoglobin in addition to sickle-cell hemoglobin, and they normally do not show signs of anemia. They are carriers of the abnormal hemoglobin S gene, which they can pass on to their children.

37. Hemoglobin concentration and hematocrit tests are performed when physicians suspect anemia.

38. A normal hemoglobin concentration of 20 g/dL is that of a newborn.

39. A high bilirubin level (present in jaundice), lipemia (fat in the blood), leukemia, and carotinemia are conditions that may cause a falsely high hemoglobin reading.

40. They each have one gene for sickle-cell hemoglobin and one gene for normal hemoglobin. Each has enough normal hemoglobin to function well under most conditions. Each inherited the sickle-cell gene from a parent who probably was also a heterozygous carrier. Other close relatives who might have inherited the gene appear to have been heterozygous as well. When two heterozygous individuals, such as the couple in question, have children, there is a good chance (25 percent) that any given child will inherit a copy of the sickle-cell hemoglobin gene from each parent. If that occurs, the child will be homozygous for the trait and will be affected by sickle-cell anemia. The couple may wish to seek genetic counseling before having children.

41. This patient has a normal hematocrit coupled with a low hemoglobin concentration. This means that she has adequate red blood cells but that the red cells have inadequate hemoglobin. It is most likely that the patient has iron-deficiency anemia, iron being necessary for hemoglobin formation. She may need to eat more foods high in iron or to take an iron supplement.

42. This hemoglobin concentration is too high for a healthy adult male, for whom the normal range is 14 to 17 g/dL. Because the patient is apparently healthy, the test result should be investigated for possible error. The most likely source of error is a dirty spectrophotometer cell. Finger smudges or other dirt on the cell can inhibit the passage of light through the cell and bias the reading upward. You should repeat the test, making sure that the cell is spotless, and compare the second result with the first.

43. Josh is right—the "white part," or buffy coat, should not be included in the hematocrit reading. The buffy coat consists of white blood cells and platelets. If it is included as part of the packed red blood-cell volume, it will produce a falsely high hematocrit reading.

44. Alberto should not consider the two results to be close enough to be in agreement because they differ from each other by more than 2 percent.

Chapter 16

1. Agglutination: a clumping together, as of red blood cells.

2. Isotonic: having the same osmotic pressure. An isotonic solution with the same osmotic pressure as red blood cells is used to prepare blood for RBC counts.

3. Leukocytosis: an abnormally high WBC count.

4. Leukopenia: an abnormally low WBC count, usually below 4,500/mm^3.

5. Polycythemia: an increase above normal in the number of red blood cells in circulation.

6. Reticulocyte: an immature red blood cell, which retains traces of endoplasmic reticula.

7. Erythrocytosis: absolute polycythemia.

8. Pseudoagglutination: the clumping together of red blood cells as in the formation of roleaux but differing from true agglutination in that the clumped cells can be dispersed by shaking.

9. Nucleated red blood cell (nuRBC): a red blood cell that contains a nucleus.

10. Rouleau: a clump of red blood cells that appear to be stacked like a roll of coins.

11. d 12. b 13. c

14. a 15. e 16. g

17. j 18. h 19. i

20. f

21. The chief functions of white blood cells are to fight infection and to provide immunity.

22. The WBC count measures the number of white blood cells per cubic millimeter of whole blood. It is performed most commonly to diagnose infection in the body.

23. The range of normal WBC count for newborns overlaps with but is higher than the normal range for adults— 9,000 to 30,000 cells/mm^3 for newborns as compared with 4,500 to 12,000 cells/mm^3 for adults.

24. Causes of normal variation in the WBC count include the patient's age, the time of day when the sample was drawn, and whether or not the patient has recently eaten, exercised strenuously, been exposed to temperature extremes, or is pregnant. Causes of abnormal variation in the WBC count include bacterial infections, leukemia, hemorrhage, sudden hemolysis of red blood cells, tumors of

the gastrointestinal tract or liver, epileptic seizures, epinephrine injections, pain, anoxia, and cigarette smoking, all of which tend to elevate the WBC count. The WBC count may be abnormally low due to viral infections; exposure to radiation, lead, or mercury; and pernicious anemia.

25. When performing a WBC count, you must add acid to the blood before counting the white blood cells in order to hemolyze the red blood cells and leave just the white blood cells intact.

26. An Adams suction apparatus is used as a safety device when performing blood counts to siphon the blood and diluting fluid into the micropipette and to prevent accidental ingestion of these liquids. It consists of an airtight rubber gasket and a stainless steel barrel with a thumbscrew at the end. The pipette is inserted into the hole in the gasket. Then, the thumbscrew is screwed out to draw the liquid into the pipette and screwed in to force the liquid out again.

27. The first three drops of fluid from the pipette always are discarded when doing a blood count to get rid of any diluting solution remaining in the stem of the pipette. Only the mixture from the bulb of the pipette should be used for the blood count.

28. When performing a WBC count, the area to be counted consists of the four 1 mm² corner squares on each side of the hemacytometer counting chamber. The total area counted on each side of the counting chamber is 4 mm².

29. The presence of nucleated red blood cells in a sample inflates the WBC count because nucleated red blood cells cannot be distinguished from white blood cells under low-power magnification. To correct for this, the number of nucleated red blood cells per 100 white blood cells must be determined on a stained blood smear under high-power magnification and then used in a formula that estimates their number per cubic millimeter. The latter number then is subtracted from the WBC count.

30. The depth factor in the WBC count formula is 10, even though the sample in the hemacytometer is only 0.1 mm deep, so that the answer will give the number of white blood cells per cubic millimeter.

31. The dilution is 1:20 in a white blood-cell pipette in which blood is drawn to the 0.5 mark and diluting fluid is drawn to the 11.0 mark because only the solution in the bulb of the pipette is used, and it contains 10 units: $\frac{0.5}{10} = \frac{1}{20}$, or 1:20.

32. RBC count includes a count of mature erythrocytes and reticulocytes. The latter usually make up about 1 percent of circulating blood cells.

33. A woman's RBC count usually is somewhat lower than the RBC count of a man. The male and female adult ranges overlap, but the female range is lower by about half a million red blood cells/mm³—4.0 to 5.5 million cells/mm³ as compared with 4.5 to 6.0 million cells/mm³ for men.

34. Causes of normal variation in the RBC count include age and sex. Causes of abnormal variation include dehydration, which increases the RBC count, and physiological states that promote erythropoiesis, such as low oxygen tension in the blood, slow circulation, and defective hemoglobin. Abnormally low RBC counts may be caused by disorders of bone marrow, such as aplastic anemia, or by certain drugs, including analgesics, like aspirin, and antihistamines, like chlorpheniramine.

35. When performing an RBC count, a solution such as normal (isotonic) saline must be added to the blood before the count is made to dilute the cells for easier counting and to prevent hemolysis of the red blood cells.

36. When performing an RBC count, the area of the hemacytometer that is counted is located within the 1 mm² center of the ruled area on each side of the counting chamber. The 1 mm² center area is divided into twenty-five smaller squares. Of these, the four corner squares and the center square are included in the red blood-cell count. The total area counted is $\frac{5}{25}$ or $\frac{1}{5}$ mm².

37. Agglutination of red blood cells on the hemacytometer may be due to low temperature of the sample. Pseudoagglutination may be due to the presence of paraprotein in the sample. The two processes can be distinguished by shaking the sample. With pseudoagglutination, the red blood cells can be dispersed by shaking. If the sample is agglutinated due to cold, discard it and then dilute another specimen, which should be warmed to body temperature before charging the hemacytometer.

38. When counting red blood cells or white blood cells, count the cells that touch the borderlines on just two sides of each square.

39. The most common reason for performing an RBC count is to diagnose anemia.

40. If a patient is taking the drug primidone, which is an anticonvulsant, his or her RBC count may be depressed. Anticonvulsants are one of many types of drugs that may lower the RBC count because they either reduce red blood-cell production or cause hemolysis of red blood cells.

41. The doctor probably will diagnose Mrs. Potts with a bacterial infection of the urinary tract. Any type of bacterial infection will produce an elevated WBC count, and Mrs. Pott's WBC count of 16,000 is somewhat higher than the normal range of variation for an adult. Urinary tract infections also may produce bleeding, which shows up in the urine, as in Mrs. Pott's case.

42. The coworker has made several errors in performing the RBC count that may endanger worker safety and jeopardize the accuracy of test results. She should have used a mechanical suction apparatus to siphon the blood and diluting fluid when using a pipette instead of her mouth and a rubber tube. Without the mechanical suction apparatus, she risks ingesting biohazardous or toxic liquids. Using a tissue or similarly absorbent material to drain the excess blood out of the pipette wicks fluid out of the pipette and may increase the blood count. Instead, she should have touched the tip of the pipette to a nonabsorbent surface, such as her gloved index finger. Tissues and other materials that may be contaminated with blood are biological hazards and should be disposed of as such. They should not have been placed in an unlabeled wastebasket or on a counter.

43. a. You should discard the sample, clean the hemacytometer, and start over again with a new sample. A difference of ten or greater in the cell tally among small squares in each corner square means that the cells are too unevenly distributed to provide an accurate WBC count. Such an uneven distribution of cells usually is caused by a dirty hemacytometer or coverslip.
    b. You should discard the sample, clean the hemacytometer, and start over again with a new sample. Air bubbles may lead to a falsely low blood count.
    c. The sample is agglutinated. You should discard the sample, clean the hemacytometer, and start over again, this time warming the specimen to body temperature before recharging the hemacytometer. If warming does not eliminate the clumping, this clumping may be caused by the presence of paraprotein in the sample, which is an indicator of an immunoglobulin disorder. In this case, you can disperse the red blood cells by shaking them.
    d. The blood sample has stood too long to be useful for a blood count. The doctor should be told what happened so that a fresh blood sample can be obtained from the patient.

44. Brad should have let the sample stand in the hemacytometer for at least three minutes before focusing the microscope and counting the cells. He also should have counted the cells on both sides of the counting chamber of the hemacy-

tometer and used the average of the two tallies to calculate the RBC count.

45. A check of the red blood-cell tallies reveals a relatively even distribution of red blood cells. None of the tallies differs by ten or more from any other. The total number of cells on the two sides of the counting chamber are 501 (100 + 99 + 103 + 95 + 104) and 505 (103 + 105 + 99 + 97 + 101), for an average number of 503 cells counted. Because the dilution is $1:200 \left(\dfrac{0.5}{100}\right)$, you can use the shorthand formula for calculating the RBC count:

$$RBC/mm^3 = \text{No. of cells counted} \times 10,000$$

Substituting, you get,

$$RBC/mm^3 = 503 \times 10,000 = 5,030,000$$

46. Anticonvulsant drugs and diuretics may reduce red blood-cell production or cause hemolysis of red blood cells, leading to a lower RBC count.

47. A WBC count of less than $1,000/mm^3$ is considered dangerously low—an action value. This should be reported to the physician immediately.

Chapter 17

1. Anisocytosis: the excessive variation in the size of cells, especially red blood cells.

2. Eosin: a red-orange acidic dye used to stain blood smears for microscopic examination.

3. Hypersegmented: having a nucleus with more than five segments, or lobes.

4. Infectious mononucleosis: an acute infectious disease in which lymphocytes are both more numerous and larger than normal and often contain vacuoles, causing them to resemble monocytes.

5. Megakaryocyte: a large bone marrow cell with large or multiple nuclei which gives rise to platelets.

6. Methylene blue: a blue alkaline dye used to stain blood smears for microscopic examination.

7. Neutropenia: a decrease below normal in the number of neutrophils in the blood.

8. Poikilocytosis: a condition in which many red blood cells have abnormal shapes.

9. Polychromatic stain: a stain containing dyes of two or more colors, such as Wright's stain.

10. Polymorphonuclear: having a multi-lobed nucleus.

11. Quick-stain method: a method of staining blood smears, in which the smear is dipped sequentially in fixative, acidic stain, and alkaline stain; also called the three-step method.

12. Wright's stain: a polychromatic stain for fixing and staining blood smears.

13. Monocytic leukemia: a form of acute leukemia in which abnormal monocytes proliferate and invade the blood, bone marrow, and other tissues.

14. Lymphocytic leukemia: predominantly a children's disease, in which the blood-forming tissues produce an excessive number of lymphocytes.

15. Endocarditis: the inflammation of the lining of the heart.

16. Granulocyte, agranulocyte—*similarities:* both are classes of white blood cells; *differences:* granulocytes make up about two-thirds of white blood cells, are polymorphonuclear, and have granules in their cytoplasm that are distinctive after staining; agranulocytes make up about one-third of white blood cells, usually are mononuclear, and most often do not have distinctive cytoplasmic granules.

17. Neutrophil, eosinophil, basophil—*similarities:* all are types of granulocytes; *differences:* neutrophils are very common, have nuclei with up to five lobes, and cytoplasm filled with fine granules that stain pink or lilac; eosinophils are relatively uncommon, have nuclei with just two lobes, and cytoplasm with large, spherical granules that stain bright red; basophils are the least common and have large, irregularly shaped cytoplasmic granules that stain blue-black and may obscure the nucleus.

18. Normochromic, hyperchromic, hypochromic—*similarities:* all are terms describing the amount of pigment in red blood cells; *differences:* normochromic refers to red blood cells with the normal amount of pigment; hyperchromic refers to red blood cells with excessive pigment; hypochromic refers to red blood cells that are relatively deficient in pigment.

19. Lymphocyte, monocyte—*similarities:* both are types of agranulocytes; *differences:* lymphocytes are much more common, are smaller, and have chromatin that is clumped; monocytes are much less common, are larger, and have chromatin that has a coarse, linear pattern.

20. Macrocyte, microcyte—*similarities:* both refer to the size of red blood cells; *differences:* macrocyte refers to an unusually large red blood cell greater than 12 micrometers (microns) in diameter; microcyte refers to an unusually small red blood cell (less than 6 micrometers in diameter).

21. Red blood cells differ from most other cells in having no nuclei and in their small size.

22. In each cubic millimeter of normal blood, there are about 5,000,000 red blood cells, 250,000 platelets, and 7,000 white blood cells. White blood cells are the largest and platelets the smallest. The smallest white blood cells are only slightly bigger than red blood cells; platelets are about half as big as red blood cells.

23. The most numerous leukocyte in adults is the neutrophil. The least numerous is the basophil.

24. A blood-smear slide should be dried by waving it in the air or blowing it with an electric fan. You should never blow on the slide because exhaled water droplets may make holes in the smear.

25. Smears that are too thin may have too few blood cells and cells that appear flattened. Smears that are too thick may have multiple layers of cells and distortion in the cells due to crowding. Both make for poor viewing of the formed elements on the smear. The spreader slide must be held at a 35 to 40 degree angle relative to the horizontal smear slide to ensure that the smear has the appropriate thickness. Too great an angle produces too thick a smear, and too small an angle produces too thin a smear.

26. A properly prepared blood-smear slide covers about two-thirds of the length of the slide and coats the slide smoothly, without grainy streaks or ridges. A correctly prepared blood-smear slide also has three different regions: the heel, the feathered edge, and the body.

27. The body of a blood-smear slide is the region examined under the microscope in a differential count because it contains numerous cells arranged in a single layer with minimal distortion from adjacent cells.

28. Cell nuclei are called basophilic because they attract basic dyes like methylene blue. Cytoplasm is called eosinophilic, or acidophilic, because it attracts acidic dyes like eosin.

29. A stained blood smear may appear too blue because the smear is too thick, the stain was left on too long, the stain was washed off inadequately, or the stain or the buffer was too alkaline. A stained blood smear may appear too pink because the staining time was too short, too much stain was washed off, or the stain or the buffer was too acidic.

30. Quick stain may be preferred to Wright's stain because it is quicker and easier to use and allows variation in the proportion of each dye used.

31. Staining affinities differ among formed elements in the blood. This characteristic, in addition to several others, helps to distinguish among the formed elements on differential smears. Cytoplasmic granules of neutrophils stain blue,

for example, while those of eosinophils stain red.

32. To differentiate among the different types of white blood cells, cell size, nuclear characteristics (shape, size, structure, and color), and cytoplasmic characteristics (amount, color, and types of inclusions) must be examined.

33. Lymphocytes can be distinguished from monocytes on the basis of several features. Lymphocytes normally are smaller than monocytes. If cytoplasmic granules are present, they tend to be smaller in monocytes. In lymphocytes, the chromatin of the nucleus is all in a clump, while in monocytes, there are light spaces between the chromatin strands, giving the chromatin a coarse, linear pattern.

34. White blood cells are counted in the body region of a differential blood-smear slide under $100 \times$ magnification, following a definite pattern to avoid counting the same area of the slide twice. A manual cell counter is used to tally the different types of white blood cells observed. The number of each type of white blood cell is expressed as a percentage of the total number of white blood cells counted.

35. A high neutrophil count usually indicates infection by pyogenic organisms, such as streptococcus and staphylococcus. A low neutrophil count may be due to certain drugs, some acute infections, radiation, and diseases of the spleen or bone marrow.

36. An increase in the number of small lymphocytes may be due to whooping cough, tuberculosis, brucellosis, infectious lymphocytosis, infectious mononucleosis, or lymphocytic anemia.

37. In a differential blood-smear slide, red blood cells are examined for their size, shape, and hemoglobin content.

38. Hemoglobin content can be assessed from the color of the red blood cells on a differential blood-smear slide. The more hemoglobin present, the darker is the red stain. The size of the pale central area of the cell also is larger in cells with less hemoglobin.

39. The biconcave disk shape of normal red blood cells assists in the transport and release of oxygen. This shape has more surface area per volume than does a spherical shape, and the relatively greater surface area helps the hemoglobin in the cells function more effectively.

40. Platelets are fragments of megakaryocytes, which are large cells formed in the bone marrow. Their function is to help blood clot.

41. Platelets are counted by counting the number of platelets in a few high-power fields and multiplying the average by 20,000.

42. A reduced platelet count may be due to acute infection, anaphylactic shock, certain hemorrhagic diseases, or anemia. An increased platelet count may be due to surgery (especially splenectomy), violent exercise, or tissue injury.

43. Several characteristics of each type of white blood cell should be pointed out to the new worker, including cell size; the shape, size, structure, and color of the nucleus; and the amount, color, and types of inclusions of the cytoplasm.

44. If the platelet count is low, you will see no more than an average of two platelets per high-power field.

45. The child has anemia. The hemoglobin concentration is likely to be low.

46. The smear is too thick. If a duplicate smear is available, stain and view it. If not, a new set of smears must be prepared for this patient.

47. When a smear is too dark it has been dipped too many times in stain, and/or it has been washed inadequately. Decrease the number of dips (to a minimum of three) for each stain solution and/or wash the smear more thoroughly until the stain has the right intensity.

48. The blood-smear slide has a precipitate. This may be caused by a dirty slide, drying during the staining period, or inadequate washing or filtering of the stain. A new slide should be prepared, avoiding these pitfalls.

Chapter 18

1. Cyanmethemoglobin: a very stable compound that results when a solution of potassium ferrocyanide and potassium cyanide is added to blood, lysing the red blood cells and releasing their hemoglobin content.

2. Electrical impedance method: the method of studying the formed elements in the blood that depends on their resistance to the flow of an electrical current.

3. Electron-optical cell counter: the automated hematology instrument that analyzes formed elements in the blood on the basis of their interruption of a beam of light from a laser lamp.

4. Hematology calibrator: a hematology control that is certified to be highly stable over its entire life. It is used to set the electronics of automated hematology instruments.

5. Photomultiplier tube (PMT): an electron multiplier in which electrons released by photoelectric emission are multiplied in successive stages by dynodes that produce secondary emission; used to detect reduction in intensity of the light beam from an electron-optical cell counter.

6. QBC (quantitative buffy coat) instrument: an automated hematology instrument that centrifuges nondiluted blood samples and estimates blood parameters, such as hemoglobin, hematocrit, platelet counts, and WBC counts, on the basis of differences in density and fluorescence.

7. Aperture: an opening, as in the probe of an electrical impedance or electron-optical cell counter, through which blood cells and other formed elements pass single file.

8. Dilution #1: the 1:250 sample dilution that is used with electrical impedance cell counters for WBC counts and hemoglobin determinations. It is made by adding 40 μL of blood to 10 mL of isotonic saline solution.

9. Electrical impedance cell counter: an automated hematology instrument, such as the Danam and Cell Dyn instruments, that analyzes formed elements in the blood on the basis of their impedance of an electrical current.

10. Light-beam method: the method of studying formed elements in the blood that depends on their interruption of a beam of light from a laser lamp.

11. The main advantages of using automated hematology instruments over using manual methods are the greater accuracy and speed of automated methods.

12. The main purposes of automated hematology instruments are to differentiate and count the formed elements in the blood and to determine hemoglobin.

13. Specific functions performed by automated hematology instruments include RBC count, WBC count, platelet count, hemoglobin determination, hematocrit, mean cell volume, mean cell hemoglobin, mean cell hemoglobin concentration, granulocyte count, percent granulocytes, nongranulocyte count, percent nongranulocytes, mid-range cell count, percent mid-range cells, lymphocyte count, percent lymphocytes, and red blood-cell distribution width.

14. Factors that should be considered when selecting an automated hematology instrument for a particular POL include the hematological tests most commonly performed, the degree of automation required, the cost of instrument and maintenance, the amount of laboratory space available, and the number of staff.

15. An electrical impedance cell counter works by counting the electrical impulses generated when blood cells pass through and momentarily impede an electrical current.

16. The electrical impedance cell counter differentiates cells on the basis of size by pulse amplitude—the larger the cell, the greater the electrical pulse created when the cell passes through the current.

17. It is necessary to dilute blood samples when performing tests using some automated cell counters because blood cells are highly concentrated, particularly red blood cells and platelets. Dilution allows the cells to be conducted in single file past the counting point. The greater the dilution, the better the separation of cells and the less likely that more than one cell will pass the counting point simultaneously and bias the count.

18. Make Dilution #1 by adding 40 μL of blood to 10 mL of 85 percent saline solution. Make Dilution #2 by further diluting 40 μL of Dilution #1 with another 10 mL of saline solution.

19. Two different dilutions are necessary when using electrical impedance cell counters because cells that are more concentrated in normal blood (red blood cells and platelets) require a greater dilution to be adequately separated when they file past the counting point. Dilution #1 is used for WBC counts and hemoglobin determinations. Dilution #2 is used for RBC counts and platelet counts.

20. A 0.85 percent saline solution is the diluent used to dilute samples for testing with electrical impedance cell counters. This diluent is used because it is isotonic with blood cells, thus preventing any alteration in cell size through the transfer of water in or out of the cells.

21. A lysing agent must be added to the blood sample for WBC counts and hemoglobin determinations when using an electrical impedance cell counter because the lysing agent destroys red blood cells, which would interfere with a WBC count, and releases hemoglobin into the plasma, where its concentration can be measured. The lysing agent used is a solution of potassium ferrocyanide and potassium cyanide.

22. A colorimetric method is used to determine hemoglobin concentration with an automated cell counter. The amount of green light absorbed by the sample, which is detected with a photodetector, has a logarithmic relationship to the concentration of hemoglobin present.

23. Electron-optical cell counters are not used commonly in POLs because they are designed to handle large volumes of blood samples and the start-up and shut-down processes are not as easy as those with more common hematology instruments.

24. An electron-optical cell counter works by measuring the reduction in intensity in a beam of light as blood cells pass through it single file.

25. Different types of blood cells are distinguished with a QBC instrument by their chemical and physical differences, which cause them to fluoresce different colors.

26. Hemoglobin concentration is estimated with a QBC instrument by noting the height of the plastic float in the hematocrit column. Red blood cells that contain large amounts of hemoglobin are more dense and cause the float to ride high. Red blood cells that are low in hemoglobin have a lower density, causing the float to sink in the column when it is centrifuged.

27. The role of quality control in the use of automated hematology instruments is to test the accuracy and precision of the instrument, the procedure, and the operator. The ways in which quality control is achieved include the regular use of calibrators to set the electronics of the instruments, the use of controls to check the stability of the settings, the use of split specimens to detect inaccurate or imprecise test results, and daily checking of reagents for quality.

28. Hematology controls are artificial bloods that include both human and animal cells. They usually are available in abnormal low values, normal values, and abnormal high values. They are used to check the stability of automated hematology instruments.

29. The hematology parameters that can be estimated with a QBC instrument include hemoglobin concentration, hematocrit, platelet count, total WBC count, total granulocyte count, percent granulocytes, total lymphocyte/monocyte count, and percent lymphocytes/monocytes.

30. If your coworker tries to run these tests on the QBC instrument, he will find that this instrument does not do RBC counts nor does it complete differential WBC counts. Instead, he could use a blood smear for a manual differential WBC count and an automated cell counter for the RBC count.

31. In acute leukemia, the percent of white blood cells rises so greatly that it affects the accuracy of the RBC count. At this stage, the white blood cells must be subtracted from the total RBC count. Normally, white blood cells are not subtracted because they are present in insignificant numbers compared to red blood cells.

32. The manual differential allows a visual inspection of all the features of the different cells. The automated differential sorts the cells into different types on the basis of size alone. It cannot identify different cells of the same size or abnormal features of cells, such as sickle-shaped cells, abnormal lymphocytes, or immature cells.

33. Because the artificial blood contains human blood components, you should handle it with the same safety precautions that apply to human blood samples.

34. The hematology instrument purchased to do erythrocyte indices should be an automated cell counter. Erythrocyte indices require accurate RBC counts, such as provided by electrical impedance and electron-optical cell counters. The QBC instrument, by contrast, does only hematocrits and hemoglobin, not RBC counts.

Chapter 19

1. j 2. c 3. b
4. g 5. d 6. e
7. f 8. h 9. a
10. i

11. Erythrocyte indices: three indicators of the size or hemoglobin content of the red blood cells that are used in the diagnosis of anemia. They include the mean cell volume (MCV), the mean cell hemoglobin (MCH), and the mean cell hemoglobin concentration (MCHC).

12. Erythrocyte sedimentation rate (ESR or sed rate): the rate at which red blood cells settle out of plasma when placed in a vertical tube.

13. Mean cell volume (MCV): the average volume of individual red blood cells in a sample.

14. Mean cell hemoglobin (MCH): the average weight of hemoglobin in individual red blood cells in a sample.

15. Mean cell hemoglobin concentration (MCHC): the average concentration of hemoglobin in a given volume of packed red blood cells in a sample.

16. The erythrocyte indices are calculated from the RBC count, hemoglobin concentration, and hematocrit.

17. The erythrocyte indices became a routine part of the complete blood count with the widespread use of automated hematology instruments. Until then, the RBC count was too prone to error for the indices to be reliable.

18. The validity of the erythrocyte indices should be checked against the appearance (size and color) of the red blood cells on a stained blood-smear slide.

19. The formula for calculating MCV is:

$$MCV = \frac{Hct \, (\%) \times 10}{RBC \, (millions)}$$

20. MCH is determined by the hemoglobin concentration and the RBC count.

21. MCHC is expressed by the ratio of the weight of hemoglobin to the volume of red blood cells.

22. The normal adult ranges for the erythrocyte indices are MCV = 82 to 102 fL or μm³, MCH = 27.0 to 33.0 pg or μμg; and MCHC = 33.0 to 38.0 g/dL.

23. A deviation of more than one unit from the normal range of an erythrocyte index usually means that the patient has some type of anemia.

24. Conditions that lead to an increase over normal in the value of MCV include vitamin B_{12} deficiency and pernicious anemia. Conditions that lead to a decrease include iron-deficiency anemia.

25. The value of MCH is likely to be greater than normal when the patient has a macrocytic anemia.

26. A very high MCHC value is suspect because it occurs only with spherocytosis, a condition in which erythrocytes assume a spheroid shape, characteristic of certain hemolytic anemias. When MCHC is above 40 percent and the other blood parameters are normal, the automated hematology instrument should be checked for malfunction.

27. The shorthand formula for the platelet count can be used whenever the dilution is 1 : 100.

28. Potential sources of error in performing manual platelet counts using the direct method include improper dilution of the sample; contaminated or cloudy reagent; clots in the blood sample or clumping of platelets (unlikely with the use of EDTA anticoagulant); overfilling or underfilling of the hemacytometer; inclusion of red blood cells or dust particles in the count; and incorrect calculations.

29. The validity of a platelet count can be checked against an estimate of the platelet count made from examination of a stained blood-smear slide. The direct count and the estimate from the slide should agree. (The slide also has the advantage of showing morphological characteristics of individual platelets.)

30. The three stages of erythrocyte sedimentation are the initial period of aggregation—the first ten minutes, during which rouleaux form and relatively slow sedimentation of red blood cells occurs; the period of rapid settling—the next half hour to two hours (depending on the length of the tube), during which sedimentation occurs at a fairly constant rate; and the third stage—the final stage, during which sedimentation slows as sedimented red blood cells are packed at the bottom of the column. The second stage, the period of rapid settling, is the most significant for the ESR.

31. Dilution of the sample by lab workers is a potential source of error in the Westergren method. The undiluted blood sample in the Wintrobe test has the added advantage of being reusable for additional tests. On the other hand, dilution of the blood sample in the Westergren method has the advantage of eliminating the need to correct for ane-

mia or polycythemia. The Westergren method is more sensitive for the serial study of chronic diseases. In terms of safety, the Sediplast Westergren system is the method of choice.

32. Sources of error that should be avoided in performing an ESR test include tilting the ESR tube; vibrations to the tube; deviation of room temperature from a constant 20 to 25 degrees Celsius; placement of the ESR rack in a draft or sunlight; use of heparin as anticoagulant; use of blood that has stood longer than two hours at room temperature; a reading time of not exactly one hour; and clots or air bubbles in the sample.

33. Red blood-cell factors that influence the sed rate include weight per unit volume; cell size; rouleau formation; and red blood-cell concentration.

34. Plasma factors that influence erythrocyte sedimentation include the levels of fibrinogen, globulin, and albumin. In most acute infections, globulins and fibrinogen are increased, while albumin is somewhat reduced. This combination increases the rate at which red blood cells settle.

35. Potential sources of error in performing reticulocyte counts include overincubation of the blood-stain mixture; use of unfiltered stains; overlooking of small amounts of reticular material in the count; counting too few cells; nonsystematic counting of the cells in the counting area; and counting artifacts as reticula.

36. The reticulocyte count is a valuable indicator of erythropoiesis because there is up to a sevenfold increase in the number of circulating reticulocytes when the production of red blood cells is increased.

37. The reticulocyte count is especially useful clinically in monitoring patient response to treatment for anemia. The reticulocyte count should increase with specific treatment. If it fails to, the cause must be investigated. A relatively small number of red blood cells may lead to an apparent reticulocytosis, which is not indicative of increased red blood-cell production. An increase in reticulocytes also may be due to premature release of reticulocytes from the bone marrow, which may follow massive hemorrhage.

38. The absolute number of reticulocytes should be reported routinely because this number can be used directly to assess bone marrow response to anemia, whereas the percent of reticulocytes must be correlated with other hematological parameters to be useful clinically.

39. The absolute number of reticulocytes, when compared to the normal average of 60,000 reticulocytes/mm³, gives phy-

sicians a direct indication of bone marrow response. A high absolute number of reticulocytes indicates increased red blood-cell production. The percentage of reticulocytes first must be correlated with other hematology results, such as erythrocyte indices, to be meaningful to physicians.

40. First find the lab manual outlining the exact procedure. Read it and collect all of the needed materials beforehand. Ask questions to clarify anything that you are unsure of. The usual procedure is to place a drop of blood and a drop of methylene blue stain side by side on a glass slide. Mix the drops together, draw them into a capillary tube, and allow the tube to stand exactly ten minutes. Deliver the blood-stain mixture to a clean slide and make a smear, following the same procedure as for a differential blood-smear slide. Air dry the smear and count the reticulocytes under the oil-immersion lens.

41. The first step should be to carefully read through the written procedure in the appropriate manual. You will need a Westergren tube, an ESR rack, and a Pasteur pipette. Alternatively, you may use a disposable Westergren kit. The anticoagulant, trisodium citrate, will be mixed with the blood. The test will require one hour. The ESR will be reported in millimeters per hour.

42. The ESR with a 50 mm/hr reading is abnormal. The reading of 5 mm/hr is normal.

43. $\text{MCV} = \dfrac{25 \times 10}{4.1} = 61 \text{ fL}$

$\text{MCH} = \dfrac{6.4 \times 10}{4.1} = 15.6 \text{ pg}$

$\text{MCHC} = \dfrac{6.4 \times 100}{25}$
$= 25.6 \text{ g/dL}$

This patient has low values for all three indices and may have iron-deficiency anemia.

44. Platelet count $= 162 \times 1,000$
$= 162,000 \text{ platelets/mm}^3$

45. Percent reticulocytes $= \dfrac{43 \times 100}{1,000}$
$= 4.3 \text{ percent}$
Absolute no. of reticulocytes $=$
$4.3\% \times 3,500,000 =$
$150,500 \text{ reticulocytes/mm}^3$

Chapter 20

1. Coagulation: the process of clotting.

2. Bleeding time: the length of time it takes a small incision to stop bleeding.

3. Cerebrovascular accident: stroke.

4. Clotting disorder: a coagulation disease in which clots form in the blood spontaneously.

5. Coagulation factor: one of the twelve compounds required for the coagulation process. Coagulation factors must be present in appropriate amounts for clotting to occur effectively.

6. Coumarin: a group of drugs, including warfarin, used to prevent and treat clotting disorders. Coumarin drugs act in the liver, where they interfere with the synthesis of vitamin K-dependent coagulation factors (II, VII, IX, and X).

7. Embolism: the sudden obstruction of a blood vessel by an embolus.

8. Fibrin: the whitish, filamentous protein formed by the action of thrombin on fibrinogen. Other formed elements in the blood become entangled in the interlacing filaments of fibrin, thus forming a blood clot.

9. Fibrinogen: coagulation factor I; a compound in plasma that is converted to fibrin by thrombin in the presence of calcium.

10. Hemophilia: one of a group of diseases in which excessive bleeding occurs because of inherited deficiencies in blood coagulation factors.

11. Hemorrhagic disease: any of several diseases in which excessive bleeding occurs because blood fails to clot.

12. Hemostasis: the arrest of bleeding.

13. Platelet plug (white thrombus): the clump of platelets that adheres to an injured vessel to help stop bleeding.

14. Prothrombin: coagulation factor II; a compound in circulating blood that is converted to thrombin by the action of thromboplastin.

15. Serotonin: a potent vasoconstrictor, which is released by platelets adhering to a wounded blood vessel.

16. Template method (Ivy bleeding time): a method of testing bleeding time. The template method standardizes the size and depth of the incision using a template device called a Simplate.

17. Thromboplastin: coagulation factor III; the immediate initiator of the blood-clotting mechanism. Thromboplastin interacts with other coagulation factors to convert prothrombin to thrombin.

18. Thrombus: a blood clot within the vascular system.

19. Vasoconstriction: the constricting, or narrowing, of a blood vessel.

20. Warfarin: one of the coumarin group of anticoagulants used to prevent and treat clotting disorders.

21. False. The mechanisms by which hemostasis comes about are coagulation, vasoconstriction, and platelet plug formation.

22. False. The process of hemostasis can be divided into three types of phenomena: intravascular, vascular, and extravascular.

23. True.

24. False. Thromboplastin interacts with other coagulation factors to convert prothrombin to thrombin.

25. False. Thrombin joins soluble fibrinogen molecules into long, hairlike molecules of insoluble fibrin.

26. False. Diseases that affect coagulation fall into two opposing categories: hemorrhagic diseases and clotting disorders.

27. False. Most cases of hemophilia are inherited.

28. False. Female hemophiliacs are extremely rare because females need two copies of the recessive gene to be affected (males need just one).

29. False. Vitamin K is the precursor from which several coagulation factors are synthesized. Therefore, it is necessary for a functioning coagulation process.

30. True.

31. Thrombosis is the formation of a blood clot or clots in the vascular system. It is treated with anticoagulant drugs that are monitored with routine lab tests of blood coagulation.

32. Myocardial infarction and cerebrovascular accident are similar in that both may be caused by a thrombus or embolus occluding an artery.

33. Heparin works to prevent clot formation by inhibiting the conversion of prothrombin to thrombin. Warfarin works to prevent clot formation by interfering with the synthesis of vitamin-K dependent coagulation factors (II, VII, IX, and X).

34. Two general tests of bleeding time are the Duke's bleeding time and Ivy bleeding time. Two specific tests of coagulation factors are the prothrombin time (PT) and the activated partial thromboplastic time (APTT).

35. A Fibrometer® or wire loop coagulation instrument detects blood clot formation with an automatic wire loop. When the clot is formed, the wire loop completes an electrical circuit, stopping the timer.

36. Quality control is maintained in blood-coagulation testing in several ways, including careful attention to sample collection and handling and other details of procedure; the use of standardized methods, such as the template method for general bleeding time; the testing of duplicate controls and patient samples for prothrombin times and activated partial thromboplastin times; and the keeping of daily quality-control records.

37. The patient's self-medication with aspirin may increase his clotting time. Before proceeding, alert the physician who ordered the test.

38. The patient is most likely taking an anticoagulant. Prothrombin times and activated partial thromboplastin times should be performed routinely on this patient's blood.

39. Your coworker should have let the sample warm up to body temperature (37 degrees Celsius) for fifteen minutes before performing the test. He also should have run a duplicate of the patient specimen. Using the cold sample will bias the results. Without testing a duplicate sample, there is less assurance that the test result is valid.

40. The tests ordered for this patient might include a platelet scan, a bleeding time, a prothrombin time, or an activated partial thromboplastin time. If the platelet scan appears abnormal, an electronic or manual platelet count might be performed.

Chapter 21

1. Beer's law: the law stating that the extent to which a light beam is absorbed as it passes through a solution depends only on the number of absorbing molecules in the light path.

2. Direct relationship: the relationship when two variables change in the same direction.

3. Dry reagent (solid-phase) chemistry: a lab test, such as a urine reagent-strip test (dip stick), in which a dry reagent on a strip is used for a chemical reaction.

4. Galvanometer: a device for measuring electric current.

5. Inverse relationship: the relationship when two variables change in opposite directions.

6. Monochromatic light: light of one color (just one or a small range of wavelengths).

7. Photocell (photoelectric cell): a device for converting light to electric current in a photometer.

8. Photometer: an instrument for measuring the intensity of light.

9. Reflectance photometer: the type of photometer that measures the amount of light reflected back from a solid, such as a reagent pad.

10. Spectrophotometer: the type of photometer that filters light with a diffraction grating device or prism.

11. Photometers are used in POLs to assess the concentration of substances, such as the concentration of hemoglobin in blood and glucose in urine.

12. Beer's law is related to the use of photometry in POLs in that it states the underlying relationship between light and the concentration of a substance, upon which colorimetry and spectrophotometry are based. Specifically, the more concentrated a substance, the more light it absorbs and the less light it transmits.

13. Colorimeters and spectrophotometers work by measuring the amount of light transmitted through a solution, from which the absorbance of light by the solution can be determined and its concentration calculated.

14. Colorimeters and spectrophotometers differ from each other in the manner in which they filter light. Colorimeters use colored glass filters to transmit light in a limited number of broad bands of wavelengths, while spectrophotometers use a diffraction grating device or prism to transmit very narrow bands of light, each of a single wavelength.

15. Reflectance photometry is based on the following principles: the amount of light reflected back from a reagent pad is inversely proportional to the amount of color change generated by the chemical reaction on the pad, which in turn is proportional to the amount of analyte present in the sample tested.

16. Reflectance photometry is used in POLs when dry reagent chemistry tests are performed, including urine reagent-strip tests (dip sticks).

17. The absorbance of light by a solution is directly proportional to the concentration of the solution. In other words, as a solution becomes more concentrated, it absorbs more light.

18. Transmittance and concentration are related inversely—the greater the concentration of a solution, the less light it transmits.

19. The reflectance of light is inversely related to the concentration of an analyte on a reagent pad; that is, the more concentrated the analyte, the more light is absorbed and the less light is reflected.

20. In photometers, photocells convert transmitted or reflected light into a small electric current.

21. A diffraction grating device or prism selects the correct wavelength of light in spectrophotometers.

22. The role of galvanometers in photometers is to measure the amount of electricity produced by the photocell.

23. In dry reagent chemistry, the color change on the reagent pad is directly proportional to the amount of analyte present. It is inversely proportional to the amount of light reflected back from the pad.

24. Quality control in the use of photometry in POLs is maintained by using a properly constructed photometer with good controls for comparisons. Daily testing of the instrument for accuracy is accomplished by running control samples with known values. When the instrument is working properly, the instrument readings for the controls are the same as the expected values provided by the manufacturer.

25. The wavelength of light is related to the use of photometry in POLs in that different substances absorb different wavelengths of light. When the wavelength most strongly absorbed by a substance is known, then the amount of transmitted or reflected light at that wavelength can be used to identify the amount of substance present.

26. The amount of light transmitted through the solution, which depends on the concentration of the solution, determines the strength of the current produced by the photocell in colorimeters or spectrophotometers.

27. Before the development of photometry, color changes were detected in analytic chemistry by visual inspection. The use of a photometer is superior to visual inspection because it provides objective, quantitative results. Visual inspection, by contrast, is subjective, and the results are not always reproducible because of individual variation in visual acuity. Because the number of color blocks for visual comparison is limited, the results are only semiquantitative.

28. If the color of a reaction is detected by visual inspection, it must fall between about 400 and 700 nm in wavelength. This is because the human eye cannot detect light of shorter or longer wavelengths.

29. The amount of light passing through a solution decreases as the concentration of the solution increases.

30. The amount of light reflected back from a reagent pad decreases as the concentration of analyte increases.

31. To read urine test strips, you should use a reflectance photometer. You cannot use the same instrument that you use to read hemoglobin tests, a spectrophotometer, because urine strips use dry reagent chemistry. Spectrophotometers measure transmission of light through solutions.

32. The reagent blank is needed to establish a zero point on the graph. Using many different concentrations of the control lessens the likelihood that one faulty solution will affect the entire graph.

33. The three levels of control that you should run include an abnormally high value, a normal value, and an abnormally low value. Compare the control test results with the expected values for the controls. If the readings are the same as the expected values, then the instrument is working properly.

Chapter 22

1. j 2. e 3. h
4. d 5. a 6. b
7. g 8. i 9. f
10. c

11. Acidosis: the condition of acidity in body fluids.

12. Diabetes mellitus: a syndrome caused by inadequate production or utilization of insulin, leading to impaired carbohydrate, protein, and fat metabolism.

13. Fructose: a simple, six-carbon sugar in fruit and honey.

14. Gestational diabetes: a transient form of diabetes that develops in response to the metabolic and hormonal changes of pregnancy in previously asymptomatic women.

15. Galactose: a simple six-carbon sugar derived from lactose, or milk sugar.

16. Hyperglycemia: an abnormally high blood-glucose level, most commonly caused by diabetes mellitus.

17. Hypertriglyceridemia: an excessive amount of triglycerides in the blood.

18. Monosaccharide: a class of simple, six-carbon sugars that is found in many foods. Monosaccharides include glucose, fructose, and galactose.

19. Standard oral glucose-tolerance test (GTT or OGTT): the glucose test in which fasting blood and urine specimens are collected before the test to serve as a baseline. Then specimens are collected over several hours after consumption of a glucose load.

20. Lipolysis: fat decomposition.

21. False. Glucagon is a hormone produced by the alpha cells of the islets of Langerhans of the pancreas.

22. True.

23. False. A blood-glucose test is based on the amount of glycosylated hemoglobin in the blood.

24. True.

25. False. When the glucose from food is not needed for energy, it is stored in the form of glycogen in liver and muscle cells.

26. In normal individuals, glucose is metabolized in the cells, where it is broken down into carbon dioxide and water, releasing stored energy for use by the cells. The pancreatic hormone insulin is required for this process because it is needed to transport glucose across cell walls.

27. Glucose is stored in liver and muscle cells in the form of glycogen.

28. The normal range of blood glucose for nonfasting samples is 70 to 110 mg/dL. The normal range for fasting samples is 70 to 90 mg/dL.

29. Hypoglycemia may be caused by hyperfunction of the islets of Langerhans or injection of excessive amounts of insulin.

30. High blood glucose may be caused by liver or adrenocortical dysfunction, but it is caused most commonly by diabetes mellitus.

31. Diabetes mellitus is caused by inadequate production or utilization of insulin.

32. NIDDM, which usually can be controlled by diet alone, is the milder form of the disease and the more common of the two, comprising 90 to 95 percent of cases. It usually has a gradual onset and generally affects adults over age forty. Patients with this form of the disease often are obese. IDDM, which requires administration of insulin to manage the disease, is more severe. It comprises only 5 to 10 percent of all cases. It is characterized by rapid onset and typically strikes before age twenty-five.

33. The clinical characteristics of IDDM include rapid weight loss; polyuria; glycosuria; polydipsia; polyphagia; drowsiness and lethargy; dehydration; vomiting; deep breathing, a sweet, fruity odor on the breath; warm but dry skin; predisposition to infection; and pruritus.

34. The biochemical characteristics of IDDM that produce the clinical features of the disease include continued secretion of free glucose by the liver, despite hyperglycemia; inhibited entry of free glucose into muscle and adipose tissue, preventing the storage of glucose as glycogen and fat; increased lipolysis; entry of uncontrolled amounts of free fatty acids into the blood; conversion of free fatty acids into ketone bodies (causing a sweet odor on the breath); severe acidosis, due to nonmetabolized ketone bodies; severe hypertriglyceridemia, due to conversion of some of the free fatty acids to triglycerides, resulting in plasma with the appearance of thick cream; and spillover of glucose into the urine from the blood, which occurs when the plasma glucose level rises above the renal threshold of about 180 mg/dL.

35. Random blood-glucose tests use samples of blood collected from nonfasting patients during routine visits to the doctor's office. The patients do not require any special preparation and the length of time since their last meal is not important. Fasting blood-sugar tests are performed on samples of blood collected when patients are in a fasting state. Patients should not smoke, eat, or drink anything other than water for eight to twelve hours before the test.

36. All three glucose-tolerance tests commonly performed in POLs assess the ability to utilize carbohydrates by measuring the body's response to a challenge load of glucose. All require that patients be in a fasting state and consume at least 150 grams of carbohydrates per day for three days prior to the test. The two-hour postprandial blood-sugar test measures blood glucose once, two hours after patients have consumed a meal that contains 100 grams of carbohydrate or drunk a 100 gram glu-

cose-load solution. The standard oral glucose-tolerance test measures blood (and urine) glucose while patients are in a fasting state for a baseline and then repeatedly (every half hour or hour) after the patients have consumed a 100 gram glucose-load solution (the dose of glucose may be tailored to the patient's body size). The Exton and Rose glucose-tolerance test measures blood (and urine) glucose while patients are in a fasting state for a baseline, followed by tests of two more samples, each thirty minutes after a 50 gram glucose load.

37. A diagnosis of diabetes mellitus is made in a standard oral glucose-tolerance test when the two-hour specimen and at least one other specimen collected after ingestion of the glucose load meet or exceed 200 mg/dL for venous plasma or 180 mg/dL for venous whole blood.

38. Glucose meters use dry reagent chemistry. The results are read by a reflectance photometer or visually by matching the color on the pad to color blocks on the reagent-strip container.

39. The test that probably is the best overall indicator of control in the management of IDDM is a fasting blood-glucose test performed in the morning, before breakfast.

40. Patient monitoring of blood glucose is extremely important in the management of IDDM because it helps patients tailor their diet and insulin dosage to their own needs, based on repeated blood-sugar readings. This in turn helps prevent wide swings in blood-glucose levels that lead to many of the deleterious consequences of diabetes.

41. Items of medical history that identify women at special risk of developing gestational diabetes include a family history of diabetes; glycosuria; previous fetal loss; and a previous birth of an unusually large infant.

42. Ms. Talbot, who is going to have a fasting blood-sugar test performed tomorrow morning, should be instructed not to smoke, eat, or drink anything other than water for eight to twelve hours before the test. Mr. Chen, who is going to have a glucose-tolerance test in three days, should be instructed to eat at least 150 grams of carbohydrates per day until the day of the test. He also should be instructed not to smoke, eat, or drink anything other than water for the last eight to twelve hours before the test.

43. A glucose concentration that remains above 200 mg/dL at the end of the second hour of the glucose-tolerance test should be interpreted as abnormal. Further readings are required to determine if a diagnosis of diabetes should be made.

44. Dark-colored reagent strips should be discarded because the dark color indicates that they have deteriorated.

45. You should tell the new patient to record the following information in the log for each blood-glucose test: the date and time; the test results; whether or not a control was run; whether or not the control was in the accepted range; the number of hours since last eating; the time of the last insulin injection or oral hypoglycemic medication; whether or not the patient is under any physical or emotional stress; and the amount of exercise performed recently by the patient.

Chapter 23

1. a   2. e   3. g
4. d   5. f   6. b
7. h   8. c

9. False. Automated blood-chemistry analyzers are based on one of two types of technology: discrete analysis or continuous flow analysis.

10. False. In continuous flow analysis systems, samples and reagents flow through the instrument, one after the other.

11. True.

12. False. The Kodak Ektachem DT analyzer is a discrete dry chemistry analyzer.

13. True.

14. False. The DTE module of the Kodak Ektachem DT analyzer has the special function of blood-electrolyte testing.

15. The major advantages of using automated blood-chemistry analyzers in POLs are increased efficiency due to rapid turnaround time and an increased amount of information attained from a single test run.

16. In selecting an automated blood-chemistry analyzer for a POL, the following questions must be addressed: Does the instrument perform tests that are needed frequently for diagnosis? How accurate are the test results? How long does each test take? Will additional staff be required? How difficult is the instrument to maintain? How difficult is the instrument to calibrate? How difficult is the quality-control program? What special training is needed to operate the instrument? How much space is needed for the instrument? How long are the reagents stable? Do the reagents require refrigeration or freezer storage? How much does the instrument cost initially? How much do the reagents cost to run each test? How much will Medicaid and Medicare reimburse for each test? Will this addition be in keeping with CLIA regulations?

17. The basic difference between continuous flow and discrete blood-chemistry analyzers is that, in the former, samples and reagents flow through the instru-

ment, one after the other, while in the latter, samples and reagents for each test are placed in separate containers, in which the tests are performed.

18. Continuous flow blood-chemistry analyzers test samples that are placed in small cups, one per test, which are placed in a circular tray. The tray rotates automatically so that the samples are introduced, reacted upon, and read by the instrument at precise time intervals.

19. Discrete blood-chemistry analyzers use wet or dry chemistry procedures.

20. For the Abbott Vision analyzer, reagents are packed in separate compartments of test-pack cassettes. For the Kodak Ektachem DT analyzer, reagents are layered on separately wrapped slides. For the Reflotron Plus analyzer, reagents are layered in reagent carriers.

21. The role of centrifugation in discrete centrifugal analyzers is to force test materials from one test-pack compartment to another in established sequences.

22. The DT60 Analyzer module of the Kodak Ektachem DT analyzer is operated as follows: a slide is loaded into the instrument; the sample is aspirated with the automatic pipette, which is placed in the spotting station where the slide is spotted with a drop of sample; the slide automatically moves into the incubator where, after five minutes, it is read automatically by reflectance photometry at the proper wavelength.

23. The DTE module of the Kodak Ektachem DT analyzer performs potentiometric tests of the concentration of electrolytes in the sample. It uses ion-selective electrodes, which are sensitive to the activity of particular ions in solution, to test the amount of sodium, potassium, chloride, and carbon dioxide.

24. The glass-fiber fleece layers in the Reflotron Plus analyzer separate plasma from erythrocytes and other cellular constituents of whole blood. Capillary forces transport the plasma to a reservoir for testing.

25. To run a test on the Reflotron Plus analyzer, press the reaction zone of the reagent carrier into the plasma reservoir. Test results are read by the reflectance photometer and printed on the printer tape.

26. Tests are read on solid-phase blood-chemistry analyzers, such as the Ektachem DT and Reflotron Plus, by reflectance photometry.

27. Recalibration of blood-chemistry analyzers should be performed whenever control values drift out of range, the lot number of the slides for a specific test changes, or the lot number of the electrolyte reference fluid changes.

28. The once-a-month self-check of the Abbott Vision analyzer checks for incubator temperature, centrifuge speed, direction of rotation, and spectrophotometer wavelength and reading time.

29. The methods of chemical analysis used by automated blood-chemistry analyzers generally do not differ from manual methods in sequence or type of chemicals.

30. Test profiles that can be performed by the Abbott Vision blood-chemistry analyzer include cardiac evaluation, lipid group, cardiac injury, hepatic group, hypertension group, renal group, metabolic group, and pancreatic group.

31. Your coworker should have placed the box of slides in the refrigerator or freezer, and she should have recalibrated the instrument after opening a new box of slides with a different lot number.

32. You should try to find the problem by consulting the troubleshooting section of the operator's manual. If you cannot find and correct the problem yourself, call the 800 phone number given by the manufacturer for technical assistance.

33. The quality-control protocol for the Abbott Vision analyzer should include guidelines for both calibration and testing of control samples. The self-check should be run once a month and any problems should be corrected by consulting the operator's manual or calling the manufacturer's technical assistance number. Controls, both normal and abnormal, should be run daily for each type of test that is performed on patient samples. Whenever control samples are out of the accepted value range for a particular test, or test packs with new lot numbers are used, the instrument should be recalibrated with calibrators supplied by the manufacturer. Proficiency-testing samples provided by the manufacturer should be analyzed and the results should be returned to Abbott Laboratories for accuracy verification.

Chapter 24

1. Albumin: the most abundant plasma protein. Albumin is responsible for maintaining osmotic pressure at the capillary membrane.

2. Amino acid: one of twenty different compounds in humans that are the building blocks of proteins. Each amino acid contains an amine group and an acidic carboxyl group.

3. Cholesterol: the sterol of primary biological significance. High levels of cholesterol are linked with increased risk of cardiovascular disease.

4. Conjugated lipid: a compound made up of fat and another compound, such as

phosphoric acid (phospholipids) or a carbohydrate (glycolipids).

5. Creatine: a nonprotein nitrogen compound found in muscle tissue. Creatine is synthesized in the liver from amino acids. It combines with phosphate to store energy for muscle contractions.

6. Creatinine: the end product of the metabolism of creatine.

7. Disaccharide: a twelve-carbon sugar. Disaccharides include sucrose, lactose, and maltose.

8. Globulin: the second most abundant type of plasma protein. Globulin has a diversity of functions, including transporting other substances and acting as a substrate.

9. High density lipoprotein (HDL): a lipoprotein that has high density because it is low in fat content. High density lipoproteins are associated with low risk for cardiovascular disease.

10. Low density lipoprotein (LDL): a protein that is low in density because it contains large amounts of fat, primarily in the form of cholesterol.

11. Oral hypoglycemic drug: a drug that decreases the amount of glucose in the blood by stimulating beta cells to secrete more insulin, inhibiting glucose production, or facilitating the transport of glucose to muscle cells.

12. Polysaccharide: a carbohydrate composed of many molecules of simple sugars. Polysaccharides include starch in plants and glycogen in animals.

13. Protein: one of a large group of complex, nitrogen-containing organic compounds, consisting of amino acids joined together by peptide bonds.

14. Triglyceride: a compound made up of fatty acids and glycerol.

15. Urea: a small molecule, formed from ammonia in the liver, which can move freely into both extracellular and intracellular fluid.

16. j   17. c   18. d
19. i   20. e   21. b
22. a   23. g   24. f
25. h

26. The hormones that regulate glucose metabolism include the pancreatic hormones insulin and glucagon, the adrenal hormone epinephrine, and the thyroid hormone thyroxine.

27. Insulin acts to lower blood-glucose levels, while the other three hormones work to raise them.

28. The major causes of hypoglycemia include, most commonly, insulin overdose in patients with unstable IDDM, and other conditions that cause high levels of circulating insulin. The latter include large tumors behind the peritoneum and tumors of the beta cells of the pancreas, called insulinomas.

29. Some of the causes of hyperglycemia include IDDM, NIDDM, hyperthyroidism, Cushing's syndrome, elevated levels of certain hormones, acromegaly, obesity, treatment with some therapeutic drugs, severe liver or kidney damage, and alcoholism.

30. Postprandial hypoglycemia, also called reactive hypoglycemia, occurs several hours after food is ingested. Symptoms generally last no more than thirty minutes, and they resolve without further carbohydrate intake. Postprandial hypoglycemia appears to be due to a delayed or exaggerated response to the insulin that is secreted when sugar is ingested. It may occur early in the development of NIDDM, but most cases have no known physiological cause. Fasting hypoglycemia is detected by measuring blood-glucose levels after a twelve or twenty-four hour fast. In contrast to postprandial hypoglycemia, fasting hypoglycemia usually is associated with recognizable anatomical changes in an organ or tissue. Causes include liver disease and pancreatic tumors.

31. The three types of biologically important lipids are neutral fats, conjugated lipids, and sterols. Neutral fats are triglycerides (fatty acids plus glycerol). Conjugated lipids are compounds made up of fat and another compound, such as phosphoric acid (phospholipids) or a carbohydrate (glycolipids). Sterols are steroid alcohols. Cholesterol is the sterol of primary biological significance.

32. Lipoproteins are classified on the basis of their density, as VLDL (very low density lipoproteins), LDL (low density lipoproteins), and HDL (high density lipoproteins).

33. Total cholesterol levels are positively correlated with risk of atherosclerosis, due to the formation of plaques, or cholesterol deposits in the arteries. More specifically, a high ratio of LDL to HDL cholesterol is linked with increased risk of atherosclerosis. Patients with low levels of HDL cholesterol are encouraged to adopt healthful life-style habits that have been found to raise HDL cholesterol levels.

34. Proteins are a large group of complex, nitrogen-containing organic compounds. The building blocks of proteins are amino acids, which are smaller molecules, each containing an amine group ($-NH_2$) and an acidic carboxyl group (COOH). Proteins consist of amino acids joined together by peptide bonds between the carbon of one amino acid and the nitrogen of the next. There are twenty different amino acids in humans, and they can be linked together in countless different combinations. As a result, there are numerous different kinds of protein molecules.

35. Structurally, proteins are the main building materials of the body, comprising three-fourths of the solid matter of the body. Proteins are the major components of muscles, blood, skin, hair, nails, and the visceral organs. Functionally, proteins are needed to form hormones, which act as chemical messengers to body organs. Enzymes help biochemical reactions occur faster and control virtually all the life processes that go on in the cells. Antibodies help protect the body against disease and transport molecules, which carry substances through the body, such as the hemoglobin protein that transports oxygen in the blood.

36. A general study of blood proteins usually measures total protein and the albumin and nonantibody globulin content of the serum. If either albumin or globulin is measured, the other can be calculated by subtraction from the total protein value. Results are given as the albumin to globulin ratio, A/G. Most protein determinations actually measure nitrogen, which is found in all amino acids. Nitrogen content then is converted to protein concentration by multiplying by a conversion factor.

37. Nonprotein nitrogen compounds found in the blood include ammonia, urea, uric acid, and creatinine.

38. The body gets most of its glucose from complex sugars and starches.

39. Cholesterol is the sterol that is most important biologically.

40. Most energy found in the body is stored in the form of triglycerides in adipose tissue.

41. LDL cholesterol is called "bad cholesterol" because high levels have been linked with greater than average risk of atherosclerosis. HDL cholesterol is called "good cholesterol" because high levels have been linked with less than average risk of atherosclerosis.

42. High levels of circulating cholesterol over a long period of time can lead to the formation of plaques, or thickened areas in the blood vessels. These may prevent blood from flowing freely, leading in turn to heart attacks and strokes.

43. Essential amino acids cannot be synthesized by humans and must be included in the diet on a regular basis. Nonessential amino acids can be synthesized by the body, so it is not necessary to include them in the diet.

44. Triglycerides can be divided into saturated fats and unsaturated fats. Unsaturated fats, such as vegetable oils, are considered to be more healthful than saturated fats, like lard and butter.

45. The three food groups that are the basis of most of the body's metabolism are carbohydrates, lipids, and proteins.

46. The physician is concerned about the patient's cholesterol level and fat intake because of potential damage to her blood vessels that may occur from the high concentration of circulating cholesterol. The development of plaques could lead to heart attack and stroke.

47. The patient most likely has diabetes. Because oral hypoglycemic drugs, diet, and exercise have been prescribed, she probably has NIDDM.

48. The patient might be tested for his serum uric acid level. It is likely to be higher than normal in a patient with gout. Deposits of uric acid crystals in the joints are a symptom of gout.

49. A possible cause of the girl's symptoms is IDDM. She might be given a glucose-tolerance test to confirm the diagnosis.

50. The likely cause of his hypoglycemia is alcoholism. Some alcoholics stop eating carbohydrates, depending instead on alcohol for their source of energy. Their glycogen stores become low and alcohol metabolites interfere with gluconeogenesis.

Chapter 25

1. f   2. b   3. h
4. j   5. c   6. d
7. a   8. g   9. i
10. e

11. False. Nonspecific immunity is the general resistance to disease that characterizes a particular species.

12. True.

13. False. Specific immunity refers to immunity acquired after exposure to a foreign invader.

14. False. Foreign substances that provoke a specific immune reaction are called antigens.

15. True.

16. True.

17. False. Specificity of a lab test for a particular disease refers to the ability of the test to identify correctly those who do not have the disease.

18. False. False negatives are people who have the disease but do not test positive.

19. True.

20. False. In determining titer, dilutions are graduated, with each dilution twice as great as the one before.

21. Four types of nonspecific immune defenses in humans are physical and anatomical barriers, physiological barriers, endocytic and phagocytic responses, and the inflammatory response.

22. In defending our bodies from microorganisms, physical and anatomical barriers are the body's first line of defense,

preventing most microorganisms from entering the body. They include the skin, mucous membranes; body secretions like tears, saliva, and mucus; and benevolent bacteria.

23. The physiological barriers of nonspecific immunity are chemical factors that kill pathogens, such as stomach acids, soluble factors, interferon, and complement.

24. The inflammatory response is a complex series of events triggered by a wound or invasion by microorganisms. It is characterized by redness, swelling, heat, and pain. This response reduces the spread of infection and promotes healing.

25. Antigens on foreign substances, such as microorganisms, elicit the production of specific antibodies. The antigens and antibodies bond and, once bonded, the antigen-antibody complex can be neutralized by precipitation or agglutination or can be tagged for destruction by phagocytes or for lysis by complement.

26. Humoral immunity refers to the formation and activity of short-lived antibodies in body fluids. It involves B-lymphocytes. Cell-mediated immunity involves T-lymphocytes, which form an army of identical cells called clones. Members of the T-cell clones perform a variety of immune functions, including producing antibodies and providing immunological memory of the foreign invader.

27. Autoimmunity refers to an inappropriate immune response to the wrong antigens—to self instead of nonself. Some possible causes include mutations, viruses, drugs, or injuries altering body tissues so they are no longer recognized as self. Normally inaccessible tissue antigens may leak into areas where they come into contact with the immune system and stimulate the production of antibodies.

28. Immunodeficiency may be due to congenital defects or acquired conditions that damage the immune system. The latter include weakening of the immune system by severe malnutrition, many types of cancer, and HIV.

29. Patients with immunodeficiency tend to have persistent or recurrent infections by organisms that do not ordinarily cause disease; incomplete recovery from infections; and undue susceptibility to certain forms of cancer.

30. Immediate and delayed hypersensitivity differ in how quickly they occur after exposure to the antigen. Immediate hypersensitivity occurs within minutes, delayed hypersensitivity after twelve to twenty-four hours. Also, immediate hypersensitivity involves Bcells, while delayed hypersensitivity involves T-cells.

31. The sensitivity of a lab test for a particular disease refers to the ability of the test to identify correctly those who have it. The specificity of the test refers to the ability of the test to identify correctly those who do not have the disease. If a test is sensitive but not specific, it will sometimes produce inaccurate results—some people who do not have the disease will test positive for it (false positives). Conversely, if a test is specific but not sensitive, it will sometimes produce inaccurate results—some people who have the disease will test negative for it (false negatives). The most accurate lab tests are both highly sensitive and highly specific. Such tests identify virtually everyone who has the disease and seldom if ever misidentify those who do not.

32. a. *ELISA test:* an antigen or antibody binds to an enzyme, which in turn produces a color change, for example, HIV and pregnancy. b. *precipitin reaction:* antigen-antibody complexes precipitate out of solution, producing a visible residue, for example, VDRL and RPR. c. *agglutinin reaction:* antigen-antibody complexes agglutinate, or clump together, in solution, for example, a screening test for mononucleosis. d. *lysin reaction:* antigen-antibody reaction causes lysis of cells, for example, a reference lab test for mononucleosis.

33. Immune reactions are measured quantitatively by determining the titer. The dilutions are graduated, with each dilution twice as great as the one before. Then, each dilution is tested and read for a positive reaction. The highest dilution that still gives a positive reaction is the titer.

34. Quality control in immunology testing in POLs involves regular testing of both positive and negative controls; making sure that the batch size is not too great; precisely following the manufacturer's instructions; taking care to avoid cross-contamination of specimens and controls; and mixing reagents correctly.

35. The ABO blood group consists of two antigens, A and B, and four different blood types: A (A antigen only), B (B antigen only), AB (both A and B antigens), and O (neither antigen).

36. Type O is the universal donor to O, A, B, and AB types. Type A may donate to another A and, in an emergency, to AB. Type B may donate to another B and, in an emergency, to AB. Type AB can donate to only another AB.

37. The Rhesus blood group consists of several antigens. The D antigen causes most of the incompatibility. The major clinically significant Rhesus blood types are Rh positive (D antigen) and Rh negative (lacking the D antigen).

38. An Rh positive patient may receive blood of both types, Rh positive and Rh negative. An Rh negative patient may receive only Rh negative blood.

39. Hemolytic disease of the newborn (HDN) may occur when an Rh negative mother bears her second (or higher order) Rh positive child if she has been sensitized in some manner to the Rh antigen. In this situation, the father must be Rh positive in order for the child to be Rh positive. HDN occurs because the D antigen in the fetal blood is attacked by antibodies to D in the blood of the sensitized mother. This may produce severe hemolysis of fetal blood.

40. Diseases or conditions tested by immunological methods include HIV, pregnancy, SLE, HDN, syphilis, infectious mononucleosis, strep throat, rheumatic fever, neonate infections, rheumatoid arthritis, respiratory infections, herpes, chlamydia, Lyme disease, hypersensitivity, autoimmune disorders, yeast infections, inflammatory conditions, and German measles.

41. Generally, blood is typed for Rh in POLs to determine if pregnant women are at risk for HDN. The father's blood is also typed if the woman is RH negative.

42. The color reaction in an ELISA test is caused by enzymes.

43. The most common sexually transmitted disease is believed to be chlamydia, a bacterial infection.

44. You should run both positive and negative controls with each batch of patient specimens that are tested.

45. The physician might order an infectious mononucleosis test to help diagnose this patient's condition.

46. The physician no doubt suspects that the child has strep throat. The physician might order a GAS (Group A Strep) test to confirm the diagnosis.

47. You will test for hCG, human chorionic gonadotropin.

48. The patient had a severe immediate hypersensitivity reaction, called anaphylaxis.

49. The patient's blood type is O negative.

Chapter 26

1. Virus: a simple organism that causes many diseases in humans, including colds and herpes. Viruses live and reproduce within the cells of a host.

2. Coccus: a spherical bacterium: Cocci include streptococcus and staphylococcus.

3. Spiral bacteria: bacteria that include those that cause syphilis and Lyme disease.

4. Gram positive: bacteria that stain deep purple with Gram stain, such as staph and strep organisms.

5. Gram negative: bacteria that stain pink or red with Gram stain, including *Escherichia coli* and *Neisseria gonorrhoeae*.

6. Fastidious bacteria: bacteria that have very precise nutritional and environmental requirements for growth, including *Neisseria gonorrhoeae*.

7. Catalase test: the lab test in which hydrogen peroxide is used in urine cultures to distinguish strep from staph infections.

8. Coagulase test: the lab test that demonstrates the presence of an enzyme produced by pathogenic staph organisms, thereby distinguishing them from nonpathogenic strains of staph.

9. Helminth: a true worm. Several species parasitize the human intestinal tract, including tapeworms and hookworms.

10. Fungus: a plant of the division *Fungi*, which lack chlorophyll. Fungi are microorganisms that include yeasts and molds, some of which cause human disease.

11. Protozoan: a single-celled animal. Several species of protozoa are pathogenic to humans, including *Giardia lamblia*.

12. Aseptic technique: a lab technique that ensures the isolation of pathogenic microorganisms by including personal protective equipment and sterilization.

13. Direct culture: a primary culture; a culture grown by inoculating patient specimens directly into the culture medium.

14. Pure culture: a culture that is grown from a single colony of bacteria, which have been taken from a direct culture. A pure culture serves to further isolate the pathogen.

15. Oxidase test: the lab test in which oxidase reagent is added to a colony of suspected *Niesseria gonorrhoeae* to confirm the presence of this organism.

16. Bacitracin: an antibiotic used in cultures to give an early indication of the presence of Group A strep.

17. Urinary tract infection (UTI): an infection of the urinary tract caused by any of several different bacteria. A UTI is diagnosed when the urine bacteria concentration is over 100,000 organisms per milliliter.

18. Microbiology: the branch of science that studies microscopic organisms.

19. Antibiotic: a drug administered to kill or inhibit the growth of bacteria.

20. Bacteria: single-celled microorganisms in the kingdom Monera. Bacteria cause many different infections in humans.

21. Types of microorganisms that cause disease in humans include viruses (AIDS), bacteria (gonorrhea), fungi (athlete's foot), protozoa (amoebic dysentery), and helminths (tapeworms).

22. Microbiology is relevant to POLs because it is necessary to isolate and identify disease-causing microorganisms and to treat many infectious diseases.

23. Infectious diseases are diagnosed by signs and symptoms; immunology tests; direct smears of patient specimens; and smears of cultures of specimens.

24. Viral diseases sometimes are difficult to diagnose because viruses are too small to be seen under a light microscope. As a result, diagnosis must depend on indirect means of detecting the organisms, such as antigen-antibody reactions.

25. Viral diseases often are difficult to treat because few drugs can kill viruses without damaging the cells of the host. Antibiotics are ineffective against them, and they often gain a foothold before they produce symptoms.

26. Gram stain is used to identify bacteria as either gram positive (deep purple) or gram negative (pink or red). The classification is useful clinically. The two types of bacteria not only react differently to chemical tests but also have different antibiotic sensitivities.

27. Species of bacteria have distinctive shapes. Some are spherical or oval (cocci), some are rod shaped (bacilli), and others are spiral (spirilla).

28. Other differences among bacterial species that aid in their identification include their metabolism, growth characteristics, and nutritional and atmospheric requirements.

29. Factors that must be appropriate for optimal growth of a given bacterial species include nutrition, atmosphere (oxygen or carbon dioxide), temperature, humidity, and pH.

30. Saprophytic bacteria consume nonliving organic material and usually are nonpathogenic. Parasitic bacteria consume living organic material and often are pathogenic.

31. Obligate anaerobes can grow only in the absence of oxygen, while facultative anaerobes prefer an atmosphere without oxygen but can grow in oxygen as well.

32. Most pathogenic bacteria prefer a temperature near 37 degrees Celsius because this is the normal body temperature of their human hosts.

33. Sensitivity testing is performed to determine which particular antibiotic will be most effective against a given bacterial pathogen. Sensitivity tests are performed by placing the antibiotics being considered for treatment in a culture medium and attempting to culture the pathogen on the medium. The same response supposedly will be produced in the patient as in the culture dish.

34. Human diseases caused by fungi include histoplasmosis, coccidioidomycosis, athlete's foot, jock itch, thrush, and vaginal yeast infections.

35. Fungal infections usually are treated with fungicidal drugs and/or antibiotics.

36. Human diseases caused by protozoa microorganisms include amoebic dysentery, giardiasis, and the STD, trichomoniasis.

37. Some helminth infestations in humans are tapeworms, hookworms, pinworms, whipworms, and roundworms.

38. Helminthic diseases are caused by worms that inhabit the human body. The diseases usually are transmitted by fecal matter in the soil or by eggs that have migrated from the anus. With poor sanitation and hygiene, risk of infection is greatly increased. This is one reason why young children are at greater risk of infection than are adults.

39. Aseptic techniques for working with microorganisms in POLs include use of personal protective gear; immediate and thorough disinfection of all nondisposable equipment and work surfaces; correct disposal of biohazardous waste, including all patient specimens and microbial samples; use of sterile equipment and supplies; and complete isolation of the microbes being studied.

40. Aseptic techniques are important when working with microbial pathogens because patients and workers must be protected from potentially serious pathogens. In addition, patient specimens must be protected from contamination with outside organisms.

41. The specimen should be examined for pinworms. The specimen should be processed by placing the scotch tape on a glass slide and then viewing the slide under low power. The worms or eggs, if present, should be readily apparent.

42. The suspected gonorrhea specimen should be processed quickly. Make a smear for a Gram stain before plating. Under the microscope, *Niesseria gonorrhoeae* appear as gram-negative diplococci within white cells. They look like two beans facing each other. Plate the specimen on the recommended media at room temperature and then incubate it in a carbon dioxide-rich atmosphere. If growth occurs, make another smear, Gram stain it, and inspect it for gram-negative diplococci.

43. You should look for evidence of beta hemolysis—a colorless translucent zone around the colonies. Disregard alpha hemolysis, which produces a green color.

44. Always follow the manufacturer's instructions for storage. After inspecting the media on arrival for any evidence of contamination or deterioration, you

should store them tightly sealed, upside down to prevent condensation on the media, in a dark refrigerator.

45. Before making the smear, you should wash your hands, put on latex gloves, and remember to follow the Universal Precautions. Make the smear by rubbing some of the specimen from the swab on a glass slide and fixing it with heat or 95 percent alcohol. Stain the smear following the Gram-stain procedure outlined in the chapter. If it is a staph infection, you should see gram-positive cocci resembling clusters of grapes.

Index

Diabetes insipidus, 132, 137
Diabetes mellitus, 405, 408
  gestational, 405, 409
  glucose in, 180
  insulin-dependent, 406, 408
  noninsulin-dependent, 406, 408
Differential white blood-cell count, 256,
    309–314, 318–322
  abnormal values for, 312–314
  counting cells and, 311–312
  differentiating cells by type and, 309–
    311
  preparing and staining blood smears
    for, 306–309, 318–322
Diluent, 67, 75
Dilution(s), 67, 75, 76–77
  making, 76–77
Dilution #1, 329, 332
Dilution #2, 329, 332
Direct culture, 483, 496
Direct relationship, 390, 391
Disaccharides, 435, 436
Discrete analysis systems, 423, 424–429
Discrete centrifugal analyzer, 423, 424–
    425
Discrete solid-phase analyzer, 423, 425–
    427
Diseases. *See also specific diseases*
  affecting coagulation, 375–377
  blood glucose and, 407–408
  of immune system, 455, 461
  of kidney, 134, 138
  of liver, hemostasis and, 375
  microorganisms causing, 485–495
  sexually transmitted, 3
  transmission of, 5, 7
Disinfection, 3, 12
Dispersion measures, 86–88
Disposable equipment, 7
Disposal, of biohazardous material, 10–
    12
Distal convoluted tubule, 132, 137
Diuretics, 161, 164
Diurnal variation, 276, 277
Dividend, 67, 71
Division
  of decimals, 71–72
  of fractions, 69
Divisor, 67, 69
Double-voided specimens, 147, 148
Drabkin's reagent, 255, 260
Drugs
  antibiotic, 483, 489–490
  anticoagulant, 230, 234, 376–377
  blood clotting and, 376
  coagulation and, 377
  diuretic, 161, 164
  oral hypoglycemic, 436, 437
Drying ovens, 55
Dry reagent chemistry, 390, 395
Duke's bleeding time, 378

Edematous sites, 230, 232
Eight-hour specimens, 147, 148
Ektachem DT system, 425–427, 429–
    430
Electrical hazards, 14
Electrical impedance cell counters, 329,
    331–333
Electrical impedance method, 329, 331–
    333

Electric incinerators, 55
Electrolytes, 132, 134
  normal values for, 522
Electronic test instruments, 57
Electron-optical cell counters, 329–330,
    333–334
Embolism, 371, 376
Embolus, 372, 376
Endocarditis, 303–304, 314
Endocrine function, detecting changes in,
    138
Endocytic and phagocytic responses,
    451, 453
Energy
  from fatty acids, 437
  sorted in glucose, 407
Engineering controls, 3, 6–7
English system, 67, 73, 74
Entamoeba histolytica, 493
Enzyme-linked immunosorbent assay
    (ELISA), 457
Eosin, 304, 307
Eosinophils, 304, 305, 310
Epinephrine, 276, 277
Epithelial cell casts, 200, 203
Equations, 67, 73
Equipment and supplies, 47–63
  adapting to, 58–59
  disposable, 7
  glass and plastic ware, 50–54
  inventory control and, 58
  for temperature maintenance, 54–55
  types of, 48–49
  for urine specimen collection, 150
Equivalent fractions, 67, 69–70
Errors, 103, 105
  in blood counts, 287
  in erythrocyte sedimentation rate
    testing, 351
  finding source of, 105–106
  in platelet counts, 347
  in reticulocyte counts, 354
Erythremia, 276, 277, 284
Erythrocyte(s). *See* Red blood cell(s);
    Red blood-cell casts; Red blood-cell
    (RBC) count
Erythrocyte count. *See* Red blood-cell
    (RBC) count
Erythrocyte indices, 342, 343–345
  calculating, 343–344, 345
  interpreting, 344
Erythrocyte sedimentation rate (ESR, sed
    rate), 342, 348–352
  as diagnostic tool, 352
  factors influencing, 351–352
  measurement of, 348–351, 356–361
  normal values for, 351, 520–521
Erythrocytosis, 274, 276, 284
Erythropoiesis, 255, 257, 352
Erythropoietin, 255, 257
Ethical issues, for record keeping, 117
Expected values, 96
Exponents, 68, 72
Exposure incidents, 3, 6
External controls, 95, 100
Exton and Rose glucose-tolerance test,
    405, 410
Eyepiece, 27, 28, 29, 30, 33

False positives, 456
Fastidious bacteria, 483–484, 488

Fasting blood-sugar (FBS) test, 405, 409
  normal values for, 521
Fats. *See also* Lipids
  saturated and unsaturated, 436–439
Fatty acids, 437
Fatty casts, 196, 200
Fetal hemoglobin, 255, 256, 259
Fibrin, 372, 374
Fibrinogen, 372, 374
Fibrometer, 372, 378
Fine adjustment, 27, 30, 33
Fire hazards, 14
Flasks, 47, 51
Flocculation, 451, 456, 457
Foam test, 161, 162
Focusing microscopes, 32–33, 37–40
Formulas, 68, 73
Fractions, 68–70
  converting to decimals, 70–71
  equivalent, 67, 69–70
  simplifying, 68, 70
Freezers, 54–55
Fructose, 405, 406
Fungi, 484, 492–493
  in urine, 203

Galactose, 176, 405, 406
  in urine, 186
Galactosemia, 176, 186
Galvanometer, 390, 394
General-policy manual, 116, 119
Genitourinary cultures, for gonorrhea,
    498–499
Gestational diabetes, 405, 409
Giardia lamblia, 493
Glassware, 50–54
  procedure for using, 60–63
Globulin, 436, 442
Glomerular filtrate, 132, 136, 137
Glomerulonephritis, 132, 136
Glomerulus, 132, 135
Glove removal technique, 10
Glucagon, 405
Gluconeogenesis, 436, 438
Glucose, 405, 406–407, 436–437. *See
    also* Blood glucose
  metabolism and storage of, 406–407
  urine, 180
Glucose meters, 405–406, 411, 413–417
Glucose-tolerance tests (GTT), 147, 148,
    409–410
  normal values for, 521
Glucosuria, 132, 137, 179, 406, 407
Glycogen, 406, 407
Glycogenolysis, 406, 407
Glycosuria, 132, 137, 179, 406, 407
Glycosylated hemoglobin (G-Hbg, G-
    hemoglobin), 406, 411
Glycosylated hemoglobin test, 406,
    410–411
Gonorrhea, genitourinary cultures for,
    498–499
Gram (g), 68, 73
Gram-negative bacteria, 484, 487
Gram-positive bacteria, 484, 487
Gram stain, 484, 487, 499–500, 504–
    509
Granular casts, 196, 200
Granulocytes, 304, 305
Granulocytic leukemia, chronic, 303,
    313

MEDICAL ASSISTANT ROLE DELINEATION CHART

Administrative

ADMINISTRATIVE PROCEDURES

- Perform basic clerical functions
- Schedule, coordinate and monitor appointments
- Schedule inpatient/outpatient admissions and procedures
- Understand and apply third-party guidelines
- Obtain reimbursement through accurate claims submission
- Monitor third-party reimbursement
- Perform medical transcription
- Understand and adhere to managed care policies and procedures
- *Negotiate managed care contracts (adv)*

PRACTICE FINANCES

- Perform procedural and diagnostic coding
- Apply bookkeeping principles
- Document and maintain accounting and banking records
- Manage accounts receivable
- Manage accounts payable
- Process payroll
- *Develop and maintain fee schedules (adv)*
- *Manage renewals of business and professional insurance policies (adv)*
- *Manage personnel benefits and maintain records (adv)*

Clinical

FUNDAMENTAL PRINCIPLES

- Apply principles of aseptic technique and infection control
- Comply with quality assurance practices
- Screen and follow up patient test results

DIAGNOSTIC ORDERS

- Collect and process specimens
- Perform diagnostic tests

PATIENT CARE

- Adhere to established triage procedures
- Obtain patient history and vital signs
- Prepare and maintain examination and treatment areas
- Prepare patient for examinations, procedures, and treatments
- Assist with examinations, procedures and treatments
- Prepare and administer medications and immunizations
- Maintain medication and immunization records
- Recognize and respond to emergencies
- Coordinate patient care information with other health care providers

General (Transdisciplinary)

PROFESSIONALISM

- Project a professional manner and image
- Adhere to ethical principles
- Demonstrate initiative and responsibility
- Work as a team member
- Manage time effectively
- Prioritize and perform multiple tasks
- Adapt to change
- Promote the CMA credential
- Enhance skills through continuing education

COMMUNICATION SKILLS

- Treat all patients with compassion and empathy
- Recognize and respect cultural diversity
- Adapt communications to individual's ability to understand
- Use professional telephone technique
- Use effective and correct verbal and written communications
- Recognize and respond to verbal and nonverbal communications
- Use medical terminology appropriately
- Receive, organize, prioritize and transmit information
- Serve as liaison
- Promote the practice through positive public relations

LEGAL CONCEPTS

- Maintain confidentiality
- Practice within the scope of education, training, and personal capabilities
- Prepare and maintain medical records
- Document accurately
- Use appropriate guidelines when releasing information
- Follow employer's established policies dealing with the health care contract
- Follow federal, state and local legal guidelines
- Maintain awareness of federal and state health care legislation and regulations
- Maintain and dispose of regulated substances in compliance with government guidelines
- Comply with established risk management and safety procedures
- Recognize professional credentialing criteria
- Participate in the development and maintenance of personnel, policy and procedure manuals
- *Develop and maintain personnel, policy and procedure manuals (adv)*

INSTRUCTION

- Instruct individuals according to their needs
- Explain office policies and procedures
- Teach methods of health promotion and disease prevention
- Locate community resources and disseminate information
- *Orient and train personnel (adv)*
- *Develop educational materials (adv)*
- *Conduct continuing education activities (adv)*

OPERATIONAL FUNCTIONS

- Maintain supply inventory
- Evaluate and recommend equipment and supplies
- Apply computer techniques to support office operations
- *Supervise personnel (adv)*
- *Interview and recommend job applicants (adv)*
- *Negotiate leases and prices for equipment and supply contracts (adv)*

* Denotes advanced skills.